ANNALS OF
THE NEW YORK ACADEMY
OF SCIENCES

Volume 1019

EDITORIAL STAFF

Director, Publishing and New Media
SARAH GREENE

Managing Editor
JUSTINE CULLINAN

Associate Editor
STEVEN E. BOHALL

The New York Academy of Sciences
2 East 63rd Street
New York, New York 10021

THE NEW YORK ACADEMY OF SCIENCES
(Founded in 1817)

BOARD OF GOVERNORS, September 2003 – September 2004

TORSTEN N. WIESEL, *Chairman of the Board*
GERALD D. FISCHBACH, *Vice Chairman*
JOHN T. MORGAN, *Treasurer*
ELLIS RUBINSTEIN, *Chief Executive Officer* [ex officio]

Honorary Life Governors
WILLIAM T. GOLDEN   JOSHUA LEDERBERG

Governors

KAREN E. BURKE	PETER B. CORR	R. BRIAN FERGUSON
RONALD L. GRAHAM	MARNIE IMHOFF	WENDY EVANS JOSEPH
JACQUELINE LEO	ROBERT W. LUCKY	PAUL MARKS
BRUCE McEWEN	RONAY MENSCHEL	JOHN F. NIBLACK
SANDRA PANEM	PETER RINGROSE	DAVID D. SABATINI

LEE G. VANCE   DEBORAH WILEY

VICTORIA BJORKLUND, *Counsel* [ex officio]   LARRY R. SMITH, *Secretary* [ex officio]

STRATEGIES FOR ENGINEERED NEGLIGIBLE SENESCENCE

Why Genuine Control of Aging May Be Foreseeable

ANNALS OF THE NEW YORK ACADEMY OF SCIENCES
Volume 1019

STRATEGIES FOR ENGINEERED NEGLIGIBLE SENESCENCE
Why Genuine Control of Aging May Be Foreseeable

Edited by Aubrey D. N. J. de Grey

The New York Academy of Sciences
New York, New York
2004

Copyright © 2004 by the New York Academy of Sciences. All rights reserved. Under the provisions of the United States Copyright Act of 1976, individual readers of the Annals are permitted to make fair use of the material in them for teaching or research. Permission is granted to quote from the Annals provided that the customary acknowledgment is made of the source. Material in the Annals may be republished only by permission of the Academy. Address inquiries to the Permissions Department (editorial@nyas.org) at the New York Academy of Sciences.

Copying fees: For each copy of an article made beyond the free copying permitted under Section 107 or 108 of the 1976 Copyright Act, a fee should be paid through the Copyright Clearance Center, Inc., 222 Rosewood Drive, Danvers, MA 01923 (www.copyright.com).

♾ The paper used in this publication meets the minimum requirements of the American National Standard for Information Sciences—Permanence of Paper for Printed Library Materials, ANSI Z39.48-1984.

Library of Congress Cataloging-in-Publication Data

International Association of Biomedical Gerontology. International Congress. (10th : 2003 : Cambridge, England)
  Strategies for engineered negligible senescence : why genuine control of aging may be foreseeable / edited by Aubrey D.N.J. de Grey.
    p. ; cm. — (Annals of the New York Academy of Sciences ; v. 1019)
  "10th Congress of the International Association of Biomedical Gerontology (IABG) held on September 19–23, 2003 in Cambridge, United Kingdom"—Contents p.
  Includes bibliographical references and index.
  ISBN 1-57331-496-X (cloth : alk. paper)— ISBN 1-57331-497-8 (pbk. : alk. paper) 1. Aging—Physiological aspects—Congresses. 2. Geriatrics—Congresses.
  [DNLM: 1. Aging—physiology—Congresses. 2. Geriatrics—Congresses. WT 104 I587s 2004] I. De Grey, Aubrey D. N. J., 1963– II. Title. III. Series.
  Q11.N5 vol. 1019
  [QP86]
  500 s—dc22
  [612.6
                            2004010880

GYAT / PCP
Printed in the United States of America
ISBN 1-57331-496-X (cloth)
ISBN 1-57331-497-8 (paper)
ISSN 0077-8923

ANNALS OF THE NEW YORK ACADEMY OF SCIENCES
Volume 1019
June 2004

STRATEGIES FOR ENGINEERED NEGLIGIBLE SENESCENCE
WHY GENUINE CONTROL OF AGING MAY BE FORESEEABLE

Editor
AUBREY D. N. J. DE GREY

This volume is the result of a conference entitled **10th Congress of the International Association of Biomedical Gerontology (IABG)** held on September 19–23, 2003 in Cambridge, United Kingdom.

CONTENTS

Preface. *By* AUBREY D. N. J. DE GREY................................. xv

Part I. The Nervous System

Challenging the Amyloid Cascade Hypothesis: Senile Plaques and Amyloid-β as Protective Adaptations to Alzheimer Disease. *By* HYOUNG-GON LEE, GEMMA CASADESUS, XIONGWEI ZHU, ATSUSHI TAKEDA, GEORGE PERRY, AND MARK A. SMITH.. 1

Combining Growth Factors, Stem Cells, and Gene Therapy for the Aging Brain. *By* SOSHANA BEHRSTOCK AND CLIVE N. SVENDSEN............ 5

The Role of Viruses and of APOE in Dementia. *By* R. F. ITZHAKI, C. B. DOBSON, S. J. SHIPLEY, AND M. A. WOZNIAK................. 15

Metabolic Substrates of Neuronal Aging. *By* E. C. TOESCU AND J. XIONG.... 19

The Biphasic Relationship between Regional Brain Senile Plaque and Neurofibrillary Tangle Distributions: Modification by Age, Sex, and *APOE* Polymorphism. *By* ELIZABETH H. CORDER, ESTIFANOS GHEBREMEDHIN, MILES G. TAYLOR, DIETMAR R. THAL, THOMAS G. OHM, AND HEIKO BRAAK.. 24

Decay of Mitochondrial Metabolic Competence in the Aging Cerebellum. *By* CARLO BERTONI-FREDDARI, PATRIZIA FATTORETTI, BELINDA GIORGETTI, MORENO SOLAZZI, MARTA BALIETTI, GIUSEPPINA DI STEFANO, AND TIZIANA CASOLI 29

Cytochrome Oxidase Activity in Hippocampal Synaptic Mitochondria during Aging: A Quantitative Cytochemical Investigation. *By* CARLO BERTONI-FREDDARI, PATRIZIA FATTORETTI, BELINDA GIORGETTI, MORENO SOLAZZI, MARTA BALIETTI, TIZIANA CASOLI, AND GIUSEPPINA DI STEFANO 33

Vitamin E Deficiency and Aging Effect on Expression Levels of GAP-43 and MAP-2 in Selected Areas of the Brain. *By* TIZIANA CASOLI, GIUSEPPINA DI STEFANO, ALESSIA DELFINO, PATRIZIA FATTORETTI, AND CARLO BERTONI-FREDDARI 37

Chronic Treatment with a Precursor of Cellular Phosphatidylcholine Ameliorates Morphological and Behavioral Effects of Aging in the Rat Hippocampus. *By* D. CRESPO, M. MEGIAS, C. FERNANDEZ-VIADERO, AND R. VERDUGA 41

Chronic Aluminum Administration to Old Rats Results in Increased Levels of Brain Metal Ions and Enlarged Hippocampal Mossy Fibers. *By* PATRIZIA FATTORETTI, CARLO BERTONI-FREDDARI, MARTA BALIETTI, BELINDA GIORGETTI, MORENO SOLAZZI, AND PAOLO ZATTA 44

Motor and Cognitive Recovery Induced by Bone Marrow Stem Cells Grafted to Striatum and Hippocampus of Impaired Aged Rats: Functional and Therapeutic Considerations. *By* CARIDAD I. FERNÁNDEZ, ESTEBAN ALBERTI, YISSEL MENDOZA, LISIS MARTÍNEZ, JAIME COLLAZO, JUAN C. ROSILLO, AND JOSÉ Y. BAUZA 48

Environmental Enrichment–Behavior–Oxidative Stress Interactions in the Aged Rat: Issues for Therapeutic Approach in Human Aging. *By* C. I. FERNÁNDEZ, J. COLLAZO, Y. BAUZA, M. R. CASTELLANOS, AND O. LÓPEZ 53

Digital Transcriptome Analysis in the Aging Cerebellum. *By* MAGDALENA C. POPESCO, ADRIENNE FROSTHOLM, KATARZYNA REJNIAK, AND ANDREJ ROTTER 58

Antiaging Treatments Have Been Legally Prescribed for Approximately Thirty Years. *By* SVETLANA V. UKRAINTSEVA, KONSTANTIN G. ARBEEV, ANATOLY I. MICHALSKY, AND ANATOLY I. YASHIN 64

Part II. The Cardiovascular System

Aging of Cardiac Myocytes in Culture: Oxidative Stress, Lipofuscin Accumulation, and Mitochondrial Turnover. *By* ALEXEI TERMAN, HELGE DALEN, JOHN W. EATON, JIRI NEUZIL, AND ULF T. BRUNK 70

Response of the Senescent Heart to Stress: Clinical Therapeutic Strategies and Quest for Mitochondrial Predictors of Biological Age. *By* FRANKLIN ROSENFELDT, FRANCIS MILLER, PHILLIP NAGLEY, ANTHONY HADJ, SILVANA MARASCO, DEAHNE QUICK, FREYA SHEERAN, MICHELLE WOWK, AND SALVATORE PEPE 78

Impairment of the Transcriptional Responses to Oxidative Stress in the Heart of Aged C57BL/6 Mice. *By* MICHAEL G. EDWARDS, DEEPAYAN SARKAR, ROGER KLOPP, JASON D. MORROW, RICHARD WEINDRUCH, AND TOMAS A. PROLLA 85

Effects of Age and Caloric Restriction on Brain Neuronal Cell Death/Survival. *By* ASIMINA HIONA AND CHRISTIAAN LEEUWENBURGH 96

Acute Coronary Syndrome, Comorbidity, and Mortality in Geriatric Patients. *By* E. TANEVA, V. BOGDANOVA, AND N. SHTEREVA 106

Differential Regulation of Telomerase in Endothelial Cells by Fibroblast Growth Factor–2 and Vascular Endothelial Growth Factor–A: Association with Replicative Life Span. *By* ELISABETH TRIVIER, DAVID J. KURZ, YING HONG, HSIU-LIN HUANG, AND JORGE D. ERUSALIMSKY .. 111

Part III. The Immune System

Interleukin-7: An Interleukin for Rejuvenating the Immune System. *By* RICHARD ASPINALL, SIAN HENSON, JEFFREY PIDO-LOPEZ, AND PA TAMBA NGOM 116

T Cell Replicative Senescence: Pleiotropic Effects on Human Aging. *By* RITA B. EFFROS 123

Zinc, Immune Plasticity, Aging, and Successful Aging: Role of Metallothionein. *By* EUGENIO MOCCHEGIANI, ROBERTINA GIACCONI, ELISA MUTI, CINZIA ROGO, MASSIMO BRACCI, MARIO MUZZIOLI, CATIA CIPRIANO, AND MARCO MALAVOLTA 127

Macrophages of the Adrenal Cortex: A Morphological Study of the Effects of Aging and Dexamethasone Administration. *By* HENRIQUE ALMEIDA, JORGE FERREIRA, AND DELMINDA NEVES 135

Looking for Immunological Risk Genotypes. *By* CALOGERO CARUSO, ALESSANDRA AQUINO, GIUSEPPINA CANDORE, LETIZIA SCOLA, GIUSEPPINA COLONNA-ROMANO, AND DOMENICO LIO 141

Part IV. Cancer

Total Deletion of *in Vivo* Telomere Elongation Capacity: An Ambitious but Possibly Ultimate Cure for All Age-Related Human Cancers. *By* AUBREY D. N. J. DE GREY, F. CHARLES CAMPBELL, INDERJEET DOKAL, LESLIE J. FAIRBAIRN, GERRY J. GRAHAM, COLIN A. B. JAHODA, AND ANDREW C. G. PORTER 147

Insights into Aging Obtained from p53 Mutant Mouse Models. *By* MELISSA DUMBLE, CATHERINE GATZA, STUART TYNER, SUNDARESAN VENKATACHALAM, AND LAWRENCE A. DONEHOWER 171

Engineering Anticancer T Cells for Extended Functional Longevity. *By* GRAHAM PAWELEC, ERMINIA MARIANI, JULIE MCLEOD, ARIE BEN-YEHUDA, TAMAS FÜLÖP, MARTIN ARINGER, AND YVONNE BARNETT 178

Telomerase Expression Is Differentially Regulated in Birds of Differing Life Span. *By* MARK F. HAUSSMANN, DAVID W. WINKLER, CHARLES E. HUNTINGTON, IAN C. T. NISBET, AND CAROL M. VLECK 186

The Role of Cellular Senescence May Be to Prevent Proliferation of Neighboring Cells within Stem Cell Niches. *By* M. D. LYNCH 191

The Aging/Precancerous Gastric Mucosa: A Pilot Nutraceutical Trial. *By* F. MAROTTA, R. BARRETO, H. TAJIRI, J. BERTUCCELLI, P. SAFRAN, C. YOSHIDA, AND E. FESCE 195

Cancer as "Rejuvenescence." *By* SVETLANA V. UKRAINTSEVA AND ANATOLY I. YASHIN 200

Part V. Protein Damage

Functional Analysis of Clusterin/Apolipoprotein J in Cellular Death Induced by Severe Genotoxic Stress. *By* IOANNIS P. TROUGAKOS AND EFSTATHIOS S. GONOS 206

Evidence of Preferential Protein Targets for Age-Related Modifications in Peripheral Blood Lymphocytes. *By* SYLVIE POGGIOLI, JEAN MARY, HILAIRE BAKALA, AND BERTRAND FRIGUET 211

Protective Effects of Mutant Ubiquitin in Transgenic Mice. *By* D. A. GRAY, M. TSIRIGOTIS, J. BRUN, M. TANG, M. ZHANG, M. BEYERS, AND J. WOULFE 215

Algae Extract Protection Effect on Oxidized Protein Level in Human *Stratum Corneum*. *By* CARINE NIZARD, SYLVIE POGGIOLI, CATHERINE HEUSÈLE, ANNE-LAURE BULTEAU, MARIELLE MOREAU, ALEX SAUNOIS, SYLVIANNE SCHNEBERT, CHRISTIAN MAHÉ, AND BERTRAND FRIGUET 219

Heat Shock Protein 47 Expression in Aged Normal Human Fibroblasts: Modulation by *Salix alba* Extract. *By* CARINE NIZARD, EMMANUELLE NOBLESSE, CÉCILLE BOISDÉ, MARIELLE MOREAU, ANNE-MARIE FAUSSAT, SYLVIANNE SCHNEBERT, AND CHRISTIAN MAHÉ 223

RAGE: A New Pleiotropic Antagonistic Gene? *By* A. SIMM, B. BARTLING, AND R-E. SILBER 228

Part VI. DNA Damage

Genetic Correction of Mitochondrial Diseases: Using the Natural Migration of Mitochondrial Genes to the Nucleus in Chlorophyte Algae as a Model System. *By* DIEGO GONZÁLEZ-HALPHEN, SOLEDAD FUNES, XOCHITL PÉREZ-MARTÍNEZ, ADRIÁN REYES-PRIETO, M. GONZALO CLAROS, EDGAR DAVIDSON, AND MICHAEL P. KING 232

Where and When Do Somatic mtDNA Mutations Occur? *By* KONSTANTIN KHRAPKO, KONSTANTIN EBRALIDSE, AND YEVGENYA KRAYTSBERG 240

Genomic Instability, Aging, and Cellular Senescence. *By* RITA A. BUSUTTIL, MARTIJN DOLLÉ, JUDITH CAMPISI, AND JAN VIJG 245

Camptothecin Sensitivity in Werner Syndrome Fibroblasts as Assessed by the COMET Technique. *By* J. LOWE, A. SHEERIN, K. JENNERT-BURSTON, D. BURTON, E. L. OSTLER, J. BIRD, M. H. L. GREEN, AND R. G. A. FARAGHER 256

Mitochondrial Dysfunction Is a Common Phenotype in Aging and Cancer. *By* KESHAV K. SINGH 260

The Extent and Significance of Telomere Loss with Age. *By* DUNCAN M. BAIRD AND DAVID KIPLING 265

Measurement of the 4,834-bp Mitochondrial DNA Deletion Level in Aging Rat Liver and Brain Subjected or Not to Caloric Restriction Diet. *By* P. CASSANO, A. M. S. LEZZA, C. LEEUWENBURGH, P. CANTATORE, AND M. N. GADALETA 269

Investigation of the Signaling Pathways Involved in the Proliferative Life Span Barriers in Werner Syndrome Fibroblasts. *By* TERENCE DAVIS, RICHARD G. A. FARAGHER, CHRISTOPHER J. JONES, AND DAVID KIPLING. 274

Mechanism of Telomere Shortening by Oxidative Stress. *By* SHOSUKE KAWANISHI AND SHINJI OIKAWA 278

Lysosomal Redox-Active Iron Is Important for Oxidative Stress–Induced DNA Damage. *By* TINO KURZ, ALAN LEAKE, THOMAS VON ZGLINICKI, AND ULF T. BRUNK 285

Low Levels of mtDNA Deletion Mutations in ETS Normal Fibers from Aged Rats. *By* JEONG W. PAK AND JUDD M. AIKEN 289

Part VII. Hormones and Signaling

Age-Related Muscle Loss and Progressive Dysfunction in Mechanosensitive Growth Factor Signaling. *By* GEOFFREY GOLDSPINK 294

What Do Hormones Have to Do with Aging? What Does Aging Have to Do with Hormones? *By* S. MITCHELL HARMAN 299

Functional Efficiency of the Senescent Cells: Replace or Restore? *By* SANG CHUL PARK, KYUNG A. CHO, IK SOON JANG, KYUNG TAE KIM, AND SUNG JIN RYU 309

Growth Hormone Alters Components of the Glutathione Metabolic Pathway in Ames Dwarf Mice. *By* HOLLY M. BROWN-BORG, SHARLENE G. RAKOCZY, AND ERIC O. UTHUS 317

Age-Related Endocrine Dysfunction in Nonhuman Primates. *By* N. D. GONCHAROVA AND B. A. LAPIN 321

Secretion of Melatonin in Healthy Elderly Subjects: A Longitudinal Study. *By* N. M. K. NG YING KIN, N. P. V. NAIR, G. SCHWARTZ, J. X. THAVUNDAYIL, AND L. ANNABLE 326

The Proinflammatory Phenotype of Senescent Cells: The p53-Mediated ICAM-1 Expression. *By* DIMITRIS KLETSAS, HARRIS PRATSINIS, GIORGOS MARIATOS, PANAYOTIS ZACHARATOS, AND VASSILIS G. GORGOULIS 330

Part VIII. Oxidative Stress

Short-Term Caloric Restriction and Sites of Oxygen Radical Generation in Kidney and Skeletal Muscle Mitochondria. *By* RICARDO GREDILLA, SHARON PHANEUF, COLIN SELMAN, SUMA KENDAIAH, CHRISTIAAN LEEUWENBURGH, AND GUSTAVO BARJA 333

Mechanism of Superoxide-Mediated Damage: Relevance to Mitochondrial Aging. *By* I. B. AFANAS'EV 343

Glutathione Metabolism during Aging and in Alzheimer Disease. *By* HONGLEI LIU, HONG WANG, SWAPNA SHENVI, TORY M. HAGEN, AND RUI-MING LIU 346

Alpha–Lipoic Acid Increases Na^+K^+ATPase Activity and Reduces Lipofuscin Accumulation in Discrete Brain Regions of Aged Rats. *By* P. ARIVAZHAGAN AND C. PANNEERSELVAM 350

The Bud Scar–Based Screening System for Hunting Human Genes Extending Life Span. *By* CUIYING CHEN AND ROLAND CONTRERAS 355

Senescence Marker Protein–30 as a Novel Antiaging Molecule. *By* DONGYUN FENG, YOSHITAKA KONDO, AKIHITO ISHIGAMI, MASASHI KURAMOTO, TAKEO MACHIDA, AND NAOKI MARUYAMA 360

Iron Accumulation during Cellular Senescence. *By* DAVID W. KILLILEA, STEPHANIE L. WONG, HENDRY S. CAHAYA, HANI ATAMNA, AND BRUCE N. AMES 365

Investigations on the Nature of the Cost of Reproduction: Susceptibility to Heat Stress in Fruitflies. *By* JALAL KOOCHMESHGI, SHADI LADONNI, AND SEYED MEHDI HOSSEINI-MAZINANI 368

Alternative Pathways Might Mediate Toxicity of High Concentrations of Superoxide Dismutase. *By* AXEL KOWALD AND EDDA KLIPP 370

No Increase in Senescence-Associated β-Galactosidase Activity in Werner Syndrome Fibroblasts after Exposure to H_2O_2. *By* JOÃO PEDRO DE MAGALHÃES, VALÉRIE MIGEOT, VÉRONIQUE MAINFROID, FRANÇOISE DE LONGUEVILLE, JOSÉ REMACLE, AND OLIVIER TOUSSAINT 375

Aging and Vitamin E Deficiency Are Responsible for Altered RNA Pathways. *By* MANUELA MALATESTA, CARLO BERTONI-FREDDARI, PATRIZIA FATTORETTI, BEATRICE BALDELLI, STANISLAV FAKAN, AND GIANCARLO GAZZANELLI 379

Senescence Marker Protein–30 Knockout Mouse as an Aging Model. *By* NAOKI MARUYAMA, AKIHITO ISHIGAMI, MASASHI KURAMOTO, SETSUKO HANDA, SACHIHO KUBO, TOSHIYUKI IMASAWA, KUNIAKI SEYAMA, TATSUO SHIMOSAWA, AND YASUSHI KASAHARA 383

Lack of Correlation between Mitochondrial Reactive Oxygen Species Production and Life Span in *Drosophila*. *By* SATOMI MIWA, KUMARS RIYAHI, LINDA PARTRIDGE, AND MARTIN D. BRAND 388

Malondialdehyde and Measures of Antioxidant Activity in Subjects from the Belfast Elderly Longitudinal Free-Living Aging Study. *By* I. M. REA, D. MCMASTER, J. DONNELLY, L. T. MCGRATH, AND I. S. YOUNG 392

Regenerative Medicine: Antagonic-Stress® Therapy in Distress and Aging. I. Preclinical Synthesis—2003. *By* D. RIGA, S. RIGA, AND F. SCHNEIDER ... 396

Prolongevity Medicine: Antagonic-Stress® Drug in Distress, Geriatrics, and Related Diseases. II. Clinical Review—2003. *By* S. RIGA, D. RIGA, AND F. SCHNEIDER 401

Part IX. Nutrition

Delaying the Mitochondrial Decay of Aging. *By* BRUCE N. AMES 406

Development of Calorie Restriction Mimetics as a Prolongevity Strategy. *By* DONALD K. INGRAM, R. MICHAEL ANSON, RAFAEL DE CABO, JACEK MAMCZARZ, MIN ZHU, JULIE MATTISON, MARK A. LANE, AND GEORGE S. ROTH 412

Interventions in Aging and Age-Associated Pathologics by Means of Nutritional Approaches. *By* KENICHI KITANI, TAKAKO YOKOZAWA, AND TOSHIHIKO OSAWA 424

Absolute versus Relative Caloric Intake: Clues to the Mechanism of Calorie/Aging-Rate Interactions. *By* R. MICHAEL ANSON 427

Acetyl-L-Carnitine Dietary Supplementation to Old Rats Increases Mitochondrial Transcription Factor A Content in Rat Hindlimb Skeletal Muscles. *By* V. PESCE, F. FRACASSO, C. MUSICCO, A. M. S. LEZZA, P. CANTATORE, AND M. N. GADALETA 430

An Appetite for Death. *By* JALAL KOOCHMESHGI 434

Reproductive Switch and Aging: The Case of Leptin Change in Dietary Restriction. *By* JALAL KOOCHMESHGI 436

Long-Lived αMUPA Transgenic Mice Exhibit Increased Mitochondrion-Mediated Apoptotic Capacity. *By* OREN TIROSH, BETTY SCHWARTZ, IGOR ZUSMAN, GEORGE KOSSOY, SHLOMO YAHAV, AND RUTH MISKIN 439

Effect of Caloric Restriction on the 24-Hour Plasma DHEAS and Cortisol Profiles of Young and Old Male Rhesus Macaques. *By* H. F. URBANSKI, J. L. DOWNS, V. T. GARYFALLOU, J. A. MATTISON, M. A. LANE, G. S. ROTH, AND D. K. INGRAM 443

Caloric Restriction Modulates Early Events in Insulin Signaling in Liver and Skeletal Muscle of Rat. *By* MIN ZHU, RAFAEL DE CABO, MARK A. LANE, AND DONALD K. INGRAM 448

Part X. Exercise

Aging, Exercise, and Phytochemicals: Promises and Pitfalls. *By* LI LI JI AND DAVID M. PETERSON 453

Aging, Exercise, and Cardioprotection. *By* SCOTT K. POWERS, JOHN QUINDRY, AND KARYN HAMILTON 462

Regular Exercise: An Effective Means to Reduce Oxidative Stress in Old Rats. *By* SATARO GOTO, ZSOLT RADÁK, CSABA NYAKAS, HAE YOUNG CHUNG, HISASHI NAITO, RYOYA TAKAHASHI, HIDEKO NAKAMOTO, AND RYOICHI ABE 471

Mechanisms in Muscle Atrophy in Immobilization and Aging. *By* MARINA BAR-SHAI, ELI CARMELI, RAYMOND COLEMAN, AND ABRAHAM Z. REZNICK 475

Effect of Physical Activity Levels on Bone Strength. *By* KAZUTOSHI KIKKAWA 479

Part XI. Exceptional Longevity

Naturally Long-Lived Animal Models for the Study of Slow Aging and Longevity. *By* DONNA J. HOLMES 483

The Extreme Aged: Sampling, Measurement, and Statistical Models in Cross-Sectional Estimation and Forecasting. *By* LARRY S. CORDER 486

Demographics of Human Supercentenarians and the Implications for Longevity Medicine. *By* L. STEPHEN COLES 490

Early-Life Programming of Aging and Longevity: The Idea of High Initial Damage Load (the HIDL Hypothesis). *By* LEONID A. GAVRILOV AND NATALIA S. GAVRILOVA 496

Cardiovascular Disease Delay in Centenarian Offspring: Role of Heat Shock Proteins. *By* DELLARA F. TERRY, MAEGAN MCCORMICK, STACY ANDERSEN, JAEMI PENNINGTON, EMILY SCHOENHOFEN, ELIZABETH PALAIMA, MARIA BAUSERO, KISHIKO OGAWA, THOMAS T. PERLS, AND ALEXZANDER ASEA 502

Testing the Free Radical Theory of Aging in Bats. *By* ANJA K. BRUNET ROSSINNI 506

The Reliability-Engineering Approach to the Problem of Biological Aging. *By* LEONID A. GAVRILOV AND NATALIA S. GAVRILOVA 509

Does Exceptional Human Longevity Come with a High Cost of Infertility? Testing the Evolutionary Theories of Aging. *By* NATALIA S. GAVRILOVA, LEONID A. GAVRILOV, VICTORIA G. SEMYONOVA, AND GALINA N. EVDOKUSHKINA 513

Emerging Area of Aging Research: Long-Lived Animals with "Negligible Senescence." *By* JOHN C. GUERIN 518

Functional Aging and Gradual Senescence in Zebrafish. *By* SHUJI KISHI 521

Part XII. Ethical and Sociological Issues

Immortal Ethics. *By* JOHN HARRIS 527

Collective Suttee: Is It Unjust to Develop Life Extension if It Will Not Be Possible to Provide It to Everyone? *By* JOHN K. DAVIS 535

Biogerontologists' Duty to Discuss Timescales Publicly. *By* AUBREY D. N. J. DE GREY 542

The Pitfalls of Planning for Demographic Change. *By* GREGORY B. STOCK 546

Report on the Open Discussion on the Future of Life Extension Research. *By* AUBREY D. N. J. DE GREY 552

Part XIII. Other Topics

Mechanisms of Hormesis through Mild Heat Stress on Human Cells. *By* SURESH I. S. RATTAN 554

The Arrest of Biological Time as a Bridge to Engineered Negligible Senescence. *By* JERRY LEMLER, STEVEN B. HARRIS, CHARLES PLATT, AND TODD M. HUFFMAN 559

Apolipoprotein E Genotype and Age at Menopause. *By* JALAL KOOCHMESHGI, SEYED MEHDI HOSSEINI-MAZINANI, SEYED MORTEZA SEIFATI, NASRIN HOSEIN-PUR-NOBARI, AND LADAN TEIMOORI-TOOLABI 564

The Molecular Chaperones and the Phenomena of Cellular Immortalization and Apoptosis *in Vitro*. *By* JENS KRØLL 568

Cirrhosis Progression as a Model of Accelerated Senescence: Affecting the Biological Aging Clock by a Breakthrough Biophysical Methodology. *By* G. MARINEO, F. MAROTTA, AND G. SISTI 572

How an Individual Fecundity Pattern Looks in *Drosophila* and Medflies. *By* V. N. NOVOSELTSEV, R. ARKING, J. R. CAREY, J. A. NOVOSELTSEVA, AND A. I. YASHIN 577

Mitochondria, Sex, and Mortality. *By* IAN K. ROSS 581

Ultrasound as an Alternative to Aspiration for Determining the Nature of Pleural Effusion, Especially in Older People. *By* FARZAD AFZALI, HAMIDREZA SAJJADIEH, VAHAB SAJJADIEH, AND AMIRREZA SAJJADIEH .. 585

Index of Contributors 593

Financial assistance was received from:
- **INTERNATIONAL SOCIETY FOR HEALTHY AGING RESEARCH AND EDUCATION**
- **HMX, INC.**
- **NOW FOODS, INC.**
- **RESEARCH INTO AGEING**
- **ELLISON MEDICAL FOUNDATION**
- **CENTER ON AGING, UNIVERSITY OF CHICAGO**
- **NATIONAL INSTITUTE ON AGING**
- **MARK MUHLESTEIN**
- **SENETEK**
- **BRITISH SOCIETY FOR RESEARCH ON AGEING**

The New York Academy of Sciences believes it has a responsibility to provide an open forum for discussion of scientific questions. The positions taken by the participants in the reported conferences are their own and not necessarily those of the Academy. The Academy has no intent to influence legislation by providing such forums.

Preface

The International Association of Biomedical Gerontology (IABG) was founded by Denham Harman in 1985, but the concept of *biomedical gerontology* is, in my view, one whose time has come only now. Biomedical gerontology fills the vacuum between basic biogerontology (the curiosity-driven study of aging for the purpose of understanding more completely how and why it occurs) and clinical gerontology (the medical field focused on identifying which currently available treatments are most effective in alleviating the health problems of old age). In biomedical gerontology the goal is to combat aging, as it is in clinical gerontology, but the technologies to be applied are still on the drawing board. As such, biomedical gerontology could not really claim legitimacy until biogerontology had progressed far enough to identify lines of exploration that were likely to succeed. Only in the past five years or so, in my view, has this become so.

The Tenth Congress mirrored this advance more than any biogerontology meeting previously held. Talks and poster presentations surveyed most of the major cellular and molecular changes that progressively accumulate during aging and for which there is a good case for eventual pathogenicity, as well as foreseeable technologies to repair them—not merely to slow their progress. The latter included numerous biomedical disciplines not traditionally associated with gerontology: not only stem cell research, whose biogerontological relevance has become abundantly clear in recent years, but also cancer research, tissue engineering, gene therapy, and even fields not normally considered biomedical at all, such as bioremediation. Additionally extensive time was allocated to discussion of social and ethical aspects of life extension.

The conference recorded in these proceedings was, in many ways, a greatly amplified version of a one-day roundtable entitled "SENS" (for Strategies for Engineered Negligible Senescence) that I held in October 2000, and which gave rise to the article that I and the other participants published in the proceedings of the Ninth IABG Congress (de Grey *et al.* 2002. Time to talk SENS: critiquing the immutability of human aging. Ann. N.Y. Acad. Sci. 959: 452–462). Two similar-sized meetings with related purposes, also giving rise to publications authored by most of the participants, were held in 2001 (de Grey *et al.* 2002. Is human aging still mysterious enough to be left only to scientists? BioEssays 24: 667–676) and 2003, the Tenth IABG Congress (de Grey *et al.* 2004. Total deletion of *in vivo* telomere elongation capacity: an ambitious but possibly ultimate cure for all age-related human cancers. Ann. N.Y. Acad. Sci. 1019: 147–170, this volume). Thus, the Tenth Congress may be considered SENS 4.

More than two-thirds of the oral and poster presentations of the Tenth IABG have resulted in papers in these proceedings. They amply cover all topics discussed at the conference, including those not traditionally featured at biogerontology meetings, such as cancer and the ethics of life extension. I am confident that this volume will substantially contribute to the accelerating effort to develop truly effective means to combat human aging in the coming decades.

—AUBREY D. N. J. DE GREY

*Department of Genetics,
University of Cambridge,
Cambridge, United Kingdom*

Past Published Proceedings of IABG Congresses

2nd Congress: Steinhagen-Thiessen, E. & D.L. Knook, Eds. 1988. Trends in Biomedical Gerontology. TNO Institute for Experimental Gerontology, Rijswijk.

4th Congress: Fabris, N., D. Harman, D.L. Knook, E. Steinhagen-Thiessen & I. Zs.-Nagy, Eds. 1992. Physiopathological Processes of Aging: Towards a Multicausal Interpretation. Annals of the New York Academy of Sciences. Vol. 673.

5th Congress: Zs.-Nagy, I., D. Harman & K. Kitani, Eds. 1994. Pharmacology of Aging Processes: Methods of Assessment and Potential Interventions. Annals of the New York Academy of Sciences. Vol. 717.

6th Congress: Kitani, K., A. Aoba & S. Goto, Eds. 1996. Pharmacological Intervention in Aging and Age-Associated Disorders. Annals of the New York Academy of Sciences. Vol. 786.

7th Congress: Harman, D., R. Holliday & M. Meydani, Eds. 1998. Towards Prolongation of the Healthy Life Span: Practical Approaches to Intervention. Annals of the New York Academy of Sciences. Vol. 854.

8th Congress: Park, S.C., E.S. Hwang, H.-S. Kim & W-Y. Park, Eds. 2001. Healthy Aging for Functional Longevity: Molecular and Cellular Interactions in Senescence. Annals of the New York Academy of Sciences. Vol. 928.

9th Congress: Harman, D., Ed. 2002. Increasing Healthy Life Span: Conventional Measures and Slowing the Innate Aging Process. Annals of the New York Academy of Sciences. Vol. 959.

Challenging the Amyloid Cascade Hypothesis

Senile Plaques and Amyloid-β as Protective Adaptations to Alzheimer Disease

HYOUNG-GON LEE, GEMMA CASADESUS, XIONGWEI ZHU, ATSUSHI TAKEDA,[a] GEORGE PERRY, AND MARK A. SMITH

Institute of Pathology, Case Western Reserve University, Cleveland, Ohio 44106, USA

[a]*Department of Neurology, Tohoku University School of Medicine, Sendai, Miyagi, Japan*

ABSTRACT: Ever since their initial description over a century ago, senile plaques and their major protein component, amyloid-β, have been considered key contributors to the pathogenesis of Alzheimer disease. However, counter to the popular view that amyloid-β represents an initiator of disease pathogenesis, we herein challenge dogma and propose that amyloid-β occurs secondary to neuronal stress and, rather than causing cell death, functions as a protective adaptation to the disease. By analogy, individuals suffering from altitude sickness nearly always have elevated levels of hemoglobin. However, while hemoglobin is toxic to cells in culture and increased erythropoiesis at sea level can be deadly, it is clear that the increases in hemoglobin occurring at altitude are beneficial. Amyloid, like hemoglobin, may also be beneficial, in this case, following neuronal stress or disease. Although controversial, a protective function for amyloid-β is supported by all of the available literature to date and also explains why many aged individuals, despite the presence of high numbers of senile plaques, show little or no cognitive decline. With this in mind, we suspect that current therapeutic efforts targeted toward lowering amyloid-β production or removal of deposited amyloid-β will only serve to exacerbate the disease process.

KEYWORDS: Alzheimer disease; amyloid-β; antioxidant; free radical; senile plaque

INTRODUCTION

To study any disease process, one generally looks at differences between normal control tissue and the diseased tissue. However, whether such differences relate directly to primary mechanisms involved in driving disease pathogenesis is something that can only be determined empirically. In Alzheimer disease (AD), the most conspicuous differences are the senile plaques, and this lesion, or its major protein component, amyloid-β, is not only a key diagnostic indicator but is also thought to play a

---

Address for correspondence: Mark A. Smith, Ph.D., Institute of Pathology, Case Western Reserve University, 2085 Adelbert Road, Cleveland, Ohio 44106. Voice: 216-368-3670; fax: 216-368-8964.

mark.smith@case.edu

key pathogenic and mechanistic role in the disease. While this notion of amyloid-β causality has now assumed the stature of dogma within the field, viewing amyloid-β as having disease-causing properties may be based upon findings that have no relevance to the disease, false interpretations, and biased logic. In fact, all of the data that is used as "evidence" for a pathogenic role for amyloid-β could equally be interpreted, and often more clearly, with very different conclusions indeed. In fact, without prior prejudice, this evidence actually points to amyloid-β having a protective role. Therefore, while we concur that amyloid-β is a crucial diagnostic indicator, we suspect that its mechanistic importance has far less to do with its consequences than with the factors that led to its formation.

AMYLOID-β: CHALLENGING THE HYPOTHESIS

Amyloid-β is the predominant mechanism thought responsible for mediating neuronal death in AD.[1] Such an assertion is primarily based on three observations that, as discussed below, have fundamental flaws.

Amyloid-β, as Senile Plaques, Are an Obligate Feature of Alzheimer Disease

Without amyloid-β there can be no diagnosis of AD. While this is true based on established diagnostic criteria, it is quite clear that such a statement has little mechanistic value and is a tautological "strawman" constructed to serve classification criteria. Interestingly, it is now apparent that the presence of amyloid-β has little bearing on other indices of disease, such as cognitive decline,[2] as one might expect if amyloid-β were playing a central pathogenic role. Additionally, and also contraindicating, a key role in disease, cell,[3] animal,[4] and human[5,6] studies all show that amyloid-β is a relatively late event in the pathogenesis of AD.

Amyloid-β Is Neurotoxic

While amyloid-β is clearly toxic in cell culture models,[1] there is little evidence supporting similar toxicity in either animal models of amyloidosis, in human aging, or in AD.[7,8] Therefore while cell culture "models" were key in formulating the amyloid hypothesis, they are not an accurate reflection of any *in vivo* or diseased conditions. A model of disease that has little bearing on the disease being modeled is a poor model, and in this regard it is now clear that the amyloid toxicity seen *in vitro* is a reflection of artifactual cell culture conditions.[9] With this in mind, and rejecting the cell culture toxicity data as artifact, the strength of the amyloid-β hypothesis is clearly diminished.

Genetic Mutations All Increase Amyloid-β

Each of the familial forms of the disease, involving either a mutation (AβPP or presenilin) or polymorphism (apolipoprotein E), leads to an increased production of amyloid-β. Since the clinical and pathological phenotype of such cases is near identical, if not identical, to all forms of AD, many have argued that increased amyloid-β is the cause of AD. However, while one interpretation of the available data is that *mutation leads to increased amyloid-β leads to disease,* an equally valid explanation is that *mutation leads to disease leads to increased amyloid-β*. Support for the latter is becoming ever apparent since mutations lead to cellular stress, which, in turn, leads to increased amyloid-β[3,4] and also because, in AD, cellular stress precedes increases in amyloid-β.[5,6] Compellingly, a reduction in stress consequentially leads to lowered levels of amyloid-β in both cell[3] and animal models.[10,11] However, of greater interest is that stress-induced increases in amyloid-β are associated with a decrease in stress,[6,12] suggesting that the upregulation of amyloid-β could play a protective function.[7,13,14] Certainly, such a notion is consistent with the upregulation of amyloid-β secondary to neuronal injury.[15] Proteins, such as amyloid-β, that are induced under oxidative conditions and act to lessen oxidative damage are typically thought of as antioxidants and, in this regard, we recently demonstrated that amyloid-β is a *bona fide* antioxidant that can act as a potent superoxide dismutase.[16]

Viewing amyloid-β as a protective response element provides a valid mechanism for why the brains of most aged individuals, when redox alterations are first manifest,[6] contain amyloid-β deposits often at loads equivalent to patients with AD.[17] While such production and deposition of amyloid-β appears to successfully stave off age-related redox imbalances in normal aging, in AD, where there is a profound and chronic redox imbalance, the presence of amyloid-β, even at high levels, proves insufficient.[8,13,18]

CONCLUSIONS

The idea that amyloid-β is protective represents a major paradigm shift to our understanding of AD. However, viewing amyloid as a response rather than cause is really not surprising since neuronal degeneration is associated with a number of responses, including the induction of antioxidants, such as heme oxygenase-1,[19] and heat shock proteins, such as ubiquitin.[20,21] Our arguments supporting amyloid-β as a crucial antioxidant defense mechanism are extremely relevant to current pharmacological efforts targeted at either removing amyloid-β or lessening amyloid-β production. Removing amyloid will likely leave neurons without one of their fundamental compensatory responses to aging and disease,[22] and therefore, we would expect that current pharmacological strategies to lower amyloid levels will actually serve to worsen the disease.[14,23–25]

ACKNOWLEDGMENTS

Work in the authors' laboratories is supported by the National Institutes of Health and the Alzheimer's Association.

REFERENCES

1. HARDY, J. & D.J. SELKOE. 2002. The amyloid hypothesis of Alzheimer's disease: progress and problems on the road to therapeutics. Science **297:** 353–356.
2. NEVE, R.L. & N.K. ROBAKIS. 1998. Alzheimer's disease: a re-examination of the amyloid hypothesis. Trends Neurosci. **21:** 15–19.
3. YAN, S.D., X. CHEN, J. FU, *et al.* 1996. RAGE and amyloid-beta peptide neurotoxicity in Alzheimer's disease. Nature **382:** 685–691.

4. PRATICÓ, D., U. URYU, S. LEIGHT, *et al.* 2001. Increased lipid peroxidation precedes amyloid plaque formation in an animal model of Alzheimer amyloidosis. J. Neurosci. **21:** 4183–4187.
5. NUNOMURA, A., G. PERRY, M.A. PAPPOLLA, *et al.* 1999. RNA oxidation is a prominent feature of vulnerable neurons in Alzheimer's disease. J. Neurosci. **19:** 1959–1964.
6. NUNOMURA, A., G. PERRY, G. ALIEV, *et al.* 2001. Oxidative damage is the earliest event in Alzheimer disease. J. Neuropathol. Exp. Neurol. **60:** 759–767.
7. ROTTKAMP, C.A., C.S. ATWOOD, J.A. JOSEPH, *et al.* 2002. The state versus amyloid-β: the trial of the most wanted criminal in Alzheimer disease. Peptides **23:** 1333–1341.
8. SMITH, M.A., G. CASADESUS, J.A. JOSEPH, *et al.* 2002. Amyloid-β and τ serve antioxidant functions in the aging and Alzheimer brain. Free Radic. Biol. Med. **33:** 1194–1199.
9. ROTTKAMP, C.A., A.K. RAINA, X. ZHU, *et al.* 2001. Redox-active iron mediates amyloid-β toxicity. Free Radic. Biol. Med. **30:** 447–450.
10. LIM, G.P., T. CHU, F. YANG, *et al.* 2001. The curry spice curcumin reduces oxidative damage and amyloid pathology in an Alzheimer transgenic mouse. J. Neurosci. **21:** 8370–8377.
11. VEURINK, G., D. LIU, K. TADDEI, *et al.* 2003. Reduction of inclusion body pathology in ApoE-deficient mice fed a combination of antioxidants. Free Radic. Biol. Med. **34:** 1070–1077.
12. NUNOMURA, A., G. PERRY, M.A. PAPPOLLA, *et al.* 2000. Neuronal oxidative stress precedes amyloid-β deposition in Down syndrome. J. Neuropathol. Exp. Neurol. **59:** 1011–1017.
13. JOSEPH, J., B. SHUKITT-HALE, N.A. DENISOVA, *et al.* 2001. Copernicus revisted: amyloid beta in Alzheimer's disease. Neurobiol. Aging **22:** 131–146.
14. SMITH, M.A., C.S. ATWOOD, J.A. JOSEPH, *et al.* 2002. Predicting the failure of the amyloid-β vaccine. The Lancet **359:** 1864–1865.
15. GENTLEMAN, S.M., M.J. NASH, C.J. SWEETING, *et al.* 1993. β-amyloid precursor protein (βAPP) as a marker for axonal injury after head injury. Neurosci. Lett. **160:** 139–144.
16. CUAJUNGCO, M.P., L.E. GOLDSTEIN, A. NUNOMURA, *et al.* 2000. Evidence that the β-amyloid plaques of Alzheimer's disease represent the redox-silencing and entombment of Aβ by zinc. J. Biol. Chem. **275:** 19439–19442.
17. DAVIS, D.G., F.A. SCHMITT, D.R. WEKSTEIN, *et al.* 1999. Alzheimer neuropathologic alterations in aged cognitively normal subjects. J. Neuropathol. Exp. Neurol. **58:** 376–388.
18. ATWOOD, C.S., S.R. ROBINSON & M.A. SMITH. 2002. Amyloid-β: redox-metal chelator and antioxidant. J. Alzheimers Dis. **4:** 203–214.
19. SMITH, M.A., R.K. KUTTY, P.L. RICHEY, *et al.* 1994. Heme oxygenase-1 is associated with the neurofibrillary pathology of Alzheimer's disease. Am. J. Pathol. **145:** 42–47.
20. MORI, H., J. KONDO & Y. IHARA. 1987. Ubiquitin is a component of paired helical filaments in Alzheimer's disease. Science **235:** 1641–1644.
21. PERRY, G., R. FRIEDMAN, G. SHAW, *et al.* 1987. Ubiquitin is detected in neurofibrillary tangles and senile plaque neurites of Alzheimer disease brains. Proc. Natl. Acad. Sci. USA **84:** 3033–3036.
22. OBRENOVICH, M.E., J.A. JOSEPH, C.S. ATWOOD, *et al.* 2002. Amyloid-β: a (life) preserver for the brain. Neurobiol. Aging **23:** 1097–1099.
23. PERRY, G., A. NUNOMURA, A.K. RAINA, *et al.* 2000. Amyloid-β junkies. The Lancet **355:** 757.
24. SMITH, M.A., J.A. JOSEPH, C.S. ATWOOD, *et al.* 2002. Dangers of the amyloid-β vaccine. Acta Neuropathol. **104:** 110.
25. SMITH, M.A., C.S. ATWOOD, J.A. JOSEPH, *et al.* 2002. Ill-fated amyloid-β vaccine. J. Neurosci. Res. **69:** 285.

Combining Growth Factors, Stem Cells, and Gene Therapy for the Aging Brain

SOSHANA BEHRSTOCK AND CLIVE N. SVENDSEN

The Waisman Center, University of Wisconsin-Madison, Madison, Wisconsin 53705-2280, USA

> ABSTRACT: Stem cells have been suggested as a possible "fountain of youth" for replacing tissues lost during aging. In the brain, replacing lost neurons is a challenge, as they have to then be reconnected with their appropriate targets. Perhaps a more realistic and practical strategy for affecting the aging process would be to prevent the loss of neurons from occurring, thus retaining intact circuitry. Glial cell line–derived neurotrophic factor (GDNF) can reverse some aspects of aging in the monkey. Additionally, we have recently shown that GDNF directly infused into the human brain has significant effects on the symptoms of Parkinson disease. Human neural stem cells can be cultured, genetically modified, and transplanted. As such, these cells are ideal for *ex vivo* gene therapy, and may be used in the future as "minipumps" to release GDNF *in vivo* to protect aging neurons. Using such an approach could delay the effects of aging in the brain, giving a better quality of life. Stem cells might not be the fountain of youth, but provide a fountain of youth through the release of growth factors such as GDNF.
>
> KEYWORDS: stem cell; GDNF; Parkinson disease; aging; gene therapy; brain

Aging is associated with impaired motor function, including decreases in movement speed, balance, spontaneous activity levels, and coordination. In part this is likely due to reduced dopaminergic transmission in the basal ganglia, a region of the brain important for coordinating movement. In the basal ganglia, the striatum—consisting of the caudate and putamen—receives dopaminergic innervation from the substantia nigra compacta. A more severe disruption of this circuitry underlies the many motor changes seen in the neurodegenerative disorder Parkinson disease (PD). In both aging and PD, loss of dopamine neurons is a key feature. Thus, one strategy for slowing the progressive neural dysfunction would be to protect or augment the remaining nigrostriatal dopaminergic circuitry. This may be achieved by administering neurotrophic factors that have potent effects on both the survival and function of neurons. One of these, glial cell line–derived neurotrophic factor (GDNF), supports midbrain dopaminergic neurons and therefore has been used to improve motor function in aged animals and has recently been used in a clinical trial for PD.[1]

Address for correspondence: Soshana Behrstock, The Waisman Center, University of Wisconsin-Madison, 1500 Highland Avenue, Madison, WI 53705-2280. Voice: 608-265-8668; fax: 608-263-5267.
 behrstock@waisman.wisc.edu

A number of studies have tested the hypothesis that GDNF would enhance motor function in aged rats and nonhuman primates. A decrease in the total number of neurons expressing tyrosine hydroxylase, the rate-limiting enzyme for dopamine production, is evident in the aged substantia nigra, and has been correlated with age-related motor impairments.[2] Following a single intranigral GDNF injection, aged rats exhibited changes in locomotor activity, including significant increases in total distance traveled and movement speed. Furthermore, there were changes in dopaminergic function, including significant increases in basal and stimulus-evoked dopamine levels and in whole tissue dopamine levels.[3]

In addition to these nigral changes, multiple age-related changes also occur in the striatum. These include decreases in the sensitivity of dopamine receptors and the levels and turnover rate of dopamine. For practical reasons, intrastriatal GDNF administration may be more feasible than intranigral application due to the accessibility of this structure. Administration of GDNF via this route has shown promising effects in aged rats and nonhuman primates. Following striatal implantation of encapsulated GDNF-producing fibroblasts, aged rats showed a significant increase in locomotor activity and bar pressing, but no significant changes in behavioral measures of balance, coordination, and skilled limb use.[4] The limited recovery observed may be due to the reported order of magnitude decrease of GDNF release from the capsules over time. Using the same rat strain and age, Bowenkamp et al.[5] showed that intrastriatal GDNF treatment significantly increased balance, though coordination and skilled limb use were not tested. While GDNF treatment affected balance in aged rats, it did not significantly change spontaneous firing rate in the striatum, striatal neuronal responses following increasing doses of dopamine receptor agonists, or the intensity of tyrosine-hydroxylase staining within the striatum and substantia nigra. This may suggest that the GDNF-mediated improvement in behavior could be located other than postsynaptically in the striatum. Alternatively, a single GDNF injection may be insufficient to elicit longer-term neurological effects such as these.

To achieve continuous exposure to GDNF, Lapchak et al.[6] used chronic intraventricular infusions to the aged rat and showed increased locomotor activity and tyrosine hydroxylase levels in the striatum and substantia nigra. More remarkable findings have been reported for monkeys. Chronic intraventricular GDNF infusion into aged primates increased fine and coarse motor performance compared with their baseline performance before GDNF and compared with vehicle recipients; indeed, the motor performance of aged GDNF recipients was comparable to young primates. Behavioral improvements were sustained over time, even during a two-month washout of GDNF. Furthermore, chronic GDNF delivery led to increased stimulus-evoked release and basal extracellular levels of dopamine.[7] In another study, chronic intraputamenal GDNF infusion into aged primates improved overall motor performance and increased dopamine levels and metabolites in the caudate nucleus, although there were no improvements in fine and coarse motor times.[8] As changes in overall motor performance only occurred after several weeks of GDNF administration and a dose increase, it is possible that behavioral changes in motor times require more than eight weeks of GDNF administration. Furthermore, there are issues when using pumps to deliver GDNF to the brain. In particular, the efficient spread of GDNF within the putamen from the tip of the catheter is still an issue to be overcome.

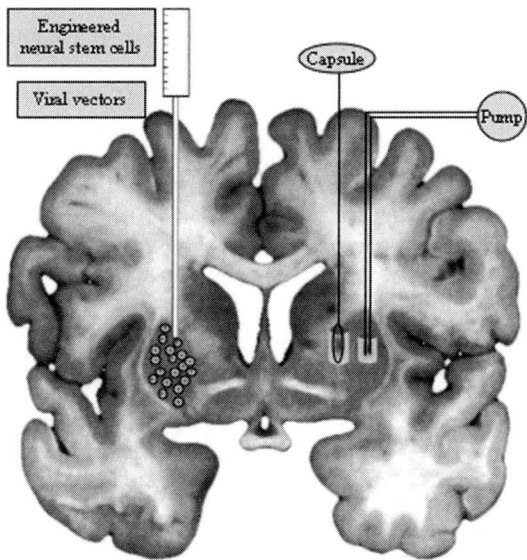

FIGURE 1. Delivery of therapeutic proteins into the brain by capsules and pumps, which provide focal delivery, compared to injected viral vectors and transplanted engineered neural stem cells, which provide more diffuse delivery.

Another approach for GDNF delivery is direct injection of live virus to the brain so that infected host cells will then express GDNF and act as "minipumps." *In vivo* gene therapy with GDNF has shown promise in aged nonhuman primates. In particular, aged monkeys receiving injections of lentivirus modified to produce GDNF showed dramatic increases in dopamine storage within the striatum, and significant functional improvement.[9] GDNF delivery can clearly delay normal age-related neuronal changes involving the nigrostriatal dopaminergic system, and thereby can reverse aspects of aging in the rodent and nonhuman primate.

While motor dysfunction is evident in normal aging, many of the most devastating changes in motor function occur in age-related neurodegenerative diseases such as PD. As with normal age-related motor changes, PD-associated motor dysfunction is due to decreases in nigrostriatal dopamine. GDNF delivery by viruses, pumps, capsules, and transplanted cells has delayed disease progression in animal studies and in a recent clinical trial (FIG. 1). Animal models of PD, including nigrostriatal lesions with 6-hydroxydopamine (6-OHDA) and 1-methyl-4-phenyl-1,2,3,6-tetrahydopryridine (MPTP), have shown that intranigral, intrastriatal, and intraventricular injections of GDNF can protect dopamine cells in the substantia nigra, and can protect and regenerate dopamine terminals in the striatum (FIG. 2A–C).

GDNF delivery into the substantia nigra or the striatum by an adenoviral vector one week before a 6-OHDA striatal lesion protected nigral dopamine cells.[10,11] Additionally, there was behavioral recovery with striatal delivery, but this was not accompanied by affects on dopamine terminals in the striatum. This discrepancy may be explained by retrograde transport of GDNF to the substantia nigra and subsequent increased dopamine release from remaining healthy dopamine nerve terminals. GDNF delivery into the substantia nigra or the striatum by lentiviral vectors before a 6-OHDA lesion also rescued nigral dopamine neurons without protection of dopamine terminals in the striatum.[12,13] There was, however, sprouting of the lesioned axons in the globus pallidus and internal capsule induced by striatal GDNF delivery. This sprouting after striatal GDNF administration is consistent with reported regional effects of GDNF delivery before a 6-OHDA lesion.[14] Striatal GDNF delivery protected nigral cell bodies, increased striatal fiber innervation, and provided behavioral recovery; in contrast, nigral delivery affected only nigral cells. While protective effects of GDNF before a lesion are promising, GDNF delivery after a lesion would be more relevant for PD since therapeutic intervention is often after significant dopamine cell loss occurs.

GDNF delivery into the striatum by an adenoviral vector one week after a 6-OHDA striatal lesion produced no protection and no behavioral recovery.[15] Similarly, Rosenblad and colleagues[16,17] showed that striatal GDNF administration after a 6-OHDA lesion produced no regeneration of striatal dopamine terminals and no behavioral recovery, though they observed protected nigral cell bodies and axonal sprouting within the globus pallidus. While these results are in contrast to the protection of striatal terminal innervation and behavioral recovery with GDNF delivery *prior* to a 6-OHDA lesion described above, other studies demonstrate that delayed GDNF infusion into the striatum can promote striatal reinnervation and recovery of motor function.[18,19] Rosenblad *et al.*[18] have shown that sustained intrastriatal GDNF administration increased nigral dopamine neuron survival and striatal reinnervation, and ameliorated functional deficits. The smaller one-site lesion and the increased total amount of GDNF administered may explain the discrepancy with Rosenblad[17] that showed no terminal regeneration and no behavioral recovery. Kirik *et al.*[19] have shown that delayed infusion of GDNF promoted recovery of motor function in a partial lesion, without striatal terminal reinnervation. A partial lesion may explain this recovery, as only 60% of nigral dopamine cell bodies are damaged compared to the 75–90% damaged by a complete lesion. Seemingly, a critical threshold of spared striatal terminals provided functional recovery after GDNF, potentially through local sprouting.

When GDNF is administered after a lesion, functional recovery is dependent on dopamine terminals in the striatum, either from sparing in a partial lesion or from reinnervation. Studies demonstrating rescue of nigral dopamine neurons without functional recovery may have used lesions where striatal fiber damage was too immediate and extensive for GDNF to promote sprouting and behavioral recovery. Indeed, discrepancies between animal models and human diseases should not be overlooked when using models to help treat disease. For example, rodent models of progressive nigrostriatal degeneration involve immediate and extensive destruction of striatal terminals. Conversely, in PD, dopaminergic fibers persist in the striatum, providing a target for GDNF-induced neuroprotection and recovery. In addition there are important anatomical differences in the striatum between rodents and primates, which may affect the outcome of these various strategies.

Nonhuman primate models of PD may better represent the disease in humans than rodent models. Indeed, GDNF delivery to parkinsonian primates, via lentiviral infection or pumps, has promoted structural and functional recovery.[9,20,21] GDNF delivered into the striatum and substantia nigra one week following an MPTP lesion reversed nigrostriatal degeneration and functional deficits.[9] GDNF preserved striatal innervation, either by prevention of fiber degeneration or by induction of sprouting from remaining fibers. Interestingly, functional recovery was absent in one monkey with the sparsest striatal reinnervation, supporting the concept that GDNF-mediated striatal reinnervation is critical for functional recovery. Additionally, GDNF delivered monthly or continuously into the lateral ventricle six weeks following an MPTP lesion partly restored the nigrostriatal dopaminergic system and motor function.[20,21] Behavioral improvements, evident in bradykinesia, rigidity, balance, and posture, were associated with increased nigral dopamine neurons and their processes innervating the striatum. Effects of GDNF were likely more restorative than protective, since delivery began six weeks following MPTP, a time when parkinsonian symptoms are more advanced. The importance of residual dopamine fibers in the striatum for GDNF-induced recovery was again emphasized, as the fiber regeneration and dopamine level increases were in regions with the highest levels of remaining fibers after MPTP lesion.

GDNF delivery in animal models of PD has prevented nigral cell death and striatal terminal degeneration and has induced fiber sprouting. The encouraging neuroprotective and neurorestorative effects initiated a clinical trial with monthly intraventricular injections of GDNF into patients with advanced PD.[22] The results, however, were disappointing with no reduction in rating scores, serious side effects, and no evidence of restoration of dopamine fibers in the striatum postmortem. This trial most likely failed as GDNF cannot penetrate into deep brain structures from the ventricular system. It is clear that in PD the caudal part of the putamen is most affected, a region that does not lie near the lateral ventricle and therefore would not be expected to receive much GDNF.

GDNF is still a promising factor to treat PD, given appropriate site-specific delivery. Local and continuous infusion of GDNF into the putamen would allow for direct protection and regeneration of the dopamine terminals affected in PD. In a recent trial, GDNF was delivered directly into the putamen using mechanical pumps.[23] Five patients showed significant clinical improvements and reductions in dyskinesias without side effects. Positron emission tomography scans showed a significant increase in dopamine storage within the putamen, suggesting a direct effect of GDNF on dopamine function (FIG. 3). Although a small and open trial, this study showed that large doses of GDNF are safe and have significant positive effects on dopamine function in patients with PD. The potential drawbacks are that pumps are complicated to implant, need constant refilling and ultimate replacement, and importantly, diffusion of GDNF from the catheter tip is limited so large areas of the putamen may not benefit from neuroprotection and neuroregeneration.

This brings up the idea of using viruses to deliver GDNF to the human brain, as discussed in the animal studies above. However, there remain serious practical and safety issues before direct gene therapy is translated to the clinic. These include (1) the inability to exactly control gene dosing following *in vivo* delivery; (2) accidental insertional mutagenesis, as described in recent reports of a gene therapy trial in France;[24] (3) forcing host cells to express a gene of interest that may compromise their normal function; (4) possible immune issues following expression of viral proteins on host cells that may stimulate an immune response; and (5) viral transport to ectopic sites that can result in aberrant, detrimental sprouting. One general caution for GDNF gene therapy is that excess production may cause downregulation of remaining tyrosine hydroxylase or extensive aberrant sprouting under certain deliv-

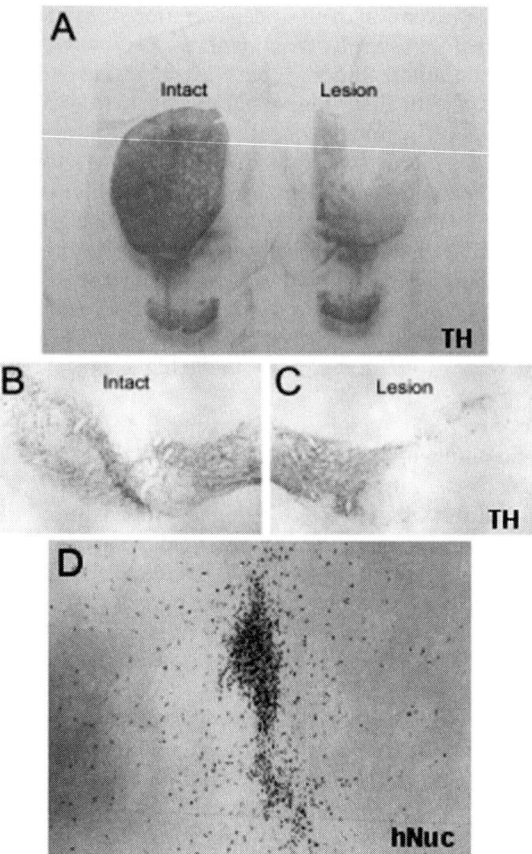

FIGURE 2. Magnitude of TH-positive terminal loss in the striatum (**A**) and cell loss in the substantia nigra (**B, C**) following a partial unilateral striatal lesion (3 injections of 7 μg 6-OHDA). A coronal section showing human neural cells in the rat striatum 8 weeks post-transplantation (**D**). Cells, detected with an antibody recognizing human nuclei, survived and migrated from the graft core to cover the striatum.

ery conditions.[25] Regulatable vectors would help circumvent this concern, and should be used for clinical trials to provide control over gene dosing and the ability to switch off GDNF given any adverse effects.

Ex vivo gene therapy is an alternative approach to direct injection of live virus to the brain. Indirect gene therapy uses viruses to transduce cells *in vitro* that can then be transplanted into the brain to release GDNF. This method of gene therapy has a number of attractive features, including that (1) cells can be selected for gene dosing (protein release) prior to transplantation; (2) the exact insertion sites can be documented from cloned cells and the disruption of normal oncogene regulation caused by the insertion can be checked; (3) healthy *ex vivo* cells, not degenerating host cells, will provide the protein delivery; and (4) because viral infection takes place *in vitro*, there is far less danger of live replication–competent virus transfer to the patient.

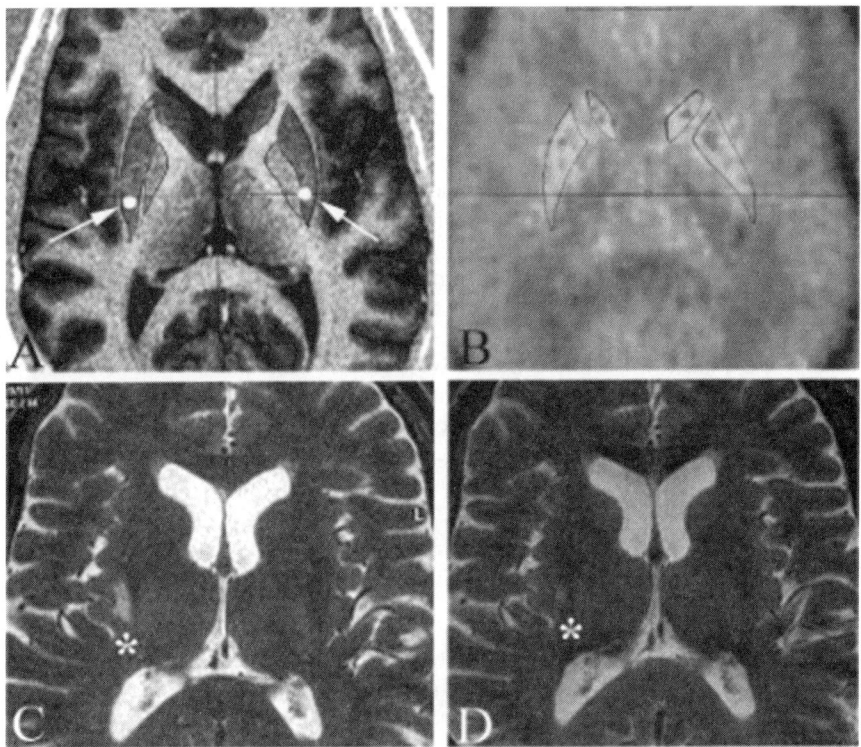

FIGURE 3. Surgical targeting and changes in MRI after chronic GDNF delivery. MRI scan showing targeted regions in the dorsal putamen (*arrows and white circles*) (**A**). The marked areas showed a low [^{18}F]dopa signal in an adjacent PET image (**B**). High signal in the area around the catheter tip 6 months after treatment with GDNF at a concentration of 43.2 μg/d at an infusion rate of 6 μL/h (*region above asterisk*) (**C**). Resolution after treatment with a lower GDNF concentration of 14.4 μg/d at a flow rate of 6 μL/h for 1 month (*region above asterisk*) (**D**).

Furthermore, in some cases, transplanted genetically engineered cells migrate to cover a large portion of the putamen, thereby providing GDNF and its trophic effects to a greater area than achievable with other delivery methods.

Different cell types can be genetically engineered *in vitro* to express GDNF and then transplanted to determine the *in vivo* effects. Transplanting engineered GDNF-producing astrocytes into the substantia nigra before a 6-OHDA lesion in the mouse prevented the loss of nigral cell bodies, provided partial protection of striatal dopaminergic fibers, and ameliorated rotational behavior.[26] While these results show promise for *ex vivo* gene therapy using GDNF-producing astrocytes, the level and pattern of GDNF expression posttransplantation into the nigra was not reported, and the function of cells transplanted into the striatum following a lesion still needs to be demonstrated. Park *et al.*[27] have shown that bone marrow cells can be genetically engineered *in vitro* to express GDNF and that after intravenous transplantation into

MPTP-lesioned mice there is protection of nigral neurons and striatal fibers. While the duration of efficacy, specific targeting of GDNF to affected brain regions, and benefit to parkinsonian-like behaviors still need to be addressed, intravenous delivery of marrow-derived GDNF-producing cells to the brain provides another proof of concept for *ex vivo* GDNF gene therapy. An immortalized neural stem cell (NSC) line genetically engineered *in vitro* to express GDNF and transplanted into a mouse model of PD engrafted well in the striatum, maintained high levels of GDNF for at least 4 months, prevented the degeneration of nigral dopamine neurons, and reduced behavioral impairment.[28] Additionally, using a lentiviral vector for *ex vivo* gene transfer, rodent NSCs have been genetically engineered to express GDNF, and following transplantation these cells were shown to increase the survival of cotransplanted dopamine neurons.[29] These cells do not have immortalizing genes and may therefore be safer candidates for clinical trials. Such studies confirm the potent effects of GDNF for PD and demonstrate the potential of NSCs for *ex vivo* gene therapy.

The manipulability *in vitro* and ability to deliver functional levels of GDNF *in vivo* make NSCs ideal for *ex vivo* gene therapy. NSCs can grow as either monolayers or free-floating aggregates termed "neurospheres" and maintain the potential to form neurons and glia. Rodent NSCs, described above, provide proof of concept for these cells as an ideal vehicle for *ex vivo* gene therapy. Ultimately, however, human cells are required for translation into the clinic. Human NSCs have been isolated from the germinal zones of postmortem fetal brain tissue, an advantage over human embryonic stem cells since fetal cells make only neural tissue and do not produce teratomas. Techniques for the growth, differentiation, and transplantation of human NSCs have now been refined.[30] These cells can be cultured for extended periods of time, induced to differentiate into various neural phenotypes, and genetically modified.[31] Furthermore, these cells survive transplantation, have extensive fiber outgrowth, and can migrate to cover a wide area of the striatum (FIG. 2D).[32,33]

It has been established that NSCs can be genetically engineered *in vitro* and that *in vivo* these cells remain healthy, disperse throughout the grafted region, stably express foreign transgenes, and deliver soluble proteins at functional levels. As such, they are an ideal candidate for *ex vivo* gene therapy. For translation into the clinic, NSCs can be derived from human fetal tissue and have been well characterized *in vitro* and *in vivo*. Currently, there are no means to delay the effects of aging in the brain. For PD, treatments include pharmacologically replacing dopamine, grafting fetal dopamine cells, and muting hyperexcited regions by lesions or high frequency stimulation. However, pharmacological intervention has decreased efficacy and increased side effects with disease progression, fetal grafts may be ineffective,[34] and altering nuclei activity can be invasive and irrevocable. Transplantation of human NSCs genetically modified to produce regulated GDNF may be the next step for neuroprotection and neuroregeneration of the degenerating nigrostriatal circuitry in normal aging and Parkinson disease.

REFERENCES

1. LIN, L.F., D.H. DOHERTY, J.D. LILE, *et al.* 1993. GDNF: a glial cell line-derived neurotrophic factor for midbrain dopaminergic neurons. Science **260:** 1130–1132.

2. EMBORG, M.E., S.Y. MA, E.J. MUFSON, et al. 1998. Age-related declines in nigral neuronal function correlate with motor impairments in rhesus monkeys J. Comp. Neurol. **401:** 253–265.
3. HEBERT, M.A. & G.A. GERHARDT. 1997. Behavioral and neurochemical effects of intranigral administration of glial cell line-derived neurotrophic factor on aged Fischer 344 rats. J. Pharmacol. Exp. Ther. **282:** 760–768.
4. EMERICH, D.F., M. PLONE, J. FRANCIS, et al. 1996. Alleviation of behavioral deficits in aged rodents following implantation of encapsulated GDNF-producing fibroblasts. Brain Res. **736:** 99–110.
5. BOWENKAMP, K.E., L. UJHELYI, E.J. CLINE & P.C. BICKFORD. 2000. Effects of intra-striatal GDNF on motor coordination and striatal electrophysiology in aged F344 rats. Neurobiol. Aging **21:** 117–124.
6. LAPCHAK, P.A., P.J. MILLER & S. JIAO. 1997. Glial cell line-derived neurotrophic factor induces the dopaminergic and cholinergic phenotype and increases locomotor activity in aged Fischer 344 rats. Neuroscience **77:** 745–752.
7. GRONDIN, R., W.A. CASS, Z. ZHANG, et al. 2003. Glial cell line-derived neurotrophic factor increases stimulus-evoked dopamine release and motor speed in aged rhesus monkeys. J. Neurosci. **23:** 1974–1980.
8. MASWOOD, N., R. GRONDIN, Z. ZHANG, et al. 2002. Effects of chronic intraputamenal infusion of glial cell line-derived neurotrophic factor (GDNF) in aged Rhesus monkeys. Neurobiol. Aging **23:** 881–889.
9. KORDOWER, J.H., M.E. EMBORG, J. BLOCH, et al. 2000. Neurodegeneration prevented by lentiviral vector delivery of GDNF in primate models of Parkinson's disease. Science **290:** 767–773.
10. CHOI-LUNDBERG, D.L., Q. LIN, Y.N. CHANG, et al. 1997. Dopaminergic neurons protected from degeneration by GDNF gene therapy. Science **275:** 838–841.
11. CHOI-LUNDBERG, D.L., Q. LIN, T. SCHALLERT, et al. 1998. Behavioral and cellular protection of rat dopaminergic neurons by an adenoviral vector encoding glial cell line-derived neurotrophic factor. Exp. Neurol. **154:** 261–275.
12. BENSADOUN, J.C., N. DEGLON, J.L. TSENG, et al. 2000. Lentiviral vectors as a gene delivery system in the mouse midbrain: cellular and behavioral improvements in a 6-OHDA model of Parkinson's disease using GDNF. Exp. Neurol. **164:** 15–24.
13. GEORGIEVSKA, B., D. KIRIK, C. ROSENBLAD, et al. 2002. Neuroprotection in the rat Parkinson model by intrastriatal GDNF gene transfer using a lentiviral vector. NeuroReport **13:** 75–82.
14. KIRIK, D., C. ROSENBLAD & A. BJORKLUND. 2000. Preservation of a functional nigrostriatal dopamine pathway by GDNF in the intrastriatal 6-OHDA lesion model depends on the site of administration of the trophic factor. Eur. J. Neurosci. **12:** 3871–3882.
15. KOZLOWSKI, D.A., B. CONNOR, J.L. TILLERSON, et al. 2000. Delivery of a GDNF gene into the substantia nigra after a progressive 6-OHDA lesion maintains functional nigrostriatal connections. Exp. Neurol. **166:** 1–15.
16. ROSENBLAD, C., D. KIRIK, B. DEVAUX, et al. 1999. Protection and regeneration of nigral dopaminergic neurons by neurturin or GDNF in a partial lesion model of Parkinson's disease after administration into the striatum or the lateral ventricle. Eur. J. Neurosci. **11:** 1554–1566.
17. ROSENBLAD, C., D. KIRIK & A. BJORKLUND. 2000. Sequential administration of GDNF into the substantia nigra and striatum promotes dopamine neuron survival and axonal sprouting but not striatal reinnervation or functional recovery in the partial 6-OHDA lesion model. Exp. Neurol. **161:** 503–516.
18. ROSENBLAD, C., A. MARTINEZ-SERRANO & A. BJORKLUND. 1998. Intrastriatal glial cell line-derived neurotrophic factor promotes sprouting of spared nigrostriatal dopaminergic afferents and induces recovery of function in a rat model of Parkinson's disease. Neuroscience **82:** 129–137.
19. KIRIK, D., B. GEORGIEVSKA, C. ROSENBLAD & A. BJORKLUND. 2001. Delayed infusion of GDNF promotes recovery of motor function in the partial lesion model of Parkinson's disease. Eur. J. Neurosci. **13:** 1589–1599.

20. GRONDIN, R., Z. ZHANG, A. YI, *et al.* 2002. Chronic, controlled GDNF infusion promotes structural and functional recovery in advanced parkinsonian monkeys. Brain **125:** 1–11.
21. GASH, D.M., Z. ZHANG, A. OVADIA, *et al.* 1996. Functional recovery in parkinsonian monkeys treated with GDNF. Nature **380:** 252–255.
22. NUTT, J.G., K.J. BURCHIEL, C.L. COMELLA, *et al.* 2003. Randomized, double-blind trial of glial cell line-derived neurotrophic factor (GDNF) in PD. Neurology **60:** 69–73.
23. GILL, S.S., N.K. PATEL, G.R. HOTTON, *et al.* 2003. Direct brain infusion of glial cell line-derived neurotrophic factor in Parkinson disease. Nat. Med. **9:** 589–595.
24. KAISER, J. 2003. Gene therapy. Seeking the cause of induced leukemias in X-SCID trial. Science **299:** 495.
25. GEORGIEVSKA, B., D. KIRIK & A. BJORKLUND. 2002. Aberrant sprouting and downregulation of tyrosine hydroxylase in lesioned nigrostriatal dopamine neurons induced by long-lasting overexpression of glial cell line derived neurotrophic factor in the striatum by lentiviral gene transfer. Exp. Neurol. **177:** 461–474.
26. CUNNINGHAM, L.A. & C. SU. 2002. Astrocyte delivery of glial cell line-derived neurotrophic factor in a mouse model of Parkinson's disease. Exp. Neurol. **174:** 230–242.
27. PARK, K., M.A. EGLITIS & M.M. MOURADIAN. 2001. Protection of nigral neurons by GDNF-engineered marrow cell transplantation. Neurosci. Res. **40:** 315–323.
28. AKERUD, P., J.M. CANALS, E.Y. SNYDER & E. ARENAS. 2001. Neuroprotection through delivery of glial cell line-derived neurotrophic factor by neural stem cells in a mouse model of Parkinson's disease. J. Neurosci. **21:** 8108–8118.
29. OSTENFELD, T., Y.T. TAI, P. MARTIN, *et al.* 2002. Neurospheres modified to produce glial cell line-derived neurotrophic factor increase the survival of transplanted dopamine neurons. J. Neurosci. Res. **69:** 955–965.
30. OSTENFELD, T. & C.N. SVENDSEN. 2003. Recent advances in stem cell neurobiology. Adv. Tech. Stand. Neurosurg. **28:** 4–61.
31. WU, P., Y. YE & C.N. SVENDSEN. 2002. Transduction of human neural progenitor cells using recombinant adeno-associated viral vectors. Gene Ther. **9:** 245–255.
32. ENGLUND, U., R.A. FRICKER-GATES, C. LUNDBERG, *et al.* 2002. Transplantation of human neural progenitor cells into the neonatal rat brain: extensive migration and differentiation with long-distance axonal projections. Exp. Neurol. **173:** 1–21.
33. OSTENFELD, T., M.A. CALDWELL, K.R. PROWSE, *et al.* 2000. Human neural precursor cells express low levels of telomerase in vitro and show diminishing cell proliferation with extensive axonal outgrowth following transplantation. Exp. Neurol. **164:** 215–226.
34. OLANOW, C.W., C.G. GOETZ, J.H. KORDOWER, *et al.* 2003. A double-blind controlled trial of bilateral fetal nigral transplantation in Parkinson's disease. Ann. Neurol. **54:** 403–414.

The Role of Viruses and of APOE in Dementia

R. F. ITZHAKI, C. B. DOBSON, S. J. SHIPLEY, AND M. A. WOZNIAK

Molecular Neurobiology Laboratory, Department of Optometry and Neuroscience, University of Manchester Institute of Science and Technology, Manchester M60 1QD, United Kingdom

ABSTRACT: The virus, herpes simplex virus type 1 (HSV1), when present in brain, acts together with the type 4 allele of the APOE gene, a known susceptibility factor in Alzheimer disease (AD), to confer a strong risk of AD; in carriers of the other two main alleles of the gene, the virus does not confer a risk. It also has been shown that the outcome of infection in the case of five diseases known to be caused by viruses is determined by APOE. It is hoped that the discovery of the involvement of HSV1 in AD will lead to future antiviral therapy and possibly to immunization against the virus in infancy.

KEYWORDS: Alzheimer disease (AD); APOE; brain; DNA; herpes simplex virus type 1 (HSV1); virus

Infectious agents often elicit diverse responses, depending on the individual host, ranging from severe to inappreciable, but in general the reasons for this are unknown. We have found that a virus, herpes simplex virus type 1 (HSV1), when present in brain, acts together with the type 4 allele of the APOE gene, a known susceptibility factor in Alzheimer disease (AD), to confer a strong risk of AD; in carriers of the other two main alleles of the gene, the virus does not confer a risk. Also, we (and another group) have shown that the outcome of infection in the case of five diseases known to be caused by viruses is determined by APOE.

HSV1 was suggested as a possible risk factor in AD many years ago. However, whether it is present in the human central nervous system (CNS), other than during the very rare acute HSV1 infection, herpes simplex encephalitis (HSE), was uncertain because the detection methods used were insufficiently sensitive. In contrast, it was well known that the virus is harbored by nearly all adults in their peripheral nervous system (PNS) in latent form: the viral DNA is present and it produces a single set of transcripts [the latency-associated transcripts (LATs)], but no viral proteins and hence no virus particles. However, it can reactivate due to, for example, stress, producing whole viruses, that is, an acute infection, which in some people (about 20–40%) causes cold sores (*Herpes labialis*), but in others is asymptomatic. Thus, another factor must interact with the virus to cause cold sores.

Address for correspondence: R.F. Itzhaki, Molecular Neurobiology Laboratory, Department of Optometry and Neuroscience, University of Manchester Institute of Science and Technology, P.O. Box 88, Manchester M60 1QD, UK. Voice: +44-(0)-161-200-3879; fax: +44-(0)-161-200-4433.

ruth.itzhaki@umist.ac.uk

We have established that HSV1 DNA is present in brains of a high proportion of elderly people (AD and normal) using polymerase chain reaction.[1] Further, we have detected antibodies to the virus in cerebrospinal fluid (these are known to be very long-lived after HSE) in a high proportion of elderly people (Wozniak, Combrinck, Wilcock & Itzhaki, submitted), including AD patients; this confirms that HSV1 is present and shows that it must have caused an acute infection in brain at least on entry there, and possibly subsequently, if reactivation occurs there as it does in the PNS.

The presence of HSV1 DNA in brains of elderly normals as well as of AD patients does not preclude its having a role in the disease: as stated above, the diverse responses to a damaging agent are presumably determined by other factors, including genetic factors. For example, although most people are infected in the PNS with HSV1, it causes cold sores only in some, and a genetic factor is indeed involved (see below).

We then discovered that, when HSV1 DNA is present in the brains of elderly people who carry an APOE-ε4 allele, it confers a strong risk of developing AD, much stronger than either factor alone.[2,3] (Our results refute alternative explanations—that AD patients or APOE-ε4 possessors are more susceptible to HSV1 infection—in that a high proportion of aged normals have HSV1 in brain, and most of these normals do not have an APOE-ε4 allele.) Subsequently, several other groups substantiated our detection of HSV1 DNA in brain, and an HSV1–APOE-ε4 association in AD was found in another study, with a second showing a similar trend. (Two other groups claimed to have found no association of HSV1 in brain and carriage of an APOE-ε4 allele in AD, but each detected HSV1 DNA in only one brain, out of 15 and 34 people, respectively, providing a rather inadequate number for detecting any correlation.) These papers are discussed in Reference 4.

We found also that a far higher proportion of sufferers from cold sores than of nonsufferers are APOE-ε4 possessors.[2,3] This provides strong and independent support for our hypothesis that the combination of HSV1 and APOE-ε4 is particularly damaging in the nervous system. Further support for the concept that APOE determines the severity of the host's response to certain viruses comes from our discovery that the damage caused by hepatitis C virus (HCV) in liver is determined by APOE;[5] we found also that susceptibility to infection by HCV, clearance of the virus, and liver damage due to other causes such as alcoholism were not affected by APOE. Another group showed a dependence on APOE in two disorders caused by HIV (in pre-AIDS patients)—dementia and peripheral neuropathy[6]—in striking parallelism to our findings on AD in the CNS and cold sores in the PNS. More recently, we found that APOE is involved in HSE.[7] Thus, the outcome of five disorders quite definitely caused by viruses—three very different viruses—is governed by APOE.

We have preliminary data indicating that APOE plays a role also in infection by the malaria protozoon: infants who are APOE-ε2 homozygotes become infected at a significantly earlier age than do infants with the other genotypes.[8]

One common factor in all these diseases, which provided the rationale for our investigating them, is that apoE and each of the pathogens share binding sites, namely, heparan sulfate proteoglycans, and/or specific receptors for apoE, on the cell surface. Thus, pathogen and apoE might compete for binding and entry into cells and, if one isoform were to compete less well than the others, it would allow more entry and spread of the pathogen and hence more damage. In fact, apoE4 binds with greater affinity to hepatoma cells in culture (see Ref. 4), so this could explain the seeming paradox that APOE-ε4 affords protection against HCV-induced damage in liver, but is harmful in respect to AD. Interestingly, the isoforms bind with similar affinity to fibroblasts, consistent with our results showing that in another HSV1 disorder, herpes simplex keratitis, in which the target tissue, the cornea, consists mainly of fibroblast-like cells, APOE genotypes do not differ statistically significantly from normals.[9] Whether there is a dependence of specific isoform affinity in other cell types has not yet been studied in detail. An alternative mechanism for the HSV1–APOE interaction in AD is a lesser extent of repair of viral damage by apoE4 in certain neural cells, but little work has been done on this aspect.

We have also sought other human herpesviruses in brain. We found human herpesvirus 6 (HHV6) DNA in a higher proportion of AD sufferers' brains than controls, suggesting that this virus might be a risk; however, the virus might be present as a consequence of AD, if the AD brain were more susceptible to infection with this virus. We found also human cytomegalovirus DNA in brain of a higher proportion of vascular dementia sufferers than aged normals, but (like HHV6 and AD) we do not know whether this virus is a cause or consequence of the disease. (Both are reviewed in Ref. 4.)

As to the mode of action of HSV1, infection of cultured human neuroblastoma cells alters the metabolism of amyloid precursor protein (APP): we found a significant increase in the levels of a 55-kDa C-terminal APP fragment, compared to uninfected cells, and concomitantly the levels of full-length APP decreased (S. Shipley, E.T. Parkin, R.F. Itzhaki & C.B. Dobson, submitted).

Three recent studies provide further indirect support for a viral role in AD: (a) AD patients showed a decline in cognitive function for at least two months after a systemic infection, associated probably with microglial cell activation;[10] (b) cognitive impairment in elderly cardiovascular patients was associated with viral pathogen burden (HSV and cytomegalovirus);[11] and (c) vaccination against various viruses was protective against AD (discussed in Ref. 4). Peripheral infection may result in cytokine production and entry into brain, leading to brain inflammation and hence reactivation of resident HSV1 (vaccination would prevent this process being initiated).

In conclusion, we hope that our discovery of the involvement of HSV1 in AD will lead to future antiviral therapy and possibly to immunization against the virus in infancy [following our study (see Ref. 4) showing the protective effect in brain of vaccination against HSV1 in infected mice].

REFERENCES

1. JAMIESON, G.A. *et al.* 1991. Latent herpes simplex virus type 1 in normal and Alzheimer's disease brains. J. Med. Virol. **33:** 224–227.
2. ITZHAKI, R.F. *et al.* 1997. Herpes simplex virus type 1 in brain and risk of Alzheimer's disease. Lancet **349:** 241–244.
3. LIN, W.R. *et al.* 1998. Alzheimer's disease, herpes virus in brain, apolipoprotein E4, and herpes labialis. Alzheimer's Rep. **1:** 173–178.
4. DOBSON, C.B., M.A. WOZNIAK & R.F. ITZHAKI. 2003. Do infectious agents play a role in dementia? Trends Microbiol. **11:** 312–317.
5. WOZNIAK, M.A. *et al.* 2002. Apolipoprotein E–epsilon 4 protects against severe liver disease caused by hepatitis C virus. Hepatology **36:** 456–463.
6. CORDER, E.H. *et al.* 1998. HIV-infected subjects with the E4 allele for APOE have excess dementia and peripheral neuropathy. Nat. Med. **4:** 1182–1184.

7. LIN, W.R. *et al.* 2001. Herpes simplex encephalitis: involvement of apolipoprotein E genotype. J. Neurol. Neurosurg. Psychiatry **70:** 117–119.
8. WOZNIAK, M.A. *et al.* 2003. Does apolipoprotein E polymorphism influence susceptibility to malaria? J. Med. Genet. **40:** 348–351.
9. LIN, W.R., A.B. TULLO & R.F. ITZHAKI. 1999. Apolipoprotein E and herpes virus diseases: herpes simplex keratitis. Eur. J. Hum. Genet. **7:** 401–403.
10. HOLMES, C. *et al.* 2003. Systemic infection, interleukin 1β, and cognitive decline in Alzheimer's disease. J. Neurol. Neurosurg. Psychiatry **74:** 788–789.
11. STRANDBERG, T.E. *et al.* 2003. Impact of viral and bacterial burden on cognitive impairment in elderly persons with cardiovascular diseases. Stroke **34:** 2126–2131.

Metabolic Substrates of Neuronal Aging

E. C. TOESCU AND J. XIONG

Department of Physiology, University of Birmingham,
Edgbaston, Birmingham B15 2TT, United Kingdom

> ABSTRACT: One mechanism proposed to explain age-dependent changes has been the "Ca^{2+} hypothesis" of aging. Data indicate that most changes in the Ca^{2+} homeostasis of the cerebellar granule neurons appear only when the aged neurons are exposed to higher levels of stimulation and that these changes are secondary to metabolic limitations imposed by altered mitochondrial function.
>
> KEYWORDS: aging; brain; $[Ca^{2+}]_i$; cerebellar granule; homeostasis; neuron

INTRODUCTION

A certain degree of impairment of neuronal activity, resulting in a decrease in memory and cognitive functions, is a normal phenotype of normal brain aging. One mechanism proposed to explain the age-dependent changes was the "Ca^{2+} hypothesis" of aging, but a thorough review of the data available revealed a number of inconsistencies.[1] Two important questions were raised: (1) Which are, if any, the most reliable age-associated changes in neuronal Ca^{2+} homeostasis? and (2) Are these changes primary, and thus determinant of the aging phenotype, or are they secondary to other changes in the physiology of the aged neurons? We approached these questions[2] by using the most physiological *in vitro* neuronal preparation—the brain slices, obtained from animals of different ages—and performing simultaneous measurements of both intracellular free Ca^{2+} ($[Ca^{2+}]_i$) and mitochondrial membrane potential in real time. Our data indicate that most of the changes in the Ca^{2+} homeostasis of the cerebellar granule neurons appear only when the aged neurons are exposed to higher levels of stimulation and that these changes are secondary to metabolic limitations imposed by altered mitochondrial function.

MATERIALS AND METHODS

Parasagittal brain slices (250 μm) from mice (C57Bl/6) of different ages were prepared as previously described.[2] For $[Ca^{2+}]_i$ and mitochondrial membrane potential measurements, the slices were loaded with 2 μM fura-2 and/or 10 μM rhodamine 123 and transferred to a perfusion bath on the stage of an Olympus BW 50I microscope. Images were taken using an intensified GenIV camera (Roper Instruments, United

---

Address for correspondence: E. C. Toescu, Department of Physiology, University of Birmingham, Edgbaston, Birmingham B15 2TT, UK. Voice: +44-121-414-6927; fax: +44-121-414-6924.
e.c.toescu@bham.ac.uk

Kingdom) with the excitation light provided by a monochromator (Cairn Research Limited, United Kingdom), controlled through the MetaFluor software (Universal Imaging, United States). The emission was set using various cutoff filters placed in a Sutter filter wheel installed in front of the camera. Images were analyzed with MetaFluor and data analysis performed off-line using Excel and Origin programs. Data are reported as the mean ± SEM.

RESULTS AND DISCUSSION

A detailed analysis of the main parameters of $[Ca^{2+}]_i$ homeostasis forms the basis of a rational assessment of the role of intracellular Ca^{2+} in mediating the effects of normal aging in neurons. Measurements, in resting conditions, of these parameters in cerebellar granule neurons in brain slices obtained from animals of various ages showed no significant age-related difference.[2] Thus, the values of resting $[Ca^{2+}]_i$ were very similar across the life span of the animals [e.g., 71 ± 4 nM Ca^{2+} for mature animals (10–15 months old; $n = 89$) and 75 ± 4 for old animals (20–24 months old; $n = 124$)]. The fact that, at rest, there are no significant differences between the aged and the mature or young neurons has important implications since the homeostatic maintenance of the resting $[Ca^{2+}]_i$ values reflects the balance between the $[Ca^{2+}]_i$ entry processes and the Ca^{2+} removal systems. If normal neuronal aging would be associated with a primary defect in any of these Ca^{2+} homeostatic mechanisms, this should result in alterations of the resting $[Ca^{2+}]_i$ values, reflecting the putative new steady-state situation.

The generation of the $[Ca^{2+}]_i$ signal of the cerebellar granule neurons in response to membrane depolarization evoked by 75 mM KCl (in the presence of 1 µM TTX) was also not affected by aging. The mean peak $[Ca^{2+}]_i$ increase in mature neurons was 512 ± 18 nM (range: 225–775 nM), compared with 527 ± 12 nM (range: 205–823 nM) in the old neurons. The mean rate of $[Ca^{2+}]_i$ increase during the rising phase of the Ca^{2+} response was also not different (167 ± 15 nM Ca^{2+}/s in the mature neurons vs. 181 ± 29 nM Ca^{2+}/s in the old neurons). This appears different from the situation in the hippocampal neurons, where aging is associated with an elevated $[Ca^{2+}]_i$ response to transynaptic stimulation.[3] A reason for this is the age-dependent increase of L-type Ca^{2+} channels in hippocampal neurons,[4] possibly associated with changes in the sensitivity of the Ca^{2+}-induced Ca^{2+} release process (CICR).[3,5] The electrophysiology of the aging cerebellar granule neuron or of the Purkinje neuron is largely unknown.

However, the young and mature neurons do not function in exactly the same regime conditions as the aged neurons, and the differences between them become apparent during periods of higher metabolic demand. We have shown previously[2] that the metabolic stress of maintaining the brain slices in *in vitro* conditions decreases the number of viable neurons in the old slices compared with the younger ones. Another difference was the type of patterns of $[Ca^{2+}]_i$ responses evoked by either chemical neuronal depolarization (with KCl) or glutamatergic stimulation. If most of the neurons (>85%) in the young and mature slices respond to a short pulse (10–30 s) of stimulation with a simple monophasic response, only about half of the neurons (55%) in the aged slices display such a pattern. The rest of the neurons showed various patterns of Ca^{2+} dysregulation following the single pulse stimulation, with aborted $[Ca^{2+}]_i$ recovery phases followed by slow, but irreversible increases in

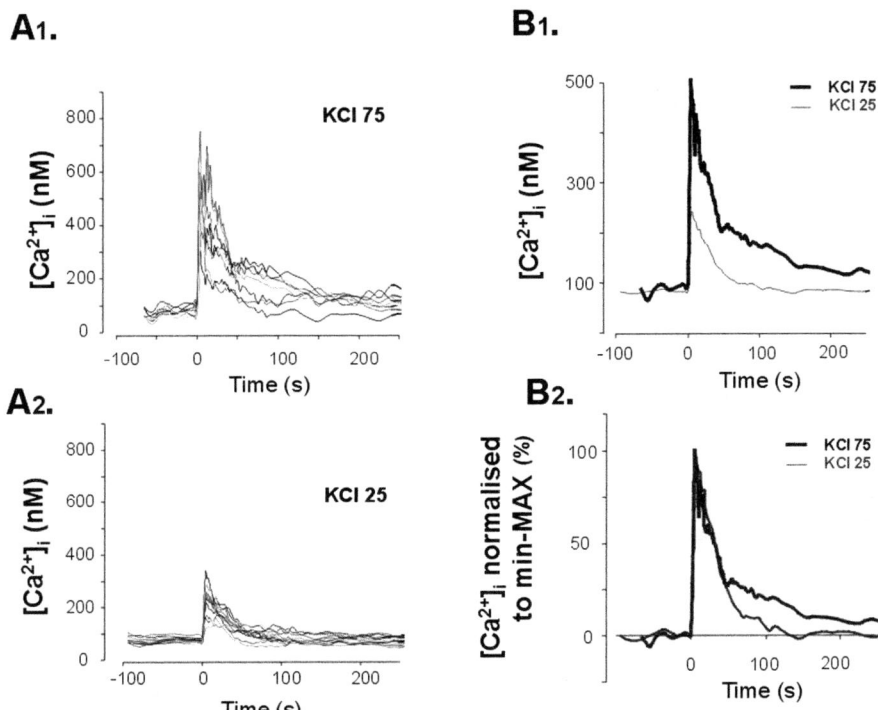

FIGURE 1. Effect of activity-induced Ca^{2+} load on the rate of $[Ca^{2+}]_i$ recovery. Cerebellar granule neurons from brain slices obtained from aged animals (20–22 months old) were exposed to different levels of chemical depolarization, evoked by perfusion with KCl. *Panel A* shows the individual traces obtained from two such experiments for each stimulation condition: 75 mM KCl (*panel A1*) and 25 mM KCl (*panel A2*). In *panel B1*, the data from several experiments were averaged for each condition and are displayed as $[Ca^{2+}]_i$ values. For ease of comparison, the data are also displayed (*panel B2*) after normalization (min-MAX normalization, with "min" being the mean of the $[Ca^{2+}]_i$ values from the last seven time points before stimulation and the "MAX" being the maximal $[Ca^{2+}]_i$ value reached during the response).

$[Ca^{2+}]_i$ (cf. Ref. 2 for KCl stimulation; and similar general patterns were observed following 100 µM glutamate or NMDA in 0 Mg^{2+}/glycine solutions).

Even for the aged neurons that respond "normally", with a monophasic $[Ca^{2+}]_i$ response, to stimulation, there are significant differences from the mature neurons in the rate of $[Ca^{2+}]_i$ recovery.[2] More recent experiments, following this observation, show that the decrease in the rate of $[Ca^{2+}]_i$ recovery is proportional to the level of stimulation. FIGURE 1A shows the individual response of aged cerebellar granule neurons from aged slices to two levels of chemical depolarization (75 and 25 mM KCl). Data are summarized in FIGURE 1B: with 75 mM KCl, the average KCl response was 510 ± 14 nM Ca^{2+} [$n = 33$ neurons (4 slices, 3 old animals)], compared with 239 ± 11 nM Ca^{2+} [$n = 25$ neurons (3 slices, 3 old animals)] for stimulation with 25 mM KCl. The differences in the recovery rate become apparent when the data are normalized, as shown in panel B2. The data points following stimulus removal were fitted, for each individual neuron, by a first-order exponential decay model generating different equations for the two stimulus protocols. For the lower level of stimulation, the time constant (τ) was 18.4 ± 1.3 s, compared with 25.7 ± 2.1 s for the higher KCl stimulation protocol ($P < .01$). Thus, these data show that the slower recovery of resting $[Ca^{2+}]_i$ values is not simply a "given" feature of the aged neurons, but a dynamic reflection of the metabolic stress experienced during activity. A similar mathematical analysis of the Ca^{2+} recovery phase in the mature neurons showed that stimulation of these neurons with either low or high KCl resulted in similar recovery kinetics, irrespective of the Ca^{2+} load induced (τ of 16.4 ± 1.1 s and 17.1 ± 1.2 s). Hence, when exposed to low levels of stimulation, the aged neurons are able to perform in a manner similar to the young neurons, implying again that the deficit is not at the level of the Ca^{2+} removal system, but most likely at the level of metabolic support for this process (or processes).

Simultaneous assessment of $[Ca^{2+}]_i$ and mitochondrial status (using rhodamine 123) indicated significant changes in the mitochondrial status in the aged neurons. These mitochondria show a small level of chronic depolarization[2,6] and significant structural and functional changes.[7] Whereas increases in cytosolic $[Ca^{2+}]_i$ determine mitochondrial Ca^{2+} loading and consequent mitochondrial depolarization,[2,8] the repolarization process is significantly delayed in the aged neurons.[2] The delay in mitochondrial repolarization correlates, on an individual neuronal level, with the degree of impairment of $[Ca^{2+}]_i$ recovery, indicating the relationship between these processes.

Overall, the picture that emerges from these studies is that the aged neurons are characterized by a decrease in their homeostatic reserve, defined as their capacity to oppose perturbations of the normal ionic homeostasis, which is most likely a consequence of the alterations in mitochondrial functions. However, whereas the mitochondrial depolarization imposes metabolic constraints on the system, which are evident especially at higher levels of stimulation, it is possible that these mitochondrial changes could represent an adaptive response of the aging neurons. This is based on the notion that the production of free radicals, which play a central metabolic role in the development of the aging phenotype,[9] is predominantly mitochondrial and is favored by a high mitochondrial membrane potential (Ψ_{mito}).[10] A decrease of Ψ_{mito} will thus reduce the production of free radicals in resting conditions.[11]

ACKNOWLEDGMENTS

The financial support of the BBSRC is gratefully acknowledged.

REFERENCES

1. VERKHRATSKY, A. & E. TOESCU. 1998. Calcium and neuronal ageing. TINS **21:** 2–7.
2. XIONG, J., A. VERKHRATSKY & E.C. TOESCU. 2002. Changes in mitochondrial status associated with altered Ca^{2+} homeostasis in aged cerebellar granule neurones in brain slices. J. Neurosci. **22:** 10761–10771.
3. THIBAULT, O., R. HADLEY & P.W. LANDFIELD. 2001. Elevated postsynaptic $[Ca^{2+}]_i$ and L-type calcium channel activity in aged hippocampal neurons: relationship to impaired synaptic plasticity. J. Neurosci. **21:** 9744–9756.

4. THIBAULT, O. & P.W. LANDFIELD. 1996. Increase in single L-type calcium channels in hippocampal neurons during aging. Science **272:** 1017–1020.
5. SOLOVYOVA, N., N. VESELOVSKY, E.C. TOESCU & A. VERKHRATSKY. 2002. Ca^{2+} dynamics in the lumen of the endoplasmic reticulum in sensory neurons: direct visualization of Ca^{2+}-induced Ca^{2+} release triggered by physiological Ca^{2+} entry. EMBO J. **21:** 622–630.
6. HAGEN, T., D. YOWE, J. BARTHOLOMEW *et al.* 1997. Mitochondrial decay in hepatocytes from old rats: membrane potential declines, heterogeneity and oxidants increase. Proc. Natl. Acad. Sci. USA **94:** 3064–3069.
7. TOESCU, E.C., N. MYRONOVA & A. VERKHRATSKY. 2000. Age-related structural and functional changes of brain mitochondria. Cell Calcium **28:** 329–338.
8. DUCHEN, M. 1999. Contributions of mitochondria to animal physiology: from homeostatic sensor to calcium signalling and cell death. J. Physiol. **516:** 1–17.
9. BARJA, G. 1999. Mitochondrial oxygen radical generation and leak: sites of production in states 4 and 3, organ specificity, and relation to aging and longevity. J. Bioenerg. Biomembr. **31:** 347–366.
10. NICHOLLS, D. & S. BUDD. 2000. Mitochondria and neuronal survival. Physiol. Rev. **80:** 315–360.
11. KOWALTOWSKI, A.J., S.S. SMAILI, J.T. RUSSELL & G. FISKUM. 2000. Elevation of resting mitochondrial membrane potential of neural cells by cyclosporin A, BAPTA-AM, and bcl-2. Am. J. Physiol. Cell. Physiol. **279:** C852–C859.

The Biphasic Relationship between Regional Brain Senile Plaque and Neurofibrillary Tangle Distributions: Modification by Age, Sex, and *APOE* Polymorphism

ELIZABETH H. CORDER,[a] ESTIFANOS GHEBREMEDHIN,[b] MILES G. TAYLOR,[c] DIETMAR R. THAL,[d] THOMAS G. OHM,[e] AND HEIKO BRAAK[b]

[a]*Center for Demographic Studies, Duke University, Durham, North Carolina 27708-0408, USA*

[b]*Department of Clinical Neuroanatomy, J.W. Goethe-University, Theodor-Stern-Kai 7, 60590 Frankfurt/Main, Germany*

[c]*Department of Sociology, P.O. Box 90088, Duke University, Durham, North Carolina 27708-0408, USA*

[d]*Institute for Neuropathology, University of Bonn Medical Center, Sigmund Freud Str. 25, 53105 Bonn, Germany*

[e]*Department of Anatomy, Medical Faculty Charite of the Humboldt University Berlin, 10098 Berlin, Germany*

ABSTRACT: Epidemiologic studies indicate that elderly women are at higher risk for Alzheimer disease compared to men. In order to pathologically verify this result, the extent of AD brain lesions (NFT and SP) was compared for men and women at each age, that is, at each decade from 25 years to 95 years, in a large sample of >5000 routine autopsy cases. Women had more affected brain regions beginning in late middle age. They also had more extensive SP depositions throughout the brain compared to men at each early NFT stage I, II, and III. At later NFT stages IV, V, and VI both men and women had extensive SP deposits. The gender gap in SPs at early NFT stages was large and specific to women who carried the *APOE4* allele ($P < .001$) and in addition to the acceleration in NFT stage also found for *APOE4*+ women.

KEYWORDS: Alzheimer disease; gender; apolipoprotein E; aging; senile plaques; neurofibrillary tangles; neuropathology; brain

Address for correspondence: Elizabeth H. Corder, Ph.D., M.P.H., Duke University, Center for Demographic Studies, 2117 Campus Drive, Durham, NC 27708-0408. Voice: 919-668-3023; fax: 919-684-5082.
beth@cds.duke.edu

Ann. N.Y. Acad. Sci. 1019: 24–28 (2004). © 2004 New York Academy of Sciences.
doi: 10.1196/annals.1297.005

INTRODUCTION

Two key neuropathologic features of Alzheimer disease (AD) are senile plaques (SPs) and neurofibrillary tangles (NFTs). Senile plaques are brain deposits that form outside cells composed primarily of beta amyloid protein. Neurofibrillary tangles are filamentous aggregates that form within nerve cells composed of hyperphosphorylated microtubule-associated *tau* protein. The regular regional brain spreading of SPs and of NFTs allows staging of AD neuropathogenesis from earliest preclinical stages to clinical stages characterized by dementia. We investigated senile plaque stage in relation to neurofibrillary tangle stage. The roles of age, gender, and apolipoprotien E (*APOE*) polymorphism in this relationship were addressed.

METHODS

The sample consisted of 5615 routine autopsy cases from eight German hospitals, 3165 men and 2450 women (age 20 to 105 years).[1] Consistent with Braak staging, three sequential SP stages (A to C), and six NFT stages (I to VI), were distinguished.[2-5] SP stages: A = low densities of plaque in the basal neocortex; B = medium densities in all isocortical-association areas, except for the primary fields with a mild involvement of the hippocampal formation; and, C = high densities in all parts of the cortex, including the primary fields.

Allocortical NFT stages are characterized by loss of projection cells beginning in the transentorhinal region (I); then the entorhinal region (II); next, modest involvement of the hippocampal formation and severe damage to the transentorhinal and entorhinal regions (III). Stages IV to VI involve the isocortex: higher-order isocortical association areas of the basal neocortex affected (IV); widespread devastation of isocortical association areas (V); and primary motor and sensory areas and unimodal secondary fields (VI). Diagnosis usually occurs in stages V and VI.

APOE *Determinations*

Apolipoprotien E (*APOE*) is a gene involved in lipid transport. Variation at two different coding sites for the three polymorphisms (ε2, ε3, ε4) determines six genotypes. The ε4 polymorphism increases the risk of AD, while ε2 is protective.[6] *APOE* genotype was ascertained by extracting genomic DNA from formaldehyde-fixed and paraffin-embedded brain, spleen, or liver specimens or from unfixed frozen brain tissue for 1323 subjects.[7]

DATA ANALYSIS

A series of linear models were constructed to predict SP stage (coded 0 to 3) given NFT stage and sex (FIG. 1). Allocortical NFT stages (I to III) were scored 0 to 3. Each isocortical stage was coded yes = 1/no = 0. A model was constructed for subjects aged 20 to 49 years, another for ages 50 to 59, 60 to 69, 70 to 79, 80 to 89, and 90 to 99. Each was age-adjusted to allow for the possibility that women were older than men within the age interval.

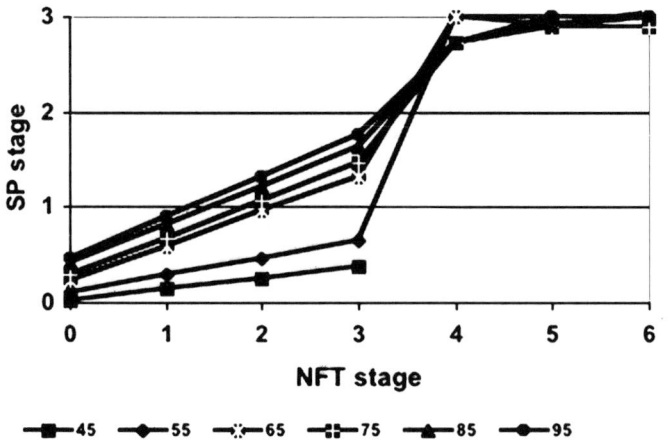

FIGURE 1. Biphasic relationship of SP and NFT stages for women. (NOTE: In late middle age, women had a rapid increase in SPs at allocortical NFT stages I to III; men had uniform age-related increases.)

To investigate the role of APOE polymorphism, subjects aged 50 to 90 having APOE information were divided into allocortical (I-III) or isocortical (IV-VI) groups. For each group, SP stage was predicted by age, sex, NFT stage, and APOE polymorphism.

RESULTS

Biphasic Relationship

We found a biphasic relationship between the staging systems (FIG. 1): allocortical NFT stages were associated with limited plaque distribution (A or B); isocortical NFT stages were associated with SP stage C.

At ages 20 to 49, an absence of tangles predicted an absence of senile plaque and small increases in expected SP stage as NFTs accumulated in transentorhinal (I), entorhinal (II), and hippocampal (III) areas. At NFT stage III there was an ~40% chance of SP stage A. With increasing age, an absence of tangles did not denote an absence of plaque: SP distribution increased with age at allocortical NFT stages. At age 85, no NFT was frequently associated with stage A, and stage III was often associated with stage B.

Men had *uniform* age-related accumulation of senile plaque at allocortical tangle stages. Women between ages 55 and 65, however, had a large increase in plaque distribution. A gender gap was found at age 65: women had 0.1 higher SP stage at NFT stage I, 0.2 higher at stage II, and 0.3 higher at stage III ($P = .006$). A small gender gap was found at age 75: 0.04 (I), 0.08 (II), and 0.12 (III).

For both genders, there was a sharp transition from SP stage A/B to stage C at NFT stage IV, denoting senile plaques in primary iscortical fields once isocortical tangles are present. The transition was marked at younger ages, when limited plaque distribution denoted limited tangle distribution. It was less evident at older ages when SP stage B was common at NFT stage III.

SP Stage in Relation to Age, Sex, NFT Stage, and APOE4

Much of the variation in SP stage at allocortical NFT stages could be explained by the combination of age and NFT stage: at NFT stage 0 (no tangles), for each decade of age there was an increment of 0.11 in SP stage. Thus, subjects age 85 (without tangles) had 0.33 higher SP stage compared to subjects age 55 (without tangles). This age-related increase could be multiplied by NFT stage to arrive at an expected age and NFT-related increases in SP stage, for example, 0.66 (I), 0.99 (II), and 1.32 (III); $P < .0001$.

APOE4 was associated with a higher plaque stage at each age and allocortical NFT stage, 0.30 for one copy of the ε4 allele (the ε2/4 or ε3/4 genotypes), 0.60 for two copies (the ε4/4 genotype) ($P = .0001$). Subjects who carried ε2 tended to have lower SP stage (0.12 lower; $P = .11$). There was an important gender difference: women aged 60 to 75 (yes = 1, others = 0) carrying one copy of ε4 had an extra 0.65 increase in SP stage—1.30 increase for ε4/4. Thus, the gender gap in SP stage for women in this age group was most evident for *APOE4+* women.

These relationships did not hold at isocortical NFT stages. SP stage was not age- or sex-related. There were small increments in SP stage related to NFT stage (0.15 higher for V vs. IV, 0.30 for VI vs. IV; $P = .002$). *APOE4* gene dose was not important (0.09 higher for each copy of ε4; $P = .15$). However, the ε2 allele was protective (0.40 lower SP stage, $P = .002$). These results indicate that once NFTs are found in the isocortex, age, sex, and *APOE4* have little importance in determining whether SP stage is B (not in primary fields) or C (primary and secondary fields). However, subjects who carried *APOE2* more often had the lower stage (B).

DISCUSSION

A biphasic relationship between NFT and SP staging systems was identified in a large routine autopsy sample, possibly the first report of this kind. Once neurofibrillary tangles were found in the isocortex, senile plaque was likely to be present in all cortical areas, including the primary cortical fields. However, *APOE2* may be protective, limiting SPs to secondary areas. At earlier allocortical tangle stages, senile plaque distribution was dictated by age and neurofibrillary involvement (transentorhinal, entorhinal, hippocampal). *APOE4* accelerated amyloid deposition,[8] especially for women in late middle age, possibly related to waning estrogen levels.[9]

Overall, there was a three-year acceleration in NFT stage for women in the sample associated with a more rapid spreading of tangles to entorhinal and hippocampal areas once found in the transentorhinal cortex, also associated with *APOE4*.[10] Thus women, especially *APOE4+* women, are at higher risk for both neurofibrillary and amyloid plaque neuropathology. These results are consistent with epidemiologic reports that women are at higher risk for AD dementia.

ACKNOWLEDGMENTS

Financial support was provided by the National Institute on Aging.

REFERENCES

1. GHEBREMEDHIN, E., C. SCHULTZ, D.R. THAL, *et al.* 2001. Gender and age modify the association between APOE and AD-related neuropathology. Neurology **56:**1696–1701.
2. BRAAK, E., K. GRIFFING, K. ARAI, *et al.* 1999. Neuropathology of Alzheimer's disease: What is new since A. Alzheimer? Eur. Arch. Psychiatry Clin. Neurosci. **249**(Suppl. 3): III/14–III/22.
3. BRAAK, H. & E. BRAAK. 1997. Frequency of stages of Alzheimer-related lesions in different age categories. Neurobiol. Aging **18:** 351–357.
4. BRAAK, H. & E. BRAAK. 1991. Neuropathological stageing of Alzheimer-related changes. Acta Neuropathol. **82:** 239–259.
5. OHM, T.G., H. SCHARNAGL, W. MARZ, *et al.* 1999. Apolipoprotein E isoforms and the development of low and high Braak stages of Alzheimer's disease-related lesions. Acta Neuropathol. **98:** 273–280.
6. CORDER, E.H., A.M. SAUNDERS, W.J. STRITTMATTER, *et al.* 1993. Gene dose of apolipoprotein E type 4 allele and the risk of Alzheimer's disease in late-onset families. Science **261:** 921–923.
7. GHEBREMEDHIN, E., H. BRAAK, E. BRAAK, *et al.* 1998. Improved method facilitates reliable APOE genotyping of genomic DNA extracted from formaldehyde-fixed pathology specimens. J. Neurosci. Methods **79***:* 229–231.
8. WALKER, L.C., J. PAHNKE, M. MADAUSS, *et al.* 2000. Apolipoprotein E4 promotes the early deposition of Aβ42 and then Aβ40 in the elderly. Acta Neuropathol. **100:** 36–42.
9. XU, H., G.K. GOURAS, J.P. GREENFIELD, *et al.* 1998. Estrogen reduces neuronal generation of Alzheimer β-amyloid peptides. Nat. Med. **4:** 447–451.
10. CORDER, E.H., E. GHEBREMEDHIN, M. TAYLOR, *et al.* 2004. Gender differences in Alzheimer's disease neuropathology. Submitted.

Decay of Mitochondrial Metabolic Competence in the Aging Cerebellum

CARLO BERTONI-FREDDARI, PATRIZIA FATTORETTI, BELINDA GIORGETTI, MORENO SOLAZZI, MARTA BALIETTI, GIUSEPPINA DI STEFANO, AND TIZIANA CASOLI

Neurobiology of Aging Laboratory, INRCA Research Department, 60121, Ancona, Italy

ABSTRACT: Cytochemically evidenced cytochrome oxidase activity was morphometrically measured in the cerebellar cortex of adult and old rats. The ratio (R) between the area of the precipitate due to the cytochemical reaction and the overall area of each mitochondrion was calculated. While in adult rats an inverse correlation between mitochondrial size and R values ($r = -.905$) was envisaged, in old animals increasing values of R were paired by increases in mitochondrial area ($r = .561$). Paired-quartile comparisons of the R values from adult and old animals documented a marked age-related impairment of the mitochondrial metabolic competence in small (I quartile: –31.6%) and medium-sized (II quartile: –26.4; III quartile: –16.4) mitochondria, while large organelles showed the lowest age-related decrease (IV quartile: –3.0%). The present findings support that a marked dysfunction of small and medium-sized mitochondria contributes to the significant decay of energy metabolism currently reported in physiological aging.

KEYWORDS: mitochondrial metabolic competence; cerebellum; mitochondrial size; megamitochondria; cytochrome oxidase activity

Although several aging theories have been proposed so far, no clear-cut causative event can be singled out among the many determinants involved in such a multifactorial process. On the basis of the available data in the literature, what can be considered a reasonable mechanism of aging is that the persistent action of even mild stressful conditions is not fully counteracted by cellular repair functions, and this leads to age-related somatic changes. In agreement with this concept, it has been documented that cellular energy metabolism progressively declines with advancing age, and there is evidence that this adverse condition is responsible for significant dysfunctions predisposing selected groups of cells and tissue compartments to age-related pathologies.[1,2]

The primary function of mitochondria is the adequate supply of adenosinetriphosphate (ATP) to respond to actual energy needs, so these organelles may play a

Address for correspondence: Dr. Carlo Bertoni-Freddari, Neurobiology of Aging Laboratory, INRCA Research Department, Via Birarelli 8, 60121 Ancona, Italy. Voice: +39-071-800-4153; fax: +39-071-206791.
c.bertoni@inrca.it

central role in the age-related decay of the cellular energy producing machinery and, in turn, mitochondrial dysfunction may constitute a very precocious alteration in the cascade of events leading to physiological and pathological aging. According to this rationale, any impairment of the mitochondrial metabolic competence (MMC), that is, the organelle's actual capacity to provide ATP, may represent a potential threat to cellular health and survival. It is currently reported that cytochrome oxidase (COX), which is the tercinal molecule (complex IV) of the mitochondrial respiratory chain, represents a reliable endogenous marker of neuronal metabolism.[3] By using diaminobenzidine (DAB) as an electron donor, COX activity can be preferentially evidenced at the inner mitochondrial membranes as a dark reaction deposit[3] (FIG. 1). The overall area of the DAB-COX cytochemical precipitate, which can be reliably measured within each mitochondrion by computer-assisted quantitative methods,[4,5] represents the surface fraction of the inner membrane of the mitochondria that is directly involved in cellular respiration and, in turn, is reported to account for COX activity.[3-5]

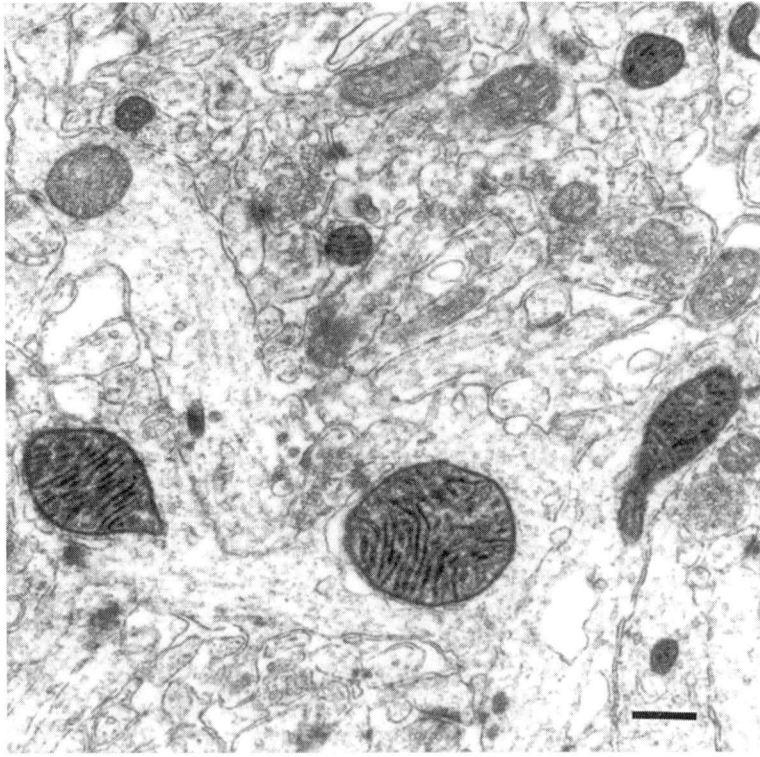

FIGURE 1. Electron microscopic picture of COX-positive mitochondria in the cerebellar cortex of an adult rat. The dark cytochemical precipitate due to the DAB-COX reaction is sharply evidenced at the inner mitochondrial membrane. *Bar:* 0.5 mm.

In the present paper, we report the results of an investigation carried out to assess MMC in aging by measuring COX activity, as evidenced cytochemically by the DAB technique, at the inner membrane of synaptic mitochondria in the cerebellar cortex of rats of different ages. The present study was performed in the cerebellar glomeruli (cell-free zones within the granule cell layer of the cerebellar cortex) of old (24–26 months of age) and adult (12 months) female Wistar rats. The animals were processed as was reported in our previous papers and as briefly described in the other chapter in this volume by Bertoni-Freddari et al. As can be clearly seen in FIGURE 1, the dark mitochondria showing COX activity can be objectively distinguished from the organelles in the same section that did not react with the DAB solution. COX-positive mitochondria were identified by the electron microscope and directly analyzed by our image analysis system (Kontron KS300). According to the equal opportunity rule,[6] we carried out a systematic random sampling on COX-positive organelles.[7] Eight glomeruli/animal were sampled, and five fields (each of 25 μm^2) were analyzed in the central zone of each glomerulus: this analysis yielded 1000 μm^2/animal and an overall sampled area of 3000 μm^2. The total area of the cytochemical precipitate due to COX activity (CPA)/mitochondrion and the area (MA) of each COX-positive organelle were the parameters semiautomatically measured by the computer program in our image analyzer. The ratio (R) between CPA and MA was also calculated and referred to as the percent of the inner membrane area of the mitochondria involved in COX activity.[4,5] The data obtained from each animal were ordered according to increasing values of MA and then divided into four quartiles. The MA and R mean values of each quartile of adult and old rats were pair compared. While there is an inverse correlation between mitochondrial size and R values ($r = -.905$) in adult rats, in old rats we found increasing values of R as the mitochondrial area increased ($r = .561$). Paired-quartile comparisons of the R values from adult and old animals documented a marked age-related impairment of MMC in small (I quartile: −31.6%) and medium-sized (II quartile: −26.4; III quartile: −16.4) mitochondria, while large organelles showed the lowest age-related decrease (IV quartile: −3.0%). By matching COX quantitative preferential cytochemistry and classic morphometric procedures, the present findings document that, within the discrete population of synaptic mitochondria, those of larger size show a lower MMC than the smaller ones. That is, we found that the R value of the enlarged mitochondria is about .28 both in adult and old rats, while the small-sized organelles showed R values of .39 in adult and .26 in old animals, respectively.

This morphofunctional difference of mitochondria of different sizes is of particular biological significance with specific reference to aging. The balance between the decrease in mitochondrial number and the increase in the size of the remaining organelles is reported by several authors, and it is considered a general trend in old organisms.[8] Mitochondrial enlargement is supposed to constitute a compensating reaction to the numeric loss of the organelles, since it extends the inner membrane area that is potentially involved in cellular respiration. This compensation has been clearly shown to be due to an increased complement of oversized mitochondria in discrete cellular or tissue compartments; however, it is still debated whether these enlarged organelles are capable of providing adequate amounts of ATP that are directly proportional to their enlarged size. In this context, our present results lend congruous support to the concept that the higher percent of oversized mitochondria consistently found in old cells[8] appears to represent a weak compensating reaction.

Considering the recent molecular biology data on mitochondrial genetics,[9] our present findings are of particular biological relevance. In the late 1980s, Linnane[10] and co-workers documented that, mainly because of the ongoing action of free radical attacks, normal and mutated mitochondrial DNA (mitDNA) molecules are present within each organelle and, as a consequence, the potential for energy provision of a given cell is in the charge of a mosaic of units with different functional capabilities. Because of this heterogeneous, though physiological, situation of the cellular bioenergetic machinery, each organelle has a very specific MMC, which can be estimated by measuring the area of the DAB-COX cytochemical precipitate against the overall mitochondrial surface.[4,5] In this context, by showing a significant reduction of the metabolic workload of the enlarged mitochondria as compared to smaller ones both in adulthood and aging, our present findings demonstrate that the increase in mitochondrial size does not appear to be matched by improvement of function. With specific reference to postmitotic cells, for example, neurons, it must be stressed that the outcome of the accumulation of mutant mitDNA with advancing age results in a marked heteroplasmy not only at the mitochondrial but also at the cellular level. This may help explain the specific vulnerability to aging and age-related pathologies of a selected populations of cells within the CNS in terms of significant impairment of cellular metabolism, which may reasonably begin with the physiological decay of MMC.

REFERENCES

1. BERTONI-FREDDARI, C., P. FATTORETTI, B. GIORGETTI, et al. 2004. Role of mitochondrial deterioration in physiological and pathological brain aging. Gerontology. In press.
2. BEAL, M.F. 2000. Energetics in the pathogenesis of neurodegenerative diseases. Trends Neurol. Sci. **23**: 298–304.
3. WONG-RILEY, M.T.T. 1989. Cytochrome oxidase: an endogenous metabolic marker for neuronal activity. Trends Neurol. Sci. **12**: 94–101.
4. BERTONI-FREDDARI, C., P. FATTORETTI, T. CASOLI, et al. 2001. Quantitative cytochemical mapping of mitochondrial enzymes in rat cerebella. Micron **32**: 405–410.
5. BERTONI-FREDDARI, C., P. FATTORETTI, R. PAOLONI, et al. 2003. Inverse correlation between mitochondrial size and metabolic competence: a quantitative cytochemical study of cytochrome oxidase activity. Naturwissenschaften **90**: 68–71.
6. COGGESHALL, R.E. 1992. A consideration of neural counting methods. Trends Neur. Sci. **15**: 9–13.
7. BERTONI-FREDDARI, C., P. FATTORETTI, T. CASOLI, et al. 1996. Age-dependent decrease in the activity of succinic dehydrogenase in rat CA1 pyramidal cells: a quantitative cytochemical study. Mech. Age. Dev. **90**: 53–62.
8. WALTER, P.B., K.B. BECKMAN & B.N. AMES. 1999. The role of iron and mitochondria in aging. In Understanding the Process of Aging. E. Cadenas & L. Packer, Eds.: 203–227. Dekker. New York.
9. MEIER-RUGE, W. & C. BERTONI-FREDDARI. 1999. Mitochondrial genome lesions in the pathogenesis of Alzheimer's disease. Gerontology **45**: 289–297.
10. LINNANE, A.W., S. MARZUKY, S. OZAWA & T. TANAKA. 1989. Mitochondrial DNA mutations as an important contributor to aging and degenerative diseases. Lancet **1**: 642–645.

Cytochrome Oxidase Activity in Hippocampal Synaptic Mitochondria during Aging: A Quantitative Cytochemical Investigation

CARLO BERTONI-FREDDARI, PATRIZIA FATTORETTI, BELINDA GIORGETTI, MORENO SOLAZZI, MARTA BALIETTI, TIZIANA CASOLI, AND GIUSEPPINA DI STEFANO

Neurobiology of Aging Laboratory, INRCA Research Department, 60121, Ancona, Italy

ABSTRACT: Synaptic mitochondria, cytochemically positive to cytochrome oxidase (COX) activity, were investigated by morphometric methods in the hippocampal dentate gyrus of adult and old rats. The number of mitochondria/μm^3 of tissue (Nv), the volume fraction occupied by mitochondria/μm^3 of tissue (Vv), the average mitochondrial volume (V), the longer mitochondrial diameter (F_{max}), and the ratio R:mitochondrial area/overall area of the cytochemical precipitate due to COX activity were measured on COX-positive organelles. In old animals, Nv, Vv, V, and F_{max} increased at a not significant extent; R was not significantly decreased. The complement (%) of longer organelles was higher in old animals. COX activity is currently considered an endogenous marker of neuronal oxidative metabolism; thus, although our findings refer to the discrete subpopulation of COX-positive organelles located at synaptic terminals, they support that changes of mitochondrial ultrastructure and metabolic competence may contribute to the age-related alterations of neuronal performances.

KEYWORDS: mitochondrial metabolic competence; morphometry; synaptic mitochondria; cytochrome oxidase activity; hippocampus

It has been reported that a significant decay of energy metabolism represents a critical condition that contributes to physiological aging and a predisposition to age-related pathologies.[1,2] With specific reference to nerve cells, an actual and adequate energy provision constitutes the necessary prerequisite for brain performances; thus, any alteration affecting the supply machinery of neuronal energy may represent a potential threat of disruptions in cell-to-cell communication. To assess the mitochondrial metabolic competence, that is, the capacity of old organelles to provide proper amounts of adenosinetriphosphate, synaptic mitochondria positive for cytochrome oxidase (COX) activity were quantitatively investigated by computer-assisted morphometric methods at the distal dendrites of the dentate gyrus granule cells in adult (12 months) and old (26–28 months) female Wistar rats. The diaminobenzidine (DAB) technique was used to represent COX activity as a sharp and dark cytochemical precipitate at the inner mitochondrial membranes and cristae. The animals were perfused with 2.5% paraformaldehyde, 1.5% glutaraldehyde in 0.1 M Sorensen buffer at pH 7.4, plus 4% sucrose. The hippocampal tissue samples (40–60 mm thick) were rinsed overnight in buffer and sucrose and then incubated (2–4 hours at 37°C in the dark) in the following solution (100 mL): 50 mg DAB, 27 mg cytochrome c, 4 g sucrose.

Postfixation in osmium tetroxide was followed by conventional inclusion, sectioning, and contrasting procedures. The following morphometric parameters were calculated on COX-positive organelles: the number of mitochondria/μm^3 of tissue (numeric density: Nv); the volume fraction occupied by mitochondria/μm^3 of tissue (volume density: Vv); the average mitochondrial volume (V); the longer mitochondrial diameter (F_{max}); and the ratio (R): mitochondrial area/overall area of the cytochemical precipitate due to COX activity. In old animals, Nv, Vv, V, and F_{max} were increased to a not significant extent, while R was significantly decreased. The percent distribution of the F_{max} values showed that the number of longer organelles is higher in old animals.

The substantial unchanged values of the parameters that were taken into account in the present study suggest that the structural plasticity of synaptic mitochondria is consistently retained by the central nervous system (CNS) in the old rats. In addition, the present findings confirm the current data in the literature documenting that the fraction of organelles of larger size in a given discrete mitochondrial population tends to increase with age,[3] and that mitochondrial elongation correlates inversely with mitochondrial metabolic competence:[4] in old rats, F_{max} increased by 5.5%, but R significantly decreased by 9.3%. A closer look at the present findings reveals that some considerations are in agreement with both the adopted cytochemical and sampling procedures, and with the critical role played by COX activity in mitochondrial functional tasks.

The DAB cytochemical method is consistently shown to be a very reliable procedure for showing COX activity, that is, to observe an accumulation of the cytochemical precipitate, the continuous oxidation of cytochrome c by COX is needed; thus, the overall area of the dark deposits at the inner membrane of each mitochondrion is proportional to the functional and actual activity of this enzyme.[5] A necessary prerequisite for performing reliable quantitative studies on the ultrastructural features of cellular organelles, as well as of positive cytochemical functional areas, is to carry out the morphometric sampling in sharply defined tissue zones easily identifiable in any biological sample.[6] In this context, it must be said that (1) although our study has been carried out on a highly selected mitochondrial population located at the nerve cell terminal regions and directly subserving synaptic performances, only the COX-positive organelles were taken into account, and (2) regarding the analyzed parameters, Nv, Vv, V, and F refer to the morphological features of the COX-positive mitochondria, while the value of R relates to the functional surface of the single mitochondrion involved in energy-providing mechanisms.[4,7]

Conceivably, while the present data provide morphofunctional information on the active fraction of synaptic mitochondria, it must be mentioned that the overall mitochondrial metabolic potential present in this specific compartment of the nerve cells

TABLE 1. Morphometric parameters of COX-positive synaptic mitochondria at the distal dendrites of hippocampal dentate gyrus granular cells

Age Group	Nv (No. Mito/μm^3)	Vv ($\mu m^3/\mu m^3$)	V (μm^3)	F_{max} (μm)	R (%)
Adult	0.9658 ± 0.0370	0.1014 ± 0.0045	0.1421 ± 0.0048	0.5907 ± 0.0272	.2972 ± .0030
Old	1.0725 ± 0.0719	0.1124 ± 0.0070	0.1327 ± 0.0071	0.6229 ± 0.0093	.2697 ± .0106*

*$P < .05$.

is higher, since the COX-negative synaptic organelles were not counted. From a functional point of view, COX, which is an integral transmembrane protein located at the inner mitochondrial membrane, is constituted by 13 subunits: 3 encoded by mitochondrial DNA, while the other 10 are nuclear encoded.[8] COX is the terminal component of the mitochondrial respiratory chain (complex IV) and catalyzes the transfer of electrons from the reduced substrate ferrocytochrome c to molecular oxygen to form water: ATP is generated during this reaction by the coupled oxidative phosphorylation process. Given these important features, COX is currently considered an endogenous marker for neuronal metabolism,[5] and quantitative assessments of its activity by biochemical and cytochemical methods may serve to map the cellular and/or tissue dynamic metabolic response to different functional demands.[4,7] On the basis of these current data from the literature, we interpret the results reported in TABLE 1 as affirmation that in the old hippocampus, despite the not significant increase of the volume fraction (Vv) as well as of the numeric density (Nv) of the COX-positive mitochondria, the organelles' metabolic competence decreases when the significant reduction of R (−9.3%) is taken into account. With reference to this last parameter, it must be stressed that it provides reliable information on the specific metabolic capabilities of the single mitochondrion as a functional unit of cellular bioenergetics. Accordingly, the lower value of R found in the old hippocampus can be considered a subtle age-related alteration that may further progress to a significant reduction of the values of the other parameters measured by us and, in turn, lead to a significant impairment of cellular metabolism. We are aware of the speculative character of our interpretation; however, it has been shown that, within the discrete population of mitochondria present in a given cellular or tissue compartment (e.g., the nerve terminal), each organelle is characterized by a different mutation load of its DNA.[9] This results in a heterogeneous mosaic of mitochondria with different functional metabolic competence.

Conceivably, the measurement of R on single organelles allows the precocious and insidious changes, which can be functionally and physiologically masked by the compensating reactions of the whole mitochondrial population, to be revealed: in the present study, the higher values of Vv and Nv found in old rats. In this context, our present findings suggest that the subtle decay of the metabolic competence of each mitochondrion may constitute one of the early steps in the age-related deterioration of the cellular bioenergetic machinery. This assumption, in addition to being in agreement with the widely documented preferential vulnerability to aging of selected populations of cells within circumscribed CNS areas (e.g., hippocampus), stresses the important role of mitochondrial alterations as critical events predisposing to typical pathologies of the senile brain, for example, Alzheimer disease.[1,7,10]

REFERENCES

1. BERTONI-FREDDARI, C. et al. 2004. Role of mitochondrial deterioration in physiological and pathological brain aging. Gerontology. In press.
2. BEAL, M.F., B.T. HYMAN & W. KOROSHETZ. 1993. Do defects in mitochondrial energy metabolism underlie the pathology of neurodegenerative diseases. Trends Neurol. Sci. **16:** 125–131.
3. WALTER, P.B., K.B. BECKMAN & B.N. AMES. 1999. The role of iron and mitochondria in aging. In Understanding the Process of Aging. E. Cadenas and L. Packer, Eds.: 203–227. Dekker. New York.
4. BERTONI-FREDDARI, C. et al. 2003. Inverse correlation between mitochondrial size and metabolic competence: a quantitative cytochemical study of cytochrome oxidase activity. Naturwissenschaften **90:** 68–71.
5. WONG-RILEY, M.T.T. 1989. Cytochrome oxidase: an endogenous metabolic marker for neuronal activity. Trends Neurol. Sci. **12:** 94–101.
6. BERTONI-FREDDARI, C. et al. 1993. Morphological plasticity of synaptic mitochondria during aging. Brain Res. **628:** 193–200.
7. BERTONI-FREDDARI, C. et al. 2001. Quantitative cytochemical mapping of mitochondrial enzymes in rat cerebella. Micron **32:** 405–410.
8. TAANMAN, J.-W. 2002. Cytochrome-c oxidase. In Wiley Encyclopedia of Molecular Medicine, 5 Vol. Wiley. New York.
9. TROUNCE, I., E. BYRNE & S. MARZUKY. 1989. Decline in skeletal muscle mitochondrial respiratory chain function: possible factor in aging. Lancet **1:** 637–640.
10. DYKENS, J.A. et al. 2003. Mitochondrial dysfunction in aging and disease: development of therapeutic strategies. In Critical Reviews of Oxidative Stress and Aging. R.G. Cutler H. Rodriguez, Eds.: 1378–1388. World Scientific. Singapore.

Vitamin E Deficiency and Aging Effect on Expression Levels of GAP-43 and MAP-2 in Selected Areas of the Brain

TIZIANA CASOLI, GIUSEPPINA DI STEFANO, ALESSIA DELFINO, PATRIZIA FATTORETTI, AND CARLO BERTONI-FREDDARI

Neurobiology of Aging Laboratory, INRCA Research Department, Via Birarelli 8, 60121 Ancona, Italy

ABSTRACT: The expression levels of GAP-43 and MAP-2, two proteins involved, respectively, in axonal and dendritic remodeling, in control adult (11 months), old (24 months), and vitamin E–deficient (11 months) rats were evaluated. mRNA levels were determined by means of a quantitative *in situ* hybridization procedure in subregions of hippocampus and cerebellum. Though a general trend can be observed indicating a reduction in GAP-43 expression in aging as compared to adult animals and an increase in vitamin E–deprived rats in comparison with adult animals, no statistically significant change was found in any region analyzed. In the same way, MAP-2 mRNA levels show an increase in vitamin E–deprived rats in comparison with other groups tested; only one variation was statistically significant, namely the increase in cerebellar cortex MAP-2 nRNA levels in vitamin E–deficient versus adult rats. These results suggest that oxidative stress and aging negatively affect neuroplasticity, showing different characteristics at the dendritic and axonal levels.

KEYWORDS: GAP-43; MAP-2; *in situ* hybridization; vitamin E; aging

GAP-43 is a presynaptic membrane phosphoprotein whose expression increases during events of axonal growth or remodeling, such as development, learning, and regeneration of an injured axon. The role of GAP-43, still to be precisely defined, may be connected to intracellular regulative events, which allows the growing axon to adapt to the changing environmental framework.[1] The microtubule-associated protein (MAP-2) is a cytoskeletal protein localized in the neuronal dendritic compartment. It is considered a marker of structural integrity and plays an important role in the growth, differentiation, and plasticity of neurons.[2] The ability of the brain to support plasticity-related phenomena declines with increasing age, and a reduction in the levels of proteins implicated in brain plasticity may be one factor contributing to this event.[3] It has been proposed that vitamin E deficiency may mimic a condition of premature aging due to the chronic lack of protection against free-radical attack of cellular components.[4] We have evaluated the effect of vitamin E deprivation on

Address for correspondence: Dr. Tiziana Casoli, Neurobiology of Aging Laboratory, "N. Masera" I.N.R.C.A. Research Department, Via Birarelli 8, 60121 Ancona, Italy. Voice: +39-71-8004203; fax: +39-71-206791.
t.casoli@inrca.it

the expression levels of GAP-43 and MAP-2 in rats and compared them to the corresponding mRNA levels in normal-fed, age-matched, and old rodents to evaluate the possible role of oxidative damage in the age-related decrease of neuronal plasticity.

Female Wistar rats were fed a standard laboratory diet or a vitamin E–deficient diet after weaning (1 month of age). Groups of rats that had received a standard diet were killed at 12 and 28 months of age (4 rats for group). The animals receiving a vitamin E–deficient diet (4 rats) were killed at 12 months of age. The vitamin E–deficient diet consisted of maize starch and sucrose 58%, extracted casein 18%, torula yeast 10%, melted filtered fat 8%, Osborne-Mendel salts 5%, and a vitamin supplement lacking vitamin E. At the end of the dietary treatment, rats were sacrificed according to the guidelines of Italian Ministry of Health regarding the use of laboratory animals. Animals were anesthetized with tribromoethanol and perfused intracardially with 400 mL of 4% paraformaldehyde. Hippocampus and cerebellum were removed, postfixed in the same fixative for 4 h at 4°C, and incubated overnight at 4°C in 30% sucrose. Brain samples were sectioned at 12 µm thickness on a cryostat, and sections were thaw-mounted on silane-coated slides. Hippocampus was permeabilized with 1 µg/mL and cerebellum with 2 µg/mL proteinase K for 15 min at 37°C followed by proteinase K inactivation at 95°C for 2 minutes. Tissue sections were dehydrated in ascending ethanol series, delipidated in chloroform (5 min), and then rehydrated in 95% ethanol (2 min). After air drying, sections were hybridized at 42°C for 18 h in a humidified chamber with a hybridization solution consisting of 50% formamide, $4 \times$ SSC, $1 \times$ Denhardt's solution, 10% dextran sulfate, 200 mM DTT, 250 µg/mL salmon sperm DNA, and 1×10^6 cpm of radiolabeled probe. Sense or antisense oligonucleotide probes to GAP-43 and MAP-2 were 3′-end labeled with ^{35}S-dATP using terminal deoxynucleotide transferase. After the hybridization step, slides were rinsed in $4 \times$ SSC buffer at room temperature for 30 min, followed by $2 \times$ SSC at room temperature (30 min), $1 \times$ SSC at 55°C (30 min), and $1 \times$ SSC at $45 \times$ C (30 min). The sections were then rinsed in double distilled water, dehydrated in ethanol solutions, and air-dried. Slides were exposed to Kodak X-OMAT for ten days and developed according to the manufacturer's instructions. Autoradiographies were analyzed by computer-assisted densitometry (KS300 image-analysis software). Films were put on a light table and images were acquired directly by a CCD camera. The area of interest was selected interactively and the mean optical density was measured. Values from sections labeled with sense probes were subtracted as a nonspecific signal. Measurements were taken over the granular layer of cerebellar cortex, dentate gyrus granule cells, and CA1 and CA3 pyramidal layer. Optical density values were determined on four sections per animal. Statistical analysis was carried out by means of one-way analysis of variance (ANOVA), followed by Newman-Keuls test for multiple comparisons.

GAP-43 mRNA expression in rat hippocampus was found at high levels in CA3 pyramidal cells, at low levels in CA1 pyramidal cells, and dentate gyrus granule cells, while MAP-2 mRNA was widely present in cell bodies and basal dendrites of dentate gyrus, CA3 and CA1 neurons. Both mRNAs were localized in the granule cell layer of the cerebellar structure. Although a general trend can be observed indicating a reduction in GAP-43 expression in aging as compared to adult animals and an increase in vitamin E–deprived rats in comparison with adult animals, no statistically significant change was found in any region analyzed (TABLE 1). In the same

TABLE 1. Quantitative evaluation of GAP-43 and MAP-2 expression in hippocampus and cerebellum of adult, vitamin E–deficient, and old rats

		Cerebeller cotex (granular layer)	Dentate gyrus (granule cell layer)	CA3	CA1
GAP-43	Adult	0.92 ± 0.6	1.31 ± 0.57	3.33 ± 1.11	1.36 ± 0.6
	−Vitamin E	1.12 ± 0.78	1.58 ± 1.14	4.7 ± 0.58	0.69 ± 0.39
	Old	0.48 ± 0.28	0.71 ± 1.19	3.28 ± 2.46	0.72 ± 0.77
MAP-2	Adult	1.22 ± 1.4	3.78 ± 0.98	3.6 ± 0.84	3.18 ± 0.88
	−Vitamin E	4.65 ± 0.17*	4.67 ± 0.32	4.55 ± 0.52	2.98 ± 0.84
	Old	1.98 ± 0.55	2.95 ± 0.66	2.73 ± 0.71	2.0 ± 0.01

NOTE: Values are expressed as mean ± SEM.
* $P < .05$ vs. adult rats.

way, MAP-2 mRNA levels show an increase in vitamin E–deprived rats in comparison with the other groups tested; only one variation resulted that was statistically significant, namely the increase in cerebellar cortex MAP-2 mRNA levels in vitamin E–deficient versus adult rats (TABLE 1).

The most widely accepted physiological function of vitamin E is its role as an important antioxidant in membranes, preventing oxidative damage to polyunsaturated lipids in the lipid bilayer. The brain is thought to be particularly vulnerable to oxidative stress due to its high rate of oxygen consumption along with its poor catalase activity and moderate amounts of superoxide dismutase and glutathione peroxidase. It has been demonstrated that vitamin E deficiency determines neurological abnormalities such as dystrophic axons, degeneration of dorsal and ventral spinocerebellar tracts, and accumulation of lipofuscin.[4] As for other cases of neuronal damage, like alcohol ingestion[8] and β-amyloid exposure,[9] we also found in this model of neurodegeneration a compensatory response of the neuronal cells to the detrimental effects elicited by the lack of antioxidant defences. Our results suggest that vitamin E deficiency may act as a stimulus to cell transcription for at least these two markers of neuronal plasticity. More experiments will be performed to definitively validate these data. Previous investigations examined GAP-43 and MAP-2 protein levels in aging and vitamin E–deficient rats in selected subfields of hippocampus and cerebellum.[5-7] Concerning the areas analyzed, GAP-43 mRNA variations parallel those of the protein in the corresponding nerve terminal. On the other hand, while MAP-2 mRNA levels do not show any change in CA1 pyramidal layer and dentate gyrus granular layer in both groups tested, protein levels in the corresponding dendrites decrease significantly both in aging and vitamin E–deficient rats vs. controls. No data are available for the other subfields. So it seems that for MAP-2 there is a lack of correlation between mRNA and protein under conditions of vitamin E deficiency and aging. These results suggest that oxidative stress and aging negatively affect neuroplasticity in the central nervous system, showing different characteristics at the dendritic and axonal levels.

REFERENCES

1. BENOWITZ, L.I. & A. ROUTTENBERG. 1997. GAP-43: an intrinsic determinant of neuronal development and plasticity. TINS **20:** 84–91.

2. SANCHEZ, C. J. DIAZ-NIDO & J. AVILA. 2000. Phosphorylation of microtubule-associated protein 2 (MAP2) and its relevance for the regulation of the neuronal cytoskeleton function. Prog. Neurobiol. **61:** 133–168.
3. HATANPAA, K., K.R. ISAACS, T. SHIRAO, et al. 1999. Loss of proteins regulating synaptic plasticity in normal aging of the human brain and in Alzheimer's disease. J. Neurophatol. Exp. Neurol. **58:** 637–643.
4. SOKOL, R.J. 1989. Vitamin E and neurologic function in man. Free Radical Biol. & Med. **6:** 189–207.
5. CASOLI, T., C. SPAGNA, P. FATTORETTI, et al. 1996. Neuronal plasticity in aging: a quantitative immunohistochemical study of GAP-43 in discrete regions of the rat brain. Brain Res. **714:** 111–117.
6. DI STEFANO, G., T. CASOLI, P. FATTORETTI, et al. 2001. Distribution of MAP2 in hippocampus and cerebellum of young and old rats by quantitative immunohistochemistry. J. Histochem. Cytochem. **49:** 1065–1066.
7. DI STEFANO, G., T. CASOLI, P. FATTORETTI, et al. 2002. Effect of vitamin E-deficiency and aging on MAP-2 and GAP-43 distribution in rat hippocampus. Free Radical Res. **36**(Suppl. 1): 61–62.
8. MASLIAH, E., M. MALLORY, I. HOUSEN, et al. 1991. Patterns of aberrant sprouting in Alzheimer's disease. Neuron **6:** 729–739.
9. CADETE-LEITE, A., M.A. TAVARES, M.M. PACHECO, et al. 1989. Hippocampal mossy fiber—CA3 synapses after chronic alcohol consumption and withdrawal. Alcohol **6:** 303–310.

Chronic Treatment with a Precursor of Cellular Phosphatidylcholine Ameliorates Morphological and Behavioral Effects of Aging in the Rat Hippocampus

D. CRESPO, M. MEGIAS, C. FERNANDEZ-VIADERO, AND R. VERDUGA

Department of Anatomy and Cell Biology, University of Cantabria, 39011-Santander, Spain

ABSTRACT: Normal aging is commonly associated with a decline in memory, mainly for that related with newly acquired information. The hippocampal formation (HF) is a brain region that has been implicated in this dysfunction. Within the HF there are several cellular types, such as pyramidal cells, granule neurons of the dentate gyrus, and astrocytes. CDP-choline is a well-known intermediate in the biosynthesis of phosphatidylcholine, a phospholipid essential for neuronal membrane preservation and function; thus, this compound would attenuate the process of neuronal aging. To test this, three groups of male mice were used in this study. An adult 12-month-old group (ACG), a 24-month-old (OCG), and an old experimental group (OEG) were administered orally a solution of CDP-choline (150 mg/kg per day) from 12 up to 24 months. Experimental observations suggest that CDP-choline has a positive effect on memory (reference errors were attenuated), and hippocampal morphology resembled that of younger animals.

KEYWORDS: hippocampus; CDP-choline; mice; memory; stereolog

INTRODUCTION

Normal aging is commonly associated with a decline in memory, mainly that related to newly acquired information and its retrieval. The hippocampal formation (HF) is a brain region that has been implicated in age-related memory dysfunction, its functional integrity is critical for normal memory function, and it is very vulnerable to the process of aging.[1] Within the HF there are several cellular types, including large principal pyramidal and nonprincipal cells of the CA regions and small granule neurons of the dentate gyrus (DG). Small neurons of the DG are added throughout life even in the aged animals.[2] Furthermore, there is an important role for HF astrocytes.

Address for correspondence: D. Crespo, Department of Anatomy and Cell Biology, Faculty of Medicine, University of Cantabria, 39011-Santander, Spain. Voice: +34-942-201927; fax +34-942-201903.
  crespod@unican.es

There is some controversy over the structural basis of memory in the hippocampus. This includes the participation of several subgroups of nonprincipal cells, mainly those neurons that synthesise nitric oxide (NO). Recent investigations reporting the involvement of NO in memory function have paved the way for the analyses of the relations between these NO–neurons and memory.

Cytidinediphosphocholine (CDP-choline) is a well-known intermediate in the biosynthesis of phosphatidylcholine (PC), a membrane phospholipid essential for membrane function. Previous studies suggested a reparative effect of CDP-choline on brain cell membranes.[3–5] For this reason, we studied the effects of chronic administration of CDP-choline on the morphology of several HF populations. Furthermore, we performed a cognitive test to evaluate the effect of this drug on memory acquisition and retrieval. Our results suggest that CDP-choline has a positive effect on memory, and induces a juvenile morphology in the HF.

MATERIALS AND METHODS

Three groups of male mice were used. An adult group of 12-month-old animals (ACG), another of 24-month-old mice (OCG), and a group of mice administered a solution of CDP-choline (150 mg/kg per day) from 12 to 24 months (OEG).

We used a histochemical technique for NADPH-d to examine age-related variations in NO neuronal activity. Astrocytes were identified using an anti-GFAP antibody. Electron microscopy was used to analyze the morphological and morphometric features of cells. The mossy fibers that are formed by axons of the DG granule cells were visualized with the Timm sulphide–silver technique. The cognitive study was performed in a radial plus maze, to test working (WM) and reference memories (RM). All animals were trained for 45 consecutive days. Comparisons among groups were performed using ANOVA. Homogeneity of variance was tested using the Bartlett's χ^2.

RESULTS

Our results revealed that the HF of the OCG animals showed some morphological characteristics of aging when compared to ACG animals. Those main features were a significant decrease in the number of NADPH-d neurons ($P < .01$) and a significant increase in the number of astrocytes ($P < .01$). In OEG animals, the number of NADPH-d positive neurons and astrocytes was not statistically different from those of the ACG animals.

The DG main feature on the OCG was the abundant presence of secondary lysosomes and nuclear inclusions (NI) on the hiliar region neurons. These NI were not noticeable in ACG animals. The neuronal preservation and mitochondrial morphology of the OEG was quite similar to the ACG. The morphometry of granular cells of the experimental group consisting of old anuimals was not statistically different when compared to old animals in the control group (83 vs. 88 μ^2). The nucleolar area of the granular cells was smaller in OCG as compared to OEG and ACG animals.

The cognitive study showed that WM errors (WME) and RM errors (RME) were increased in the ACG when compared to OCG. The OEG performed their task faster than any other group ($P < .05$). Our results indicate that only reference memory errors could be significantly attenuated by administration of CDP-choline.

DISCUSSION

The term *neuroprotection* implies amelioration of neuronal degeneration upon normal aging and/or injury to the nervous system. A variety of agents have been studied and proposed as neuroprotective drugs.[6] Among these molecules are NMDA receptor antagonists, free radical scavengers, and CDP-choline. There is some evidence that CDP-choline has a positive effect on memory and behavior, at least in the short term.[1] Our observations suggest some improvement in the long term both at the microscopic and behavioral levels. Thus, CDP-choline acts as a neuroprotector in these experiments.

ACKNOWLEDGMENTS

This work was supported in part by Grants BSA2001-0803-C02-01 and PR2002-0392 from MECD, Spain.

REFERENCES

1. ALVAREZ, X.A., C. SAMPEDRO, R. LOZANO, *et al.* 1999. Citicoline protects hippocampal neurons against apoptosis induced by brain beta-amyloid deposits plus cerebral hypoperfusion in rats. Methods Find. Exp. Clin. Pharmacol. **8:** 535–540.
2. CRESPO, D., B. STANDFIELD & W.M. COWAN. 1986. Evidence that late-generated granule cells neurons do not simply replace earlier formed neurons in the rat dentate gyrus. Exp. Brain Res. **3:** 541–548.
3. ZWEIFLER, R.M. 2002. Membrane stabilizer: citicoline. Curr. Med. Res. Opin. **18**(Suppl 2): s14–s17.
4. ZHENG, C. & M. HOUWELING. 2002. Phosphatidylcholine and cell death. Biochim. Biophys. Acta **2–3:** 87–96.
5. DEMPSEY, R.J. & V.L. RAGHAVENDRA-RAO. 2003. Cytidinediphosphocholine treatment to decrease traumatic brain injury-induced hippocampal neuronal death, cortical contusion volume, and neurological dysfunction in rats. J. Neurosurg. **98:** 867–873.
6. HICKENBOTTOM, S.L & J. GROTTA. 1998. Neuroprotective therapy. Semin. Neurol. **18:** 485–492.

Chronic Aluminum Administration to Old Rats Results in Increased Levels of Brain Metal Ions and Enlarged Hippocampal Mossy Fibers

PATRIZIA FATTORETTI,[a] CARLO BERTONI-FREDDARI,[a] MARTA BALIETTI,[a] BELINDA GIORGETTI,[a] MORENO SOLAZZI,[a] AND PAOLO ZATTA[b]

[a]*Neurobiology of Aging Laboratory, INRCA Research Department, Ancona, Italy*
[b]*CNR-Institute for Biomedical Technologies, Padova Unit "Metalloproteins," Department of Biology, University of Padova, Padova, Italy*

ABSTRACT: The effect of chronic aluminium administration (2 g/L/6 months) was investigated in the central nervous system (CNS) of old rats. The content of Al^{3+}, Cu^{2+}, Zn^{2+}, and Mn^{2+} was measured in prosencephalon + mesencephalon, pons-medulla, and cerebellum. The area occupied by the mossy fibers in the hippocampal CA3 zone was also measured. In Al-treated rats the contents of Al^{3+}, Cu^{2+}, Zn^{2+}, and Mn^{2+} were significantly increased in prosencephalon + mesencephalon and pons-medulla, while no change was observed in the cerebellum except a Cu^{2+} decrease. The area occupied by the mossy fibers in the CA3 field was significantly increased (+32%) in Al-treated rats. Taken together, the present findings document that the aging CNS is particularly susceptible to aluminum toxic effects that may be responsible for a consistent rise in the cell load of oxidative stress. This may contribute, as an aggravating factor, to the development of neurodegenerative events, as observed in Alzheimer disease.

KEYWORDS: aluminum administration; brain metal ions; hippocampus; Timm's reaction; Alzheimer disease

There is evidence that chronic intake of aluminum with the diet represents a critical causative event in the pathogenesis of neurodegenerative pathologies. Many experimental results and epidemiological studies stress both Al toxicity and the susceptibility of the mammalian central nervous system (CNS) to this metal ion.[1] Despite the wealth of data in the literature, a direct link between Al(III) toxicity and typical neurodegenerative diseases of the senile brain, for example, Alzheimer disease (AD), remains elusive.[1,2] Among the proposed mechanism(s) of action through which Al(III) may be detrimental for nerve cells, it has been proposed that, particularly in old individuals, chronic dietary aluminum intake may exacerbate oxidative stress[3] and, in

Address for correspondence: Dr. Patrizia Fattoretti, Neurobiology of Aging Laboratory, INRCA Research Department, Via Birarelli 8, 60121 Ancona, Italy. Voice: +39-071-80-4153; fax: +39-071-206791
p.fattoretti@inrca.it

turn, lead to neuropathological events.[2] To test this assumption, high doses of Al(III) were administered in the drinking water of 28-month-old rats, and the levels of this metal ion as well as those of copper, zinc, and manganese (as ions linked to the two antioxidant enzymes superoxide dismutases (SOD)) were measured in different CNS areas. Taking the reported susceptibility to aging of the hippocampal formation into account,[4] and considering that damaged nerve terminals may accumulate Zn ions,[5] the area occupied by the mossy fibers in the CA3 subfield was also measured by computer-assisted morphometric methods by using Timm's preferential staining to visualize zinc-positive terminals.

Two groups (12 animals each) of male Wistar rats (22 months of age) were used. Group 1 was treated with a dose of 2 g/L $AlCl_3 \times 6\ H_2O$ in the drinking water for 6 months, while group 2 was used as the control. Six controls and six Al-treated rats were sacrificed by decapitation, the brain was immediately removed and transferred to polystyrene test tubes prewashed with a diluted solution of HNO_3. Samples were then mineralized in HNO_3 at 70°C for two days until the solutions were clear. Al^{3+}, in digested biological samples, was determined by inductively coupled plasma atomic emission spectrometry on a Perkin-Elmer plasma 40-emission spectrometer. Copper, zinc, and manganese were measured by flame atomic absorption after tissue mineralization, as reported earlier.

Six controls and six Al-treated rats were used to perform Timm's staining in the hippocampal CA3 subfield (FIG. 1), as reported in detail in our previous paper.[6] Briefly, following anesthesia, the rats were decapitated and the region of the telencephalon approximately 4000 µm caudal to bregma was excised. Timm's staining was carried out on tissue samples snap-frozen in isopentane cooled by liquid nitrogen. The tissue sections were mounted on gelatin-coated slides, air dried, and covered with a physical developer containing 60 mL of 33% arabic gum, 10 mL of citrate buffer (25.5 g citric acid, 23.5 g trisodium citrate $\times\ 2H_2O$, 100 mL of distilled water), 15 mL of 5.67% hydrochinone, and 15 mL of 0.73% silver lactate. The staining was carried out in the dark at 26°C for one hour. The slides were washed in distilled water, air-dried, contrasted with methyl green, rinsed in distilled water, dehydrated, and mounted with Biomount. In the CA3 subfield, the area occupied by the mossy fibers that showed positive to Timm's staining (FIG.1) was measured by a computer-assisted image analyzer connected to a light microscope. Twenty-five consecutive hippocampal sections/animal were sampled and analyzed. Statistical comparisons were performed by the Student's t-test.

The analytical measurements (µg/g fresh tissue) of aluminum, zinc, copper, and manganese were carried out in three discrete zones of the CNS: prosencephalon + mesencephalon (PME), pons-medulla (PMD), and cerebellum. Al concentration significantly increased by 94% and 53% in PME and PMD, respectively, while it was the same in the cerebellum of control and treated animals. In PME: copper, zinc, and manganese concentrations were significantly increased by 32%, 41%, and 50%, respectively. In PMD, the concentrations of these metal ions were also increased by 46% (Cu), 46% (Zn), and 41% (Mn). In the cerebellum, no significant change was observed in the concentrations of copper, zinc, and manganese. The area occupied by the mossy fibers in the hippocampal CA3 subfield was increased by 47% in the Al-treated rats.

Our results show that the chronic intake of high doses of aluminum with the diet causes significant alterations in the CNS of old animals. Although the clear-cut

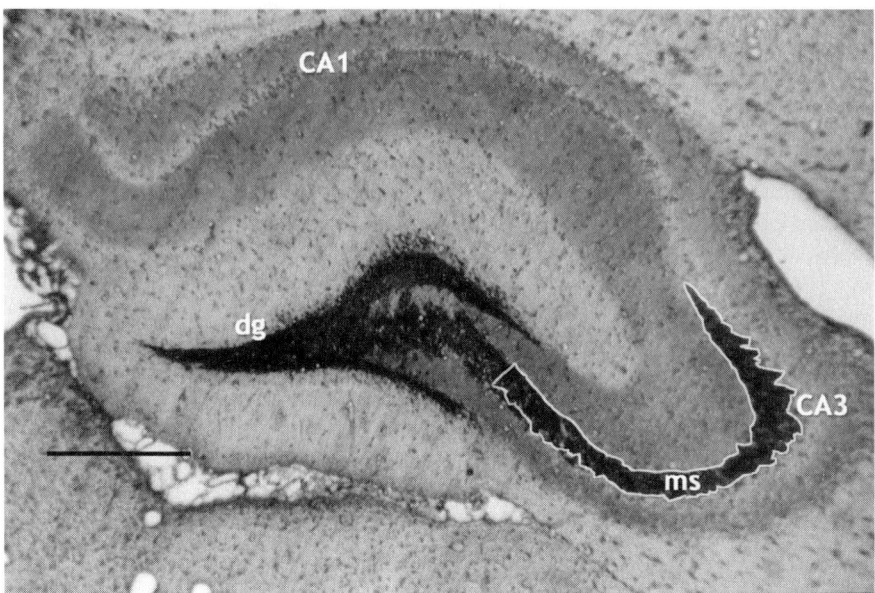

FIGURE 1. Al-treated hippocampal frozen section stained by Timm technique. The Timm-positive mossy fiber area is outlined by a *white line*: d.g.: granular cells of dentate gyrus; CA1: neuronal pyramidal cells of CA1 sector; CA3: neuronal pyramidal cells of CA3 area; m.s.: mossy fibers. *Bar*: 500 μm.

mechanism(s) of aluminum toxicity have not been identified, recent studies suggest that this metal ion is responsible for subtle rearrangements of membrane lipids[7] and cholesterol,[8] which may facilitate the peroxidative action of other redox ions.[1] This hypothesized process of membrane destabilization is reliably supported by *in vitro* experiments documenting the potentiation of iron-induced membrane lipid peroxidation when aluminum is added to the culture medium.[7] In agreement with this rationale, we interpret the increase of Cu, Zn, and Mn in PME and PMD of Al-treated rats to witness an increased genetic expression and/or turnover of both cytosolic and mitochondrial SOD. We are aware of the speculative character of our assumption; however, the overexpression of these antioxidant enzymes may have been sustained for the whole period of time that Al was administered, thus resulting in higher levels of their specific metal ions. Moreover, increased Al intake has been recently reported to be responsible of an increased SOD activity.[9]

Al is shown to accumulate preferentially in the hippocampus where it is thought to cause aging-like alterations.[4] The enlarged area of the mossy fibers that show positive to the Timm's reaction for Zn ions, which we found in the hippocampal CA3 subfield of Al treated rats, lends consistent support to this assumption. It is well demonstrated that Zn ions are located within the vesicles at presynaptic terminals, where they play an important role in synaptic transmission. It has been reported that dishomeostasis of Zn ions, due to defective Zn movement from pre- to postsynaptic neurones, represents a marker of cell damage.[10] When nerve cell injury occurs, Zn is lost from the neuropil and is accumulated by most damaged neurones. These Zn ions are free or loosely bound, and are histochemically detectable by Timm's reaction.[5] This rationale and the increase of Zn ions in PME and PMD reliably suggest that increased nerve cell damage may have occurred in Al-treated rats.

Taken together, the present findings support the concept that aging seems to represent a condition in which the CNS (and to a greater extent the hippocampal formation) is particularly susceptible to a chronic intake of aluminum with the diet. As reported by several experiments from different laboratories, increased Al intake may lead to an exacerbation of oxidative stress and to the development of a typical neurodegenerative disease of the senile brain, for example, Alzheimer disease.

REFERENCES

1. GRANT, W.B. et al. 2002. The significance of environmental factors in the etiology of Alzheimer's disease. Alzheimer's Dis. **4:** 179–189.
2. SCOTT, C.W. et al. 1993. Aggregation of tau protein by aluminum. Brain Res. **628:** 77–84.
3. PRATICÒ, D. et al. 2002. Aluminum modulates brain amyloidosis through oxidative stress in APP transgenic mice. FASEB J. **16:** 1138–1140.
4. DELONCLE, R. et al. 2001. Ultrastructural study of rat hippocampus after chronic administration of aluminum L-glutamate: an acceleration of the aging process. Exp. Gerontol. **36:** 231–244.
5. FREDERICKSON, C.J. & G. DANSCHER. 1990. Zinc-containing neurons in hippocampus and related CNS structures. *In* Progress in Brain Research. J. Storm-Mathisen, J. Zimmer, and O.P. Ottersen, Eds.: 71–84/ Elsevier. New York.
6. FATTORETTI, P. et al. 2003. The effect of chronic aluminum(III) administration on the nervous system of aged rats: clues to understand its suggested role in Alzheimer's disease. J. Alzheimer's Dis. **5:** 437–444.
7. GUTTERIDGE, J.M. et al. 1985. Aluminium salts accelerate peroxidation of membrane lipids stimulated by iron salts. Biochim. Biophys. Acta **835:** 441–447.
8. SARIN, S., V. GUPTA & K.D. GILL. 1997. Alterations in lipid composition and neuronal injury in primates following chronic aluminium exposure. Biol. Trace Elem. Res. **59:** 133–143.
9. MICIC, D.V., N.D. PETRONIJEVIC & S.S. VUCETIC. 2003. Superoxide dismutase activity in the Mongolian gerbil brain after acute poisoning with alumiunum. J. Alzheimer's Dis. **5:** 49–56.
10. SUH, S.W. et al. 2000. Evidence that synaptically-released zinc contributes to neuronal injury after traumatic brain injury. Brain Res. **852:** 268–273.

Motor and Cognitive Recovery Induced by Bone Marrow Stem Cells Grafted to Striatum and Hippocampus of Impaired Aged Rats

Functional and Therapeutic Considerations

CARIDAD I. FERNÁNDEZ,[a] ESTEBAN ALBERTI,[a] YISSEL MENDOZA,[b] LISIS MARTÍNEZ,[a] JAIME COLLAZO,[a] JUAN C. ROSILLO,[a] AND JOSÉ Y. BAUZA[a]

[a]*Basic Division, International Center of Neurological Restoration (CIREN), Havana 11300, Cuba*

[b]*Center of Genetic Engineer and Biotechnology (CIGB), Havana 11300, Cuba*

ABSTRACT: Impairments in motor coordination and cognition in normal and pathological aging are often accompanied by structural changes, that is, loss of synapses and neurons. Also, it has been shown recently that bone marrow stem cells can give origin to cells of different tissues, including neural cells. Given the therapeutic implications of increasing health and functional possibilities in the aged brain, we have tested the effects of rat femur bone marrow stem cells (rBMSCs) grafting to the striatum hippocampus of aged rats with motor or cognitive deficits, respectively. Bone marrow cells were transduced with an adenovirus driving the expression of green fluorescence protein (GFP) and other classic stains to determine their migration, engraftment, differentiation, and associated behavioral recovery. Five weeks after it, control and grafted rats were re-evaluated with the Morris Water Maze test, Passive avoidance, open-field, motor coordination, and Marshall tests and perfused. Brains were processed and analyzed for fluorescent protein expression. GFP was detected in cells with some differentiation degree into neural-like cells. Their exact phenotype is yet to be determined. A significant functional recovery was observed 6 weeks after grafting, suggesting a trophic interaction between rBMSCs and the aged/dystrophic host brain, or with the host brain progenitor cells and/or by increasing the number of functional cells at striatum or hippocampus, suggesting that the aging brain keeps its functional plasticity as well as that BMSCs are interesting candidates for cell replacement therapies in neurodegenerative disorders.

KEYWORDS: bone marrow stem cells; brain aging; cognition; motor coordination; behavioral recovery; grafting; green fluorescent protein

Address for correspondence: Caridad I. Fernández, Basic Division, International Center of Neurological Restoration (CIREN), Ave 25 No. 15805. Playa, Havana 11300, Cuba. Voice: +537-271-5353; fax: +537-332420.
  ivettefer@yahoo.es

Impairments in motor coordination and cognition in normal aging and age-associated neurodegenerative disorders often are accompanied by functional and structural changes, that is, increased oxidative stress and neuronal atrophy.[1] The ability to replace these loss/malfunctioning cells using stem cells and the origin of new ones have been the subject of recent intensive research.[2] Also, it has been shown recently that bone marrow stem cells can give origin to cells of different tissues, including neural cells.[3] Given its potential therapeutic implications to the aged/dystrophic brain, we have evaluated the functional evidence (regarding motor and cognitive improvement, if any) of rat bone marrow mesenchymal cells grafting to the striatum or hippocampus of aged rats.

Old Sprague-Dawley rats (male, 20–22 months old) were defined as motoric or cognitively impaired using Morris Water Maze (MWM) task and Transverse Bridges test performances, respectively, according to previously defined criteria.[4,5] Open-field behavior, passive avoidance test, and Marshall test also were conducted (data no shown). Rat bone marrow mesenchymal cells (BMMCs) were isolated from femurs of adult rats. The "*ex vivo*" manipulation included infection with an adenovirus which codified for green fluorescent protein (GFP). Each rat received 2 µL of cell suspension (1.5×10^5 cells/mL) into the striatum (A = +1.0 mm, L = ±2.5 mm, V = 3.5 mm below dura, N = 10) or hippocampus (A = +3.0 mm, L = ±3.8 mm, V = 3.7 mm below dura, N = 10) on each side of the brain. Control rats (N = 5/group) received medium without cells. Five weeks later, control and grafted rats were re-evaluated at MWM test, passive avoidance, open-field, motor coordination, and Marshall tests and perfused (saline, 4% phosphate-buffered paraformaldehyde). Brains were removed and postfixed. Coronal sections (20-µm tissue thickness) were cut on a sliding knife freezing microtome. Alternate sections were assigning to cresyl violet and immunohistochemistry. Observations for GFP expression were performed immediately after cutting using an optic microscope with blue filter. Magnification was ×62.5. Intragroup comparisons included Wilcoxon test. For comparisons, intergroup ANOVA tests were used. Those analyses with $P < .05$ were considered statistically significant.

Overall, the experimental paradigm and behavioral tests were well tolerated by all of the rats. Control or grafted groups (S or H) were not significantly different from each other during the first evaluation (PRE), ANOVA tests. Spontaneous exploratory activity indicates that grafting procedures either at hippocampus or striatum did not modify the habituation pattern within trial/day as well as intertrials/day for all groups. Grafting of BMMCs to the striatum significantly improved functional recovery on swimming abilities according to the Marshall scale for vigor and success, as well as on motor coordination tested with the transverse bridges test (with different cross-section and diameter) (TABLE 1) similar to previous results using fetal tissue.[4] Analysis of the inhibitory avoidance behavior and MWM execution as index of mnesic functions showed differences between pre- versus postperformances in hippocampus-grafted rats for specific tests; meanwhile, control groups persisted in their initial behavioral condition. Thus, data from them are not shown so that results presentation is simplified (TABLE 1).

In general, animals with striatum graft showed a specific and significant melioration in motor functions. Meanwhile, their cognitive performance was unchanged or not significantly improved in relation to their initial performance. Also, the opposite situation was observed in the H-graft group, indicating that the observed

TABLE 1. Performance of aged rats before and after grafting treatment at hippocampus or striatum during cognitive and motor tests

Test/parameter		Hippocampus		Striatum	
MWM task	Total latency (s)	22.40 ± 1.40	7.94 ± 1.09^a	20.22 ± 1.16	18.76 ± 3.79
	Crossing occurrence	1.16 ± 0.98	5.35 ± 2.4^a	1.33 ± 1.03	1.83 ± 0.75
Bridge test (latency to fall)	Square (2 × 2 cm)	98.33 ± 15.09	101.71 ± 0.16	101.03 ± 11.9	113.83 ± 5.10^a
	Rounded (Ø = 2 cm)	82.66 ± 27.89	79.53 ± 41.61	69.66 ± 45.23	98.33 ± 15.83^a

^{a}Pre- vs. postcomparison with Wilcoxon matched pairs test. Significant at $P < .05$.

improvement is specific and sensitive to the "cell-replaced area;" that is, the functional recovery is mediated by a selective effect of grafted cells on the target region and consequently to the associated functions,[6] suggesting that interactive signals have taken place between host and grafted tissue and that those signals are probably tissue specific or generic to injury.[7]

Tracking of grafted cells was conducted successfully using GFP as a marker. Cells were well integrated into the tissue structure, but if there was morphological distinction from their host-derived neighbors it remains to be determined. However, it could be observed that some cells exhibited a lengthening, remembering a "bipolar neuron" (FIG. 1). Surprisingly, the infused cells did not aggregate as it has been reported with infusion of fibroblasts and other stem cells.[8] Instead, the cells integrated and migrated along 2–3 mm from the injected site. GFP fluorescent cells were not seen in other structures. The same pattern of integration and migration has been reported by others in both rat and human BMMCs infused into the brains of adult rats,[3,9] but grafted tissue did not appear to reestablish the normal cytoarchitecture at 6 weeks after grafting. Thus, it is highly likely that the ability of grafted cells to induce functional changes (such as the described motor and cognitive recovery) in response to appropriate stimulus (such as the dystrophic host) would be associated with an exchange of signals between host and grafted cells, similar to a positive feedback, rather than by replacement or integration of BMMCs to neural circuits: signals from the targeted tissue (microenvironment) can elicit the pluripotentiality expression by those cells[10] as well as which genes will be activated or modified into them, and, consequently, these molecular signals could promote synthesis of proteins (trophic factors, cytokines, specific neurotransmitters) able to modify the neuronal activity in the host.[6,9]

It is concluded that, first, rodent BMMCs can survive and exert some trophic effect on the age-impaired rat brain and modify the course of age-associated motor or cognitive deterioration. Second, considering the observed recovery in impaired functions, it could be suggested that rat BMMCs could work as "functional neurons" or inductors of neural functions in the targeted tissue, suggesting that intrinsic genomic mechanisms of lineage restriction and cell function are mutable. It is suggested that an exchange of signals and positive interaction between grafted BMMCs and the host took place. In addition, the grafted cells could activate the brain's stem cells, which probably could migrate to make new neurons in the injected site and

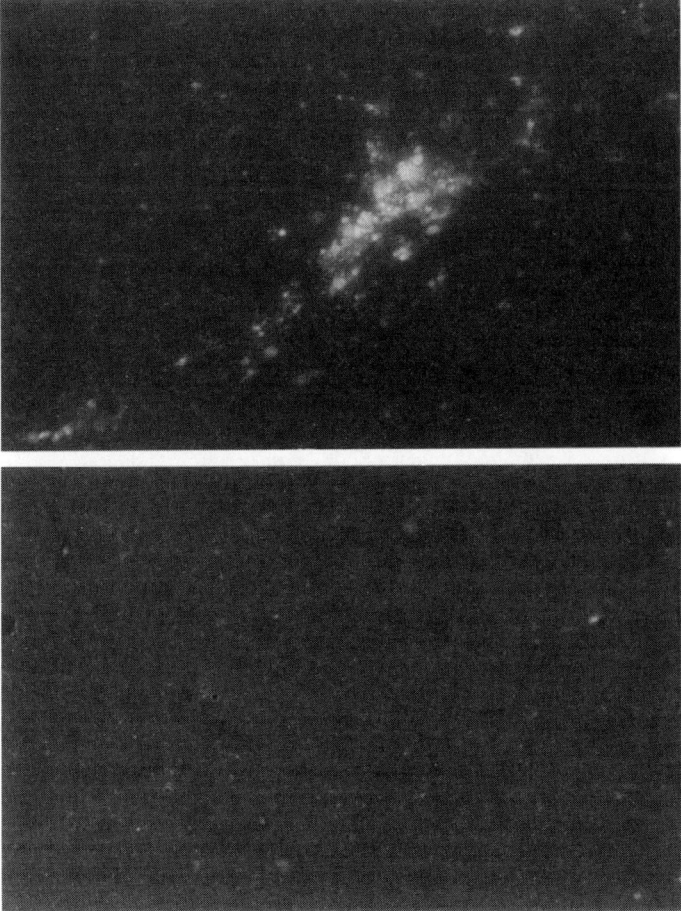

FIGURE 1. Photomicrographs show the grafted GFP-expressing cells into the caudate-putamen region in the recipient rat brain (*top*) or their absence in control rats that received medium without cells (*bottom*).

additional locations. Although it remains to be demonstrated, it is another interesting possibility that cannot be left out of discussion. The induction of existent neural stem cells to produce useful numbers of functional nerve cells in chosen parts of the brain could be a new cell replacement modality in degenerative disorders involving neuronal damage and death, among them Alzheimer disease, Parkinson disease, stroke, and trauma. Finally, there are very limited studies on peripheral mesenchymal cells grafted to the brain of aged, behaviorally impaired rats in which functional recovery had been detected or described. BMMCs may be useful in the treatment of a wide variety of neurological diseases, offering significant advantages (e.g., no immunological rejection, and greater availability) over other "stem" cells or fetal tissue as donors.

REFERENCES

1. MATTSON, M.P., W. DUAN, J. LEE & Z. GUO. 2001. Suppression of brain aging and neurodegenerative disorders by dietary restriction and environmental enrichment: molecular mechanisms. Mech. Ageing Dev. **122:** 757–778.
2. FILIP, S., J. MOKRY & I. HRUSKA. 2003. Adult stem cells and their importance in cell therapy. Folia Biol. **49:** 9–14.
3. MEZEY, E., S. KEY, G. VOGELSANG, et al. 2003. Transplanted bone marrow generates new neurons in human brains. Proc. Natl. Acad. Sci. USA **100:** 1364–1369.
4. FERNÁNDEZ, C.I., J. SOTO, O. GONZÁLEZ, et al. 1994. Brain aging and neurotransplantation. I. Nigral cell suspension graft to aged rodent striatum and motor disabilities. Arch. Gerontol. Geriatr. **4:** 51–58.
5. FERNÁNDEZ, C.I., J. SOTO, O. GONZÁLEZ, et al. 1994. Brain aging and neurotransplatation. II. Effects of septal cell suspension grafts to hippocampus of aged rodents on learning and memory impairments. Arch. Gerontol. Geriatr. **4:** 59–65.
6. CHEN, J., Y. LI, L. WANG, et al. 2001. Therapeutic benefit of intracerebral transplantation of bone marrow stromal cells after cerebral ischemia in rats. J. Neurol. Sci. **189:** 49–57.
7. ABOODY, K.S., A. BROWN, N.G. RAINOV, et al. 2000. Neural stem cells display extensive tropism for pathology in adult brain: evidence from intracranial gliomas. Proc. Natl. Acad. Sci. USA **97:** 12846–12851.
8. LIMKE, T.L. & M.S. RAO. 2002. Neural stem cells in aging and disease. J. Cell. Mol. Med. **6:** 475–496.
9. LI, Y., J. CHEN, X.G. CHEN, et al. 2002. Human marrow stromal cell therapy for stroke in rat. Neurotrophins and functional recovery. Neurology **59:** 514–523.
10. MARSHAK, D.R., R.L. GARDNER & D. GOOTLIEB. 2001. Stem Cells Biology. Cold Spring Harbor Laboratory Press. Cold Spring Harbor, NY.

Environmental Enrichment–Behavior–Oxidative Stress Interactions in the Aged Rat

Issues for a Therapeutic Approach in Human Aging

C. I. FERNÁNDEZ, J. COLLAZO, Y. BAUZA, M. R. CASTELLANOS, AND O. LÓPEZ

Basic Division, International Center of Neurological Restoration (CIREN), Havana 11300, Cuba

ABSTRACT: The effects of environment enrichment on motor activity, exploration, and cognitive performances were studied in aged rats. Both nonimpaired (NI) and impaired (I) rats were submitted to daily training in a complex-enriched environment (cEE) for 60 days. Animals were examined at spatial water maze task, passive avoidance test, open-field test, and sensorimotor coordination tasks (bridges test and Marshall scales). At the end of experiments, animals were killed for brain biochemical determinations (gluthatione content and specific-ChAT activity). Results after the first evaluation (before training) corroborate that the aged rat population showed a heterogeneity in behavioral patterns like that observed in humans. Also, cEE modified exploration activity, cognition, motor functions, and biochemical markers in both NI and I groups, but changes reached significant relevance for the last group. It is significant that neurotrophins, "novo" synthesis of neurotransmitters, and oxidative stress levels may mediate the observed changes, indicating that the aged brain still has appreciable plasticity in response to well-manipulated environmental stimulation. Finally, our results also support the novel concepts and programs in prevention/reduction both in incidence/severity and outcome of age-associated neurodegenerative conditions.

KEYWORDS: environmental enrichment; brain aging; cognition; motor coordination; behavioral recovery; ChAT activity; glutathione; GSH

Several studies support the concept that multimodal activation of the brain may contribute to the restoration of several aspects of cognition and other central functions.[1] The aged brain is subjected to multiple factors that result in damage to its cellular constituents and the neural networks that form the bases of behavior. Also, neuronal activity can be affected not only by genetic and age-related factors but also by multiple environmental factors.[2] Recent advances in neuroscience have led to the development of psychophysical methods that can ameliorate the effects of those factors.[3] By altering the balance between neuronal injury and repair/reposition, we can delay

---

Address for correspondence: C. I. Fernández, Basic Division. International Center of Neurological Restoration (CIREN), Ave 25 No. 15805, Playa, Havana 11300, Cuba. Voice: +537-271-5353; fax: +537-332420.
ivette.fdez@infomed.sld.cu

the expression and progression of the neurodegenerative processes of brain aging and related neurodegenerative disorders.[1,4]

Male Sprague-Dawley rats (20 months old) were used in this study. Morris Water Maze (MWM) and Bridge's test performances were used for defining cognitive and motor impairment criteria.[4] Open-field behavior, passive avoidance test, and Marshall test also were conducted. Experimental conditions for environmental enrichment (EE) included a large cage (0.8 m^2), social interaction (up to 10 rats, both sexes), stimulation of exploratory behavior (voluntary running, tunnels, toys, with daily change), and food and water dispenser set at different places and positions (frequently upstairs 45° or throughout narrow bridges).

Groups of impaired (I) and nonimpaired (NI) rats were submitted to 60 days of EE (n = 15/group). After it, they were retested and killed for biochemical studies, specific-ChAT activity (Fonnum method, expressed as nmol acetylcholine (Ach)/mg protein/min), and glutathione content (GSH) in different brain regions. Each half of control groups for both I and NI status (n=30/group) living under standard conditions were sacrificed at different moments of the experiment (beginning/end) for biochemical determinations. Data were expressed as mean ± SEM and analyzed using Wilcoxon test for pre- vs. postintragroup comparisons (behavioral studies). A t test was used for biochemical data. A significant level of .05 was assumed.

Housing under EE induced positive modifications of the recipient's behavior in both I and NI rats, but the most relevant modifications were seen in the I group. The "relative" reduction of exploratory activity during the first day at open-field test observed in rats in standard housing conditions (pre-EE) was restored by a novel and complex environment (TABLE 1). Differences between initial and ending performances also were observed for the ability of the rat to pass through different transverse bridges when tasks were made more challenging, that is, square versus rounded bridges and a diminished cross-section. Results shown in TABLE 1 confirm the behavioral heterogeneity previously described in aged rodents[4] and additionally provide evidence that environmental factors contribute significantly to cognitive and motor aging. The acquisition rate expressed as latency of a spatial learning task (MWM) and retention as counting of crossing occurrence during trial 36 in the same test were significantly improved by EE. These results and those not shown from avoidance response and Marshall scale indicate an increment in the behavioral "flexibility" for motor and cognitive function induced by a novel and complex environment.[4]

Sixty days of exposition in an EE improves not only the behavioral concerns. The distribution pattern of specific ChAT activity and the glutathione content in brain regions varied from I versus NI rats at the standard conditions (Pre-EE in Section B, TABLE 1). After EE housing, both I and NI groups exhibit modifications in this biochemical marker, significantly relevant at the I group. EE significantly increased ChAT activity in the following order: striatum > septum > hippocampus > cortex (P < .05, TABLE 1), which is in accordance with previous results, associating these modifications with arousal mechanisms and selective attentional functions.[5] It also provides evidence that senile impairment of the cholinergic system in rats is related to decrease in ChAT-protein expression rather than an acute degeneration of neuronal cell bodies.

The glutathione content distribution was increased in NI versus I rats (data not shown) under standard conditions. EE promoted a significant recovery in GSH levels

TABLE 1A. Behavioral studies

Test	Nonimpaired		Impaired	
Latency (s)	Pre-EE	Post-EE	Pre-EE	Post-EE
Open-field activity. All visited squares during first day.	41.66 ± 1.21	56.33 ± 0.48	29.49 ± 4.33	45.32 ± 2.73^a
MWM task total latency	9.16 ± 1.94	6.68 ± 2.57ns	36.24 ± 5.99	12.87 ± 3.62^a
Crossing occurrence trial 36	4.32 ± 2.05	5.01±1.86ns	1.48±0.02	4.74±2.45^a
Bridges test square 2 × 2 cm	86.74 ± 11.20	105.41 ± 9.18^a	16.04 ± 29.63	65.00 ± 6.22^b
Round (Ø=2 cm)	69.51 ± 1.47	79.86 ± 0.5^a	33.43 ± 5.30	81.82 ± 6.8^b

^{a}Pre-EE vs. Post-EE, $P<.05$, Wilcoxon test.
^{b}Pre-EE vs. Post-EE, $P<.01$, Wilcoxon test.

TABLE 1B. Biochemical determinations (impaired rats)

	Pre-EE	Post-EE	Percent Variation
Glutathione content (GSH) (mol/g wet weight)			
Hippocampus	1.0407 ± 0.071	1.329902 ± 0.056^a	126
Total cortex	1.101 ± 0.078	1.188054 ± 0.298ns	107
Striatum	0.346 ± 0.067	0.839424 ± 0.132^b	242
Specific ChAT activity (nmol Ach/mg protein/min)			
Septum	0.0010 ± 0.001	0.0028 ± 0.003^b	280
Striatum	0.0074 ± 0.001	0.022 ± 0.005^b	301
Hippocampus	0.0086 ± 0.002	0.012 ± 0.005^b	139
Total cortex	0.0063 ± 0.0004	0.0063 ± 0.002ns	101

$^a P<.05$, t test.
$^b P<.01$, t test.
NOTE: Pre-EE refers to the housing conditions at the beginning of the experiment.

in brains from impaired animals in the following order: striatum > hippocampus > cortex ($P < .05$). Reduced glutathione plays an important role in cellular protection against damage from reactive oxygen species (ROS). A GSH level is also important in the regulation of brain functions.[6,7] The high susceptibility of striatum and hippocampus to cumulative oxidative stress is reduced after EE, indicating that the combination of physical activity plus sensorial and cognitive stimulation provides protection against age-related oxidative stress.

Environmental enrichment consists of many components, such as expanded learning opportunities, increased social interaction, more physical activity, and larger housing. So then a possible synergism among all of them could take place, promoting a selective and prolonged neuroprotection response. We could not separate their relative contribution to the observed changes, neither the practice nor training effects. Our complex enrichment paradigm was conceived with all those elements that could permit us a possible extrapolation of results to humans.

It is now clear that exercise and EE can increase levels of neurotrophic factors, increase resistance to brain insult, and improve learning and mental performance.[7] Among neurotrophins, the nerve growth factor (NGF) is a good candidate. NGF has been associated with cognitive functions and shown to improve the performance of aged rats in spatial learning and memory task. Also, atrophy of cholinergic neurons is strongly correlated with learning and memory impairments.[4] Furthermore, it has been demonstrated that EE and exercise mobilizes gene expression profiles that would be predicted to benefit brain plasticity processes and the neurotrophins production.[8] In addition, EE induces the production of proteins that suppress the oxyradical production, such as glutathione and stabilizes cellular calcium homeostasis and inhibits apoptotic biochemical cascades.[6,7] It is suggested that EE protects the brain against ROS by upregulation of glutathione and/or activates other enzymes involved in this process, maybe through astroglial activation.[7] Interestingly, EE also increases newly generated neural cells in the adult brain, suggesting that this environment manipulation can increase the brain's capacity for plasticity and self-repair.[9,10] Therefore, in rats, particularly in those with cognitive impairment, signs of neuronal aging can be diminished by a sustained active and challenging life, even if this stimulation started only at middle age. Several studies have demonstrated that gene expression and morphological and biochemical indices in the brain undergo alterations in response to environmental influences.[9,11] Our results corroborate previous evidence.

Considering the observed beneficial effects of EE on behavior, the increased protection against oxidative injury, and the recovery of cholinergic neurotransmission in cognitively impaired aged rats, as well as different social factors, have been taken into account as factors with predictable value in the course of AD. First, EE could be a factor that modifies the magnitude and temporal course of age-associated motor and cognitive disabilities. Second, a complex and novel environment would be a useful therapeutic/preventive strategy toward restimulation of neuronal activity rate in older/mature people. Third, our results support the novel concepts and programs in prevention/reduction of both incidence/severity and outcome of age-associated neurodegenerative conditions.

REFERENCES

1. COTMAN, C.W. & N.C. BERCHTOLD. 2002. Exercise: a behavioral intervention to enhance brain health and plasticity. Trends Neurosci. **25:** 295–301.
2. SWAAB, D.F., E.J. DUBELAAR, M.A. HOFMAN, et al. 2002. Brain aging and Alzheimer's disease; use it or lose it. Prog. Brain Res. **138:** 343–373.
3. CHURCHILL, J.D., R. GALVEZ, S. COLCOMBE, et al. 2002. Exercise, experience and the aging brain. Neurobiol. Aging **23:** 941–955.

4. CACABELOS, R., C.I. FERNANDEZ, E. GIACOBINI & M. TAKEDA. 1999. Basic and clinical neurosciences: brain aging and Alzheimer's disease. 1999. Prous Science. Barcelona, Spain.
5. GIOVANNINI, M.G., A. RAKOVSKA, R.S. BENTON, et al. 2001. Effects of novelty an habituation on acetylcholine, GABA, and glutamate release from the frontal cortex and hippocampus of freely moving rats. Neuroscience **106:** 43–53.
6. DRINGEN, R., J.M. GUTTERER & J. HIRRLINGER. 2000. Glutathione metabolism in brain: metabolic interaction between astrocytes and neurons in the defense against reactive oxygen species. Eur. J. Biochem. **267:** 4912–4916.
7. MATTSON, M.P., W. DUAN, J. LEE & Z. GUO. 2001. Suppression of brain aging and neurodegenerative disorders by dietary restriction and environmental enrichment: molecular mechanisms. Mech. Ageing Dev. **122:** 757–778.
8. PHAM, T.M., B. ICKES, D. ALBECK, et al. 1999. Changes in brain NGF levels and NGF receptors in rats exposed to environmental enrichment for one year. Neuroscience **94:** 279–286.
9. KEMPERMANN,G., D. GAST & F.H. GAGE. 2002. Neuroplasticity in old age: sustained fivefold induction of hippocampal neurogenesis by long-term environmental enrichment. Ann. Neurol. **52:** 135–143.
10. PRAAG, H., G. KEMPERMANN & F.H. GAGE. 2000. Neural consequences of environmental enrichment. Neuroscience **1:** 191–198.
11. DIAMOND, M.C. 2001. Response of the brain to enrichment. An. Acad. Bras. Cienc. **73:** 211–220.

Digital Transcriptome Analysis in the Aging Cerebellum

MAGDALENA C. POPESCO, ADRIENNE FROSTHOLM, KATARZYNA REJNIAK, AND ANDREJ ROTTER

Department of Pharmacology and the Mathematical Biosciences Institute, The Ohio State University, Columbus, Ohio 43210, USA

> ABSTRACT: Serial analysis of gene expression (SAGE) was used to identify and quantify all expressed cerebellar genes in the adult (P92) and aged (P810) C57BL/6J mouse cerebellum. A "closest-neighbor" algorithm was used to differentiate low abundance tags from possible sequencing errors in both libraries. Unique tags were categorized into four groups: (1) novel genes; (2) ESTs; (3) RIKEN, KIA, and hypothetical genes; and (4) known genes. Known genes were further subdivided into functional categories based on the gene ontology classification, using a web-based program developed in this laboratory (MmSAGEClass). Comparison of adult and aged cerebellar libraries revealed several genes that were differentially expressed, including growth hormone and prolactin, both of which were markedly decreased in the aged cerebellum. In addition, several tags showing differential expression were not identified in the Unigene database and are likely to represent novel genes. The present SAGE data on the aged cerebellar transcriptome may reveal candidate genes involved in the aging process.
>
> KEYWORDS: digital transcriptome analysis; cerebellum; SAGE

The major function of the cerebellum is to integrate sensory input and motor output, thus modulating movement and balance. The cerebellar cortex of aged mice has a reduced number of Purkinje, basket, and stellate cells; granule cell numbers are retained relatively intact.[1] Senescent cerebellar cells also display dendritic atrophy,[2] reduction in somatic volume,[3] and alterations in electrophysiological properties[4] and microstructural features.[5] In recent studies, DNA microarrays were used to examine gene expression profiles in the aging mouse cerebellum;[6,7] the results suggested that senescence was accompanied by an inflammatory response, oxidative stress, and reduced neurotrophic support, all aspects of human neurodegenerative diseases.

Whereas DNA microarray technology is a "closed" system capable of detecting known genes, Serial Analysis of Gene Expression (SAGE) is an "open" system that detects and quantifies both known, and previously unknown, genes. The basic prin-

---

Address for correspondence: Department of Pharmacology and the Mathematical Biosciences Institute, The Ohio State University, Columbus, OH 43210. Voice: 614-292-7747.
rotter.1@osu.edu

ciple of SAGE is the isolation of a short cDNA sequence (tag) from a specific and invariable position within a given mRNA. This 14–15-bp tag is located immediately adjacent to the 3' proximal *Nla*III restriction site; its sequence varies according to the particular mRNA from which it was derived. Each tag contains enough nucleotides to identify each transcript and thus is a unique marker for any expressed gene. The frequency with which any particular tag is detected is directly proportional to the number of mRNAs originally present in the cell or tissue being studied. Therefore, the number of identical tags detected is a measure of the abundance of the corresponding mRNAs in the original tissue. Each unique SAGE tag is matched with tags derived from the Unigene database. In the current study, serial analysis of gene expression was conducted in the adult and aged mouse cerebellum.

METHODS

SAGE libraries were constructed from the cerebellum of postnatal day (P) 92 and 810 mice. The aged mouse (C57BL/6Jnia) was purchased from the National Institute of Aging colony. The adult C57BL/6J animal was bred from Jackson Laboratories stocks. Animals were killed, cerebella were removed rapidly, and total RNA was prepared.[8] SAGE (I-SAGE kit) was performed as described by the manufacturer (Invitrogen). Sequence trace files were analyzed with the *Phred* base-calling software (Applied Biosystems). The SAGE2000 analysis software[8] was used to extract and analyze the primary sequence data from the electrophoretic trace files. The software extracts tag sequences from the sequence files, counts each tag, and provides a report containing the occurrence of each tag and its expression level and *P* value. Tag sequences were compared with the National Center for Biotechnology Information (NCBI) mouse SAGE tag-to-gene mapping reference database (ftp://ftp.ncbi.nih.gov/pub/sage/map/Mm/NlaIII/).

RESULTS AND DISCUSSION

Tag frequency in each SAGE library reflects the relative abundance of the corresponding cerebellar mRNA, a feature that allows digital comparisons between independently generated libraries. Both libraries were calculated to contain more than 100,000 tags, indicating that they were sufficiently large to obtain a good representation of expressed genes. The actual number of tags sequenced (total tags) was much smaller: 16,430 for the P92 library and 18,581 for the P810 library. This cutoff was arbitrary, based primarily on sequencing cost. Because the original libraries were retained, it is possible to obtain additional tags by sequencing more clones. Additional sequencing will permit the detection of additional low-frequency tags and more accurate quantitation of low-abundance tags. The tag sequences and counts were deposited in the SAGE database accessible via the NCBI Web site.

Although the majority of tags in both libraries were present in multiple copies, a significant number of tags were present once only. In most studies, these single tags are discounted because it is assumed that many could arise through errors due to base substitution, deletion, or addition. However, this process tends to eliminate genuine tags corresponding to genes expressed at very low levels. To compromise between the two extremes of either retaining or discounting all single tags, we developed an algorithm ("closest neighbor") that substitutes, deletes, or adds bases to determine whether any tag in the SAGE library is related to another. In the event that such a tag is found, it is deleted from the list of total tags. This adjustment reduced the number of tags to 14,128 in the P92 library and 13,131 in the P810 library. All duplicate tags and genes were consolidated to obtain the number of unique tag sequences: the P92 library contained 4,842, and the P810 library had 5,094 unique tags.

Unique tags were further categorized into four groups: (1) novel genes, (2) ESTs, (3) RIKEN, KIA and hypothetical genes, and (4) known genes. The percentage of tags in each group was (1) 11 and 20, (2) 26 and 27, (3) 25 and 21, and (4) 38 and 32, for P92 and P810 mice, respectively. The high percentage of novel genes is surprising because they represent relatively abundant transcripts, which it might be assumed would have been detected previously. It is also notable that the percentage of novel tags is almost twice as high in the aged cerebellar library, suggesting that during the aging process novel genes become active. The known genes were further subdivided into functional categories based on the Gene Ontology classification (http://www.geneontology.org) using a Web-based program developed in our laboratory (http://mbi.osu.edu/~rejniak/MmSAGEClass.html). For both young adult and aged libraries, among the most numerous identifiers were enzyme activity (~6%), binding activity (~5%), transporter activity (~4%), signal transducer activity (~1%), and structural molecule activity (~1%). A notable feature of the classification scheme is that the sizes of the functional gene classes expressed in the two libraries were conserved. This indicates that there are no major shifts in the categories of abundantly expressed genes during aging, but changes do occur in the expression of individual genes within the larger functional categories.

The three hundred most abundant genes in the P92 and P810 libraries were compared. The results (TABLE 1) are listed in decreasing order of fold change (>5). This calculation takes into consideration the total tags in each group. The two libraries represent gene expression in neurons and glia of the entire cerebellar cortex and deep cerebellar nuclei, as well as in blood vessels, choroid plexus, and pia arachnoid membrane. Because granule cells compose the majority of all cerebellar cells, the SAGE transcriptome is presumably heavily weighted to this cell type. Genes demonstrating a large upregulation in the P810 cerebellum included testis-specific protein, dcd8; tumor rejection antigen, gp96; macrophage activation 2; olfactomedin 1 and several ESTs, RIKEN, and novel genes. Genes exhibiting a large downregulation included prolactin, Smt3h2, ribosomal protein S3a, glucose-regulated protein 58, growth hormone, a RIKEN gene, and a novel gene.

In this study, we have used the most stringent controls and data acceptance criteria to provide a conservative estimate of genes that may participate in cerebellar aging. We have demonstrated substantial changes in several transcripts in young adult and aged mouse cerebellum, the most striking of which was a strong downregulation in prolactin and growth hormone. Both are signal transduction molecules that interact with cognate receptors activating the JAK2/STAT5 signaling pathway.[9] Furthermore, growth hormone and prolactin influence the insulin growth factor–1 signaling pathway via IRS-1 and Shc,[9] respectively. Reduced activity of the IGF-1 pathway greatly increases life span in *C. elegans*.[10]

TABLE 1. Differentially expressed transcripts in a young adult (P92) and aged (P810) mouse cerebellum[a]

Tag Sequence	Unigene ID No.	Gene Name	Tag count P92	Tag count P810	Fold Change	P Chance
Increase in gene expression						
ATAAATACAT	41973	testis-specific protein, Ddc8	0	24	21.22	<2.3E-05
TATTAAATAC	34715; 131660	RIKEN cDNA 1700026N20 gene; ESTs	0	15	13.26	2.3E-05
ATAATACAAT		novel	0	15	13.26	2.3E-05
AATAATACAT	127042	EST	0	15	13.26	2.3E-05
TGTATAAAAA	4526; 227099	tumor rejection antigen gp96; tubulin, beta 2	1	14	12.38	5.6E-04
ATAATACATT	5057	macrophage activation 2	0	13	11.50	2.2E-04
ATAATACCAT	218873	RIKEN cDNA 3110054G10 gene	0	11	9.73	9.5E-04
ATAATAACAT	10735	calcium/calmodulin-dependent serine protein kinase	0	11	9.73	9.5E-04
AATACTGACA		novel	0	11	9.73	9.5E-04
ATTAATACAT		novel	0	10	8.84	0.002
TAACTTTAAG	43278	olfactomedin 1	2	12	5.31	0.012
CCCTTCTTCT	196110; 89136	hemoglobin alpha, adult chain 1; H3 histone, family 3A	9	52	5.11	<2.3E-05

TABLE 1. (continued) Differentially expressed transcripts in a young adult (P92) and aged (P810) mouse cerebellum[a]

Tag Sequence	Unigene ID No.	Gene Name	Tag count P92	Tag count P810	Fold Change	P Chance
Decrease in gene expression						
CTTGGGTGCA	1270	prolactin	29	2	−16.40	<2.3E-05
TAGGGCAATC	29923	SMT3 (suppressor of mif two, 3) homologue 2 (*S. cerevisiae*)	11	1	−12.44	4.0E-04
GGGAAGGCGG	6957	ribosomal protein S3a	11	1	−12.44	4.0E-04
GGCTGCATTC	29703; 709	DNA segment, Chr 7, expressed; glucose regulated protein	11	0	−12.44	9.0E-04
GGGTTGTTCA	74363	transient receptor cation channel, subfamily C, member 3	10	1	−11.31	9.0E-04
AAGTGTCGCC	1240	growth hormone	37	4	−10.46	<2.3E-05
TGTCATCTAG	4071; 5163	laminin receptor 1; Ras-like without CAAX 2	9	1	−10.18	0.004
GCTGCCCTAG	197515; 196396	tubulin, alpha 2; tubulin, alpha 1	8	1	−9.05	0.007
GAGCGTTTTG	5246	peptidylprolyl isomerase A	13	2	−7.35	5.2E-04
GACAAAGGGG	38576	DNA segment, Chr 11, Brigham	13	2	−7.35	5.2E-04
AGGAGGACTT	14534	RIKEN cDNA 9130221H12 gene	19	3	−7.16	2.0E-05
AACAATTTGG	14244	ribosomal protein L9	18	3	−6.79	2.3E-05
CCGCCCCTTT	29846	N-myc downstream regulated 4	6	1	−6.79	0.026
GATGTGGCTG	2718; 90587	eukaryotic translation elongation factor 1 beta 2; enolase 1, alpha	11	2	−6.22	0.002
GCCCCCTCT	44101	hypothetical protein MGC27631	16	3	−6.03	1.5E-04
ATGACTGATA		novel	53	10	−5.99	<2.3E-05
GAGAGAAGAG	1287	microtubule-associated protein tau	15	3	−5.65	2.2E-04
TGTGTGAGGA	141230; 21086	1-acylglycerol-3-phos O-acyltransferase 3; elongation factor 1	10	2	−5.65	0.003

[a]Transcripts listed show greater than 5-fold increases.

ACKNOWLEDGMENTS

This work was supported by NIH Grants AG021698 and AA014422.

REFERENCES

1. STURROCK, R.R. 1989. Changes in neuron number in the cerebellar cortex of the ageing mouse. J. Hirnforsch. **30:** 499–503.
2. HADJ-SAHRAOUI, N., F. FREDERIC, H. ZANJANI, et al. 2001. Progressive atrophy of cerebellar Purkinje cell dendrites during aging of the heterozygous staggerer mouse ($Rora^{+/sg}$). Dev. Brain Res. **126:** 201–209.
3. MONTEIRO, R.A.F., R.M.F. HENRIQUE, E. ROCHA, et al. 1998. Age-related changes in the volume of somata and organelles of cerebellar granule cells. Neurobiol. Aging **19:** 325–332.
4. ROGERS, J., M.A. SILVER, W.J. SHOEMAKER & F.E. BLOOM. 1980. Senescent changes in a neurobiological model system: cerebellar Purkinje cell and correlative anatomy. Neurobiol. Aging **1:** 3–11.
5. ROGERS, J., S.F. ZORNETZER, F.E. BLOOM & R.E. MERVIS. 1984. Senescent microstructural changes in the rat cerebellum. Brain Res. **292:** 23–32.
6. LEE, C.-K., R. WEINDRUCH & T.A. PROLLA. 2000. Gene-expression profile of the ageing brain in mice. Nat. Genet. **25:** 294–297.
7. WEINDRUCH, R., T. KAYO, C.K. LEE & T.A. PROLLA. 2002. Gene expression profiling of aging using DNA microarrays. Mech. Aging Dev. **123:** 177–193.
8. VELCULESCU, V.E., L. ZHANG, B. VOGELSTEIN & K.W. KINZLER. 1995. Serial analysis of gene expression. Science **270:** 484–487.
9. CARTER-SU, C., A.P. KING, L.S. ARGETSINGER, et al. 1996. Signalling pathways of GH. Endocrinol. J. **43:** S65–S75.
10. MURPHY, C.T., S.A. MCCARROLL, C.I. BARGMANN, et al. 2003. Genes that act downstream of DAF-16 to influence the lifespan of *Caenorhabditis elegans*. Nature **424:** 277–284.

Antiaging Treatments Have Been Legally Prescribed for Approximately Thirty Years

SVETLANA V. UKRAINTSEVA,[a,c] KONSTANTIN G. ARBEEV,[a,c] ANATOLY I. MICHALSKY,[b] AND ANATOLY I. YASHIN[a,c]

[a]*Max Planck Institute for Demographic Research, 18057 Rostock, Germany*
[b]*Institute of Management Problems, Moscow, Russia*
[c]*Duke University, Center for Demographic Studies, Durham, North Carolina, USA*

ABSTRACT: There is an interesting divergence between the achievements of geriatrics and gerontology. On the one hand, during the last 30 years physicians in many developed countries have successfully prescribed several medicines to cure various symptoms of senescence. On the other hand, the influence of such medicines on human life span practically has not been studied. The most common of the relevant medicines are nootropic piracetam, gamma-aminobutyric acid (GABA), selegiline, *Ginkgo biloba*, pentoxifylline, cerebrolysin, solcoseryl, ergoloid, vinpocetin, sertraline, and estrogens, among others. Available data from human clinical practices and experimental animal studies indicate that treatments with these drugs improve learning, memory, brain metabolism, and capacity. Some of these drugs increase tolerance to various stresses such as oxygen deficit and exercise, stimulate the regeneration of neurons in the old brain, and speed up the performance of mental and physical tasks. This means that modern medicine already has "antiaging" treatments at its disposal. However, the influence of such treatments on the mean and maximal life span of humans, and on the age trajectory of a human survival curve has been poorly studied. The increase in human life expectancy at birth in the second half of the last century was mostly caused by the better survival at the old and oldest old rather than at the young ages. In parallel, the consumption of brain protective and regenerative drugs has been expanding in the elderly population. We provide evidence in support of the idea that the consumption of medicines exerting antiaging properties may contribute to the increase in human longevity.

KEYWORDS: antiaging drugs; longevity; cognitive functioning

HIDDEN ANTIAGING INTERVENTIONS

The prescription and consumption of nootropic, brain protective, and regenerative drugs is increasing in the elderly population. During the last three decades, geriatricians in the developed countries have successfully used these drugs to cure

Address for correspondence: Svetlana V. Ukraintseva, Ph.D., Duke University Center for Demographic Studies, 2117 Campus Drive, Box 90408, Durham, NC 27708-0408. Voice: 919-682-9759, ext. 224.
ukraintseva@cds.duke.edu

various symptoms of senescence. The most common of relevant medicines are nootropic piracetam, gamma-aminobutyric acid (GABA), ergoloid, estrogens, pentoxifylline, vinpocetin, *Ginkgo biloba*, cerebrolysin, solcoseryl, semax, sertraline, aspirin, and selegiline. There is strong evidence from human clinical practice and experimental animal studies that some of the brain protective and regenerative drugs significantly improve learning, memory, brain metabolism, and capacity. They are shown to increase the tolerance to various stresses such as oxygen deficit and exercise. Several agents may even stimulate the regeneration of neurons in the old brain and speed up the performance of mental and physical tasks.[1–21] The latter is very important because the age-related decline in the rate of information processing is a key feature of mammalian aging, and a potential antiaging intervention, in principle, should aim to reverse this decline. Thus, the therapeutic effect of several modern medicines is, in fact, an antiaging one. Some of these drugs are officially prescribed medications both in the United States and Europe. Hydergine (ergoloid mesylates), Trental (pentoxifylline), and Zoloft (sertraline) are examples. Others (e.g., piracetam and vinpocetin) have a long history (of up to 30 years) of successful prescription in Europe for the treatment of age-associated cognitive impairment and brain restoration after serious damage (e.g., after a stroke). However, they are used only as dietary supplements or drug compounds in the United States.

BRAIN PROTECTIVE DRUGS AND OLD AGE SURVIVAL: IS THERE A CAUSAL ASSOCIATION?

Curiously, the achievements of practical geriatrics and experimental gerontology diverge. On the one hand, the modern medicine unwittingly offers therapies with physiological "antiaging" effects. On the other hand, the impact of such "antiaging" treatments on the healthy life span, the age trajectory of a survival curve, and the longevity of humans have been poorly studied. In the second half of the last century, human life expectancy at birth increased owing to the better survival of the old and the oldest old rather than the young ages. Similarly, the prevalence of severe cognitive impairment in the elderly has declined in the last two decades in some developed countries.[22] In parallel, the consumption of medicines exerting antiaging properties has increased in the elderly population. It may have been one of the factors that contributed to both the increase in survival and the decrease in disabilities at oldest old ages. Indirect indicators of such an influence may be found in human and animal studies.

GABA and Piracetam

GABA and its chemical relative piracetam (Nootropil) are probably today's most common nootropic agents. GABA is a natural neuromediator transmitting inhibitory signals between neurons. It is used to treat the age-related memory impairment and the consequences of brain ischemia in the elderly. It has recently been shown to improve the cortical function in senescent monkeys.[1] In numerous studies, piracetam significantly improved learning, the performance of perceptual-motor tasks, and mental alertness.[2–5] Piracetam has been shown to regenerate neurons and increase neuronal receptor density.[3,4] Three randomized, double-blind, placebo-controlled, clinical trials and one large population-based survey measured the influence of piracetam on the activities of daily living (ADL) of 6,000 elderly demented patients in Italy, Austria, and Belgium as well as on the basic nursing and therapeutic costs. It was found that piracetam treatment significantly decreased dependency, compared with placebo.[5]

Gingko biloba

Another common drug with nootropic action is a plant extract, namely, *Ginkgo biloba* (Tanakan). It has been shown to enhance memory and the speed of information processing in elderly and middle-aged individuals.[6–9] It also improves spatial learning, reduces indices of oxidative stress in brain tissue, diminishes cumulative oxidative changes, and accelerates functional recovery from hemiplegia in aged rats.[10–12] In a recent case–control study, treatment with *Ginkgo biloba* reduced the risk of developing Alzheimer dementia in a cohort of 1,462 community-dwelling elderly women aged 76 years and older.[13]

Deprenyl

Some of the brain-protective drugs provide protection against the age-related depletion of the dopaminergic nervous system. Deprenyl (selegiline) is probably the best example. This selective inhibitor of MAO-B is commonly used in clinical practices to treat symptoms of Parkinson disease. In animal studies, Deprenyl substantially increased survival of rodents and dogs up to twofold.[14,15] Named as Anipryl, it has been recently approved by the FDA (1999) for the treatment of cognitive dysfunction syndrome in aging dogs. The effects of the long-term use of deprenyl in healthy aging individuals, however, have yet to be studied.

Trental

Most of the nootropic drugs also improve the blood circulation in the brain. Separate agents such as pentoxifylline (Trental) do it preferably. This leads to the regression of age-associated circulatory insufficiency. Trental has been shown to reduce symptoms of vascular dementia and improve cognitive function and psychointellectual performance in elderly patients.[16,17]

Hydergine

A popular adrenergic nootropic agent in the United States, Hydergine (ergoloid mesylates) has been used to treat the impairment of mental function in the elderly. It has a modest effect related to improved performance and reduced retardation. An advantage of this drug is that it is very well tolerated and can be used for long-term treatment.[18]

Estrogens

Although estrogens are not prescribed directly as an antiaging treatment, many studies suggest such an effect, particularly on cognitive functioning.[19,20] Conjugated estrogens were shown to promote neuronal survival as well as reverse skin aging in preclimacteric women. Ashcroft and colleagues (1999) have found that delays in wound healing in the elderly can be significantly diminished by topical estrogen in both male and female patients.[21] Unlike many other drugs, there are plenty of studies demonstrating improved survival among the long-term female estrogen users (relative risk of death from all causes varies 0.5–0.6 in most cases).[23–26] The FDA is currently reviewing new information on the neuroprotective characteristics of estrogens and will determine whether labeling should be respectively updated.

Aspirin

The association of aspirin use with cognitive performance in middle-aged adults has been shown to be modest. However, in persons 75 years and older, the positive effect of aspirin on the memory retention is significant.[27] The daily intake of low-dose aspirin also significantly improved survival in a Finnish centenarian cohort with a parallel shift of the survival curve to the right.[28] Such a pattern of the survival improvement resembles what we have observed recently in the general population.

Vitamin E

There are several "questionable" substances approved as dietary supplements in both the United States and Europe. These show some "antiaging" effect; however, available data do not allow a definite conclusion. Vitamin E could be example. It has been shown in an EPES (Established Populations for Epidemiologic Studies of the Elderly) study of 11,178 persons aged 67 to 105 years that the use of vitamin E significantly reduces the risk of all-cause mortality ($RR = 0.66$) and particularly the risk of coronary disease mortality ($RR = 0.53$).[29] At the same time, other studies suggest that supplementary vitamin E may worsen acute infections in the elderly.[30] Vitamin E protects tissues from oxidative damage that accumulates with age. However, the excessive antioxidative action may weaken immunity because some immune cells need oxidative agents to fight infection. Thus, it seems that dose-dependent effects of the vitamin E should be seriously taken into account in future studies of this agent.

Our Research in Progress and Preliminary Results

We are currently analyzing information on regularly taken medicines in aged (65+) noninstitutional individuals from the NLTCS (National Long Term Care Survey) (the USA) and the LSADT (Longitudinal Study of Aging Danish Twins) (Denmark) longitudinal studies of human aging. We are interested in the long-term effects of individual exposure to these medicines on the indices of health, aging, longevity, and cognitive functioning. Our preliminary results indicate that drugs that improve survival at old ages may do so via increasing the rate of information processing in brain. For example, the regular use of vitamin A alone significantly decreased five-year risk of death at ages 65+ ($RR = 0.7$) in association with enhanced mental alertness in the NLTCS sample. The regular use of iron supplementary tabs showed *negative* effect also on both old age survival and cognitive functioning. It significantly increased the chances of death ($RR = 1.3$) along with a decline in the mental alertness. The regular intake of multivitamins did not show any profitable outcome for the elderly subjects in our study.

CONCLUDING REMARKS

Taken together, the data suggest that some of the brain protective and regenerative drugs may decelerate and even reverse aging-related changes in an old organism, particularly in the brain. There is limited evidence about their positive influence on human survival and risk of disabilities in the old. An important question arises about the contribution of these medicines to the contemporary increase in human longevity. Our study in progress aims to answer this question at least in part.

REFERENCES

1. LEVENTHAL, A.G. *et al.* 2003. GABA and its agonists improved visual cortical function in senescent monkeys. Science **300:** 812–815.
2. MINDUS, P. *et al.* 1976. Piracetam-induced improvement of mental performance. A controlled study on normally aging individuals. Acta. Psychiatr. Scand. **54:** 150–160.
3. SCHEUER, K. *et al.* 1999. Piracetam improves cognitive performance by restoring neurochemical deficits of the aged rat brain. Pharmacopsychiatry **32** (Suppl. 1): 10–16.
4. MULLER, W.E. 1988. Restoration of age-related receptor deficits in the central nervous system, a common mechanism of nootropic action? Methods Find. Exp. Clin. Pharmacol. **10:** 773–783.
5. VLIETINCK, R. *et al.* 1993. Retrospective estimate of the nursing cost of autonomy impairment and cost benefit in clinical trials: feasibility and application of piracetam in demented elderly patients. Adv. Ther. **10:** 226–244.
6. RAI, G.S., C. SHOVLIN & K.A WESNES. 1991. A double-blind, placebo controlled study of *Ginkgo biloba* extract ("tanakan") in elderly outpatients with mild to moderate memory impairment. Curr. Med. Res. Opin. **12:** 350–355.
7. ALLAIN, H. *et al.* 1993. Effect of two doses of ginkgo biloba extract (EGb 761) on the dual-coding test in elderly subjects. Clin. Ther. **15:** 549–558.
8. SEMLITSCH, H.V. *et al.* 1995. Cognitive psychophysiology in nootropic drug research: effects of Ginkgo biloba on event-related potentials (P300) in age-associated memory impairment. Pharmacopsychiatry **28:** 134–142.
9. SIMANYI, M. 1999. [Use of special Ginkgo biloba extract for cognitive disorders in the elderly]. Wien Med. Wochenschr. **149:** 231–234. German.
10. BRAILOWSKY, S. & T. MONTIEL. 1997. Motor function in young and aged hemiplegic rats: effects of a Ginkgo biloba extract. Neurobiol. Aging **18:** 219–227.
11. AL-ZUHAIR, H., A. ABD EL-FATTAH & M.I. EL-SAYED. 1998. The effect of meclofenoxate with ginkgo biloba extract or zinc on lipid peroxide, some free radical scavengers and the cardiovascular system of aged rats. Pharmacol. Res. **38:** 65–72.
12. TOPIC, B. *et al.* 2002. Enhanced maze performance and reduced oxidative stress by combined extracts of zingiber officinale and ginkgo biloba in the aged rat. Neurobiol. Aging. **23:** 135–143.
13. ANDRIEU, S. *et al.* 2003. EPIDOS study. Association of Alzheimer's disease onset with ginkgo biloba and other symptomatic cognitive treatments in a population of women aged 75 years and older from the EPIDOS study. J. Gerontol. A Biol. Sci. Med. Sci. **58:** 372–377.
14. RUEHL, W.W. *et al.* 1997. Treatment with L-deprenyl prolongs life in elderly dogs. Life Sci. **61:** 1037–1044.
15. MILGRAM, N.W. *et al.* 1990. Maintenance on L-deprenyl prolongs life in aged male rats. Life Sci. **47:** 415–420.
16. PARNETTI, L. *et al.* 1986. The role of haemorheological factors in the ageing brain: long-term therapy with pentoxifylline ("Trental" 400) in elderly patients with initial mental deterioration. Pharmatherapeutica **4:** 617–627.
17. SHA, M.C. & C.M. CALLAHAN. 2003. The efficacy of pentoxifylline in the treatment of vascular dementia: a systematic review. Alzheimer Dis. Assoc. Disord. **17:** 46–54.
18. HUBER, F. *et al.*1986. Effects of long-term ergoloid mesylates ("Hydergine") administration in healthy pensioners: 5-year results. Curr. Med. Res. Opin. **10:** 256–279.

19. LEBLANC, E.S. et al. 2001. Hormone replacement therapy and cognition: systematic review and meta-analysis. JAMA 285: 1489–1499.
20. YAFFE, K. et al. 1998. Estrogen therapy in postmenopausal women: effects on cognitive function and dementia. JAMA 279: 688–695.
21. ASHCROFT, G.S. et al. 1999. Topical estrogen accelerates cutaneous wound healing in aged humans associated with an altered inflammatory response. Am. J. Pathol. 155: 1137–1146.
22. MANTON, K.G. & X. GU. 2001. Changes in the prevalence of chronic disability in the United States black and nonblack population above age 65 from 1982 to 1999. Proc. Natl. Acad. Sci. USA 98: 6354–6359.
23. PETITTI, D.B., J.A. PERLMAN & S. SIDNEY. 1987. Noncontraceptive estrogens and mortality: long-term follow-up of women in the Walnut Creek Study. Obstet. Gynecol. 70 (3 Pt 1): 289–293.
24. HENDERSON, B.E., A. PAGANINI-HILL & R.K. ROSS. 1991. Decreased mortality in users of estrogen replacement therapy. Arch. Intern. Med. 151: 75–78.
25. ETTINGER, B. et al. 1996. Reduced mortality associated with long-term postmenopausal estrogen therapy. Obstet. Gynecol. 87: 6–12.
26. CAULEY, J.A. et al. 1997. Estrogen replacement therapy and mortality among older women. The study of osteoporotic fractures. Arch. Intern. Med. 157: 2181–2187.
27. JONKER, C., H.C. COMIJS & J.H. SMIT. 2003. Does aspirin or other NSAIDs reduce the risk of cognitive decline in elderly persons? Results from a population-based study. Neurobiol. Aging 24: 583–588.
28. AGUERO-TORRES, H. et al. 2001. The effect of low-dose daily aspirin intake on survival in the Finnish centenarians cohort. J. Am. Geriatr. Soc. 49: 1578–1580.
29. LOSONCZY, K.G., T.B. HARRIS & R.J. HAVLIK. 1996. Vitamin E and vitamin C supplement use and risk of all-cause and coronary heart disease mortality in older persons: the Established Populations for Epidemiologic Studies of the Elderly. Am. J. Clin. Nutr. 64: 190–196.
30. MILLER, S.M. 2002. Vitamin E may worsen acute respiratory tract infections in the elderly. J. Fam. Pract. 51: 925.

Aging of Cardiac Myocytes in Culture

Oxidative Stress, Lipofuscin Accumulation, and Mitochondrial Turnover

ALEXEI TERMAN,[a] HELGE DALEN,[a] JOHN W. EATON,[b] JIRI NEUZIL,[c] AND ULF T. BRUNK[a]

[a]*Division of Pathology II, Faculty of Health Sciences, Linköping University, SE-58185, Linköping, Sweden*

[b]*James Graham Brown Cancer Center, University of Louisville, Louisville, Kentucky, USA*

[c]*Heart Foundation Research Center, School of Health Sciences, Griffith University, Southport, Queensland, Australia*

ABSTRACT: Oxidative stress is believed to be an important contributor to aging, mainly affecting long-lived postmitotic cells such as cardiac myocytes and neurons. Aging cells accumulate functionally effete, often mutant and enlarged mitochondria, as well as an intralysosomal undegradable pigment, lipofuscin. To provide better insight into the role of oxidative stress, mitochondrial damage, and lipofuscinogenesis in postmitotic aging, we studied the relationship between these parameters in cultured neonatal rat cardiac myocytes. It was found that the content of lipofuscin, which varied drastically between cells, positively correlated with mitochondrial damage (evaluated by decreased innermembrane potential), as well as with the production of reactive oxygen species. These results suggest that both lipofuscin accumulation and mitochondrial damage have common underlying mechanisms, likely including imperfect autophagy and ensuing lysosomal degradation of oxidatively damaged mitochondria and other organelles. Increased size of mitochondria (possibly resulting from impaired fission due to oxidative damage to mitochondrial DNA, membranes, and proteins) also may interfere with mitochondrial turnover, leading to the appearance of so-called "giant" mitochondria. This assumption is based on our observation that pharmacological inhibition of autophagy with 3-methyladenine induced only moderate accumulation of large (senescent-like) mitochondria but drastically increased numbers of small, apparently normal mitochondria, reflecting their rapid turnover and suggesting that enlarged mitochondria are poorly autophagocytosed. Overall, our findings emphasize the importance of mitochondrial turnover in postmitotic aging and provide further support for the mitochondrial–lysosomal axis theory of aging.

KEYWORDS: aging; heart; lipofuscin; lysosomes; mitochondria; oxidative stress

Address for correspondence: Alexei Terman, Division of Pathology II, Faculty of Health Sciences, Linköping University, SE-58185, Linköping, Sweden. Voice: +46-13-221529; fax: 46-13-221529.
 alete@inr.liu.se

INTRODUCTION

Macromolecular damage by reactive oxygen species (ROS) is considered a major contributor to aging.[1,2] Age-related alterations are most evident in long-lived postmitotic cells, such as neurons, cardiac myocytes, skeletal muscle fibers, and retinal pigment epithelial cells.[3–5] Mitochondrial changes and lipofuscin deposition are the most characteristic features of aged cells.[2,6,7]

Senescent mitochondria are usually enlarged, sometimes substantially (so-called "giant" mitochondria), and show structural alterations such as swelling, partial loss of cristae, or almost complete destruction of mitochondrial components.[8–11] These changes are combined with mitochondrial DNA (mtDNA) mutations, disturbed energy metabolism, and consequent decrease of ATP production.[2,6,12,13]

Lipofuscin (age pigment) is an undegradable, autofluorescent, electron-dense intralysosomal material, composed basically of oxidatively modified protein and lipid residues.[7] Autophagocytosed mitochondria, rich in oxidized macromolecular compounds, constitute an important source of lipofuscin. Within lysosomes, which contain low-molecular weight redox active iron, autophagocytosed material undergoes further oxidative modification, resulting in macromolecular crosslinking and resistance to hydrolytic enzymes.[7,14]

As assumed in the mitochondrial–lysosomal axis theory of aging,[5] defective mitochondria progressively accumulate because not all of them are removed by autophagy. This occurs even in young, initially undamaged cells. Mitochondrial turnover, however, worsens in aged cells, whose autophagic capacity is depressed because of lipofuscin overload of lysosomes still receiving a good part of newly produced lysosomal enzymes, failing to degrade the undegradable pigment.[15] Nonrecycled, effete mitochondria continue to produce ROS and contribute to lipofuscin formation, thus closing the vicious circle.

From the perspective of the mitochondrial–lysosomal axis theory, mitochondrial changes and lipofuscin accumulation are interrelated and therefore are likely to show corresponding alterations with age and dependence of ROS formation. In this study, using cultured neonatal rat cardiac myocytes as a model system, we demonstrate that intracellular lipofuscin content positively correlates with both production of ROS and mitochondrial damage, thus supporting the proposed hypothesis. We also show that insufficient turnover of mitochondria may arise partially from initial mitochondrial enlargement which, in turn, would potentially complicate autophagy.

MATERIALS AND METHODS

Neonatal rat ventricular myocytes, prepared according to a previously described technique,[16] were used in all experiments. Cell cultures were maintained in a humidified atmosphere of 8% O_2, 87% N_2, and 5% CO_2. A subset of the cultures was continuously exposed to 5 mM 3-methyladenine to suppress autophagic sequestration. For experiments requiring high-resolution vital microscopy, cells were cultivated in Petriperm dishes (Sartorius) with 25-µm-thick Teflon bottoms.

To assess lipofuscin-related cellular autofluorescence, we examined live cultures in an LSM-410 laser scanning microscope (Carl Zeiss) using a 543-nm helium-neon laser and a 590-nm barrier filter. Laser scanning images then were used for detection of intracellular lipofuscin content.[15]

For evaluation of the mitochondrial innermembrane potential, cultured cells were exposed to 5 µM of the mitochondrial tracker JC-1 (Molecular Probes) for 30 minutes at 37°C, washed, and examined in an Axiovert S100 TV inverted fluorescence microscope (Carl Zeiss) using blue excitation light. Active mitochondria with high innermembrane potential exhibit orange fluorescence, whereas damaged or inactive mitochondria with low membrane potential display green fluorescence.[17] Images were recorded using an ORCA-100 color digital camera (Hamamatsu). For quantification of green JC-1 fluorescence (indicative of mitochondrial damage), images were taken with an LSM-410 laser scanning microscope using a 488-nm argon laser and two channels with 515 to 565-nm bandpass and 590-nm barrier filters, respectively.

Intracellular ROS production was estimated by exposing cells to 5 µM dihydroethidium (Molecular Probes) for 30 minutes. The formation of oxidized product (ethidium) was detected in an LSM-410 microscope using a 543-nm laser and a 590-nm barrier filter.

To study the relationship between lipofuscin content and mitochondrial damage or ROS production, we first examined cells in marked areas of the dishes (circles approximately 1 mm in diameter) for lipofuscin content using an LSM-410 microscope. Images of the same cells then were taken after staining with JC-1 or dihydroethidium, respectively, as described above. Because the fluorescence of JC-1 and ethidium were much brighter than lipofuscin autofluorescence, it allowed the attenuation of laser light to a level when lipofuscin was undetectable.

Transmission electron microscopy specimens were prepared according to a previously described protocol[15] and examined in a 1200-EX electron microscope (JEOL).

Image analysis was performed using the National Institutes of Health Image program (http://rsb.info.nih.gov/nih-image/). All experiments were repeated at least three times. The relationship between groups was evaluated using Pearson's correlation coefficient.

RESULTS AND DISCUSSION

Consistent with our earlier observations,[16,18] cultured cardiac myocytes gradually accumulated lipofuscin pigment (FIG. 1) and showed progressive mitochondrial changes, such as enlargement, decreased innermembrane potential, and altered ultrastructure (FIG. 2). Both lipofuscin content and mitochondrial alterations, however, drastically varied between cardiac myocytes. As is clear from FIGURE 3A–C, showing strong positive correlation between lipofuscin content and decrease of mitochondrial membrane potential, these changes in cardiac myocytes occurred in parallel; that is, those cells that had accumulated larger quantities of lipofuscin also displayed more mitochondrial damage. Moreover, because lipofuscin content also positively correlated with ROS production (FIG. 3D–F), it is reasonable to suppose that a similar relationship exists between mitochondrial membrane potential and formation of ROS. These observations suggest that the progress of age-related changes

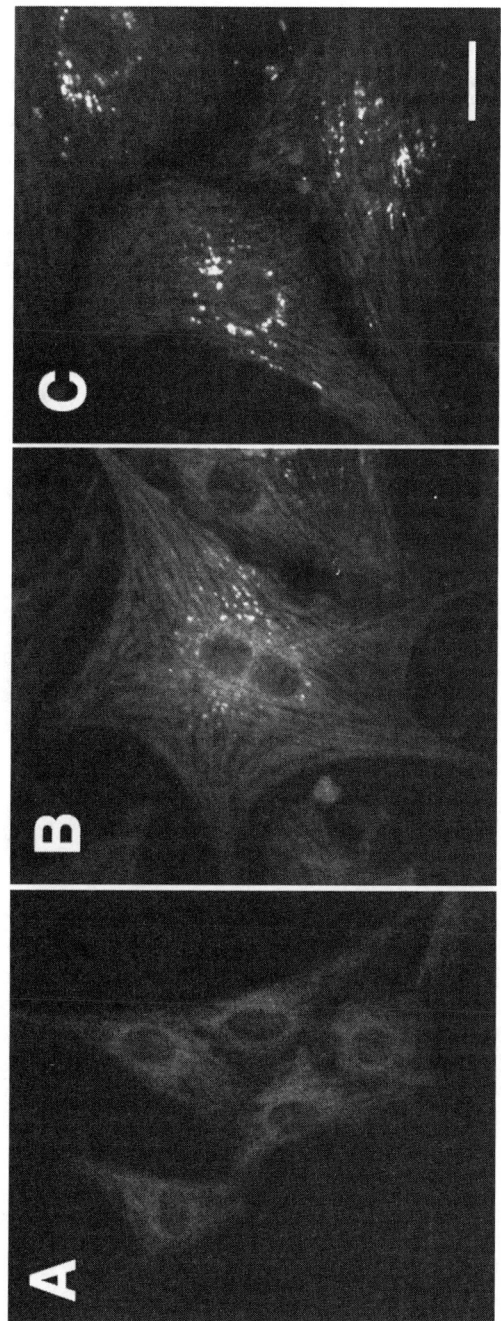

FIGURE 1. Lipofuscin accumulation in cultured neonatal rat cardiac myocytes. (A–C) Confocal laser scanning images of cells cultured for 1, 14, and 28 days, respectively. Bar = 20 µm.

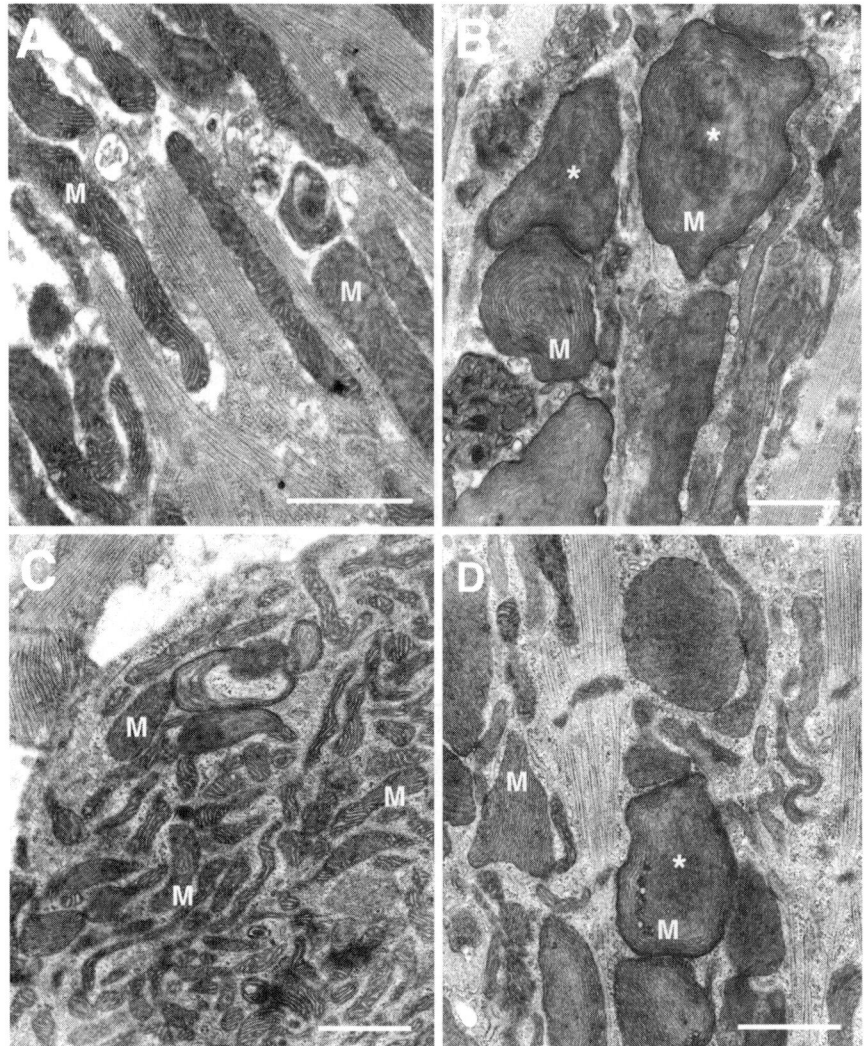

FIGURE 2. Mitochondria of neonatal rat cardiac myocytes exposed to 3-methyladenine display senescent-like ultrastructural changes. (**A**) Untreated 17-day-old cells show predominantly normal mitochondria with clearly visible cristae; (**B**) untreated cells aged 3 months (senescent) contain enlarged mitochondria with concentrically arranged, partially homogenized cristae; and (**C, D**) 17-day-old cells exposed to 3-methyladenine for 12 days contain numerous small mitochondria with minor alterations (C), as well as clearly senescent-like enlarged mitochondria (D; compare with **B**). M, mitochondria; asterisks indicate amorphous material replacing destroyed cristae. Bar = 1 µm.

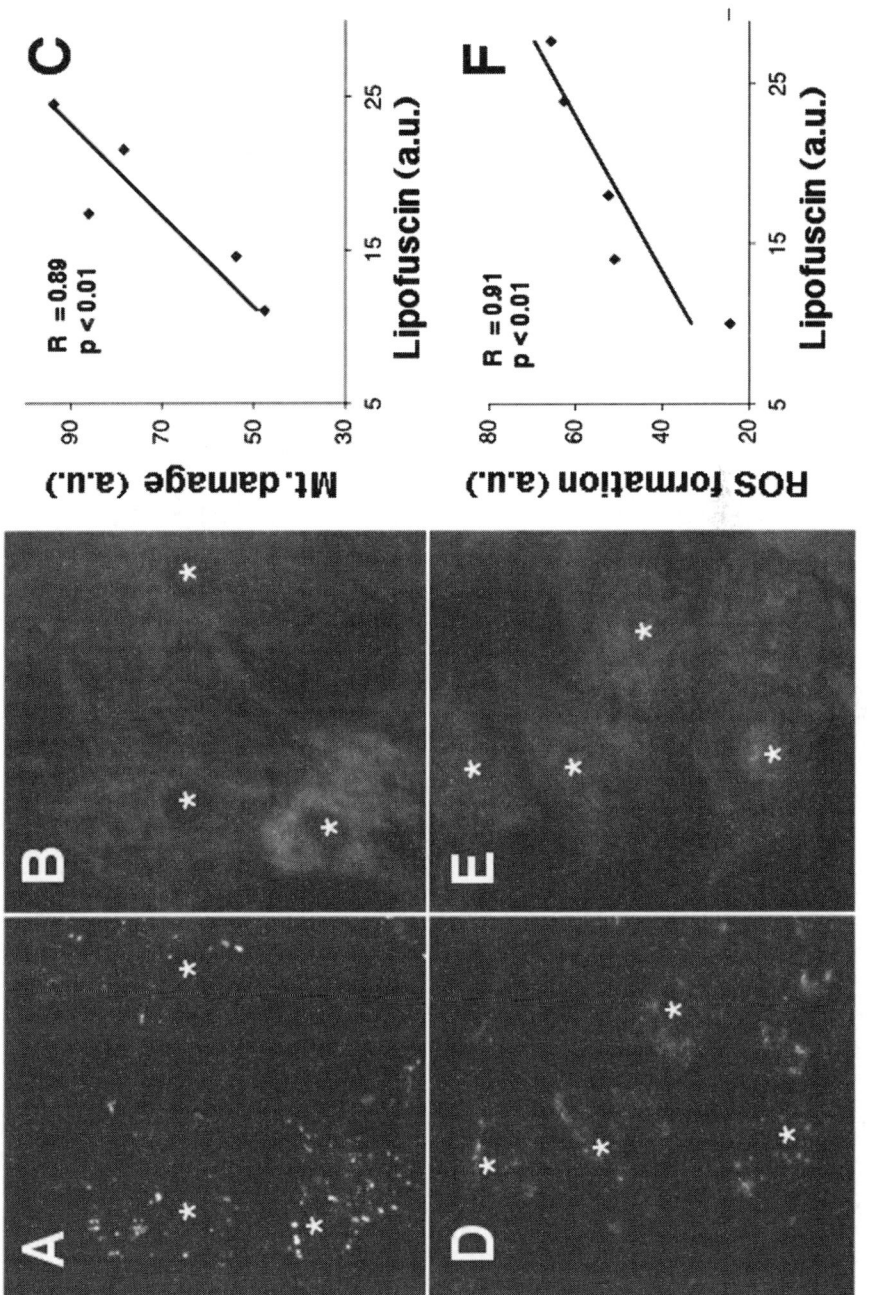

FIGURE 3. *See following page for legend.*

differs in various cells and that mitochondrial injury and lipofuscin accumulation are interrelated and apparently are both dependent on oxidative stress.

Whether lipofuscin loading of lysosomes is responsible for additional mitochondrial damage in senescent cells due to compromised autophagy (see above) remains to be investigated.

There are, however, good reasons to believe that lysosomes are indeed important for maintaining a healthy mitochondrial population and that decreased autophagy due to lipofuscin overload[15] contributes to age-related mitochondrial damage. When autophagic degradation in neonatal rat cardiac myocytes was blocked with 3-methyladenine, cells accumulated large quantities of mitochondria, resulting in the premature death of the cultures within less than 20 days versus over 3 months for controls.[18] Mitochondria that accumulated because of suppressed autophagy had decreased innermembrane potential and often displayed a senescent-like morphology (FIG. 2). Interestingly, the exposure of cells to 3-methyladenine induced a much more pronounced accumulation of small mitochondria than of large ones, suggesting that small mitochondria are normally recycled with a higher rate. This is reasonable, considering that the autophagy of a large mitochondrion should be more energy consuming than that of a small one, and that there seems to be an upper limit to the possible size of an autophagosome. Mitochondrial enlargement potentially can result from disturbed fission due to oxidative damage to mitochondrial components, which is consistent with hampered DNA synthesis in large mitochondria.[18]

In summary, these data support the mitochondrial–lysosomal axis theory of aging,[5] which considers progressive mitochondrial damage in long-lived postmitotic cells to a large extent dependent on imperfect autophagic turnover. Extreme lipofuscin overload of senescent cells makes mitochondrial turnover insufficient for life maintenance and leads to cell death.

ACKNOWLEDGMENTS

This work was supported by grant 4481 from the Medical Branch of the Swedish Research Council (Vetenskapsrådet).

REFERENCES

1. HARMAN, D. 1972. The biologic clock: the mitochondria? J. Am. Geriatr. Soc. **20:** 145–147.
2. BECKMAN, K.B. & B.N. AMES. 1998. The free radical theory of aging matures. Physiol. Rev. **78:** 547–581.

FIGURE 3. Amount of lipofuscin in aged (60 days old) cardiac myocytes positively correlates with ROS production and mitochondrial damage. (**A, B**) Fluorescence images of live unstained cells and cells exposed to JC-1 for detection of mitochondrial membrane potential, respectively; (**C**) the relationship between lipofuscin content and mitochondrial damage assessed by green JC-1 fluorescence indicative of low mitochondrial potential. (**D, E**) Fluorescence images of live unstained cells and cells exposed to dihydroethidium for detection of ROS, respectively; (**F**) the relationship between lipofuscin content and ROS formation. The graphs shown in **C** and **F** are based on median values of 50 cells distributed into five quantiles. *Asterisks* indicate the nuclei of corresponding cells.

3. STREHLER, B.L. 1977. Time, cells, and aging. Academic Press. New York.
4. COMFORT, A. 1979. Ageing: the biology of senescence. Elsevier. New York.
5. BRUNK, U.T. & A. TERMAN. 2002. The mitochondrial-lysosomal axis theory of aging: accumulation of damaged mitochondria as a result of imperfect autophagocytosis. Eur. J. Biochem. **269:** 1996–2002.
6. OZAWA, T. 1997. Genetic and functional changes in mitochondria associated with aging. Physiol. Rev. **77:** 425–464.
7. BRUNK, U.T. & A. TERMAN. 2002. Lipofuscin: mechanisms of age-related accumulation and influence on cell functions. Free Radic. Biol. Med. **33:** 611–619.
8. SACHS, H.G., J.A. COLGAN & M.L. LAZARUS. 1977. Ultrastructure of the aging myocardium: a morphometric approach. Am. J. Anat. **150:** 63–71.
9. VANNESTE, J. & P. VAN DEN BOSCH DE AGUILAR. 1981. Mitochondrial alterations in the spinal ganglion neurons in ageing rats. Acta Neuropathol. **54:** 83–87.
10. COLEMAN, R. et al. 1987. Giant mitochondria in the myocardium of aging and endurance-trained mice. Gerontology **33:** 34–39.
11. BEREGI, E. et al. 1988. Age-related changes in the skeletal muscle cells. Z. Gerontol. **21:** 83–86.
12. KADENBACH, B. et al. 1995. Human aging is associated with stochastic somatic mutations of mitochondrial DNA. Mutat. Res. **338:** 161–172.
13. WALLACE, D.C. 1997. Mitochondrial DNA in aging and disease. Sci. Am. **277:** 22–29.
14. BRUNK, U.T., C.B. JONES & R.S. SOHAL. 1992. A novel hypothesis of lipofuscinogenesis and cellular aging based on interactions between oxidative stress and autophagocytosis. Mutat. Res. **275:** 395–403.
15. TERMAN, A., H. DALEN & U.T. BRUNK. 1999. Ceroid/lipofuscin-loaded human fibroblasts show decreased survival time and diminished autophagocytosis during amino acid starvation. Exp. Gerontol. **34:** 943–957.
16. TERMAN, A. & U.T. BRUNK. 1998. On the degradability and exocytosis of ceroid/lipofuscin in cultured rat cardiac myocytes. Mech. Ageing Dev. **100:** 145–156.
17. DI LISA, F. et al. 1995. Mitochondrial membrane potential in single living adult rat cardiac myocytes exposed to anoxia or metabolic inhibition. J. Physiol. **486:** 1–13.
18. TERMAN, A. et al. 2003. Mitochondrial recycling and aging of cardiac myocytes: the role of autophagocytosis. Exp. Gerontol. **38:** 863–876.

Response of the Senescent Heart to Stress

Clinical Therapeutic Strategies and Quest for Mitochondrial Predictors of Biological Age

FRANKLIN ROSENFELDT,[a] FRANCIS MILLER,[a] PHILLIP NAGLEY,[b] ANTHONY HADJ,[a] SILVANA MARASCO,[a] DEAHNE QUICK,[a] FREYA SHEERAN,[a] MICHELLE WOWK,[a] AND SALVATORE PEPE[a]

[a]*Cardiac Surgical Research Unit, Alfred Hospital and Baker Heart Research Institute (Wynn Domain), Melbourne, Australia*

[b]*Department of Biochemistry and Molecular Biology, Monash University, Melbourne, Australia*

ABSTRACT: The aging heart has an impaired response to many kinds of stress. In clinical practice, there is a need for senescence-specific therapies to protect against stress and for biochemical markers of senescence to identify those patients most in need of therapy. In isolated rat hearts, in human tissues, and in a clinical trial, we have shown previously that coenzyme Q_{10} has the ability to protect the heart against stress especially in senescence. We recently have devised a regimen of therapy to protect the senescent heart against stress, combining metabolic therapy (coenzyme Q_{10}, alpha lipoic acid, magnesium orotate, and omega 3 polyunsaturated fatty acids) with physical exercise and mental stress reduction. The preliminary results of this program are promising. In an endeavor to predict the likely response of individual senescent hearts to stress, we correlated the tissue load of mitochondrial DNA deletions and total cellular mitochondrial DNA copy number in human cardiac tissue with recovery of the same tissue from ischemia/reperfusion stress. We found that these mitochondrial markers actually were less predictive of impaired response to stress than age alone. We conclude that the aging heart has a diminished capacity to recover from stress that is not readily predictable by cardiac content of intact mitochondrial DNA and that this recovery can be improved by metabolic therapy combined with physical exercise and mental stress reduction.

KEYWORDS: cardiovascular surgery; exercise; mitochondria; aging; coenzyme Q_{10}; metabolic therapy

INTRODUCTION

Multiple clinical trials have demonstrated that the mortality after myocardial infarction, balloon coronary angioplasty, and cardiac surgery in patients older than 70 years is three times that in younger age groups.[1–4] Myocardial failure is the most

Address for correspondence: Franklin Rosenfeldt, Cardiac Surgical Research Unit, Alfred Hospital and Baker Heart Research Institute, Commercial Road, Prahran Victoria 3181, Australia. Voice: +61-3-9276-3684; fax: +61-3-9276-2317.

f.rosenfeldt@alfred.org.au

common cause of death in these elderly patients, suggesting that the aged myocardium is more sensitive to ischemia and other stresses. Thus, in clinical practice there is a need for special strategies to protect the aging heart during major cardiac stress. It would also be useful to have cellular markers that could identify those individuals who were particularly likely to demonstrate an impaired response to stress.

METABOLIC PHYSICAL AND MENTAL PREPARATION FOR STRESS

Metabolic therapy involves adding an excess of a component in a specific metabolic pathway so as to drive a reaction, usually involving energy production, in a desired direction. Applying metabolic treatment such as coenzyme Q_{10} (CoQ_{10}) to a normal heart with normal metabolism has no effect (FIG. 1). However, if the heart is stressed as with cardiac surgery, metabolism is disturbed and metabolic therapy may normalize metabolism and improve function, particularly in the elderly patient. We previously demonstrated in rats that CoQ_{10} has a senescence-specific protective effect on the heart.[5] We also showed in human cardiac tissue strips that the cardioprotective effect of CoQ_{10} increases with age.[6] In a previous clinical trial, we demonstrated that CoQ_{10} therapy given for two weeks before cardiac surgery increases CoQ_{10} content in atrial trabeculae and in cardiac mitochondria, improves efficiency of mitochondrial energy production, and improves *in vitro* posthypoxic myocardial contractile function.[7] Additional factors that have a negative impact on the ability of the patient to recover from stress are physical unfitness, anxiety, and depression.

There is good evidence of the beneficial effect of physical exercise in preparation for cardiac surgery. A Canadian trial tested the effect of a six-week program of physical exercise before coronary bypass surgery.[8] A randomized comparison with an untreated control group showed that physical exercise resulted in a shorter hospital stay and an improved physical quality of life before surgery. This difference was maintained two months and six months after surgery. Exercised patients on average had a one-day shorter hospital stay than nonexercised controls.

Interventions designed to reduce mental stress have been shown in patients with ischemic heart disease to retard the progression of lesions in the coronary arteries and to reduce the frequency and duration of angina. Blumenthal and colleagues

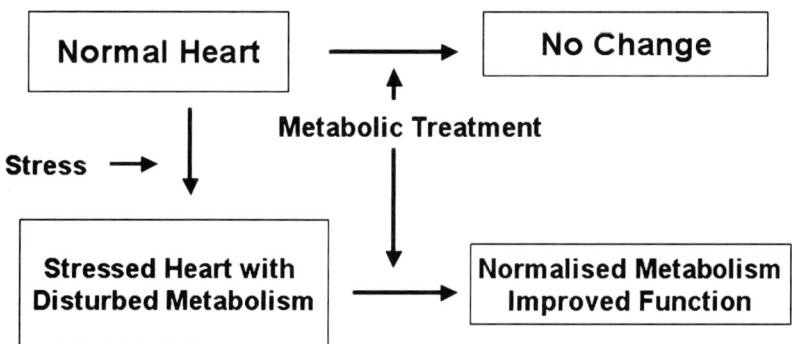

FIGURE 1. Principles of metabolic therapy.

found that stress management, as part of a cardiac rehabilitation program, lowered the risk of a major cardiac event.[9] A meta-analysis by Linden *et al.* also concluded that the addition of psychological treatments to standard cardiac rehabilitation regimes reduced mortality, morbidity, and psychological distress.[10] Patients presenting for cardiac surgery and indeed all major surgery are often anxious about the outcome of their operation. Given that behavioral and psychological factors play such a significant and independent role on the symptoms of coronary artery disease and its complications, methods of reducing stress and improving the mental health and well-being before surgery should be beneficial. We therefore designed a program, the MPM (Metabolic Physical and Mental) Program, of preparation for cardiac surgery incorporating metabolic protection, physical exercise, and mental stress reduction.

Methods

For the metabolic component, we used our previously validated regime of 300 mg of CoQ_{10} per day[7] combined with added alpha-lipoic acid (150 mg per day), magnesium orotate (1.2 gm per day) and omega-3 fatty acids (3 gm per day). Alpha-lipoic acid is an antioxidant and cofactor for enzymes involved in energy production that has been shown to have beneficial effects on the heart.[11] We previously have validated the beneficial effects on the heart of orotate[12] and omega-3 fatty acids.[13] Patients in the MPM program undertook a two-week regimen of modest physical exercise before surgery under the supervision of a physiotherapist. This involved a gentle, non-symptom-producing program of stretching, treadmill exercise, bicycle exercise, and training with light weights.

Patients were taught techniques of mental stress reduction, meditation, and relaxation. The techniques were learned in one or two instruction sessions run by the hospital occupational therapist and subsequently performed by patients in their own homes.

We conducted a feasibility and quality assurance study to assess the impact of the MPM program on the outcomes from surgery using improvements in quality of life (QoL) measured by the SF36 questionnaire. The questionnaire was administered before enrollment in the program, at the completion of 2–10 weeks on the program immediately before cardiac surgery, and again one month after surgery. Because this was a feasibility study and not a clinical trial, there was no randomized control group. However, for a control group we used a historical control group, comprising 64 patients who had quality-of-life assessments performed before and one month after surgery in a previous study in our unit.[14] In a subgroup of the MPM group, to assess oxidative stress, measurements of the lipid preoxidation product, malondialdehyde, were made in blood sampled before and after the program, immediately before surgery.

Results

Quality-of-life assessments conducted before and after the program (but before surgery) ($N = 16$) showed an increase in the physical quality of life assessment scores from 33.5 ± 4.12 before to 41.0 ± 4.5 after the program ($P = .005$; FIG. 2). Similarly

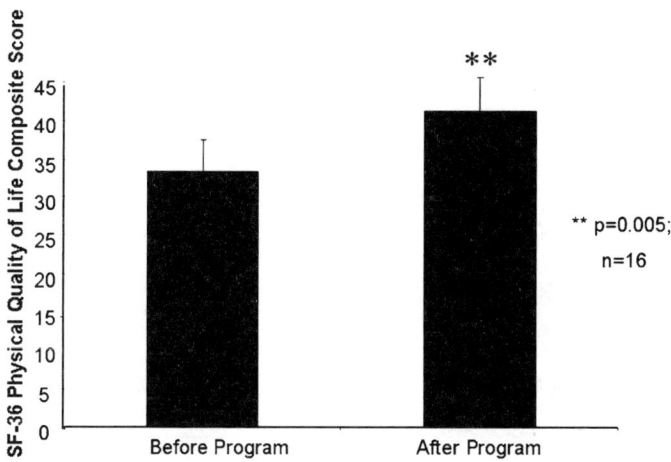

FIGURE 2. Effect of MPM program on physical quality of life before surgery.

mental quality-of-life scores also showed an improvement from 44.3 ± 4.5 before to 54.1 ± 5.3 afterward ($P = .006$). The quality-of-life assessments, conducted before and one month after surgery, also showed a significant improvement in the physical quality of life in the MPM group from 37.7 ± 5.0 before to 56.5 ± 7.0 afterward ($P = .01$; FIG. 3) This was in contrast with the control group that showed a deterioration ($P = .05$). For mental quality-of-life scores, there was a similar pattern, with improvement in the MPM group from 48.4 ± 6.2 to 65.0 ± 5.7 ($P = .048$) and a deterioration in the control group ($P = .05$). Malondialdehyde levels decreased from 23.9 ± 2.5 before the MPM program to 13.2 ± 2.1 µM/mL afterward ($P = .026$).

Conclusion

A program of combined metabolic, physical, and mental preparation before major surgery has the potential to reduce oxidative stress and improve the quality of life of the patient immediately before and one month after surgery.

MITOCHONDRIAL PREDICTORS OF BIOLOGICAL AGE

Mitochondrial function, especially oxidative phosphorylation, declines with age. Also with age there is an accumulation of damage to and mutations of mitochondrial DNA.[15,16] Major accumulation of mutated mitochondrial DNA (50% or more) is associated with overt mitochondrial diseases such as Kearn Sayre syndrome. These data led us to ask the question, Could the abundance of mitochondrial DNA mutations or the total cellular content of mitochondrial DNA be clinically useful predictors of reduced tolerance to stress such as cardiac surgery in the aging heart, that is, a measure of biological age? To answer this question, we measured the recovery of strips of human cardiac tissue after a stress of simulated ischemia and correlated the

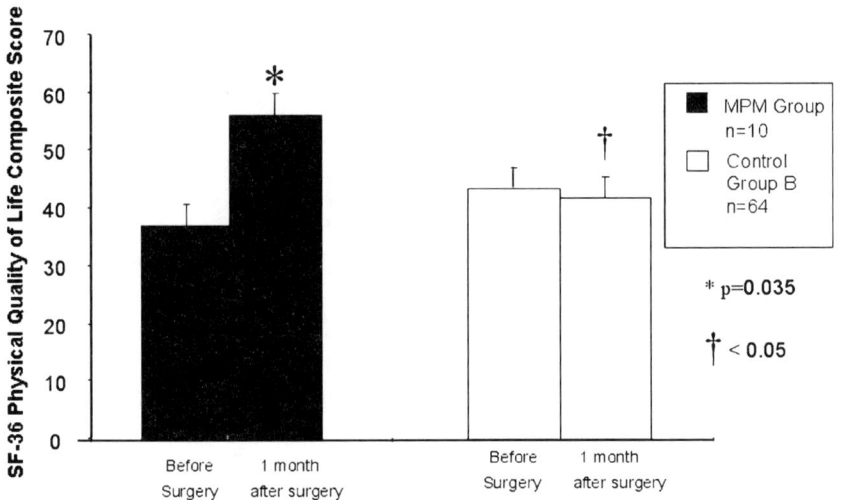

FIGURE 3. Effect of MPM program on physical quality of life before and after surgery compared with usual care controls.

magnitude of recovery with the abundance of mutated mitochondrial DNA and with the total cellular content of mitochondrial DNA in the same tissue samples.

Methods

Cardiac myocardial tissue was obtained from atrial appendages discarded at the time of open heart surgery. The mitochondrial (common) deletion mtDNA^{4977} was measured using a technique of a quantitative polymerase chain reaction (PCR).[17] Total cellular content of mitochondrial DNA was measured for copy number of mitochondrial DNA genomes per diploid nuclear gene complement using a technique of quantitative PCR.[18] This technique used a dual insert plasmid as a standard. This plasmid contained a section of mitochondrial DNA containing the single-copy beta-globin gene and a sequence of normal mitochondrial DNA in the region of the cytochrome *b* gene. Samples of the same muscle strips on which the PCRs had been performed were subjected to simulated ischemic stress by removing oxygen and organ bath fluid for 30 minutes. Recovery of contractile function was measured after reoxygenation and reperfusion. Correlations were performed between the recovery of the atrial strips from ischemic stress and the abundance of the mtDNA^{4977} deletion or the mitochondrial DNA copy number.

Results

Recovery of developed force after ischemia/reperfusion showed a negative correlation with age ($R^2 = .21$, $P < .001$). The abundance of mtDNA^{4977} increased with age ($R^2 = 0.78$, $P < .001$). However, it was notable that the absolute value for the abundance of mtDNA^{4977} was small (<.001% of total mitochondrial cellular DNA).

TABLE 1. Predictors of recovery of force: multivariate analysis

	MtDNA^{4977}	Copy number	Age
P value	0.86	0.73	0.0001
Slope	−0.36	−1.04	−0.76

When recovery of developed force was related to mitochondrial DNA deletional abundance, the relationship was found to be significant but weak ($R^2 = .08$, $P = .047$). Mitochondrial DNA copy number showed no change with age ($R^2 = .01$, $P = .56$). The average mitochondrial DNA copy number in the myocardium, 7,000 per diploid nuclear DNA gene complement, was greater than that in skeletal muscle, 3,700 ($P = .006$). There was no relationship between recovery of developed force and mitochondrial DNA copy number ($R^2 = .01$ $P = .46$). We performed a multivariate analysis to assess the relative importance of all these predictors of postischemic recovery in myocardial tissue. This analysis indicated that only age was a significant predictor ($P = .0001$), whereas mitochondrial DNA deletional abundance ($P = 0.86$) and mitochondrial DNA copy number ($P = .73$) were not significant (TABLE 1).

CONCLUSIONS

Combined metabolic mental and physical therapy shows promise as an inexpensive holistic preparation for elderly and high-risk patients undergoing cardiac and other major surgery. Data from the aging human heart do not support a major role for mitochondrial DNA deletions or copy number as a marker of biological age in the myocardium.

REFERENCES

1. LINDSAY, J. JR., V. REDDY, E. PINNOW, et al. 1994. Morbidity and mortality rates in patients undergoing percutaneous coronary transluminal angioplasty. Am. Heart J. **128:** 697–702.
2. STONE, G., C. GRINES, K. BROWNE, et al. 1995. Predictors of in-hospital and 6-month outcome after acute myocardial infarction in the reperfusion era: the primary angioplasty in myocardial infarction (PAMI) trial. J. Am. Coll. Cardiol. **25:** 370–377.
3. JAEGER, A., M. HLATKY, S. PAUL & S. GORTNER. 1994. Functional capacity after cardiac surgery in elderly patients. J. Am. Coll. Cardiol. **24:** 104–108.
4. CALDARONE, C., I. KRUKENCAMP, P. BURNS, et al. 1995. Blood cardioplegia in the senescent heart. J. Thorac. Cardiovasc. Surg. **109:** 269–274.
5. ROWLAND, M.A., P. NAGLEY, A.W. LINNANE & F.L. ROSENFELDT. 1998. Coenzyme Q_{10} treatment improves the tolerance of the senescent myocardium to pacing stress in the rat. Cardiovasc. Res. **40:** 165–173.
6. ROSENFELDT, F.L., S. PEPE, A. LINNANE, et al. 2002. The effects of ageing on the response to cardiac surgery: protective strategies for the ageing myocardium. Biogerontology **3:** 37–40.
7. ROSENFELDT, F.L., S. MARASCO, W. LYON, et al. Coenzyme Q_{10} therapy before cardiac surgery improves mitochondrial function and in-vitro contractility of myocardial tissue. J. Thorac. Cardiovasc. Surg. In press.
8. ARTHUR, H.M., C. DANIELS, R. MCKELVIE, et al. 2000. Effect of a preoperative intervention on preoperative and postoperative outcomes in low-risk patients awaiting

elective coronary artery bypass graft surgery: a randomised controlled trial. Ann. Intern. Med. **133:** 253–262.
9. BLUMENTHAL, J.A., J. WEI, M.A. BABYAK, *et al.* 1997. Stress management and exercise training in cardiac patients with myocardial ischaemia: effects on prognosis and evaluation of mechanisms. Arch. Intern. Med. **157:** 2213–2223.
10. LINDEN, W., C. STOSSEL & J. MAURICE. 1996. Psychological interventions for patients with coronary artery disease. Arch. Int. Med. **156:** 745–752.
11. ZIMMER, G., T.K. BEIKLER, M. SCHNEIDER, *et al.* 1995. Dose-response curves of lipoic acid R and S forms in the working rat heart during reoxygenation: superiority of the R-enatiomer in enhancement of aortic flow. J. Mol. Cell. Cardiol. **27:** 1895–1903.
12. NEWMAN, M.A.J., X.-Z. CHEN, M. RABINOV, *et al.* 1989. Sensitivity of the recently infarcted heart to cardioplegic arrest. J. Thorac. Cardiovasc. Surg. **97:** 593–604.
13. BURR, M.L., A.M. FEHILY, J.F. GILBERT, *et al.* 1989. Effect of changes in fat, fish, and fibre intakes on death and myocardial reinfarction: diet and reinfarction trail (DART). Lancet **2:** 757–761.
14. MYLES, P.S., J.O. HUNT, H.O. HOLDGAARD, *et al.* 1999. Clonidine and cardiac surgery: haemodynamic and metabolic effects, myocardial ischaemia and recovery. Anaesth. Intensive Care **27:** 137–147.
15. HAYAKAWA, M., K. TORII, S. SUGIYAMA, *et al.* 1991. Age-associated accumulation of 8- hydroxydeoxyguanosine in mitochondrial DNA of human diaphragm. Biochem. Biophys. Res. Commun. **179:** 1023–1029.
16. LINNANE, A.W., A. BAUMER, R.J. MAXWELL, *et al.* 1990. Mitochondrial gene mutation: the ageing process and degenerative diseases. Biochem. Int. **22:** 1067–1076.
17. ZHANG, C., A. BAUMER, R.J. MAXWELL, *et al.* 1992. Multiple mitochondrial DNA deletions in an elderly human individual. FEBS Lett. **291:** 34–38.
18. MILLER, F.J., F.L. ROSENFELDT, C. ZHANG, *et al.* 2003. Precise determination of mitochondrial DNA copy number in ageing human myocytes by a PCR-based assay: lack of change of copy number with age. Nucleic Acids Res. **31:** e61.

Impairment of the Transcriptional Responses to Oxidative Stress in the Heart of Aged C57BL/6 Mice

MICHAEL G. EDWARDS,[a] DEEPAYAN SARKAR,[b] ROGER KLOPP,[c] JASON D. MORROW,[d] RICHARD WEINDRUCH,[c,e] AND TOMAS A. PROLLA[a]

[a]*Department of Genetics and Medical Genetics, University of Wisconsin, Madison, Wisconsin 53706, USA*

[b]*Department of Statistics, University of Wisconsin, Madison, Wisconsin 53706, USA*

[c]*Veterans Administration Hospital, University of Wisconsin, Madison, Wisconsin 53706, USA*

[d]*Department of Pharmacology and Medicine, Vanderbilt University, Nashville, Tennessee 37232-6602*

[e]*Department of Medicine and Wisconsin Primate Research Center, University of Wisconsin, Madison, Wisconsin 53706, USA*

ABSTRACT: To investigate the transcriptional response to oxidative stress in the heart and how it changes with age, we examined the cardiac gene expression profiles of young (5 months old), middle-aged (15 months old), and old (25 months old) C57BL/6 mice treated with a single intraperitoneal injection of paraquat (50 mg/kg). Mice were killed at 0, 1, 3, 5, and 7 hours after paraquat treatment, and the gene expression profile was obtained with high-density oligonucleotide microarrays. Of 9,977 genes represented on the microarray, 249 transcripts in the young mice, 298 transcripts in the middle-aged mice, and 256 transcripts in the old mice displayed a significant change in mRNA levels (ANOVA, $P < .01$). Among these, a total of 55 transcripts were determined to be paraquat responsive for all age groups. Genes commonly induced in all age groups include those associated with stress, inflammatory, immune, and growth factor responses. Interestingly, only young mice displayed a significant increase in expression of all three isoforms of GADD45, a DNA damage-responsive gene. Additionally, the number of immediate early genes found to be induced by paraquat was considerably higher in the younger animals. These results demonstrate that, at the transcriptional level, there is an age-related impairment of specific inducible pathways in the response to oxidative stress in the mouse heart.

KEYWORDS: aging; paraquat; gene expression

Address for correspondence: Tomas A. Prolla, Department of Genetics and Medical Genetics, University of Wisconsin, Madison, WI 53706. Voice: 608-265-5205; fax: 608-262-2976.
taprolla@facstaff.wisc.edu

INTRODUCTION

Although the increased susceptibility of older animals to various forms of stress has been well documented, little is known about the genetic basis underlying this change.[1] There is also evidence to suggest that longevity and the ability to resist oxidative and metabolic stress are related processes. Several long-lived mutants have been identified in *Saccharomyces cerevisiae*,[2] *Drosophila*,[3] and *Caenorhabditis elegans*[4] that exhibit increased resistance to a wide range of physiological and pharmacological insults. The basic molecular defense systems used by these organisms are very similar to those used in mammals,[5] suggesting that stress responses also may play a role in aging of longer lived species. The endogenous production of reactive oxygen species (ROS), a byproduct of cellular respiration, may contribute to the aging phenotype.[6] The heart is an organ that is likely to be particularly vulnerable to increases in oxidative stress, because cardiomyocytes depend heavily on mitochondrial function. The ability to cope with cardiovascular injury has been shown to decline with age,[7] and many heart-related stresses, such as myocardial ischemia and reperfusion, generate ROS that may contribute to pathology.[8]

Previous studies using high-density oligonucleotide arrays have characterized the basal transcriptional response to the aging process in skeletal muscle,[9] brain,[10] and heart[11] of mice. However, this technology has not been used to characterize the transcriptional response to acute oxidative stress as a function of age. Accordingly, we investigated the transcriptional response to oxidative damage in the heart by challenging 5-month (young), 15-month (middle-aged), and 25-month-old mice with paraquat. Paraquat is a toxin that reacts with molecular oxygen *in vivo* to generate ROS in several tissues and has been used previously to elicit oxidative stress in rodents.[12] To identify genes that have differential expression levels between young and old animals after paraquat treatment, we used oligonucleotide arrays that can simultaneously measure mRNA levels of thousands of genes.

MATERIALS AND METHODS

Animal Treatments

Details on the methods used to house and feed male inbred C57BL/6NHsd mice, which have an average life span of ~30 months in our colony, have been described.[13] Mice were individually housed and, from 2 months on, fed 84 kcal per week which is ~5–20% less than the range of individual *ad libitum* intakes. Animals were given a single intraperitoneal injection of paraquat at a dose of 50 mg/kg body weight dissolved in phosphate-buffered saline 24 hours after their last feeding and death by cervical dislocation 1, 3, 5, and 7 hours after injection. Three different animals were used for each time point and age group. All collected hearts then were dissected, placed in a microcentrifuge tube, flash-frozen in liquid nitrogen, and stored at –80°C.

Tissue Preparation, Oligonucleotide Array Hybridization, and Data Analysis

Polyadenylate [poly(A)+] RNAs were extracted from frozen heart tissue and used to generate array image data as previously described.[11] Because for each gene we are more interested in the fold changes than in the absolute intensities, the raw image data were normalized by dividing all raw measurements for each gene by the mean raw signal intensity for the same gene as measured in the three control animals (nontreated) for that particular age group to give the normalized signal intensity.

Statistical Analysis

Each gene was considered separately when attempting to classify it as paraquat responsive. All genes considered absent as determined by Affymetrix software for all measured time points in all age groups were eliminated from our analysis (4,463 probe sets from a total of 9,977 were eliminated based on these criteria). A gene was classified as paraquat responsive in young mice as follows: a one-way analysis of variance (ANOVA) model was fit to the intensities obtained for that gene from the young mice, with five treatment conditions, namely, 0, 1, 3, 5, and 7 hours after paraquat, and three replicates for each condition. Genes that had a small P value ($<.01$) and had at least one present call, as determined by Affymetrix software, for one of the time points were categorized as paraquat responsive. This procedure also was used to classify a gene as paraquat responsive in middle-aged and old mice. For a gene to be considered paraquat responsive in all age groups, its P value, as determined by ANOVA for each specific age group, had to be less than .01 in two of the three ages, and less than .05 in the remaining age group.

RESULTS

Paraquat-Responsive Genes

Of 9,977 genes probed on the oligonucleotide microarray, we identified 249 genes in the young mice, 298 genes in the middle-aged mice, and 256 genes in the old mice with differential expression levels in response to paraquat over the 7-hour time course (ANOVA, $P < .01$). Among these induced genes, a total of 55 transcripts were determined to be paraquat responsive for all age groups (TABLE 1). Among these 55 common genes, the FK506 binding protein 5 (Fkbp5) encoding gene had the largest fold change in both the young and old groups (12.2- and 24.5-fold in young and old respectively). The FK506-binding protein is tightly associated with the cardiac sarcoplasmic reticulum Ca^{2+}-release channel (ryanodine receptor type 2 [RyR2]), and it is likely that Fkbp5 inhibits the signaling of calcineurin through its association with this receptor.[14] Paraquat induced metallothionein 1 and 2, two low molecular mass proteins that bind to free metal ions and regulate cellular copper and zinc metabolism. Metallothionein, which protects cells against oxidative insults, can be induced by a variety of stressors, including glucocorticoids,[15] heavy metals,[16] ischemia-reperfusion,[17] and ionizing and UV irradiation.[18]

The observed induction of several genes appears to be associated with a protective metabolic stress response in the heart. Bcl-XL is a antiapoptotic protein that allows cells to maintain oxidative metabolism during cellular stress by allowing continued transport of metabolites across the outer mitochondrial membrane.[19] 5' nucleotidase activity controls the production of adenosine in the heart through dephosphorylation of AMP.[20] Adenosine receptors may play a key role in the adap-

TABLE 1. Common paraquat-responsive genes in young (5 months old), middle-aged (15 months old), and old (25 months old) C57B16/J mouse hearts[a]

		Greatest change (Time)			
Identifier	Gene Name	Young	Middle-aged	Old	Function
Stress, Immune or Inflammatory Response					
U16959	FK506 binding protein 5 (51 kDa)	12.2 (7)	2.3 (5)	24.5 (7)	calcium release
L00039	Myelocytomatosis oncogene	11.4 (3)	5.4 (3)	17.2 (5)	immediate early response
K02236	Metallothionein 2	10.0 (7)	11.5 (7)	12.6 (7)	antioxidant response
AW048937	Cyclin-dependent kinase inhibitor 1A (P21)	5.6 (7)	2.3 (7)	6.5 (7)	cell cycle
L35049	Bcl2-like	3.9 (7)	1.9 (7)	3.0 (7)	apoptosis
V00835	Metallothionein 1	3.5 (7)	5.3 (7)	6.6 (7)	antioxidant response
X14678	Zinc finger protein 36	2.9 (5)	3.2 (5)	3.1 (3)	immediate early response
M61007	CCAAT/enhancer binding protein (C/EBP), beta	2.8 (3)	1.7 (7)	4.3 (7)	immediate early response
AW046181	Serum/glucocorticoid-regulated kinase	2.7 (5)	2.2 (7)	2.7 (5)	immediate early response
AI846938	Herpud1	2.4 (7)	1.7 (7)	2.7 (7)	unfolded protein response
M74570	Alcohol dehydrogenase family 1, subfamily A2	2.2 (7)	1.4 (7)	3.2 (7)	antioxidant response
AI843106	p53 regulated PA26 nuclear protein	2.0 (7)	2.2 (7)	2.4 (7)	genotoxic response
U52073	N-myc downstream regulated-like	1.8 (7)	1.7 (5)	1.5 (7)	stress response
U40930	Oxidative stress induced	1.7 (7)	1.9 (7)	2.2 (7)	oxidative stress response
AF103875	ATP-binding cassette, sub-family G (WHITE), member 2	1.6 (7)	1.7 (7)	2.0 (7)	drug resistance
M63801	Gap junction membrane channel protein alpha 1	0.4 (7)	0.4 (7)	0.4 (7)	ion transporter
Growth Factor Response/Signaling					
AF064748	S3-12 protein	5.7 (7)	3.0 (7)	3.2 (7)	growth factor response
M70642	connective tissue growth factor	4.6 (3)	5.2 (5)	7.2 (5)	immediate early gene
U50413	Phosphatidylinositol 3-kinase, regulatory subunit, polypeptide 1	3.5 (7)	2.0 (7)	2.3 (7)	adipocyte differentiation

TABLE 1. (*continued*) Common paraquat-responsive genes in young (5 months old), middle-aged (15 months old), and old (25 months old) C57B16/J mouse hearts[a]

		Greatest change (Time)			
Identifier	Gene Name	Young	Middle-aged	Old	Function
AF009246	RAS, dexamethasone-induced 1	3.2 (7)	3.1 (7)	9.5 (7)	GTP binding
AF051945	Cardiac morphogenesis	2.5 (7)	2.1 (7)	2.1 (5)	growth factor response
U28656	Eukaryotic translation initiation factor 4E binding protein 1	2.0 (7)	1.9 (7)	1.8 (7)	IGF response
U58992	MAD homolog (*Drosophila*)	1.8 (7)	1.9 (7)	2.6 (7)	TGF-beta super-family pathway
AW049372	Transforming growth factor alpha regulated gene 4	1.7 (7)	1.4 (7)	1.7 (7)	unknown
L29441	Tumor differentially expressed 1	1.5 (7)	1.6 (7)	1.8 (7)	oncogenesis
U85259	Estrogen related receptor, alpha	0.7 (7)	0.9 (7)	0.6 (7)	steriod receptor
AF084466	Ras-like GTP-binding protein rad	0.2 (7)	0.3 (5)	0.2 (7)	isulin signal transduction
Metabolic/Catabolic					
AJ001418	Pyruvate dehydrogenase kinase 4	6.5 (7)	4.4 (5)	10.4 (7)	glucose metabolism
L12059	5' nucleotidase	2.8 (5)	1.9 (7)	1.9 (3)	AMP catabolism
Y08027	ART3 gene	2.6 (7)	2.2 (7)	2.2 (7)	NAD(+) ADP-ribosyltransferase
AF020185	Dynein, cytoplasmic, light chain 1	0.4 (5)	0.4 (7)	0.5 (5)	nitric oxide biosynthesis
Transcription Regulation					
D49473	SRY-box containing gene 17	3.7 (7)	4.0 (5)	4.1 (7)	embryogenesis
AF072240	Methyl-CpG binding domain protein 1	3.4 (7)	2.4 (7)	4.1 (7)	DNA methylation
D42124	V-maf, protein K	1.6 (7)	1.9 (7)	1.7 (5)	induction of iron-regulating genes
Miscellaneous					
AF015790	Phospholipid scramblase 2	2.8 (3)	2.9 (7)	3.6 (5)	calcium ion binding
L02914	Aquaporin 1	2.1 (7)	1.9 (7)	1.7 (7)	water transport
AW123904	GABA(A) receptor-associated protein like 1	2.0 (7)	1.9 (7)	1.8 (7)	unknown
AF022992	Period homolog (*Drosophila*)	2.0 (7)	1.9 (7)	2.6 (7)	biological rhythm

TABLE 1. (*continued*) Common paraquat-responsive genes in young (5 months old), middle-aged (15 months old), and old (25 months old) C57B16/J mouse hearts[a]

Identifier	Gene Name	Greatest change (Time)			Function
		Young	Middle-aged	Old	
AI844532	splicing factor 3b, subunit 1, 155 kDa	1.9 (7)	1.6 (7)	1.6 (5)	mRNA processing
AI846077	pleckstrin homology, Sec7 and coiled/coil domains 3	1.8 (3)	1.8 (7)	1.6 (5)	vesicular transport
U71205	RAS-like protein expressed in many tissues	1.7 (7)	1.8 (7)	1.6 (7)	calmodulin binding
AF085192	Hippocalcin-like 1	1.5 (5)	1.1 (5)	1.5 (7)	calcium binding
D50527	Ubiquitin C	1.4 (3)	1.7 (5)	1.6 (3)	protein degradation
X98475	Vasodilator-stimulated phosphoprotein	0.6 (7)	0.6 (7)	0.6 (7)	platelet inhibition
	Unknown				
AI553024		7.7 (7)	1.8 (7)	13.9 (7)	unknown
AI849939		5.2 (7)	2.5 (7)	4.7 (7)	unknown
AI853531		3.2 (1)	2.7 (1)	2.9 (5)	unknown
AI225296		3.0 (5)	1.8 (3)	2.2 (5)	unknown
C85523		2.6 (3)	2.4 (7)	3.0 (7)	unknown
AW212475		2.5 (1)	2.6 (1)	3.8 (5)	unknown
AW122893		1.8 (7)	3.3 (7)	2.9 (5)	unknown
AI849135		1.6 (5)	1.5 (3)	1.9 (7)	unknown
AW124678		1.4 (7)	1.7 (7)	1.7 (5)	unknown
AW125272		0.6 (5)	0.7 (5)	0.6 (7)	unknown
AA958903		0.4 (7)	0.5 (7)	0.4 (5)	unknown

[a]The 55 common genes that changed significantly in response to paraquat at all ages. The largest or smallest normalized measurement is shown in the table along with the corresponding time point in which it occurs for that particular age group. There were 48 common genes that increased and 7 common genes that decreased in mRNA levels for the majority of the paraquat time course.

tive response to altered O_2 delivery or increased metabolic activity.[21] Pyruvate dehydrogenase kinase 4 (PDK4) is a key element involved in fuel selection. PDK4 inhibits pyruvate dehydrogenase and thus minimizes carbohydrate oxidation by preventing the flow of glycolytic products into the tricarboxylic acid cycle.[22]

Aging Is Associated with Altered Transcription of Immediate Early Genes after Oxidative Stress

We found that young mice displayed a greater number of immediate early response genes (IEGs) induced as compared with middle-aged and old mice (12 genes in the young, 7 genes in the middle-aged, and 5 genes in the old), suggesting age-

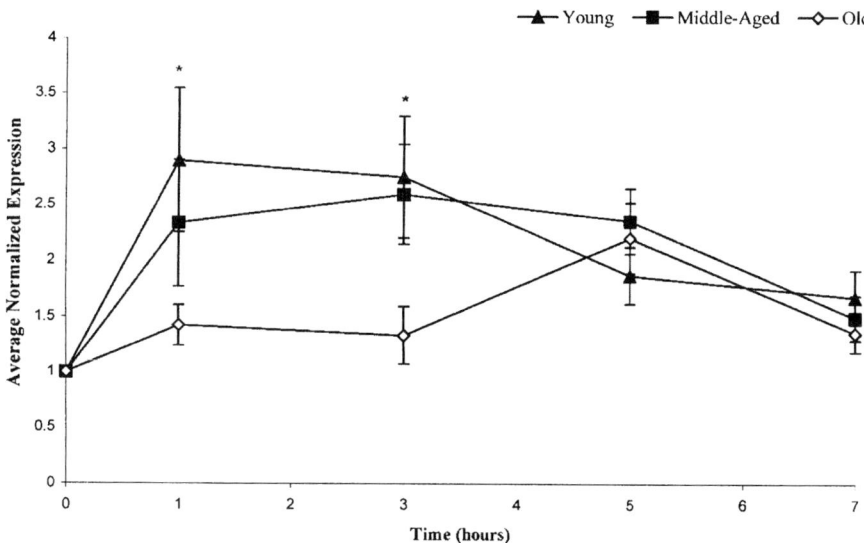

FIGURE 1. Age-associated changes in expression profiles of MAPKK-dependent IEGs in the hearts of young and old mice after induced oxidative stress. Lines represent the averaged normalized expression ±SE for six paraquat-responsive IEGs in the young (*zfp36, btg2, ptpn16, cyr61, nr4a1,* and *atf3*) and three other IEGs measured on this microarray (*junb, krox-24,* and *ptgs2*) shown to be dependent on MAPKK signaling for expression[23,24] in the hearts of young, middle-aged, and old mice. No significant differences were found in the constitutive levels of these genes when comparing the average raw intensity levels for young control versus old control mice. The averaged normalized expression for these genes is significantly higher (*Wilcoxon signed rank test, $P < .05$ for young mice vs. old mice) in the heart of young animals 1 and 3 hours after paraquat treatment, but similar to old hearts by the 5-hour time point. *c-fos*, another IEG whose transcription is stimulated by MAPKK signaling, is not measured on our array and therefore not included in the graph.

related impairment in this response (TABLE 2). Interestingly, many of the IEGs that showed age-related impairment in the transcriptional response have been shown to be dependent on mitogen-activated protein kinase kinase (MAPKK) signaling for expression including *zfp36, btg2, cyr61, nr4a1, ptpn16,*[23] and *atf3*.[24] The average normalized expression of the MAPKK-dependent IEGs increased significantly in the young and middle-aged hearts 1 hour after paraquat injection and then returned to similar levels of normalized expression as found in the old animals 5 hours after the initial oxidative insult (FIG. 1).

Aging Is Associated with an Impairment in the Induction of Stress-Response Genes: GADD45, MAP3K6, and JunB

The levels of the three GADD45 transcripts (GADD45α, GADD45β, and GADD45γ) increased significantly in the young hearts after paraquat treatment, two of which were also significantly induced in the middle-aged hearts (GADD45α and GADD45γ), but no induction was found in the old hearts (FIG. 2). The only MAPK-

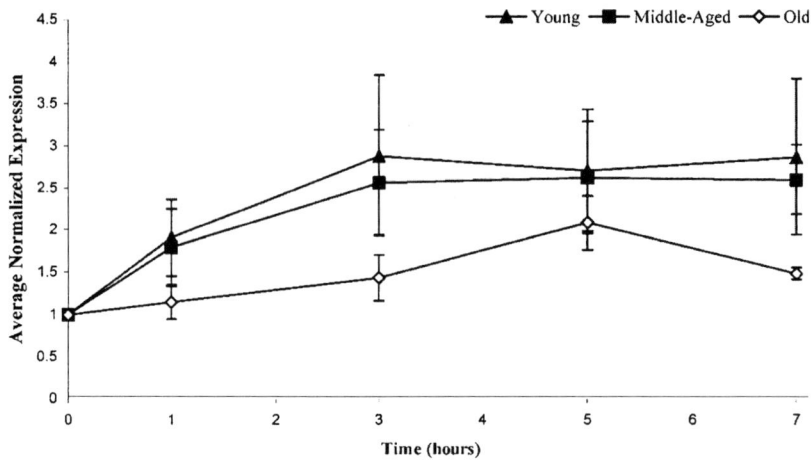

FIGURE 2. GADD45 gene expression in young and old mice after paraquat treatment. Average normalized expression of all three GADD45 isoforms (alpha, beta, and gamma) measured on our microarray for all ages of mice. Each point on the graph represents the mean ± SE for all measurements generated for the three GADD45 isoforms for each individual age group at that time point.

TABLE 2. IEGs identified as paraquat-responsive (ANOVA, $P < .05$)[a]

		Paraquat Responsive		
	Immediate Early Gene	Young	Middle-aged	Old
Cebpb	CCAAT/enhancer binding protein (C/EBP), beta	Yes	Yes	Yes
c-myc	Myelocytomatosis oncogene	Yes	Yes	Yes
Ctgf	Connective tissue growth factor	Yes	Yes	Yes
Sgk	Serum/glucocorticoid regulated kinase	Yes	Yes	Yes
Zfp36	**Zinc finger protein 36**	Yes	Yes	Yes
Btg2	**B cell translocation gene 2, antiproliferative**	Yes	Yes	No
Cyr61	**Cysteine-rich protein 61**	Yes	Yes	No
Atf3	**Activating transcription factor 3**	Yes	No	No
Gadd45b	Growth arrest and DNA damage–inducible 45 beta	Yes	No	No
Tieg	TGFB-inducible early growth response	Yes	No	No
Nr4a1	**Nuclear receptor subfamily 4, group A, member 1**	Yes	No	No
Ptpn16	**Protein tyrosine phosphatase, nonreceptor type 16**	Yes	No	No

[a] All immediate early genes (IEGs) were paraquat responsive in young mice, and this number declined with age. Genes in bold represent IEGs dependent on MAPKK signaling for expression.

encoding gene found to be paraquat responsive by our ANOVA criteria was *map3k6*. MAP3K6 is a member of a MAPK cascade that is known to activate two closely related but distinct stress-responsive parallel pathways; the c-Jun N-terminal kinase (JNK) or stress-activated kinase (SAPK) pathway and the p38 kinase pathway. Overexpression of MAP3K6 has been shown to activate the JNK but not the p38 kinase pathway.[25] This gene, found to be significantly induced in young animals only, had the highest normalized expression of all paraquat-responsive genes (20-fold). Levels of *c-jun* and *jund* expression remained constant over the experimental time course for both age groups, whereas levels of *junb* mRNA increased considerably in all age groups after paraquat. *Junb* expression in the young and middle-aged group had a peak normalized expression of 7.9 and 6.7, respectively, 1 hour after paraquat (ANOVA, $P < .05$). The increase in *junb* expression was reduced (3.6-fold) and more variable (ANOVA, $P < .20$) in older mice, and its peak normalized expression was delayed (5 hours after injection) when compared with the young and middle-aged animals.

DISCUSSION

Our study provides the first gene expression profile associated with oxidative stress in the heart and suggests that aging is associated with defects in the transcriptional induction of specific cellular signaling pathways. Specifically, we observed an impaired transcriptional activation of IEG genes dependent on MAPKK signaling which also includes the JNK pathway. The lack of MAPKK-dependent IEG induction in the old mouse hearts suggests an attenuated response in this pathway, which is likely to result in less induction of downstream targets. Additionally, only young and middle-aged mouse hearts display significant changes in the expression of *GADD45*-like genes which are mediators of stress-activated protein kinase signaling (JNK).[26] Further evidence for an age-related change in paraquat-induced JNK signaling in the heart comes from examining the expression levels of components and targets of this pathway. *Map3k6* (a signal-regulated kinase of the JNK pathway) and *junb* (a downstream target of stress-activated signaling) both exhibit higher levels of normalized expression after paraquat injection in the young mice when compared with the old. Previous studies agree with our findings, having shown reduced levels of expression of the IEGs *c-fos*, *c-myc*, and *c-jun* in aged rat hearts after hemodynamic stress.[27,28] It is conceivable that the observed early increase in expression of JNK-related genes in the young animals provides increased protection in the heart against induced oxidative stress as compared with that of their old counterparts. One possibility is that the response to oxidative damage is already activated in the older mice and therefore signaling pathways, such as the MAPK pathways, are chronically activated and display less induction after exogenous oxidative stress. We did not find evidence to support this hypothesis at the transcriptional level, because the basal level of IEGs and GADD45 mRNA is similar in young and old animals. We also note that our data reveal several paraquat-inducible genes that were not previously known to respond to oxidative stress. These include several genes involved in metabolic adaptation, signal transduction, and cell growth. Other genes that respond to paraquat have no known homology or function (TABLE 1). Eventual elucidation of the roles of these genes as components of the antioxidant response may increase our understanding of cellular oxidative damage defense mechanisms in the heart. We also note that our study represents a first step in understanding transcriptional mechanisms of age-related inability to cope with oxidative stress in the heart. Future studies will involve characterization of specific pathways at the biochemical and cellular level to identify the cell type specificity and the molecular basis of the age-related transcriptional impairment described here.

ACKNOWLEDGMENTS

This research was supported in part by NIH Grants DK48831, GM15431, CA77839, R01AG18922, U24DK058776, and NSF#0090286. J.D.M. is the recipient of a Burroughs Welcome Fund Clinical Scientist Award in Translational Research.

REFERENCES

1. PAPACONSTANTINOU, J., P.D. REISNER, L. LIU & D. KUNNINGER. 1996. Mechanisms of altered gene expression with aging. In Handbook of the Biology of Aging. E.L. Schneider & J.W. Rowe, Eds.: 150–183. Academic Press. San Diego.
2. FABRIZIO, P. et al. 2001. Regulation of longevity and stress resistance by Sch9 in yeast. Science **292**: 288–290.
3. LIN, Y.J., L. SEROUDE & S. BENZER. 1998. Extended life-span and stress resistance in the Drosophila mutant methuselah. Science **282**: 943–946.
4. MURAKAMI, S. & T.E. JOHNSON. 1998. Life extension and stress resistance in *Caenorhabditis elegans* modulated by the tkr-1 gene. Curr. Biol. **8**: 1091–1094.
5. WASKIEWICZ, A.J. & J.A. COOPER. 1995. Mitogen and stress response pathways: MAP kinase cascades and phosphatase regulation in mammals and yeast. Curr. Opin. Cell Biol. **7**: 798–805.
6. HARMAN, D. 1981. The aging process. Proc. Natl. Acad. Sci. USA **78**: 7124–7128.
7. MARIANI, J., et al. 2000. Tolerance to ischemia and hypoxia is reduced in aged human myocardium. J. Thorac. Cardiovasc. Surg. **120**: 660–667.
8. DAS, D.K., N. MAULIK & I.I. MORARU. 1995. Gene expression in acute myocardial stress. Induction by hypoxia, ischemia, reperfusion, hyperthermia and oxidative stress. J. Mol. Cell. Cardiol. **27**: 181–193.
9. LEE, C.K. et al. 1999. Gene expression profile of aging and its retardation by caloric restriction. Science **285**: 1390–1393.
10. LEE, C.K., R. WEINDRUCH & T.A. PROLLA. 2000. Gene-expression profile of the ageing brain in mice. Nat. Genet. **25**: 294–297.
11. LEE, C.K. et al. 2002. Transcriptional profiles associated with aging and middle age-onset caloric restriction in mouse hearts. Proc. Natl. Acad. Sci. USA **99**: 14988–14993.
12. SUNTRES, Z.E. 2002. Role of antioxidants in paraquat toxicity. Toxicology **180**: 65–77.
13. PUGH, T.D., R.G. KLOPP & R. WEINDRUCH. 1999. Controlling caloric consumption: protocols for rodents and rhesus monkeys. Neurobiol. Aging **20**: 157–165.
14. BANDYOPADHYAY, A. et al. 2000. Calcineurin regulates ryanodine receptor/Ca(2+)-release channels in rat heart. Biochem. J. **352**: 61–70.
15. GHOSHAL, K. et al. 1998. Metallothionein induction in response to restraint stress. Transcriptional control, adaptation to stress, and role of glucocorticoid. J. Biol. Chem. **273**: 27904–27910.
16. ALI, M. et al. 2002. Induction of metallothionein by zinc protects from daunorubicin toxicity in rats. Toxicology **179**: 85.
17. CAMPAGNE, M.V. et al. 2000. Increased binding activity at an antioxidant-responsive element in the metallothionein-1 promoter and rapid induction of metallothionein-1 and -2 in response to cerebral ischemia and reperfusion. J. Neurosci. **20**: 5200–5207.

18. CAI, L. et al. 1999. Metallothionein in radiation exposure: its induction and protective role. Toxicology **132:** 85–98.
19. VANDER HEIDEN, M.G. et al. 2000. Outer mitochondrial membrane permeability can regulate coupled respiration and cell survival. Proc. Natl. Acad. Sci. USA **97:** 4666–4671.
20. LLOYD, H.G. et al. 1988. The transmethylation pathway as a source for adenosine in the isolated guinea-pig heart. Biochem. J. **252:** 489–494.
21. HEADRICK, J., K. CLARKE & R.J. WILLIS. 1989. Adenosine production and energy metabolism in ischaemic and metabolically stimulated rat heart. J. Mol. Cell. Cardiol. **21:** 1089–1100.
22. BUCK, M.J., T.L. SQUIRE & M.T. ANDREWS. 2002. Coordinate expression of the PDK4 gene: a means of regulating fuel selection in a hibernating mammal. Physiol. Genomics **8:** 5–13.
23. INUZUKA, H. et al. 1999. Differential regulation of immediate early gene expression in preadipocyte cells through multiple signaling pathways. Biochem. Biophys. Res. Commun. **265:** 664–668.
24. CAI, Y. et al. 2000. Homocysteine-responsive ATF3 gene expression in human vascular endothelial cells: activation of c-Jun NH(2)-terminal kinase and promoter response element. Blood **96:** 2140–2148.
25. WANG, X.S. et al. 1998. MAPKKK6, a novel mitogen-activated protein kinase kinase kinase, that associates with MAPKKK5. Biochem. Biophys. Res. Commun. **253:** 33–37.
26. TAKEKAWA, M. & H. SAITO. 1998. A family of stress-inducible GADD45-like proteins mediate activation of the stress-responsive MTK1/MEKK4 MAPKKK. Cell **95:** 521–530.
27. SHIDA, M. & S. ISOYAMA. 1993. Effects of age on c-fos and c-myc gene expression in response to hemodynamic stress in isolated, perfused rat hearts. J. Mol. Cell. Cardiol. **25:** 1025–1035.
28. TAKAHASHI, T. et al. 1992. Age-related differences in the expression of proto-oncogene and contractile protein genes in response to pressure overload in the rat myocardium. J. Clin. Invest. **89:** 939–946.

Effects of Age and Caloric Restriction on Brain Neuronal Cell Death/Survival

ASIMINA HIONA AND CHRISTIAAN LEEUWENBURGH

University of Florida, Biochemistry of Aging Laboratory, Gainesville, Florida 32611, USA

ABSTRACT: Aging may pose a challenge to the central nervous system, increasing its susceptibility to apoptotic events. Recent findings indicate that caloric restriction (CR) may have a profound effect on brain function and vulnerability to injury and diseases, by enhancing neuroprotection, stimulating the production of new neurons, and increasing synaptic plasticity. Apoptosis and apoptotic regulatory proteins in the brain frontal cortex of 6-month-old *ad libitum* fed (6AD), 26-month-old *ad libitum* fed (26AD), and 26-month-old caloric-restricted (26CR) male Fischer 344 rats (40% restriction compared to *ad libitum* fed) were investigated. Levels of Poly-ADP ribose polymerase (PARP–DNA repair enzyme; its cleaved 89 kDA fragment is a marker of apoptosis), cytoplasmic histone-associated DNA fragments, and X chromosome–linked inhibitor of apoptosis (XIAP—an endogenous apoptosis inhibitor) were determined. A significant age-associated increase in PARP was found, which was ameliorated in the frontal cortices of the CR rats. No significant differences in cytoplasmic histone-associated DNA fragments with age or with CR were observed. XIAP levels significantly increased with age in the brains of the *ad libitum* animals, while CR animals exhibited the highest levels of this inhibitor compared to all groups. Our findings suggest that caloric restriction may provide neuroprotection to the aging brain by preserving DNA repair enzymes in their intact form, and/or upregulating specific antiapoptotic proteins involved in neuronal cell death.

KEYWORDS: aging; apoptotic events; caloric restriction; neurons; apoptosis

INTRODUCTION

Neuronal apoptosis is the cardinal feature of both acute and chronic neurodegenerative diseases,[1] but its role during normal brain aging needs to be further substantiated. Multiple molecular, cellular, structural, and functional alterations occur in the brain as a result of aging. Increased oxidative damage to lipids, nucleic acids, and aggregation of oxidatively damaged proteins, promote dysfunction of various metabolic and signaling pathways.[2,3] Neurons may also face energy deficits due to cerebral vasculature alterations or mitochondrial dysfunction, with age.[3,4] Examples of

---

Address for correspondence: Christiaan Leeuwenburgh, Ph.D., University of Florida, Biochemistry of Aging Laboratory, Center for Exercise Science, 25 FLG, P.O. Box 118206, Gainesville, FL 32611. Voice: 352-392-9575, ext. 1356; fax: 352-392-0316.
cleeuwen@ufl.edu

Ann. N.Y. Acad. Sci. 1019: 96–105 (2004). © 2004 New York Academy of Sciences.
doi: 10.1196/annals.1297.018

such signaling mechanisms affected by the aging process include protein phosphorylation,[5] protein folding and proteolysis,[6,7] cellular calcium homeostasis,[8] and gene transcription.[9,10] In the normally aging brain, oxidative stress may activate mitochondrial-mediated apoptotic pathways, since mitochondria of aged neurons produce more oxidants, accumulate calcium, and exhibit increased oxidative damage, all known stimuli for apoptosis.[11–14] Moreover, experimental evidence suggests that neuronal loss due to apoptosis may play a role within the brain during normal aging.[14–16] On the other hand, multiple mechanisms exist to maintain the integrity of nerve cell circuits and promote recovery of function after injury. These mechanisms include production of neurotrophic factors and cytokines as well as expression of various cell survival–promoting proteins, for example, Bcl-2 family proteins and inhibitor of apoptosis proteins (IAP), antioxidant enzymes, and protein chaperones.[17]

Interestingly, caloric restriction, a dietary manipulation that increases life span and resistance to various age-related diseases in rodents, also exerts beneficial effects on the brain, including enhanced learning and memory and increased resistance of neurons to excitotoxic, oxidative, and metabolic insults.[18,19] Recently in our laboratory, we demonstrated that CR significantly attenuated the age-associated decline in ARC levels (an apoptosis repressor, which inhibits caspase-2 activity and also attenuates cytochrome c release from the mitochondria) in the brain frontal cortex.[14] We also recently determined that CR had important benefits to skeletal muscle function. Specifically, long-term CR opposed the age-associated decline in muscle mass-to-body mass ratio, and strength-to-body mass ratio in the extensor digitorum longus. Importantly, muscle-specific force of 28-month-old rats was equal to that of 12-month-old AD rats.[20] Moreover, the age-associated increase in extracellular space was reduced with CR. In gastrocnemius muscle, we found that CR suppressed the age-associated rise in the levels of pro- and cleaved caspace-3, and procaspase-12.[21]

Age-related changes in the expression of genes that encode proteins involved in energy metabolism, oxidative stress, and innate immunity, are counteracted by CR.[17] For example, CR attenuates age-related deficits in learning and memory ability and motor function in rodents.[19,22] Furthermore, it can stabilize mitochondrial function and reduce oxidative stress in brain cells.[17,23] Importantly, CR can induce the expression of neurotrophic factors as well as the expression of specific genes that encode proteins that promote neuronal survival and synaptic plasticity, such as Bcl-2 and IAP family proteins, heat shock protein 70 (HSP-70), and glucose regulated protein 78 (GRP-78).[24,25] This amelioration of brain aging at the molecular level may underlie the preservation of brain function during aging in animals maintained on CR.[17]

In the following experiment we examined whether CR could prevent the accumulation of DNA fragmentation in the brain and induce the expression of antiapoptotic regulatory proteins. The proteins investigated are PARP and XIAP. PARP is a 113-kDa multifunctional enzymatic protein involved in numerous biological functions, all of which are associated with the breaking and rejoining of DNA strands, including DNA repair, DNA replication, and genetic recombination.[26–28] This enzyme covalently attaches to and elongates homopolymers of poly-ADP-ribose to a number of nuclear proteins, using NAD, an abundant nucleotide in eukaryotic nuclei, as a substrate.[29] During the execution phase of apoptosis PARP is proteolytically cleaved, and inactivated, by caspases (primarily caspase-3, but also caspase-7) into two fragments, the 24-kDa fragment, containing the N-terminal DNA binding site, and the 89-kDa peptide, comprising the central automodification domain, the C-terminal NAD binding site, and the catalytic domain.[30] XIAP is a member of the IAPs. Among the IAPs, the XIAP is regarded as the most potent suppressor of mammalian cell death through direct binding and inhibition of caspases. Specifically, the BIR12 region of XIAP is a potent and specific inhibitor of caspases-3 and -7, whereas the BIR3 domain is specific for caspase-9.[31]

Apoptosis and CR in the brain have not been extensively investigated, and in light of the capabilities just discussed, the present study attempted to determine the mechanisms of neuronal cell death and survival with age and life-long caloric restriction.

MATERIALS AND METHODS

Animals

Ad libitum fed and caloric-restricted (CR) male Fischer 344 rats were obtained from the National Institute of Aging (NIA) colony (Indianapolis, IN). In the present study, we used 6-month-old *ad libitum* fed (6AD, $n = 8$), 26-month-old *ad libitum* fed (26AD, $n = 7$), and 26-month-old caloric-restricted animals (26CR, $n = 10$). The animals were housed individually at the University of Florida Animal Care Services (Gainesville FL) in a temperature-controlled (18–22°C) environment, under a photoperiod of 12L/12D. For all the CR animals, caloric restriction (10% restriction) started at 3.5 months of age, increased to 25% restriction at 3.75 months, and was maintained at 40% from 4 months of age throughout the animal's life. After 2 weeks of acclimation, the animals were anesthetized with an i.p. injection of sodium pentobarbital solution (Abbot Laboratories, Abbott Park, IL; 5-mg/100-g body weight). The heart was removed first, and immediately after the brain was removed and the frontal cortex was isolated. Body and organ mass were recorded for all animals prior to sacrifice. Nuclear, cytosolic, and mitochondrial proteins were obtained using differential centrifugation.[14] In brief, for cytosolic and mitochondrial extraction, the tissues were homogenized on ice, in a Potter-Elvehjem glass–glass homogenizer (1:10 wt/vol) of ice-cold buffer A (20 mM hepes-KOH [pH 7.5], 250 mM sucrose, 10 mM KCl, 1.5 mM $MgCl_2$, 1 mM EGTA, 1 mM EDTA, 1 mM DTT, and 0.1 mM PMSF). The homogenate was centrifuged at 4000 rpm for 16 min at 4°C. The supernatant was then centrifuged at 13,700 rpm for 11 min. The resulting pellet (mitochondrial fraction) was resuspended in ice-cold buffer A without sucrose and apportioned into several aliquots. The supernatant (cytosol) was also apportioned into several aliquots. Both cytosol and mitochondria were stored at −80°C for further analysis. To obtain nuclear proteins the tissue (~300 mg) was homogenized in 35 mL of ice-cold buffer 1 (10 mM HEPES, [pH to 7.5], 10 mM $MgCl_2$, 5 mM KCl, 0.1 mM EDTA [pH to 8], 0.1% Triton X-100). On the day of extraction, 1 mM DTT, 0.1 mM PMSF, 2 µg/mL aprotinin, and 2 µg/mL leupeptin were added fresh to 500 mL of buffer 1. The homogenate was centrifuged for 5 min at 4000 rpm at 4°C. The resulting pellet was resuspended in 500–1000 µL of ice-cold buffer 2 (20 mM HEPES, [pH to 7.9], 25% glycerol, 500 mM NaCl, 1.5 mM $MgCl_2$, 0.2 mM EDTA, [pH to

8.0]—on the day of extraction, 0.5 mM DTT, 0.2 mM PMSF, 2 μg/mL aprotinin, and 2 μg/mL leupeptin were added fresh to 500 mL of buffer 2), and centrifuged for another 5 min at 4000 rpm. The supernatant (nuclear extract) was transferred to a 5000 nominal molecular weight limit, 4 mL Ultrafree Filter Unit (Millipore, Bedford, MA) and centrifuged for 30 min at 8000 rpm at 4°C. This step concentrates the nuclear protein in the sample.

Determination of PARP Levels, XIAP Content, and Levels of Cytoplasmic Histone-Associated DNA Fragments

Apoptotic DNA fragmentation was quantified by measuring the amount of cytosolic mono- and oligonucleosomes using a "Cell Death Detection ELISA" (Roche diagnostics, GmbH, Germany). All samples were run in triplicate and the means expressed as arbitrary OD units normalized to mg of cytosolic protein, with sample protein concentrations determined by the Bradford method. For quantification of the 89-kDa cleaved fragment of PARP, and XIAP by Western blot analysis, nuclear, and cytosolic proteins, respectively, were separated using 4–20% PAGEr® Gold precast tris-glycine gels (BioWittaker Molecular Applications, Rockland, ME) under denaturing conditions, and transferred to nitrocellulose membranes (0.2 μm, Trans-Blot® Transfer Medium, Bio-Rad Laboratories, Hercules, CA). Membranes were blocked overnight using a blocking solution containing PBS and 5% milk. Protein concentration was determined using the Bradford assay, and subsequently normalized so that the protein content among samples, within a gel, was identical. Subsequently, 20 μL of sample was loaded to each well. A 10-μL HeLa cell lysate sample (Stressgen, Victoria, British Columbia, Canada) was used as a positive control. In this study, we only compared protein bands within an individual gel; therefore, we did not make any across gel comparisons. Membranes were incubated at room temperature for 120 min in the 5% blocking solution containing either the monoclonal mouse primary antibody: PARP (1:200, Oncogene Research Products, Cambridge, MA), or XIAP (1:200, Medical and Biological Laboratories Co., Nagoya City, Japan). Membranes were then incubated for 90 min at room temperature with antimouse Ig horseradish peroxidase-linked whole secondary antibody (1:1000, Amersham Biosciences UK Ltd., Amersham, UK). Specific protein bands were visualized using ECL reagent (Amersham Pharmacia Biotech, Amersham, UK). The resulting Western blots were exposed to film (Hyperfilm™ ECI™, Amersham Pharmacia Biotech, Amersham, UK) and analyzed using the Kodak Imaging System (Kodak 440CF). Values were expressed as arbitrary OD units calculated by multiplying the area of each band by its optical density. Triplicate measurements were taken and the resulting means were used for analysis.

Statistical Analysis

All analyses were performed in triplicate and the means obtained were used for independent t tests. Statistical analyses were carried out using a Graph-pad Prism statistical analysis program (San Diego, CA). Statistical significance was set at $P < .05$. All data are reported as mean ± SEM.

TABLE 1. Body weight and brain mass of male Fischer 344 rats

	6AD	26AD	26CR	P value
Body weight (g)	367.5 ± 5.32	410.4 ± 9.67*	307.1 ± 2.3$^{\#}$	(*P = .0015) ($^{\#}$P < .0001)
Brain mass (g)	1.95 ± 0.015	2.014 ± 0.04	1.93 ± 0.01$^{\#}$	($^{\#}$P = .035)

NOTE: Male Fischer 344 rats (6-month, 6AD, $n = 8$; 26-month 26AD, $n = 7$ *ad libitum* fed; and 26-month calorie-restricted, 26CR $n = 10$).
(*Significantly different from 6AD; # significantly different from 26AD.)

RESULTS

Body and Organ Weight

The body weight of the animals was significantly increased with age (6AD vs. 26AD, $P = .0015$) and significantly decreased by caloric restriction (26AD vs. 26CR, $P < .0001$) (TABLE 1). Brain mass did not alter significantly with age (6AD vs. 26AD, $P = .106$). However, brain weights were significantly lower (~5%) in the 26CR group compared to the age-matched *ad libitum* group, $P = .035$) (TABLE 1).

Mono- and Oligonucleosome Content in Brain with Age and Caloric Restriction

Apoptosis results in the activation of endonucleases that cleave double-stranded DNA between nucleosomes, resulting in cytoplasmic histone-associated DNA fragments (mono- and oligonucleosomes). We quantified the amount of DNA fragmentation in the frontal cortex of 6-month-old AD, 26-month-old AD, and 26-month-old CR animals. No significant differences in cytosolic mono- and oligonucleosome levels were observed with age (6AD vs. 26AD, 1.51 ± 0.22, $n = 8$ vs. 1.02 ± 0.15, $n = 7$, $P = .091$), or with caloric restriction (26AD vs. 26CR, 1.02 ± 0.15, $n = 7$, vs. 0.96 ± 0.098, $n = 9$, $P = .756$). Results (mean ± SEM) are reported as OD/mg of protein.

PARP and XIAP Levels

PARP, a highly conserved nuclear DNA-repair enzyme and marker of apoptosis (the 89-kDa cleaved fragment), as well as XIAP, an inhibitor of apoptosis, specifically caspase-3 and -7, were quantified by Western blotting. Cleaved PARP was significantly elevated in the frontal cortex with age (6AD vs. 26AD, $P = .0056$), while CR significantly attenuated this increase (26AD vs. 26CR, $P = .0015$) (FIG. 1). XIAP levels were significantly increased with age, as well as with caloric restriction (FIG. 2). Older animals expressed higher levels of the inhibitor compared to their younger counterparts (6AD vs. 26AD, $P = .0275$). Similarly, the 26-month-old CR animals exhibited the highest XIAP levels, being significantly different from the 26-month-old AD rats (26AD vs. 26CR, $P = .0496$) (FIG. 2).

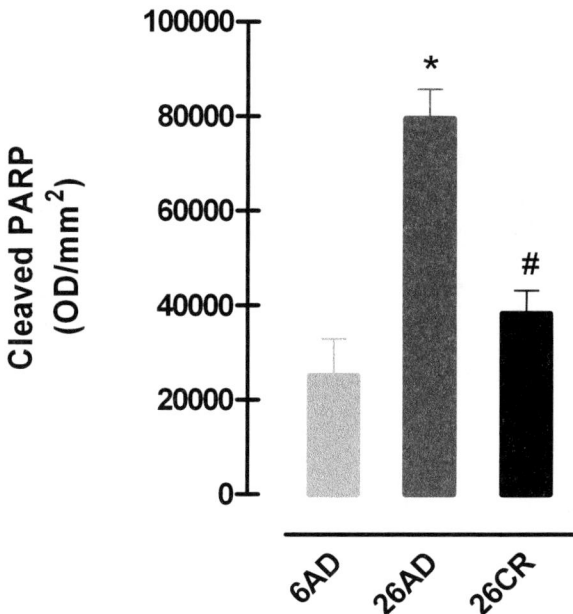

FIGURE 1. Nuclear PARP content (the 89-kDa cleaved fragment) was determined in the frontal cortex of 6-month-old (6AD, $n = 3$), 26-month-old (26AD, $n = 3$) *ad libitum* fed, and 26-month-old caloric-restricted (26CR, $n = 6$) male Fischer 344 rats. PARP content was determined by Western blot analysis, and results (mean ± SEM) are reported as OD/mm^2. 6AD vs. 26AD, *$P = .0056$ ($25,080 \pm 7893$, $n = 3$ vs. $79,450 \pm 6167$, $n = 3$), and 26AD vs. 26CR, #$P = .0015$ ($79,450 \pm 6167$, $n = 3$ vs. $38,290 \pm 4877$, $n = 6$). (*Significantly different from 6AD; #significantly different from 26AD.)

DISCUSSION

Neuronal apoptosis plays an important role in neurodegenerative diseases,[1] yet its contribution to normal brain aging is not clearly defined. On the other hand, caloric restriction has been shown to counteract age-associated changes on gene expression and protein levels that otherwise would be detrimental to brain function, thereby providing greater protection to the central nervous system (CNS).[17] In the present study we examined the effects of age and long-term caloric restriction, compared to *ad libitum* controls, on markers and inhibitors of apoptosis, as well as on direct DNA fragmentation in the brain frontal cortex. The frontal cortex and parts of the hippocampus area, regions involved in learning, memory, and motor coordination, appear to be especially affected by age.[16]

To quantify apoptosis we chose the ELISA technique because of its greater sensitivity in quantifying DNA fragmentation as compared with DNA laddering or the TUNEL method. Moreover, apoptosis is a fairly rapid process in cell culture, but it is unknown how fast this process occurs *in vivo*, and is probably dependent on the cell type, and may take a day or even several days before the entire cell is removed.[14] Therefore, the accuracy of the two latter assays is questionable, since both of them

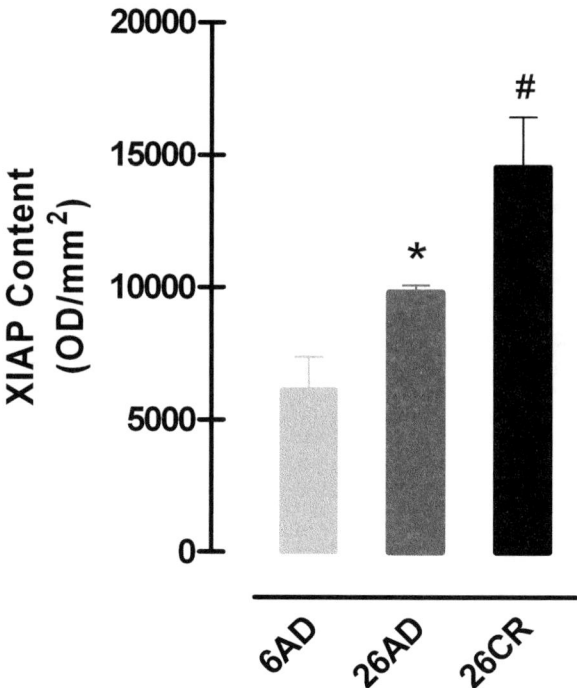

FIGURE 2. We determined cytosolic XIAP content in the frontal cortex of 6-month-old (6AD, $n = 4$), 26-month-old (26AD, $n = 4$) *ad libitum* fed, and 26-month-old caloric-restricted (26CR, $n = 4$) male Fischer 344 rats. XIAP content was determined by Western blot analysis, and results (mean ± SEM) are reported as OD/mm^2. 6AD vs. 26AD, *$P = .0275$ (6125 ± 1244, $n = 4$ vs. 9815 ± 276.6, $n = 4$), and 26AD vs. 26CR, #$P = .0496$ (9815 ± 276.6, $n = 4$ vs. 14,530 ± 1904, $n = 4$). (*Significantly different from 6AD; #significantly different from 26AD.)

indicate a rate of apoptosis so fast that all the cells should have been removed within a few months had that rate persisted.[14] However, we found no significant differences with age or caloric restriction in the levels of cytosolic mono- and oligonucleosomes. A possible explanation for this would be the fact that changes in the rate of apoptosis, as a consequence of aging, are expected to be very small and therefore very difficult to detect, even using the ELISA method. In addition, because apoptosis is a transient phenomenon, and there is evidence of some neuronal regenerative capacity,[32,33] determining the actual rate of apoptosis in a "snap-shot" is a very difficult task. Furthermore, since the entire cortex was homogenized and used to quantify apoptosis, it is very possible that types of neurons not likely to undergo apoptosis may have obscured the results in the direction of nonsignificance in terms of DNA fragmentation. Therefore, the ELISA, although a sensitive tool for the assessment of apoptosis, it may not have been sensitive enough for our purposes. A more sensitive tool may probably be immunohistochemical analysis, staining for specific neurons more prone to apoptosis. This is a possibility we intend to pursue in our laboratory in the near future. On the other hand, there is always the possibility that after development and the early post-natal period, apoptotic levels remain fairly stable throughout the animal's life span, and are probably very little affected, if at all, by caloric restriction. However, the preceding hypothesis still needs to be substantiated.

In light of the limitations just discussed, we examined an indicator–marker of apoptosis, PARP, as well as alterations in the antiapoptotic signaling protein XIAP. PARP appears to be among the earliest death substrates to be cleaved upon induction of apoptosis, and both the 89- and the 24-kDa fragments are used as apoptotic markers.[30] The site of PARP cleavage is located within the nuclear localization signal and is highly conserved. We measured the 89-kDa fragment of PARP in the nuclear fraction. Our results demonstrate a significant elevation in the levels of this fragment in the brain with age, while CR attenuated this increase. While we were not able to detect significant differences in direct DNA fragmentation, the PARP data indicate that DNA damage and programmed cell death are probably induced much more frequently in the old AD animals compared to their young AD or CR counterparts. Thus, one of the ways by which caloric restriction applies its neuroprotective effect may be through maintaining this DNA repair enzyme in its intact, active form.

Further, we investigated XIAP, a member of the IAPs. XIAP applies its protective effect by blocking the activation of caspases (-3, -7, and -9). Besides inhibiting caspases, this protein has been reported to induce active signal transduction pathways mediated by nuclear factor-kB (NFkB), c-Jun aminoterminal kinase, and SMAD-dependent transcription.[34] We found an increase in the XIAP content in the brain with age, which is in agreement with previous findings in our laboratory, in skeletal muscle of old compared to young animals.[21] It appears that increases in oxidative stress and apoptotic events with aging pose the need for increased protection, especially in tissues where cell regeneration is limited.[35–37] Moreover, since both the extrinsic (receptor-mediated pathway) and intrinsic (mitochondrial pathway) cell death pathways require the executioner caspase-3, XIAP can be effective in preventing the induction of either apoptotic pathway. Interestingly, the CR animals exhibited the highest levels of this inhibitor, suggesting an added protection conferred upon caloric restriction on these animals. A possible explanation for this is that neuronal survival factors and neurotrophic factors such as brain-derived neutrophic factor (BDNF), nerve growth factor (NGF), HSP-70, GRP-78, could influence the expression of apoptotic regulatory proteins in the brain, and are upregulated by CR.[18,24,25,38,39] Indeed, mice and rats maintained on dietary restriction have demonstrated increased levels of BDNF,[18,39] NGF,[18] and glial cell line–derived neurotrophic factor in several brain regions.[38] BDNF, NGF, and other neurotrophic factors induced by CR can initiate signal transduction pathways that involve mitogen activated protein kinases (MAPK) and phosphatidyl inositol-3 kinase (PI3 kinase).[38] Activation of such proteins can induce the expression of transcription factors such as NFkB, as well as other genes that encode proteins that suppress oxidative stress (antioxidant enzymes, HSPs), stabilize cellular calcium homeostasis (calcium-regulating proteins), and inhibit apoptosis (IAP and Bcl-2 family proteins).[38] Therefore, the induction of one of the preceding by CR can have as a direct result the upregulation of XIAP in the brain. In fact, it has been shown that the expression of XIAP is under the control of NFkB.[40]

The present study strongly suggests that CR induces neuroprotection in the brain by bolstering the action of antiapoptotic regulatory proteins that could prevent neuronal death. Since the mechanisms of neuroprotection are likely to be intricate, further investigations into those mechanisms, using transgenic models, senescent accelerated animals, and caloric restriction mimetics, need to be conducted to allow targeted interventions for the attenuation of age-related neuronal loss and possibly for the prevention of neurodegenerative diseases.

ACKNOWLEDGMENTS

This research was supported by grants from The National Institute of Health, and the National Institute of Aging AG17994, AG 10485, and AG 21042. We thank Dr. Suma Kendaiah for her technical assistance and expertise and Dr. Barry Drew for a critical reading and editing of the manuscript.

REFERENCES

1. YUAN, J. & B.A. YANKNER. 2000. Apoptosis in the nervous system. Nature **407:** 802–809.
2. LEBEL, C.P. & S.C. BONDY. 1992. Oxidative damage and cerebral aging. Prog. Neurobiol. **38:** 601–609.
3. MATTSON, M.P. *et al.* 2002. Neuroprotective and neurorestorative signal transduction mechanisms in brain aging: modification by genes, diet and behavior. Neurobiol. Aging **23:** 695–705.
4. HOYER, S. 1995. Age-related changes in cerebral oxidative metabolism. Implications for drug therapy. Drugs Aging **6:** 210-218.
5. JIN, L.W. & T. SAITOH. 1995. Changes in protein kinases in brain aging and Alzheimer's disease. Implications for drug therapy. Drugs Aging **6:** 136–149.
6. GRUNE, T. *et al.* 2001. Age-related changes in protein oxidation and proteolysis in mammalian cells. J. Gerontol. A Biol. Sci. Med. Sci. **56:** B459–B467.
7. KUMAR, V.B. *et al.* 2000. Identification of age-dependent changes in expression of senescence-accelerated mouse (SAMP8) hippocampal proteins by expression array analysis. Biochem. Biophys. Res. Commun. **272:** 657–661.
8. MATTSON, M.P. 1992. Calcium as sculptor and destroyer of neural circuitry. Exp. Gerontol. **27:** 29–49.
9. PROLLA, T.A. 2002. DNA microarray analysis of the aging brain. Chem. Senses **27:** 299–306.
10. LEE, C.K., R. WEINDRUCH & T.A. PROLLA. 2000. Gene-expression profile of the ageing brain in mice. Nat. Genet. **25:** 294–297.
11. SOHAL, R.S. & U.T. BRUNK. 1992. Mitochondrial production of pro-oxidants and cellular senescence. Mutat. Res. **275:** 295–304.
12. SOHAL, R.S. *et al.* 1994. Oxidative damage, mitochondrial oxidant generation and antioxidant defenses during aging and in response to food restriction in the mouse. Mech. Ageing Dev. **74:** 121–133.
13. POLLACK, M. *et al.* 2002. The role of apoptosis in the normal aging brain, skeletal muscle, and heart. Ann. N.Y. Acad. Sci. **959:** 93–107.
14. SHELKE, R.R. & C. LEEUWENBURGH. 2003. Lifelong caloric restriction increases expression of apoptosis repressor with a caspase recruitment domain (ARC) in the brain. FASEB J. **17:** 494–496.
15. MORRISON, J.H. & P.R. HOF. 1997. Life and death of neurons in the aging brain. Science **278:** 412–419.
16. MATTSON, M.P. 2000. Apoptosis in neurodegenerative disorders. Nat. Rev. Mol. Cell Biol. **1:** 120–129.
17. MATTSON, M.P., S.L. CHAN & W. DUAN. 2002. Modification of brain aging and neurodegenerative disorders by genes, diet, and behavior. Physiol. Rev. **82:** 637–672.

18. DUAN, W., Z. GUO & M.P. MATTSON. 2001. Brain-derived neurotrophic factor mediates an excitoprotective effect of dietary restriction in mice. J. Neurochem. **76**: 619–626.
19. INGRAM, D.K. et al. 1987. Dietary restriction benefits learning and motor performance of aged mice. J. Gerontol. **42**: 78–81.
20. PAYNE, A.M., S.L. DODD & C. LEEUWENBURGH. 2003. Life-long calorie restriction in Fischer-344 rats attenuates age related loss in skeletal muscle specific force and reduces extracellular space. J. Appl. Physiol. **96**: 938-942.
21. DIRKS, A. & C. LEEUWENBURGH. 2004. Aging and life-long calorie restriction result in adaptations of skeleteal muscle apoptosis repressor (ARC), apoptosis inducing factor (AIF), X-linked inhibitor-of-apoptosis (XIAP), caspase-3 and caspase-12. Free Radic. Biol. Med. **36**: 27–39.
22. STEWART, J., J. MITCHELL & N. KALANT. 1989. The effects of life-long food restriction on spatial memory in young and aged Fischer 344 rats measured in the eight-arm radial and the Morris water mazes. Neurobiol. Aging **10**: 669–675.
23. GUO, Z. et al. 2000. Beneficial effects of dietary restriction on cerebral cortical synaptic terminals: preservation of glucose and glutamate transport and mitochondrial function after exposure to amyloid beta-peptide, iron, and 3-nitropropionic acid. J. Neurochem. **75**: 314–320.
24. YU, Z.F. & M.P. MATTSON. 1999. Dietary restriction and 2-deoxyglucose administration reduce focal ischemic brain damage and improve behavioral outcome: evidence for a preconditioning mechanism. J. Neurosci. Res. **57**: 830–839.
25. DUAN, W. & M.P. MATTSON. 1999. Dietary restriction and 2-deoxyglucose administration improve behavioral outcome and reduce degeneration of dopaminergic neurons in models of Parkinson's disease. J. Neurosci. Res. **57**: 195–206.
26. BURKLE, A. 2001. Physiology and pathophysiology of poly(ADP-ribosyl)ation. Bioessays **23**: 795–806.
27. JEGGO, P.A. 1998. DNA repair: PARP—another guardian angel? Curr. Biol. **8**: R49–R51.
28. SIMBULAN-ROSENTHAL, C.M. et al. 1998. Transient poly(ADP-ribosyl)ation of nuclear proteins and role of poly(ADP-ribose) polymerase in the early stages of apoptosis. J. Biol. Chem. **273**: 13703–13712.
29. ROSENTHAL, D.S. et al. 1997. Detection of DNA breaks in apoptotic cells utilizing the DNA binding domain of poly(ADP-ribose) polymerase with fluorescence microscopy. Nucleic Acids Res. **25**: 1437–1441.
30. KANKOFER, M. & L. GUZ. 2003. Is poly(ADP-ribose) polymerase involved in bovine placental retention? Domest. Anim. Endocrinol. **25**: 61–67.
31. WU, T.Y. et al. 2003. Development and characterization of nonpeptidic small molecule inhibitors of the XIAP/caspase-3 interaction. Chem. Biol. **10**: 759–767.
32. GAGE, F.H. 2000. Mammalian neural stem cells. Science **287**: 1433–1438.
33. SONG, H.J., C.F. STEVENS & F.H. GAGE. 2002. Neural stem cells from adult hippocampus develop essential properties of functional CNS neurons. Nat. Neurosci. **5**: 438–445.
34. SALVESEN, G.S. & C.S. DUCKETT. 2002. IAP proteins: blocking the road to death's door. Nat. Rev. Mol. Cell Biol. **3**: 401–410.
35. PHANEUF, S. & C. LEEUWENBURGH. 2002. Cytochrome c release from mitochondria in the aging heart: a possible mechanism for apoptosis with age. Am. J. Physiol. Regul. Integr. Comp. Phy siol. **282**: R423–R430.
36. POLLACK, M. & C. LEEUWENBURGH. 2001. Apoptosis and aging: role of the mitochondria. J. Gerontol. A Biol. Sci. Med. Sci. **56**: B475–B482.
37. DIRKS, A. & C. LEEUWENBURGH. 2002. Apoptosis in skeletal muscle with aging. Am. J. Physiol. Regul. Integr. Comp. Physiol. **282**: R519–R527.
38. MATTSON, M.P., W. DUAN & Z. GUO. 2003. Meal size and frequency affect neuronal plasticity and vulnerability to disease: cellular and molecular mechanisms. J. Neurochem. **84**: 417–431.
39. LEE, J. et al. 2000. Dietary restriction increases the number of newly generated neural cells, and induces BDNF expression, in the dentate gyrus of rats. J. Mol. Neurosci. **15**: 99–108.
40. STEHLIK, C. et al. 1998. Nuclear factor (NF)-kappaB-regulated X-chromosome-linked iap gene expression protects endothelial cells from tumor necrosis factor alpha-induced apoptosis. J. Exp. Med. **188**: 211–216.

Acute Coronary Syndrome, Comorbidity, and Mortality in Geriatric Patients

E. TANEVA, V. BOGDANOVA, AND N. SHTEREVA[a]

Clinic of Cardiology, Intensive Care, Medical University, Sofia1431, Bulgaria
[a]Department of Ethics, Faculty of Public Health, Medical University, Sofia, Bulgaria

ABSTRACT: Morbidity and mortality rates from heart diseases are highly represented in geriatric-aged patients, but these patients also have supporting diseases. Acute coronary syndrome includes unstable angina and acute myocardial infarction with and without ST elevation. The aim of this study was to make a retrospective morbidity analysis of patients admitted to the emergency department. The study is made for a period of three years (from 1998 to 2000). It includes 588 patients divided by age (395 were 65–75 years old; 193 were older than 75 years) and sex (there were 326 men and 262 women). Comorbidity and mortality were investigated. Patients with one, two, three, and more than three supporting diseases were 6.29%, 23.13%, 68.53%, and 2.04%, respectively, of the total number. The most frequent geriatric patients had heart failure, followed by endocrinological diseases (type 2 diabetes, obesity, struma), neurological diseases (insultus, paresis), and chronic kidney diseases (pielonephritis, nephrolithiasis). The combination of hypertension, heart failure, and type 2 diabetes had the highest comorbidity frequency. The mortality rate for 1998 was 8.81%, for 1999 7.74%, and for 2000 13.41%. The mortality rate at the first 12 hours at the beginning of the acute coronary syndrome was 66.6%. Geriatric patients suffer from many diseases, and at the beginning of the onset of acute coronary syndrome they have multiorganal failure. Elderly patients are a high-risk contingent in intensive coronary care units.

KEYWORDS: geriatrics; acute coronary syndrome; morbidity; comorbidity; mortality

Acute coronary syndrome (ACS) is a major healthcare problem and represents a large number of the annual hospitalizations in Bulgaria. ACS includes unstable angina (UA) and myocardial infarction with or without ST elevation. There are degenerative changes with the advance in age that are connected with the aging of the organism. These changes are mostly seen in cardiovascular and nervous systems, also in kidneys and liver. Morbidity and mortality rates from ACS are increased in geriatric patients, because of the presence of already existed abnormalities, which complicate the proceeding of the disease and its outcome. Because of demographic changes and the increased prevalence of coronary artery disease in adults and elderly patients, the number of those at risk is increasing. The geriatric patients with ACS and certain comorbidities require special attention and follow-up by a clinician.

Address for correspondence: E. Taneva, Clinic of Cardiology, Intensive Care, Medical University, 1, Georgi Sofiiski strasse, Sofia1431, Bulgaria.
etaneva_md@yahoo.com

The aim of this study was to make a retrospective analysis of the geriatric patients with ACS, comorbidity, and mortality.

MATERIALS AND METHODS

The study was for a period of three years (1998–2000) in the Intensive Coronary Care Unit of the Medical University, Sofia. It included 588 geriatric patients with ACS (42.86% for 1998, 47.06% for 1999, and 45.79% for 2000) from the total number of registered patients. They are divided by age, sex, and diagnosis as is shown in TABLE 1.

The patients were admitted to the emergency department with chest pain, electrocardiogram, repeat measurements of markers of myocardial necrosis (creatininkinase–MB) for ACS. All patients received antiischemical, anticoagulation, and antiplatelet therapy. An additional and symptomatic (sedatives, antianxyolitics) therapy was used according to comorbidity. In patients with ST elevation and those being hospitalized in the first 12 hours of the syndrome's beginning, a fibrinolythic therapy with streptokinase and invasive treatment for revascularization was made in six patients. The correlation of morbidity rates from ACS between male and female patients was examined. The type and number of already existing diseases were investigated on the basis of the anamnesis, clinical examinations, and other investigations (e.g., echocardiography, angiography). The mortality rate of geriatric patients from each age group was noted as was the mortality rate at the first 12 hours after entrance into the hospital.

RESULTS

The geriatric patients had pre-existing and supporting diseases, divided into types: hypertension, heart failure, arrhythmias and disarrhythmias, recurring myocardial infarction, patients with chronic pulmonary disease, endocrinological diseases (type 2 diabetes, struma, obesity), cardiogenic shock, nervous diseases (insultus, paresis, morbus Parkinson), nephrological diseases (nephrolithiasis, pielonephritis), orthopedic diseases (ankylosis, endoprosthesis, kiphoscoliosis), oncological diseases, ophthalmologic diseases (glaucoma, cataracta), and other.

Although these symptoms might not appear in the prehospital condition of the patients, during the disease course, arrhythmias, dysarrhythmias, recent type 2 diabetes, and hypertension may present themselves.

TABLE 1 shows the number of geriatric patients and the number of comorbid diseases. It is obvious that there are fewer patients with more than three accompanying diseases. Those with three diseases (hypertension, heart failure, and type 2 diabetes) are the most frequently seen patients. From our results, we conclude that the total number of geriatric patients and of those with three accompanying diseases has expanded.

The frequency of the comorbidity is shown in TABLE 1 as percentages; those with two diseases were 23.13%, with one disease 6.29%, and with more than three diseases 2.04%. The geriatric patients with ACS and three supporting diseases made up

TABLE 1. Division of patients according to demographic indices, number of comorbidity patients, and frequency of comorbidity and mortality

Year	Diagnosis Age	Acute Coronary Syndrome							Ratio	Total geriatric patients	Comorbidity				Mortality percentage
		Unstable angina		MI without ST elevation		MI with ST elevation		M:F		1 disease	2 diseases	3 diseases	< 3 diseases	
		M	F	M	F	M	F							
1998	Over 65	35	27	14	9	3	2	1.41	159	12	45	98	4	8.81%
	Over 75	18	8	16	12	4	1	1.26						
1999	Over 65	24	21	25	20	7	3	1.27	168	10	40	116	2	7.74%
	Over 75	18	17	13	11	6	3	1.19						
2000	Over 65	47	37	33	28	12	10	1.23	261	15	51	189	6	13.41%
	Over 75	34	24	11	10	8	7	1.29						
Total		17 6	14 4	112	90	40	26	1.275	588	37	136	403	12	9.98%

68.53% of all geriatric patients. The highest comorbidity frequency was for the combination of hypertension, heart failure, and type 2 diabetes.

Geriatric mortality rates are shown in TABLE 1 as percentages. There was no significant difference in the analysis of the mortality rates in adults (older than 65 years) and elderly patients (older than 75 years), so the mortality rates are displayed in general. Note that for the last year of our investigation (2000) the mortality rate was almost doubled.

The calculated mortality rate at the first 12 hours after the hospitalization of the geriatric patient is significant, at an average of 66.67%. There was no significant difference in the analysis of the mortality rates during the single years of the investigated period.

DISCUSSION

According to the number of diseases, pre-existing abnormalities, and mortality rates,[1,5,7,8,10] there was no important difference in the patient groups (adults older than 65 and elderly adults older than 75) in our investigation. They are more likely to have cardiac and noncardiac comorbidities. These include a diminished beta-sympathetic arterial compliance and arterial hypertension, cardiac hypertrophy, and ventricular dysfunction, especially systolic dysfunction.

Hypertension occurs in the more than two thirds of individuals after the age of 65.[4,9] This is also the population with the lowest rates of blood pressure control. The highest comorbidity rates are in geriatric patients with ACS. Most of the patients in our country have long-lasting arterial hypertension, systematically untreated because of financial and health-related problems (preparedness and the beginning of health reform in our country was in 2000).

Heart failure is an increasing problem. Of patients with ACS, 37.62% also suffer from heart failure, determined clinically and with Ro-graphy and echocardiography. Heart failure is presumed to be caused by systolic dysfunction (ejection fraction is <50%). The results indicate that the main etiological factor for heart failure was coronary heart disease, a finding that is expected and is in keeping with other studies.[6] Hypertension was still an important factor, being the second most common underlying cause.

In geriatric patients with ACS and type 2 diabetes, inflammation and infection of atheromatous plaque and plaque rupture occurs that can cause angina or myocardial infarction. Patients with diabetes mellitus represent a higher risk group of patients after both percutaneous and surgical coronary revascularization and the decision regarding the choice of revascularization procedure.

Mortality rates in both groups (older than 65 and older than 75 years) were almost equal, so they were represented as a general mortality rate. When adjusted for these risk factors,[2–4] age (i.e., a comparison of patients older than 75 years with those from 65 to 74 years old) is not a significant risk factor. There is greater likelihood of comorbidity and mortality rates for cardiac events and interventions in this population. The high mortality rate in geriatric patients during the first 12 hours is defined from ACS and severity and number of the comorbidity.

CONCLUSIONS

Geriatric patients suffer from many diseases, and at the beginning of onset of ACS they experience multiorganal failure. Elderly patients are a high-risk contingent in the intensive coronary care unit.

Although there are many scores and different types of indices that are used to diagnose ACS in geriatric patients, there is no index in which presence or absence may define the sure outcome of this disease in each patient. Of course, the geriatric patients are in a high-risk category, because of their age.

With so many mechanistically different approaches to the management of ACS, clinicians have reason for optimism that continued progress will further reduce the morbidity, comorbidity, and mortality in the coming years.

REFERENCES

1. ALLEN, K.B. et al. 1999. Comparison of transmyocardial revascularization with medical therapy in patients with refractory angina. N. Engl. J. Med. **341**: 1029–1030.
2. BARRABES, J.A., J. FIGUERAS, C. MOURE, et al. 2003. Prognostic value of lead aVR in patients with a first non-ST-segment elevation acute myocardial infarction. Circulation **108**: 814–819.
3. BARTHEL, P., R. SCHNEIDER, A. BAUER, et al. 2003. Risk stratification after acute myocardial infarction by heart rate turbulence. Circulation **108**: 1221.
4. BRAUNWALD, E. et al. 2002. ACC/AHA Guideline update for the management of patients with unstable angina and non-ST-segment elevation myocardial infarction. A Report of the American College of Cardiology/American Heart Association Task Force on Practice Guidelines (Committee on the Management of Patients with Unstable Angina).
5. CHEN, E.W. et al. 2003. Relation between hospital intra-aortic balloon contarpulsation volume and mortality in acute myocardial infarction complicated by cardiogenic shock. Circulation **108**: 95.
6. CHEN, Y.-T., V. VACCARINO, C.S. WILLIAMS, et al. 1999. Risk factors for heart failure in the elderly: a prospective community-based study. Am. J. Med. **106**: 605–612.
7. NASH, D.T. 2003. Outcome of medical vs invasive therapy for elderly patients with angina. JAMA **289**: 1117–1123.
8. KENCHAIAH, S. et al. 2002. Obesity and the risk of heart failure. N. Engl. J. Med. **347**: 303–313.
9. PSATY, B.M., T.A. MANOLIO, N.L. SMUTH, et al. 2002. Time trends in high blood pressure control and the use of antihypertensive medications in older adults. Arch. Intern. Med. **162**: 2325–2332.
10. MANSON, J.E., G.A. COLDITZ, M.J. STAMPFER, et al. 1990. A prospective study of obesity and risk of coronary heart disease in women. N. Engl. J. Med. **322**: 882–889.

Differential Regulation of Telomerase in Endothelial Cells by Fibroblast Growth Factor–2 and Vascular Endothelial Growth Factor–A

Association with Replicative Life Span

ELISABETH TRIVIER,[a] DAVID J. KURZ,[b] YING HONG,[a] HSIU-LIN HUANG,[a] AND JORGE D. ERUSALIMSKY[a]

[a]*Cell Biology Group, Department of Medicine, University College London, London, United Kingdom*

[b]*Cardiovascular Research, Institute of Physiology, University of Zurich, and Cardiology, University Hospital, Zurich, Switzerland*

ABSTRACT: In cultured human umbilical vein endothelial cells (HUVECs), fibroblast growth factor–2 (FGF-2), but not vascular endothelial growth factor–A (VEGF-A), upregulates telomerase activity. Here, we examined the functional significance of this differential regulation on the replicative life span of HUVECs. HUVECs were serially passaged until senescence under four different conditions: (1) EGM-2, a medium containing both VEGF-A and FGF-2; (2) basal medium (BM), consisting of EGM-2 devoid of FGF-2 and VEGF-A; (3) BM supplemented with FGF-2; and (4) BM supplemented with VEGF-A. Cells cultured in BM demonstrated decreased growth rate and ceased to proliferate at ~15 population doublings (PDs), whereas those cultured with VEGF-A alone initially proliferated vigorously but arrested growth abruptly at a PD level comparable with cultures grown in BM. In contrast, cells maintained in EGM-2 or in BM/FGF-2 attained a normal replicative life span (~40 PDs). These differences in replicative behavior were reflected by the early appearance of a senescent phenotype in cultures grown in BM or BM/VEGF-A. HUVECs grown in the presence of VEGF-A alone have a decreased life span compared with cultures maintained with FGF-2. This suggests that the upregulation of telomerase activity by FGF-2, an effect not achieved with VEGF-A, plays a functional role in preventing the early onset of senescence.

KEYWORDS: endothelial cell; senescent cell; β-galactosidase

Like most other somatic cells, normal human endothelial cells (ECs) are endowed with a limited replicative capacity, a property that is manifested on serial passage in culture. When this potential is exhausted, ECs enter into a permanent nondividing state referred to as replicative senescence. Human ECs have been reported to prolif-

Address for correspondence: Jorge D. Erusalimsky, Department of Medicine, UCL, 5 University Street, London WC1E 6JJ, UK. Voice: +44-0-2076796613; fax: +44-0-2076796212.
j.erusalimsky@ucl.ac.uk

erate vigorously in culture for up to 30 to 50 population doublings before their growth rate slows down and senescence begins to occur.[1] ECs undergoing senescence in culture show characteristic changes in morphology, such as an increase in size, polymorphic nuclei, and vacuolization,[1,2] as well as alterations in gene expression reminiscent of a proinflammatory/prothrombotic phenotype.[3,4] Furthermore, in common with other senescent cell types,[5] ECs show positive staining for senescence-associated β-galactosidase (SA-β-gal), a result of an increase in their lysosomal mass.[2] Because a similar pattern of morphological and functional alterations is also found in ECs from human atherosclerotic plaques, the occurrence of endothelial cell senescence *in vivo* is thought to directly contribute to the progression of atherosclerosis and its clinical sequelae.[6]

At the mechanistic level, replicative senescence has been linked to the erosion of telomeric DNA.[7] The G-rich strand of telomeric DNA is synthesized by a specialized reverse transcriptase called telomerase.[7] Telomerase activity plays an important role in determining the onset of replicative senescence by counteracting telomere erosion. In addition, there is evidence to suggest that the elongation of telomeres is not the only function of telomerase. Its binding to the telomere could be essential to form a complete telomere cap and could also signal for cell survival in replicating cells.[7] Furthermore, very low levels of telomerase appear to fulfill an active role in maintaining cellular replicative capacity by a mechanism that preserves telomere function independently of telomere length maintenance.[8]

In human postnatal life, besides its pathological upregulation in many tumor cells, telomerase activity can be readily detected in the germ line, in activated lymphocytes, and in some somatic tissues that undergo proliferative renewal. In most other somatic cells, however, telomerase is repressed or expressed at very low levels. Conflicting views exist as to whether human endothelial cells express telomerase,[9,10] probably because activity levels are low. In our own studies, we have shown that telomerase activity is virtually absent in cells freshly isolated from the aortic or umbilical vein endothelium, where the cells are normally maintained in a quiescent state, but is markedly upregulated when the same cells are placed in culture and stimulated to proliferate.[10] While cells are actively growing, telomerase activity is maintained at a relatively constant level, whereas culture conditions leading to quiescence result in a significant and completely reversible downregulation of telomerase activity.[10] Examination of the impact of individual endothelial mitogens with known proangiogenic properties demonstrated that fibroblast growth factor–2 (FGF-2), but not vascular endothelial growth factor–A (VEGF-A), was able to restore telomerase activity in human endothelial cells in a time- and dose-dependent manner. Reverse transcriptase polymerase chain reaction analysis revealed that this differential regulation of telomerase activity occurred primarily at the transcriptional level, with FGF-2, but not VEGF-A, upregulating the mRNA levels of hTERT (the catalytic subunit of telomerase), and of the *hTERT* gene transactivation factor Sp1. In contrast, mRNA levels for c-Myc, a second important *hTERT* transactivation factor, were equally upregulated by FGF-2 and VEGF-A, whereas mRNA levels of Max and Mad1, a repressor of *hTERT* expression, were not influenced by the proliferative status of endothelial cells.[10] These findings suggest that Sp1 and c-Myc both must be upregulated and need to cooperate at their respective binding sites in the *hTERT* core promoter region to enable successful *hTERT* transactivation. Whether the upregulation of telomerase by FGF-2 plays a role in the maintenance of EC replicative capacity is currently unclear. Here, we report the functional significance of the differential effects of FGF-2 and VEGF-A on the growth kinetics and replicative life span of normal human ECs.

Human umbilical vein endothelial cells (HUVECs) were serially passaged in culture until the onset of senescence under several culture conditions: (1) endothelial growth medium-2 (EGM-2, Biowhittaker), a commercially available complete medium consisting of modified CCMD130 medium supplemented with 2% fetal calf serum, hydrocortisone, R^3-insulin-like growth factor–1, human epidermal growth factor, heparin, ascorbic acid, gentamycin, amphotericin B, VEGF-A, and FGF-2; (2) basal medium (BM) consisting of EGM-2 devoid of FGF-2 and VEGF-A but containing all the other supplements; (3), BM supplemented with 20 ng/mL FGF-2; and (4) BM supplemented with 20 ng/mL VEGF-A. At each passage, population doublings (PDs) were calculated using the formula PD = $\log_2$ ([number of cells harvested]/[number of cells seeded × attachment efficiency]). Cytochemical staining for SA-β-gal was performed as previously described.[1]

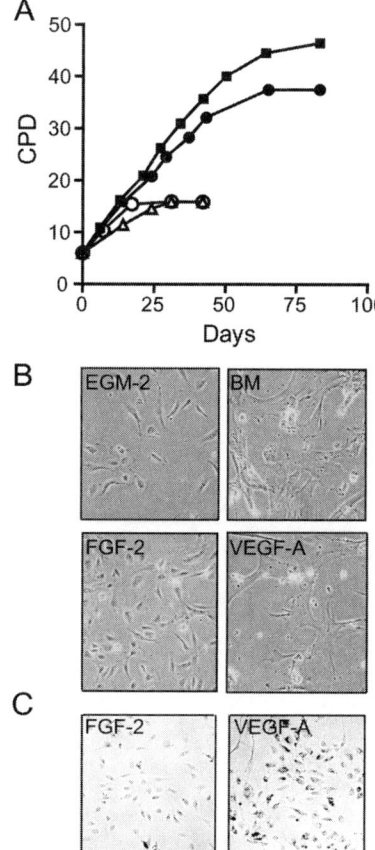

FIGURE 1. Effect of FGF-2 and VEGF-A on the replicative life span of HUVECs. (**A**) Cumulative population doublings (CPDs) of serially passaged HUVECs in EGM-2 (●, complete endothelial growth medium), BM (△, EGM-2 without FGF-2 and VEGF-A), FGF-2 (■, BM + 20 ng/mL FGF-2), and VEGF-A (○, BM + 20 ng/mL VEGF-A). (**B**) Phase contrast photomicrographs (original magnification ×200) of HUVECs cultured as in **A**. Cells in BM and VEGF-A underwent ~15 CPDs, and cells in EGM-2 and FGF-2 underwent ~30 CPDs. (**C**) Bright-field photomicrographs showing SA-β-gal staining of HUVECs cultured in BM + 20 ng/mL FGF-2 (FGF-2) or BM + 20 ng/mL VEGF-A (VEGF-A) at 31 CPDs and 16 CPDs, respectively.

As shown in FIGURE 1A, cultures grown in the absence of FGF-2 and VEGF-A (BM) demonstrated a markedly decreased rate of replication and ceased to proliferate at an early replicative age. Consistent with the mitogenic properties of VEGF-A, HUVECs treated with saturating concentrations of this growth factor proliferated vigorously during initial passages, with a rate comparable to that of cultures grown in EGM-2 or in BM + FGF-2. However, after this initial stage proliferation ceased abruptly, so that VEGF-A –treated cultures reached the same replicative life span as those grown in BM. In contrast, cells maintained in EGM-2 or in BM supplemented with 20 ng/mL FGF-2 attained a normal replicative life span (35–45 PDs). These differences in replicative behavior were accompanied by substantial morphological differences between the four culture conditions (FIG. 1B). Thus, cells grown in media containing FGF-2 (either EGM-2 or FGF-2) still retained a typical cobblestone morphology when the cultures reached ~30 PDs. In contrast, at ~15 PDs, cultures grown in BM or in the presence of VEGF-A displayed characteristic features of senescence such as an increase in cell size, an irregular veil-like cell shape, and numerous binucleated cells. Furthermore, in cultures treated with BM or BM + VEGF-A, a large proportion of cells stained positive for SA-β-gal, whereas cultures grown in the presence of EGM-2 or FGF-2 showed a low frequency of SA-β-gal–positive cells (FIG. 1C and data not shown).

In this work, we have shown that cultures grown in the presence of VEGF-A alone, in contrast with FGF-2, rapidly accumulate cells displaying a senescent phenotype. This suggests that the upregulation of telomerase activity by FGF-2, an effect not achieved with VEGF-A, plays a functional role in preventing the early onset of senescence. This association may be the mechanistic basis for the long-known observation that human umbilical vein endothelial cells are more fastidious in their growth requirements than other large-vessel endothelial cells and require the presence of FGF-2 to maintain long-term culture. Furthermore, our findings are consistent with results from other laboratories showing that (1) FGF-2 prolongs the life span of endothelial cells in culture,[11] (2) overexpression of telomerase enables normal human cells, including endothelial cells, to delay or escape senescence,[9] and (3) disruption of endogenous telomerase in normal human fibroblasts induces premature senescence.[8]

ACKNOWLEDGMENTS

Drs. Trivier, Hong, and Erusalimsky received grant support from the British Heart Foundation. Dr. Kurz received grant support from the Swiss National Science Foundation and the Swiss Heart Foundation.

REFERENCES

1. VAN DER LOO, B., M.J. FENTON & J.D. ERUSALIMSKY. 1998. Cytochemical detection of a senescence-associated β-galactosidase in endothelial and smooth muscle cells from human and rabbit blood vessels. Exp. Cell Res. **241:** 309–315.
2. KURZ, D.J., S. DECARY, Y. HONG, et al. 2000. Senescence-associated β-galactosidase reflects an increase in lysosomal mass during replicative ageing of human endothelial cells. J. Cell Sci. **113:** 3613–3622.

3. MAIER, J.A.M., M. STATUTO & G. RAGNOTTI. 1993. Senescence stimulates U937-endothelial cell interactions. Exp. Cell Res. **208:** 270–274.
4. COMI, P., R. CHIARAMONTE & J.A.M. MAIER. 1995. Senescence-dependent regulation of type 1 plasminogen activator inhibitor in human vascular endothelial cells. Exp. Cell Res. **219:** 304–308.
5. DIMRI, G.P., X. LEE, G. BASILE, et al. 1995. A biomarker that identifies senescent human cells in culture and in aging skin in vivo. Proc. Natl. Acad. Sci. USA **92:** 9363–9367.
6. MINAMINO, T. & I. KOMURO. 2002. Role of telomere in endothelial dysfunction in atherosclerosis. Cur. Opin. Lipidol. **13:** 537–543.
7. BLACKBURN, E.H. 2001. Switching and signalling at the telomere. Cell **106:** 661–673.
8. MASUTOMI, K., E.Y. YU, S. KHURTS, et al. 2003. Telomerase maintains telomere structure in normal human cells. Cell **114:** 241–253.
9. YANG, J., E. CHANG, A.M. CHERRY, et al. 1999. Human endothelial cell life extension by telomerase expression. J. Biol. Chem. **274:** 26141–26148.
10. 10. KURZ, D.J., Y. HONG, E. TRIVIER, et al. 2003. Fibroblast growth factor-2, but not vascular endothelial growth factor, upregulates telomerase activity in human endothelial cells. Arterioscler. Thromb. Vasc. Biol. **23:** 748–754.
11. AUGUSTIN-VOSS, H.G., A.K. VOSS & B.U. PAULI. 1993. Senescence of aortic endothelial cells in culture: effects of basic fibroblast growth factor expression on cell phenotype, migration, and proliferation. J. Cell Physiol. **157:** 279–288.

Interleukin-7

An Interleukin for Rejuvenating the Immune System

RICHARD ASPINALL, SIAN HENSON, JEFFREY PIDO-LOPEZ,
AND PA TAMBA NGOM

*Department of Immunology, Faculty of Medicine, Imperial College,
London SW10 9NH, United Kingdom*

ABSTRACT: Infection of an individual (aged 20–30 years) by a virus will cause a response from the T (thymus derived) lymphocytes of which there are approximately 3×10^{11}. If the individual has not met the virus before, the response will come from the naive T cell subset (50 ± 10% of the total T cell pool at this age) containing recent thymic emigrants produced from the thymus at approximately 10^8 per day. Their antigen-specific receptor has a defined specificity governed by the conformation of its two chains (α and β), and the repertoire of specificities is somewhere in the region of 2×10^7 to 10^8. A successful response leads to clonal expansion and the generation of memory T cells to the infecting agent.

KEYWORDS: aging; antigen-specific receptor; T cell

Aging is accompanied by thymic atrophy, a reduction in thymic output, and a consequent reduction in the naive T cell pool. This is not accompanied by a reduction in the absolute number of T cells because of the expansion of the memory T cell subset. Successive rounds of division within this subset may be responsible for the accrual of defects and the accumulation of senescent cells. Within the thymus, age-related thymic atrophy is accompanied by a decline in the production of interleukin-7 (IL-7), a cytokine known to have an essential role in T cell development. Therapeutic intervention with IL-7 in old mice increases both the size of the thymus and its subsequent output benefiting the functional performance of the T cells in the peripheral T cell pool.

COMPONENTS OF A SUCCESSFUL IMMUNE RESPONSE

An infectious agent once breaching the defenses of the body may be picked up by an antigen-presenting cell (probably a dendritic cell), which will migrate to secondary lymphoid tissue (local lymph nodes) and present peptides held in the cleft of the expressed MHC molecule from the infectious agent to T cells. A T cell with the receptor with the correct configuration will interact strongly with this peptide + MHC

Address for correspondence: Richard Aspinall, Department of Immunology, Faculty of Medicine, Imperial College, London SW10 9NH, UK.
r.aspinall@ic.ac.uk

complex and, providing a costimulatory signal is received, will become activated. This state of activation is accompanied by cell enlargement, a change in the expression of surface proteins, alteration in gene expression, and the production of several cytokines. Successful activation is followed by clonal expansion, providing more cells with the appropriate receptor specific for the infectious agent. The activation cascade leads to the activation and expansion of effector lymphocytes, which may be cytotoxic T cells, responsible for killing cells in which the infective agent has become housed, or B cells, which may produce antibody, an essential requirement for containing the spread of a virus during acute infection. Two major points are clear from this brief description. The first is that the T lymphocyte is a central component of the immune system orchestrating the immune response, and the second is that proliferation ensuring clonal expansion of antigen-specific lymphocytes is a key factor in a successful immune response.

The T cells are produced by the thymus from where they exit and join the peripheral T cell pool. The cells become part of a subset of T cells that recirculate around the body moving from the blood through the lymphoid organs and back to the blood again to maximize their chance of encountering an antigen specific for their receptor. Failure to meet their specific antigen eventually will lead to their loss from this pool. However, success is met with the process detailed above and the eventual production of memory T cells. These are specific for the peptide + MHC that initiated their activation, thus providing protection should there be repeat exposure to the potential pathogen. The memory cell pool can be viewed as a history of exposure and provides protection from these potential pathogens in the environment. Exposure to a new possible pathogenic agent is covered by the range of receptor specificities present in the T cell population produced by the thymus.

AGE-RELATED CHANGES, CHARACTERIZATION, AND CONSEQUENCES

The complex relationship between the thymic and the peripheral T cell pool is further changed by the reduction in the rate of export from the thymus. When the rate of export of T cells decreases with age, the potential reduction in T cell numbers within the pool is made up by proliferation of constituent members, and so the total number of cells in the pool is kept within closely defined limits. Because of the restrictions placed on the activation of cells within the naive T cell pool, this proliferation comes from members of the memory T cell pool. Aging of the immune system is accompanied by an increase in the memory T cell subset,[1] which because of its rather restricted antigen repertoire, leads to a possible limitation in the range of potential pathogenic organisms that the individual can recognize. A second consequence of maintaining T cell numbers by the proliferation of memory T cells is that unless there is high-fidelity replication of the memory T cells there are likely to be an accumulation of defects. Several experimental studies have shown that aging is associated with an increase in the number of cells showing defects in signaling pathways,[2] cell cycle progression,[3] cytokine production,[4] and the expression of key cell surface molecules.[5] A third consequence is that like other somatic cells T cells have a limited proliferative life span,[6] which is a problem when proliferation is at the core of a successful immune response.[7]

TABLE 1. Deaths from pneumonia and influenza (ICD-9 code 480–487) in 2000

Gender	<1	1 to 14	15 to 44	45 to 64	65 to 74	>75	Total
Males	22	30	277	1474	3217	18038	23058
Females	15	23	205	959	2393	30185	33780
Sum	37	53	482	2433	5610	48223	56838
Percent of P & I deaths	0.1	0.1	0.8	4.3	9.9	84.8	100

(Age Range (years))

TABLE 2. Total deaths in 2000

Gender	<1	1 to 14	15 to 44	45 to 64	65 to 74	>75	Total
Males	1886	836	11899	41265	60593	139068	255547
Females	1491	581	6412	26725	42174	202734	280117
Sum	3377	1417	18311	67990	102767	341802	535664
Percent of P & I deaths	0.6	0.3	3.4	12.7	19.2	63.8	100

(Age Range (years))

This combination of narrowed repertoire, increased incidence of defects, and reduced replicative ability will result in a decline in the efficient functioning of T cells from elderly individuals. Clinically this would lead to a reduction in the ability of aged individuals to cope with potentially pathogenic organisms producing an increased incidence and severity of infection. This inference is supported by reports that urinary tract infections, lower respiratory tract infections, skin and soft tissue infections, intraabdominal infections, infective endocarditis, bacterial meningitis, tuberculosis, and herpes zoster have a higher incidence in the elderly and show a higher mortality rate compared with younger adult patients with the same disease.[8] Although the dysfunctional immune response may not be wholly responsible for the increase in mortality seen with these diseases in the elderly, it may make a significant contribution.

Comparison of the effectiveness of the immune response to infective agent can be seen from the mortality statistics for England and Wales from the Office for National Statistics. If we look at the deaths in the year 2000 from pneumonia and influenza (ICD-9 code 480-487, TABLE 1), we see that as a cause of death, pneumonia and influenza are age related, with almost 85% of all the deaths within the population in persons older than age 75. The suggestion that pneumonia and influenza is a hazard for this age group is shown in TABLE 2 in which we show that of all the deaths in the year 2000 only approximately 64% were in the older than 75 age group.

Clearly, a therapy directed at reversing the senescence seen in the immune system with age would have to be a multihit therapy to be effective on the peripheral T cell pool. A more rational approach may be to direct a therapy at the involuting thymus and determine whether the atrophy seen with age can be reversed.

LOCATION OF AN AGE-RELATED LESION IN THYMOPOIESIS: DOES IT RESULT FROM A DEFICIENCY IN THE PROGENITOR OR THE MICROENVIRONMENT?

The thymus is seeded during adult life by cells derived from the bone marrow, which can be identified by their phenotype of $CD44^+CD25^-CD3^-CD4^{lo}CD8^-$.[9] Maintenance of the numbers of the multipotential $CD44^+CD25^-$ population within the early stages of the pathway, but an age-associated reduction in the numbers of all downstream populations, suggested that there was deficiency either in these thymocyte progenitors or in the thymic environment.[10] If the $CD44^+CD25^-$ cells have an intrinsic deficiency preventing their differentiation, then this would become evident in a simple comparative experiment looking at T cell development of young and old multipotential stem cells *in vitro*. Culture of 14-day fetal thymic lobes from C57/Bl mice with 2-deoxyguanosine removes the $CD44^+CD25^-$ cells of host origin, and these cells can be replaced with equivalent cells from the thymus of either old or young animals that can be allowed to differentiate in the permissive environment provided by fetal thymic organ cultures to produce all of the thymic subsets in the developmental pathway. The experiment showed that from the same number of multipotential $CD44^+CD25^-$ cells derived from either young or old animals produced numbers of progeny within each thymic subsets that were not significantly different. Thus, the functional capacity of the multipotential $CD44^+CD25^-$ cell is independent of the age of the animal from which they were obtained.[11]

The possibility of a differential step in the pathway being compromised leads to the option to determine the potential cause of the deficiency to remedy it. Analysis of the events surrounding this stage of T cell development suggests several factors are important, but here we will deal with just two of them, IL-7 and stem cell factor (SCF). Evidence that the presence of SCF and IL-7 are obligatory in early T cell development is shown most clearly by the $c\text{-}kit^{-/-}\gamma c^{-/-}$ mice, which show complete abrogation of T cell development.[12] There is clearly some overlap in the function of these factors because there is limited thymopoiesis present in the single deficiency transgenics.[12,13] Although there is a marked reduction in thymic cellularity in the single deficiency transgenics, there is permissive T cell development, suggesting that SCF/c-*kit* interactions can support T cell development in the absence of IL-7/IL-7R interaction and vice versa. The similarity between the stages of T cell development affected by aging and those affected by either IL-7 or SCF prompted experiments to link age-related thymic atrophy with potential deficiencies in either of these factors. Because IL-7 is so closely linked to cell survival within the early stages of the thymocyte development pathway, we set out to establish whether any changes in apoptosis within this pathway occurred with age.

As mentioned above, the cells seeding the thymus from the bone marrow are $CD44^+CD25^-CD3^-CD4^{lo}CD8^-$, and differentiation within the thymus is associated with expression of CD25 ($CD44^+CD25^+$) and then loss of CD44 ($CD44^-CD25^+$) followed by loss of CD25 ($CD44^-CD25^-$). Analysis of these population in old mice revealed that aging was associated with a significant increase in the percentage of apoptotic cells within the $CD44^+CD25^+$ and $CD44^-CD25^+$ subpopulations, thus locating the age-associated increase in apoptosis to the stages of the pathway associated with initiation of TCRβ chain rearrangement.[14] To determine whether SCF or IL-7 were effective *in vivo* in this process, we treated old mice for 4 days with either

IL-7 or SCF or a combination of both or saline vehicle alone and then analyzed them the following day. The results revealed that compared with the saline vehicle–treated group, treatment with IL-7 produced increases in the number of live cells within each of the early subsets, something that treatment with SCF alone failed to achieve. Furthermore IL-7 and SCF together failed to significantly improve thymopoiesis above that shown by IL-7 alone.[14]

IL-7 AND RENEWED THYMOPOEISIS

Having shown that IL-7 could induce the production of new thymocytes, we next determined whether such treatment could translate into increasing thymic output (and possibly immune function) in old mice. We were aware that administration of IL-7 under conditions associated with repopulation of the peripheral T cell pool is known to proceed via both thymic-dependent as well as thymic-independent pathways of T cell expansion.[15] The major problem has been to discriminate between the contribution of the thymus and the contribution from peripheral expansion mechanisms.

Changes in thymic output in humans have been easier to follow after the introduction of the TREC assay. The $\alpha\beta^+$ T cells in humans undergo a process whereby the TCRα chain is produced by excision of the TCRδ locus from between the flanking δrec and ψJα genes. The precise nature of the excision generates a unique nucleotide sequence that allows for the design of primers that lead to the production of a PCR product across the joint region that is specific for $\alpha\beta^+$ T cells. This extrachromosomal circle is of a defined size, is nonreplicating, and therefore present in higher amounts in populations of recent thymic emigrants, whereas its dilution by division means it is present at lower numbers in memory T cell populations. Such characteristics are useful in the quantitative TREC assay used to analyze thymic output under different pathological conditions.[16] In a similar manner in the mouse, the δrec and ψJα loci flank the δ locus and excision of this locus from within the TCRα locus also occurs before TCRα chain gene rearrangement producing circular extrachromosomal DNA.[17] However, unlike humans, the murine δrec deleting element is more promiscuous, binding to other Jα gene segments as alternative acceptor sites to the ψJα gene making the equivalent TREC assay less precise. The murine episomal DNA fragments produced, however, have one salient feature in common: the presence of the TCRδ constant gene (Cδ) that is retained in TCR$\alpha\beta^+$ T cells, and we have shown that measurement of this locus within $\alpha\beta^+$ T cells can be used for the measurement of change in thymic output in mice.

Using this δEC assay, we were able to study the effect of IL-7 administration on the thymic function of old mice. We allowed a rest period of 3 weeks before analysis after treatment to permit the decay of recombinant IL-7 used for therapy (a half-life of 115 minutes *in vivo* has been reported[18]) and allowing the basal levels of IL-7 to return to pretreatment levels. Our findings revealed that when analyzed there was no significant difference in the total number of T cells in the peripheral T cell pool of mice treated with IL-7 when compared with the control group treated with saline. Similarly, there was no difference in the total numbers of either naive T cells in either the CD4 or CD8 subset nor in the total number of memory T cells in either the CD4 or CD8 subsets when the IL-7–treated animals were compared with the saline-treated animals. Despite this apparent failure to identify changes in the thymic output using phenotypic analysis, our analysis using the δEC assay revealed a different outcome. Analysis of $\alpha\beta^+$ T cells from both the IL-7– and saline-treated animals revealed levels of δECS in all IL-7–treated mice to be significantly higher than those of the saline-treated controls, indicating an increased thymic output.[19] This disparity between the δECS and phenotype analysis results may be explained in view of recent work revealing that recent thymic migrants in old mice rapidly take on the phenotype of memory cells.[20] In old animals, the naive T cell pool is much reduced, and any recent thymic entry into the naive T cell pool may be induced to proliferate and hence change phenotype. Thus, these old animals may possess naive T cells masquerading as phenotypic memory T cells. Under these conditions, the δECS assay will prove to be a more accurate, more sensitive, and a more reliable measure of thymic output than phenotypic analysis.

Studies on the capacity of T cells from IL-7–treated animals to respond in functional tests revealed that IL-7 therapy leads to enhanced T cell responsiveness. Because the amount of IL-7 used in the treatment would be less than one molecule per animal at the time of assay, a direct effect of IL-7 upon peripheral T cells would seem unlikely. A more likely scenario is that the improved response in functional tests comes from the increased number of recent thymic emigrants in the peripheral T cell pool after therapy.

CONCLUSION

If intervention in the aging process is to work, then the approach to be taken must be through hypothesis-led experimentation. We believe it is important that the approach should be to define the cause of the aging process within a specific organ or system and determine what rationale can be used to prevent or reverse the process. We have set a goal for ourselves to define a simple interventionist technique that will reverse the age-related changes seen in the immune system. A good therapeutic agent must have several key features. First, it must work and work safely. It must be predictable in its action (i.e., it must act against a specific target, with little or no side effects) and must have a defined and measurable effect. It should achieve this effect within a broad range of concentrations in the tissue, and these levels should be easy to monitor and to maintain. Finally and most importantly, its use must have a rational basis.

In tackling the problem of reversing age-associated changes in the immune system, it becomes clear that directing a therapy at peripheral T cells would be complex because of the many problems that affect peripheral T cells in older individuals. Directing a therapy at the thymus, where a potential defect in an early stage of thymocyte differentiation leads to a reduction in thymic output could prove more fruitful. We have shown that one likely candidate to use as a therapeutic agent is IL-7. This molecule is produced in the thymus by MHC class II$^+$ epithelial cells, and production of IL-7 appears to decline with age, leading to reduced survival within early thymic subsets.

Treatment of old animals with IL-7 reverses thymic atrophy, improves thymopoiesis, and subsequently results in increased thymic output to the peripheral T cell pool. Treated animals show better response in assays of T cell function than untreated animals.

This finding suggests a potential and promising role for a therapy based on the use of IL-7 for the restoration of immunocompetence in the elderly population.

REFERENCES

1. KURASHIMA, C., M. UTSUYAMA, M. KASAI, et al. 1995. The role of thymus in the aging of Th cell subpopulations and age-associated alteration of cytokine production by these cells. Int. Immunol. **7:** 97–104.
2. UTSUYAMA, M., A. WAKIKAWA, T. TAMURA, et al. 1997. Impairment of signal transduction in T cells from old mice. Mech. Ageing Dev. **93:** 131–144.
3. QUADRI, R.A., A. ARBOGAST, M.A. PHELOUZAT, et al. 1998. Age-associated decline in cdk1 activity delays cell cycle progression of human T lymphocytes. J. Immunol. **161:** 5203–5209.
4. HOBBS, M.V., W.O. WEIGLE, D.J. NOONAN, et al. 1993. Patterns of cytokine gene expression by CD4+ T cells from young and old mice. J. Immunol. **150:** 3602–3614.
5. VALLEJO, A.N., J.C. BRANDES, C.M. WEYAND & J.J. GORONZY. 1999. Modulation of CD28 expression: distinct regulatory pathways during activation and replicative senescence. J. Immunol. **162:** 6572–6579.
6. WENG, N.P., B.L. LEVINE, C.H. JUNE & R.J. HODES. 1995. Human naive and memory T lymphocytes differ in telomeric length and replicative potential. Proc. Natl. Acad. Sci. USA **92:** 11091–11094.
7. EFFROS, R.B. & G. PAWELEC. 1997. Replicative senescence of T cells: does the Hayflick limit lead to immune exhaustion? Immunol. Today **18:** 450–454.
8. YOSHIKAWA, T.T. 2000. Epidemiology and unique aspects of aging and infectious diseases. Clin. Infect. Dis. **30:** 931–933.
9. WU, L., R. SCOLLAY, M. EGERTON, et al. 1991. CD4 expressed on earliest T-lineage precursor cells in the adult murine thymus. Nature **349:** 71–74.
10. ASPINALL, R. 1997. Age-associated thymic atrophy in the mouse is due to a deficiency affecting rearrangement of the TCR during intrathymic T cell development. J. Immunol. **158:** 3037–3045.
11. ASPINALL, R. & D. ANDREW. 2001. Age-associated thymic atrophy is not associated with a deficiency in the CD44(+)CD25(–)CD3(–)CD4(–)CD8(–) thymocyte population. Cell. Immunol. **212:** 150–157.
12. RODEWALD, H.R., M. OGAWA, C. HALLER, et al. 1997. Pro-thymocyte expansion by c-kit and the common cytokine receptor gamma chain is essential for repertoire formation. Immunity **6:** 265–272.
13. DI SANTO, J.P., I. AIFANTIS, E. ROSMARAKI, et al. 1999. The common cytokine receptor gamma chain and the pre-T cell receptor provide independent but critically overlapping signals in early alpha/beta T cell development. J. Exp. Med. **189:** 563–574.
14. ANDREW, D. & R. ASPINALL. 2001. Il-7 and not stem cell factor reverses both the increase in apoptosis and the decline in thymopoiesis seen in aged mice. J. Immunol. **166:** 1524–1530.
15. FRY, T.J. & C.L. MACKALL. 2001. Interleukin-7: master regulator of peripheral T-cell homeostasis? Trends Immunol. **22:** 564–571.
16. DOUEK, D.C., R.D. MCFARLAND, P.H. KEISER, et al. 1998. Changes in thymic function with age and during the treatment of HIV infection [see comments]. Nature **396:** 690–695.
17. SHUTTER, J., J.A. CAIN, S. LEDBETTER, et al. 1995. A delta T-cell receptor deleting element transgenic reporter construct is rearranged in alpha beta but not gamma delta T-cell lineages. Mol. Cell. Biol. **15:** 7022–7031.
18. BUI, T., C. FALTYNEK & R.J. HO. 1994. Differential disposition of soluble and liposome-formulated human recombinant interleukin-7: effects on blood lymphocyte population in guinea pigs. Pharm. Res. **11:** 633–641.
19. PIDO-LOPEZ, J., N. IMAMI, D. ANDREW & R. ASPINALL. 2002. Molecular quantitation of thymic output in mice and the effect of IL-7. Eur. J. Immunol. **32:** 2827–2836.
20. THOMAN, M.L. 1997. Effects of the aged microenvironment on CD4+ T cell maturation. Mech. Ageing Dev. **96:** 75–88.

T Cell Replicative Senescence

Pleiotropic Effects on Human Aging

RITA B. EFFROS

Department of Pathology and Laboratory Medicine, David Geffen School of Medicine at UCLA, Los Angeles, California 90095-1732, USA

ABSTRACT: Long-term culture studies using CD8 T cells, the immune cells responsible for control of viral infection, have identified the major features of replicative senescence. Aging is associated with increased proportions of CD8 T cells with similar characteristics, such as absence of expression of the CD28 costimulatory molecule and reduced antiviral effector functions. Proinflammatory cytokines produced by senescent CD8 T cells also may exert pleiotropic suppressive effects on overall immune function and bone homeostasis. Thus, modulation of T cell replicative senescence may provide a comprehensive therapeutic strategy to prevent multiple age-associated pathologies.

KEYWORDS: T cells; replicative senescence; aging; immune system

INTRODUCTION

The characteristics of replicative senescence have been explored in a variety of cell types, but only recently has this experimental paradigm been applied to the immune system. Limited proliferative potential may be particularly deleterious for immune cells, because massive clonal expansion is essential to their function. The drastic decline in immunity during aging suggests that T cells might be an ideal model system to further elucidate the process of replicative senescence itself and also to assess its multifaceted physiological consequences.[1]

PROLIFERATION IS ESSENTIAL FOR LYMPHOCYTE FUNCTION

The intricate genetic mechanism by which lymphocyte antigen receptors are generated allows a limited number of genes to create an immune system with an enormous range of specificities. In brief, during a lymphocyte's development, a random series of juxtapositions forming a sequence of gene segments, and the subsequent combinatorial pairing of two different chains, results in an antigen receptor molecule that is unique to that cell. By these mechanisms, a small amount of genetic material is used to generate $\sim 10^{16}$ different T cell specificities.

Address for correspondence: Rita B. Effros, Ph.D., Department of Pathology and Laboratory Medicine, David Geffen School of Medicine at UCLA, 10833 Le Conte Avenue, Los Angeles, CA 90095-1732.

reffros@mednet.ucla.edu

The exquisite specificity of each lymphocyte results in the ability of the organism to respond to a nearly infinite number of foreign antigens. However, because of the enormous repertoire of responding immune cells, the number of cells that can recognize and respond to any *single* antigen is extremely low. Thus, to generate a sufficient quantity of specific effector cells to fight an infection, an activated lymphocyte must proliferate extensively before its progeny differentiate into effector cells. Repeated or chronic exposure to that antigen requires additional rounds of proliferation. Therefore, a limitation on the process of cell division potentially could have devastating consequences on immune function, particularly by old age.

CELL CULTURE STUDIES OF T CELL REPLICATIVE SENESCENCE

To characterize the process of replicative senescence in the so-called "CD8" or "cytotoxic" T cells, the class of lymphocytes that controls viral infection, cultures established from peripheral blood of healthy young-adult donors are propagated by repeated rounds of antigenic stimulation until they reach irreversible cell cycle arrest. Senescent CD8 T cells show a variety of genetic and functional changes that are reminiscent of fibroblasts, including altered patterns of protein secretion, apoptosis resistance, and reduced stress-induced upregulation of *hsp70* gene expression.[1]

Certain changes associated with replicative senescence are unique to T cells. For example, the high level of telomerase activity induced during antigen-driven activation undergoes progressive decline with each subsequent antigenic stimulation. By the fourth encounter with antigen, CD8 T cells show no detectable telomerase activity, despite continued proliferation.[2] The second major genetic change associated with T cell senescence is the complete and permanent loss of expression of a critical costimulatory molecule, known as "CD28," whose signaling is essential for full T cell activation.[3] CD28 signal transduction results in interleukin (IL)–2 gene transcription, expression of the IL-2 receptor, and the stabilization of a variety of cytokine messenger RNAs. CD28 has additional biologic functions which include influencing glucose metabolism,[4] modulating T cell migration and homing, and, importantly, enhancing telomerase activity.[2]

T CELL REPLICATIVE SENESCENCE OCCURS *IN VIVO*

The Holy Grail of replicative senescence studies has been to demonstrate that aging *in vivo* is accompanied by the accumulation of cells showing characteristics of replicative senescence identified in cell culture. Our documented suppression of CD28 gene expression as a marker of T cell senescence *in vitro* therefore provided an unparalleled opportunity to test whether similar cells accumulate during aging *in vivo*.

Analysis of CD28 expression on T cells derived from donors of different ages has shown that there is a progressive increase with age in the proportion of CD8 T cells that lack CD28 expression.[1] In fact, in some elderly persons, more than 50% of the peripheral blood CD8 T cell pool consists of cells that do not express CD28. Moreover, by flow cytometric cell sorting of T cells derived from peripheral blood samples into $CD28^+$ and $CD28^-$ fractions, we and others have shown that $CD28^-$ T cells have shorter telomeres, and minimal proliferative potential, compared with CD28+ T cells from the same donor, indicating a distinct replicative history for the two cell populations.[5] Finally, CD8 T cells lacking CD28 expression that are isolated immediately *ex vivo* are resistant to certain types of apoptotic stimuli.[6] Thus, *in vivo* aging is associated with a progressive increase in a population of T cells with the key characteristics of senescent T cell cultures, namely, loss of CD28 expression, shortened telomeres, apoptosis resistance, and inability to proliferate.

PHYSIOLOGICAL CONSEQUENCE OF T CELL REPLICATIVE SENESCENCE

Both aging and chronic HIV infection, which has been proposed to represent accelerated immunological aging, are associated with high proportions of CD8 T cells with characteristics suggestive of replicative senescence.[5] In addition to compromising the immune control over certain viruses, senescent T cells are associated with other deleterious effects. First, based on their abundance alone, the clonally expanded populations of senescent CD8 T cells effectively reduce the repertoire of antigen specificities available in elderly persons. In addition, clinical studies have shown a significant correlation between high proportions of CD8 T cells that lack CD28 expression and poor antibody response to influenza vaccination in the elderly.[7] This observation is consistent with numerous studies showing that CD8+CD28− T cells exert suppressive effects on a variety of other immune cell types.

Senescent T cells also may influence other organ systems. CD8 T cells that reach replicative senescence in cell culture secrete high titers of two proinflammatory cytokines (TNF-α and IL-6) that are known to enhance bone absorption. Interestingly, clinical studies have shown a correlation between osteoporotic fractures in the elderly and high proportions of CD8 T cells expressing senescent markers and secreting TNF-α.[8] Finally, high proportions of CD8 T cells lacking CD28 expression are also part of the "immune risk phenotype," an immune profile that is associated with early mortality in the elderly.[9] Thus, replicative senescence of CD8 T cells may have pleiotropic effects on multiple organ systems during aging, thereby modulating life span itself.

FUTURE DIRECTIONS

Given the broad physiological consequences of T cell replicative senescence, prevention or reversal of this process may provide a comprehensive therapeutic strategy to correct multiple age-associated pathologies. Indeed, gene transduction with the catalytic component of human telomerase (hTERT) leads to enhanced proliferation, telomere length stabilization, and improved antiviral immune function in CD8 T cells.[10] Nevertheless, several aspects of the replicative senescence program are not corrected, including loss of CD28 expression and certain cytokine changes. Future research directed at improving transfection protocols, inclusion of additional genes, and hormonal-based strategies that have an impact on the senescence pathway are approaches that may prove to be more effective in correcting the multifaceted outcomes of T cell replicative senescence.

ACKNOWLEDGMENTS

This work was supported by the NIH and the UCLA Center on Aging. Dr. Effros holds the Thomas and Elizabeth Plott Endowed Chair in Gerontology.

REFERENCES

1. EFFROS, R.B. & G. PAWELEC. 1997. Replicative senescence of T lymphocytes: does the Hayflick Limit lead to immune exhaustion? Immunology Today **18:** 450–454.
2. VALENZUELA, H.F. & R.B. EFFROS. 2002. Divergent telomerase and CD28 expression patterns in human CD4 and CD8 T cells following repeated encounters with the same antigenic stimulus. Clin. Immunol. **105:** 117–125.
3. EFFROS, R.B. 1997. Loss of CD28 expression on T lymphocytes: a marker of replicative senescence. Dev. Comp. Immunol. **21:** 471–478.
4. FRAUWIRTH, K.A., J.L. RILEY, M.H. HARRIS, et al. 2002. The CD28 signaling pathway regulates glucose metabolism. Immunity **16:** 769–777.
5. EFFROS, R.B., R. ALLSOPP, C.P. CHIU, et al. 1996. Shortened telomeres in the expanded CD28-CD8+ subset in HIV disease implicate replicative senescence in HIV pathogenesis. AIDS **10:** F17–F22.
6. POSNETT, D.N., J.W. EDINGER, J.S. MANAVALAN, et al. 1999. Differentiation of human CD8 T cells: implications for in vivo persistence of CD8+ CD28– cytotoxic effector clones. Int. Immunol. **11:** 229–241.
7. SAURWEIN-TEISSL, M., T.L. LUNG, F. MARX, et al. 2002. Lack of antibody production following immunization in old age: association with CD8(+)CD28(–) T cell clonal expansions and an imbalance in the production of Th1 and Th2 cytokines. J. Immunol. **168:** 5893–5899.
8. PIETSCHMANN, P., J. GRISAR, R. THIEN, et al. 2001. Immune phenotype and intracellular cytokine production of peripheral blood mononuclear cells from postmenopausal patients with osteoporotic fractures. Exp. Gerontol. **36:** 1749–1759.
9. WIKBY, A., B. JOHANSSON, J. OLSSON, et al. 2002. Expansions of peripheral blood CD8 T-lymphocyte subpopulations and an association with cytomegalovirus seropositivity in the elderly: the Swedish NONA immune study. Exp. Gerontol. **37:** 445–453.
10. DAGARAG, M.D., H. NG, R. LUBONG, et al. 2003. Differential impairment of lytic and cytokine functions in senescent HIV-1-specific cytotoxic T lymphocytes. J. Virol. **77:** 3077–3083.

Zinc, Immune Plasticity, Aging, and Successful Aging

Role of Metallothionein

EUGENIO MOCCHEGIANI, ROBERTINA GIACCONI, ELISA MUTI, CINZIA ROGO, MASSIMO BRACCI, MARIO MUZZIOLI, CATIA CIPRIANO, AND MARCO MALAVOLTA

Immunology Center (Section Nutrition, Immunity and Ageing) Research Department, I.N.R.C.A., Ancona, Italy

ABSTRACT: The capacity of the remodeling immune responses during stress (immune plasticity) is fundamental to reach successful aging. We herein report two pivotal models to demonstrate the relevance of the immune plasticity in aging and successful aging. One model is represented by the circadian rhythms of immune responses; the other one is the immune responses during partial hepatectomy/liver regeneration (pHx). The latter is suggestive because it mimics the immunosenescence and chronic inflammation 48 hours after partial hepatectomy in the young through the continuous production of IL-6, which is the main cause of immune plasticity lack in aging. The constant production of IL-6 leads to abnormal increments of zinc-bound metallothionein (MT), which is, in turn, unable in zinc release in aging. As a consequence, low zinc ion bioavailability appears for thymic and extrathymic immune efficiency, in particular, of liver NKT cells bearing TCR gd. The remodeling during the circadian cycle and during pHx of zinc-bound MT confers the immune plasticity of liver NKT γδ cells and NK cells in young and very old age, not in old age. Therefore, zinc-bound MT homeostasis is crucial in conferring liver immune plasticity with subsequent successful aging.

KEYWORDS: NKT cells; NKT αβ and γδ cells; zinc; metallothionein; IL-6; gp130; PARP-1; immune plasticity; liver extrathymic T cell pathway; circadian cycle; partial hepatectomy; liver regeneration; aging; successful aging

INTRODUCTION

Immune plasticity is a condition "sine qua non" for healthy aging. The absence of the plasticity leads the organism to be a "low responder" to oxidative stress with subsequent appearance of age-related diseases. The remodeling of the immune sys-

---

Address for correspondence: Dr. Eugenio Mocchegiani, Immunology Center (Section Nutrition, Immunity and Ageing) Research Department I.N.R.C.A., Via Birarelli 8, 60121, Ancona, Italy. Voice: +39-071-800-4216; fax: +39-071-206-791.
e.mocchegiani@inrca.it

tem to various harmful stimuli allows a prompt immune response and the organism becomes a "high responder." Therefore, the capacity for remodeling can be considered the plasticity of the immune system against oxidative stress. The lack of this capacity leads the cells of the immune system to undergo cell death or necrosis triggered by oxidative stress.[1] Such a plasticity is a common event in young-adult age during transient stress-like conditions. During aging, the capacity of the remodeling of the immune system is very limited because the stress-like condition is chronic.[2] This phenomenon allows reduced immune responses to oxidative stress and a low cellular capacity in DNA repair.[3] As a consequence, the risk of the appearance of age-related diseases, that is, cancer and infections, is high.[3] On the other hand, the "free radical theory," which takes into account the production of free radicals by oxidative stress, is the more common theory of the aging process.[4] The molecular basis of the absence of immune plasticity in aging is poorly understood, and, at the same time, was also poorly studied 10 years ago when the scientific community had seen many centenarians among elderly people. Indeed, healthy centenarians differ from "normal" aged individuals for their optimal metabolic compensation and immune response and for the ability to efficiently counter the alteration of the oxidative status typical of aging. In this context, various hypotheses have been proposed to reach successful aging. Limited inflammation, higher homing of stem cells to substitute the damaged cells, an increased capacity in DNA repair, and, finally, a major genomic integrity are characteristics of oldest individuals.[5] However, the capacity of the remodeling of the immune system also can be pivotal in these exceptional individuals and, as such, an improved immune plasticity. In this context, the role played by zinc and metallothioneins (MTs) may be crucial for the following reasons. First, zinc is a trace element indispensable for the efficiency of the immune system in both thymic and extrathymic T cell pathways, and this latter is fundamental to compensate thymic failure in aging.[2] Second, MT is relevant in zinc sequestering and in zinc release for the immune efficiency during transient stress. The zinc release by MT does not occur in aging because stress-like condition is chronic, leading to low zinc ion bioavailability for immune efficiency and for zinc-dependent biological functions, such as enzyme antioxidant activity and DNA repair.[6] Third, the gene expression of MT is induced by proinflammatory cytokines (IL-1, IL-6, and TNF-α) during inflammation.[7] The increment of these cytokines in aging leads to abnormal increase of MT coupled with low zinc ion bioavailability and impaired immune response.[6] Consistent with these findings, zinc and MT homeostasis is crucial in conferring immune plasticity during aging taking also into account that satisfactory zinc ion bioavailability is observed in centenarians.[1] In this article, two relevant models are reported to demonstrate the relevance of the immune plasticity in aging: the variations of the immune functions (1) during the circadian cycle and (2) during the compensatory liver growth after partial hepatecomy. The choice of these two models is based by previous findings showing the impact that thymic circadian variation[8] and the liver extrathymic T cell pathway[1] have in the economy of the immune response in aging and successful aging. In addition, the model of young partial hepatectomy/liver regeneration is very interesting because, other than a good model for the study of acute and chronic inflammation, it mimics the aging process in thymic failure and in impaired peripheral immune efficiency at 48 hours after partial hepatecomy in young pHx mice.[9] Young, old, and very old mice were used in both models. A parallelism with elderly, nonagenarians, and old infected patients is reported.

IMMUNE PLASTICITY: MODEL OF THE CIRCADIAN CYCLE

Young mice display fluctuating variations in plasma zinc and in thymic endocrine activity during the circadian cycle with nocturnal peaks.[8] In contrast, no significant variations occur in old mice during the circadian cycle with an absence of nocturnal peaks.[8] This absence also is observed in peripheral immune efficiency. In particular, the low natural killer (NK) cell activity observed in old mice during the light period also are maintained during the dark with no significant variations during the whole circadian cycle.[1,8] Such a defect in old mice is closely related to the appearance of age-related diseases (cancer and infection) and subsequent death.[8] Conversely, immune peripheral variations occur in young-adult mice coupled with the capacity of young mice to respond to external antigenic stimuli and, subsequently, in avoiding diseases triggered by the oxidative stress. Indeed, an interleukin, such as IL-2 that is relevant for NK cell activity, displays nocturnal peaks in young mice.[1] Nocturnal peaks of thymic and peripheral immune functions also occur in very old mice.[1] These findings are clear evidence that the immune variations during the circadian cycle are fundamental in maintaining the immune efficiency and plasticity, which are indispensable for health longevity.[1] In this context, an interesting aspect of the immune system, that is, the liver extrathymic T cell pathway deputed to compensate the thymic failure in aging,[2] shows variations during the circadian cycle in young and very old mice, but not in old ones.[1] The liver NKT cells bearing TCR αβ or γδ play an intriguing role. These cells are the first sentinels for the host defense against viruses and bacteria because secreting IL-2 and IFN-γ, which, in turn, affect the activity of classic NK cells.[10] These particular liver NKT cells display a circadian rhythm in young and very old mice with significant modifications between the light and dark period. In particular, the number of NKT γδ cells increases in young and very old mice during the dark, whereas it remains unmodified in old mice. The num-

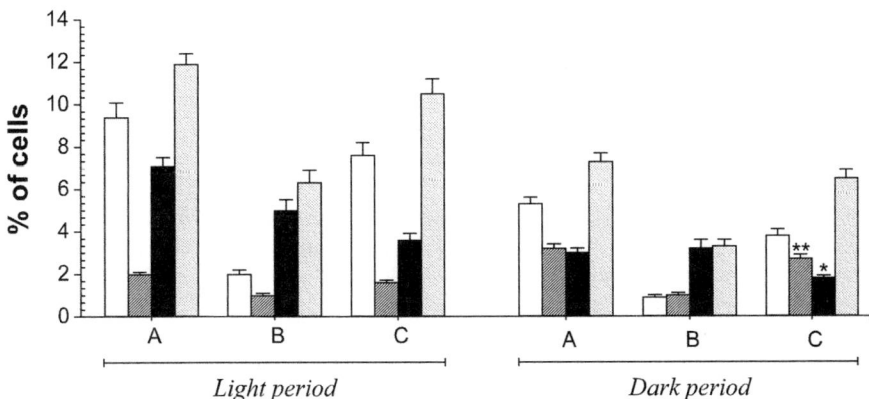

FIGURE 1. Percentage of NKT cells (NK 1.1+CD3+) (*gray bars*), NKT αβ (*white bars*), and γδ (*striped bars*) cells and NKT cells expressing Fas (CD95) (*black bars*) in young (**A**), old (**B**), and very old mice (**C**) during the circadian cycle. **P < .01 in comparison with B mice in the dark; *P < .05 in comparison with B mice in the dark. (E. Mocchegiani, unpublished results.)

ber of NKT $\alpha\beta$ cells displays an opposite trend with a decrement in young, old, and very old mice during the dark as compared with the light period (FIG. 1). These findings suggest that NKT $\gamma\delta$ cells may be more involved in the maintenance of liver extrathymic immune plasticity during aging leading to successful aging. This maintenance may be because of a better preservation by cell death of NKT $\gamma\delta$ cells than $\alpha\beta$ because of low Fas expression (CD95) in NKT $\gamma\delta$ cells in oldest individuals.[12] On the other hand, a significant decrement in liver NKT cells expressing Fas (CD95) occurs in very old mice in the dark as compared with old mice during the same period (FIG. 1). In contrast, old mice display low numbers of NKT $\gamma\delta$ cells for the whole circadian cycle with no fluctuations (FIG. 1), impaired NKT $\gamma\delta$ cell cytotoxicity, or decreased production of IL-2 and IFN-γ in comparison with very old mice.[1] Similar phenomena occur in centenarians. Although no data are available during the dark in centenarians but exclusively in the light period, the major preservation of NKT $\gamma\delta$ cells in centenarians[12] is also coupled with satisfactory NKT cell citotoxicity[13] and IL-2 production.[11] Thus, the functionality and the number of these cells, in particular, of liver origin, are pivotal to reach successful aging because some age-related diseases, such as infections, might be avoided. Indeed, old infected patients display a still lower number of NKT $\gamma\delta$ cells than elderly,[11] giving further support to the relevance of liver T$\gamma\delta$ cells for host defense against viruses and bacteria.[10]

IMMUNE PLASTICITY: MODEL OF THE PARTIAL HEPATECTOMY/LIVER REGENERATION

Partial hepatectomy/liver regeneration (pHx) is a good model for the study, other than the liver regeneration, of acute and chronic inflammation in aging because of the likeness with aging in impaired thymic endocrine activity, low zinc ion bioavailability, and peripheral immune efficiency (NK cell activity and IL-2 production) in young pHx mice at 48 hours after pHx.[2,9] A complete remodeling of zinc ion bioavailability and immune efficiency, however, occurs in the late period of compensatory liver growth (7th and 15th day) in young pHx mice. In contrast, no remodeling occurs in old mice displaying the same low zinc ion bioavailability and impaired immune functions for the whole period of the compensatory liver growth (time 0, 48 hours, 7th and 15th day).[9] These findings are intriguing because they suggest that pHx is also a good model to show the immune plasticity and, at the same time, the relevance of this plasticity in liver extrathymic T cell pathway during aging. This assumption is supported by the fact that very old pHx mice show the same pattern in zinc ion bioavailability and liver NKT cell activity observed in young pHx mice (FIG. 2). In other words, both zinc ion bioavailability and liver NKT cell activity are not lost during the compensatory liver growth in very old mice, but a remodeling occurs in the late period of the liver regeneration (15th day), as occurring in young pHx mice (FIG. 2). These findings in very old mice, whereas on one hand demonstrate the presence of the immune plasticity in very old age, on the other hand they pinpoint that very old mice are still capable of responding to a great inflammation, such as partial hepatectomy, with a remodeling of the liver immune efficiency.

This fact is very important in the oldest individuals because it means that many age-related diseases may be avoided. As a consequence, very old individuals become

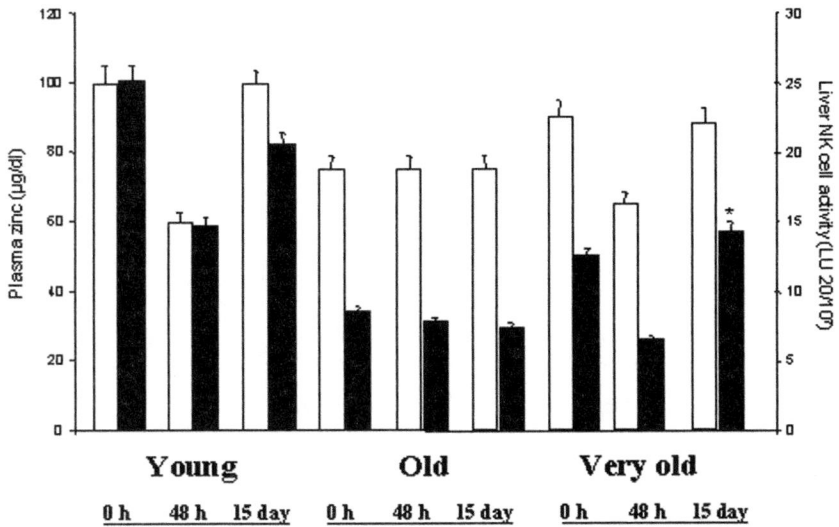

FIGURE 2. Plasma zinc (μg/dL) (*white bars*) and liver NKT cell activity (L.U. 20/10^7) (*black bars*) during the compensatory liver growth after partial hepatectomy in young, old, and very old mice. (0 h = sham controls). *$P < .01$ as compared with old (15th day). (Redrawn from Cipriano et al.[14] with permission.)

"high responders" to oxidative stress, as occurring in the young.[1] Indeed, the lack of response to a great inflammation (such as partial hepatectomy) in old age provokes a shorter survival in old pHx mice in comparison with old sham controls.[14] Indeed, old pHx mice display a greater incidence of cancer and infections.[14] Thus, a good functioning of liver immune plasticity is pivotal to reach successful aging.

MECHANISMS OF ACTION IN THE MAINTENANCE OF THE IMMUNE PLASTICITY

It has been demonstrated that the zinc ion bioavailability is fundamental for the efficiency of the immune system.[2] The loss of zinc ions by intestinal malabsorption or by reduced food intake provokes a zinc deficiency with damage in cell-mediated immunity, including thymic efficiency, NK cell activity, and cytokine production. In particular, anti-inflammatory cytokines, such as IL-2, IL-12, IFN-α, IFN-γ, decrease whereas proinflammatory cytokines, such as TNF-α, IL-1, IL-6, increase.[2] In this context, zinc more affects the cytokine production by Th1 than Th2 cells.[2] That zinc has a beneficial effect on IFN-α production by Th1 cells is supported by the recent discovery in virus transfected cells showing a protein Staf-50 involved in a new family of IFN-α production that contains two zinc finger motifs.[15] This fact suggests an unbalance of Th1/Th2 paradigm during zinc deficiency toward Th2 cytokine production,[2] which leads to the induction of some proteins deputed in fighting the oxidative

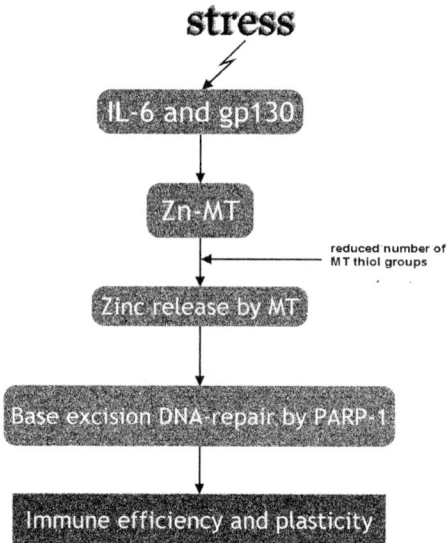

FIGURE 3. Schematic mechanism of action in conferring immune efficiency and plasticity in young and very old age involving the interrelationships among stress, IL-6, and MT (for explanations, see text).

stress. In this context, MT plays a pivotal role because it sequesters and dispenses zinc. MT acts as antioxidant against wide spectrum of stressor agents, because the zinc-sulfur cluster is sensitive to changes of cellular redox state and oxidizing sites in MT (reduced number of thiol groups) induce the transfer of zinc from its binding sites in MT to those of lower affinity in other proteins.[16] This transfer occurs in conferring biological activity to antioxidant metalloenzymes, such as superoxide dismutase,[6] in the base excision DNA repair by PARP-1, in the genomic stability by telomerases, and, finally, in conferring directly or indirectly, via zinc finger motifs, the immune efficiency[6] (FIG. 3). Therefore, the redox properties of MT and their effect on zinc in the clusters are crucial for the biological functions of MT. Indeed, MT is peculiar in cellular proliferation and in protecting cells against cytotoxic effects of reactive oxygen species, ionizing radiations, electrophilic anticancer drugs, and mutagens and heavy metals.[2] A peculiar role of MT is played during partial hepatectomy/liver regeneration, with a strong MT induction that is useful, other than in facilitating the liver regeneration by various hepatocyte growth factors, in protecting the cells by the inflammation after partial hepatectomy. It has been shown that high MT, either as gene expression or protein, is present in young pHx mice at 48 h from pHx coupled with low zinc ion bioavailability, high IL-6, and impaired thymic and extrathymic T cell pathways.[9,14] A complete downregulation of MT and IL-6 followed by a restoration of the immune efficiency occurs in the late period of the compensatory liver growth (7th and 15th day from pHx).[14] In contrast, the high MT and IL-6 gene expressions as well as the low zinc ion bioavailability and the impaired immune functions, already present in old mice, are not modified during the liver regeneration in old pHx mice.[14] An intriguing aspect is the complete remodeling of MT, zinc ion bioavailability, and immune function in very old pHx mice at 7th and 15th day from partial hepatectomy.[14] These findings further demonstrate that MT is not protective against chronic inflammation, like in aging, because it is unable in release zinc, whereas its protective role occurs during young-adult age.[1] Therefore, MT turns from role of protection in young age to harmful one in aging because of its inability in zinc release.[1,6] This phenomenon in aging provokes low zinc ion bioavailability for zinc-dependent enzyme antioxidant activity, for base excision DNA repair by PARP-1, and for thymic and extrathymic T cell pathways. Therefore, MT plays a pivotal role in zinc turnover in aging and consequently in conferring the immune plasticity.[6] Such an assumption is supported during the circadian cycle in which the high nocturnal peaks of zinc and immune efficiency observed in young and very old mice are related to low MT either as gene expression or as protein.[1] No circadian variation of MT occurs in old mice.[1] In addition, low MT gene expression and good zinc ion bioavailability also are observed in lymphocytes from centenarians.[1] This phenomenon of MT in regulating zinc turnover is closely dependent by the inflammatory status, in particular, by the gene expression and induction of proinflammatory cytokines, such as IL-6, and of its subunit receptor gp130. As IL-6 and gp130 are constantly high in aging,[2] this fact leads to continuous increase of MT followed by the stealing of intracellular zinc ions and no subsequent zinc release by MT. As a consequence, low zinc ion bioavailability appears in the maintenance of the immune plasticity in aging.[1,2,6] It is not a simple coincidence that both very old mice and centenarians display low gp130 despite IL-6 being high.[11] This fact leads to low MT induction, good zinc ion bioavailability, satisfactory immune efficiency, and an increased capacity in base excision DNA repair by PARP-1 in very old age.[1,14] In contrast, high MT, IL-6, and gp130 coupled with reduced capacity in base excision DNA repair are present in elderly and in old infected patients.[11] In these latter, alterations in DNA repair and in MT are still more severe. Indeed, abnormal high expression of MT is an index of unfavorable prognosis in cancer and infections.[2,11] Therefore, zinc-bound MT homeostasis, via IL-6 and gp130, is a fundamental mechanism in conferring immune plasticity to reach successful aging. In conclusion, MT can be considered a potential biological and genetic marker of immunosenescence upstream affecting functional biochemical cascade involved in the maintenance of the immune plasticity, in particular, liver NKT gd cells, with subsequent successful aging.

ACKNOWLEDGMENTS

This work was supported by INRCA and the Italian Health Ministry (R.F. n. 216/02 to E.M). We thank G. Mazzarini for graphic design and N. Gasparini and G. Bernardini for technical assistance.

REFERENCES

1. MOCCHEGIANI, E., R. GIACCONI, C. CIPRIANO, et al. 2002. MtmRNA gene expression, via IL-6 and glucocorticoids, as potential genetic marker of immunosenescence: lessons from very old mice and humans. Exp. Gerontol. **37:** 349–357.

2. MOCCHEGIANI, E., M. MUZZIOLI, C. CIPRIANO, *et al.* 1998. Zinc, T-cell pathways, aging: role of metallothioneins. Mech. Ageing Dev. **106:** 183–204.
3. PAWELEC, G. & R. SOLANA. 1997. Immunosenescence. Immunol. Today **18:** 514–516.
4. ASHOK, B.T. & R. ALI. 1999. The aging paradox: free radical theory of aging. Exp. Gerontol. **34:** 293–303.
5. FRANCESCHI, C., M. BONAFE & S. VALENSIN. 2000. Human immunosenescence: the prevailing of innate immunity, the failing of clonotypic immunity, and the filling of immunological space. Vaccine **18:** 1717–1720.
6. MOCCHEGIANI, E., M. MUZZIOLI & R. GIACCONI. 2000. Zinc and immunoresistance to infection in aging: new biological tools. Trends Pharmacol. Sci. **21:** 205–208.
7. DAVIS, S.R. & R.J. COUSINS. 2000. Metallothionein expression in animals: a physiological perspective on function. J. Nutr. **130:** 1085–1088.
8. MOCCHEGIANI, E., L. SANTARELLI, A. TIBALDI, *et al.* 1998. Presence of links between zinc and melatonin during the circadian cycle in old mice: effects on thymic endocrine activity and on the survival. J. Neuroimmunol. **86:** 111–122.
9. MOCCHEGIANI, E., D. VERBANAC, L. SANTARELLI, *et al.* 1997. Zinc and metallothioneins on cellular immune effectiveness during liver regeneration in young and old mice. Life Sci. **61:** 1125–1145.
10. BIRON, C.A. & L. BROSSAY. 2001. NK cells and NKT cells in innate defense against viral infections. Curr. Opin. Immunol. **13:** 458–464.
11. MOCCHEGIANI, E., M. MUZZIOLI, R. GIACCONI, *et al.* 2003. Metallothioneins/PARP-1/IL-6 interplay on natural killer cell activity in elderly: parallelism with nonagenarians and old infected humans. Effect of zinc supply. Mech. Ageing Dev. **124:** 459–468.
12. ROMANO, G.C., M. POTESTIO, G. SCIALABBA, *et al.* 2000. Early activation of gammadelta T lymphocytes in the elderly. Mech. Ageing Dev. **121:** 231–238.
13. MIYAJI, C., H. WATANABE, H. TOMA, *et al.* 2000. Functional alteration of granulocytes, NK cells, and natural killer T cells in centenarians. Hum. Immunol. **61:** 908–916.
14. CIPRIANO, C., R. GIACCONI, M. MUZZIOLI, *et al.* 2003. Metallothionein (I+II) confers, via c-myc, immune plasticity in oldest mice: model of partial hepatectomy/liver regeneration. Mech. Ageing Dev. **124:** 877–886.
15. TISSOT, C. & N. MECHTI. 1995. Molecular cloning of a new interferon-induced factor that represses human immunodeficiency virus type 1 long terminal repeat expression. J. Biol. Chem. **270:** 14891–14898.
16. MARET, W. & B.L. VALLEE. 1998. Thiolate ligands in metallothionein confer redox activity on zinc clusters. Proc. Natl. Acad. Sci. USA **95:** 3478–3482.

Macrophages of the Adrenal Cortex

A Morphological Study of the Effects of Aging and Dexamethasone Administration

HENRIQUE ALMEIDA, JORGE FERREIRA, AND DELMINDA NEVES

Instituto de Histologia e Embriologia, Faculdade de Medicina do Porto, 4200-319 Porto, Portugal

Instituto de Biologia Molecular e Celular da Universidade do Porto (IBMC), Rua do Campo Alegre, 4150-180 Porto, Portugal

ABSTRACT: Macrophages are present throughout the adrenal cortex, particularly in the deeper layers. They locate next to parenchyma cells, which secrete glucocorticoids under the regulation of the pituitary adrenocorticotropic hormone (ACTH). Blockade of ACTH secretion is followed by adrenocortical cell atrophy and apoptosis, an effect likely to cause an increase in local macrophage number and phagocytic activity. The purpose of the current study was to verify this effect and ascertain its age-related variation after ACTH blockade. Male rats at five different ages ranging from 2 to 24 months were divided into two groups, which were injected with dexamethasone phosphate or saline for 3 days. The adrenals were processed for morphological and morphometric study. The age-related increase in macrophage number seen in a survey of the sections was confirmed in the quantitative study: a significant increase in volume density (Vv), numerical density (Nv), and cell volume was found in both groups; Vv and Nv were higher in treated rats. These findings in the deeper layers of the cortex suggest a continuous process of phagocytosis, likely of parenchyma dead cells or their debris, which increases further after ACTH blockade. An additional modulatory effect of macrophages also may occur because of their secretory role.

KEYWORDS: adrenal; macrophage; age-related; dexamethasone; apoptosis

INTRODUCTION

The adrenal cortex (AC) is the site of synthesis and secretion of various steroid hormones. Its structure comprises the outer zone (or zona glomerulosa [ZG]) and the inner zone (IZ, further divided into zona fasciculata [ZF] and reticularis [ZR]), arranged in cords of parenchyma cells. Among these, macrophages are also present. They occur throughout the AC but are specially numerous at the ZR, located deeply in the IZ.

Address for correspondence: Henrique Almeida, Instituto de Histologia e Embriologia, Faculdade de Medicina do Porto, 4200-319 Porto, Portugal. Voice: +351-22-509-1468; fax: +351-22-550-5728.
almeidah@med.up.pt

Ann. N.Y. Acad. Sci. 1019: 135–140 (2004). © 2004 New York Academy of Sciences.
doi: 10.1196/annals.1297.024

When the IZ is stimulated by the adrenocorticotropic hormone (ACTH), of pituitary origin, the cells synthesize glucocorticoids and secrete them to the blood. Conversely, blockade of ACTH secretion by hypophysectomy or corticosteroid administration is followed by depression of steroid secretion, AC atrophy and the appearance of apoptosis,[1,2] notably at ZR and the transition ZF/ZR. Such findings were observed in newborn and young adult rats; however, the consequences of ACTH blockade by steroid administration at the ZR of aged animals are unknown. In particular, it is lacking structural data related to macrophages, which are likely to present modifications at this apoptotic setting.[3]

To ascertain this point, we performed a quantitative study.

MATERIALS AND METHODS

Wistar male rats were obtained from the former colony of the Gulbenkian Institute of Science, Oeiras, Portugal, now bred at the IBMC. The animals were kept with free access to water and laboratory diet. At 2, 6, 12, 18, and 24 months, eight apparently healthy animals were selected and randomly divided into two groups. The first group was injected with 4 mg/kg of dexamethasone phosphate (Decadron,® Merck Sharp & Dhome, Portugal), intramuscularly, for 3 consecutive days; the second group (controls), received a similar volume of saline. At the fourth day, the animals were sacrificed by decapitation and the adrenals were processed for ultrastructural morphology and cytochemistry using previously described procedures.[4] For the morphometric study, Epon sections 1 μm thick, stained with Azur II were used. In randomly selected areas of the ZR, a morphometric study was made to determine macrophage volume density (V_v), numerical density (N_v), and cellular volume (CV).[5]

ANOVA was used to compare the means of the measurements at the different ages. The statistical significance of differences between individual pairs of means was assessed using the least significant difference procedure of Fisher (LSD test).

RESULTS

Observations

In control animals, the general structure of the AC and parenchyma cells was conserved throughout aging and presented previously described features.[4]

Macrophages had a subendothelial location and displayed elongated, frequently notched nuclei. In many of them, at all ages, the cytoplasm was filled with coarse azurophilic or cyano colored and round or irregularly shaped granules (FIG. 1A). At

---

FIGURE 1. (**A**) ZR of an 18-month-old rat displaying parenchymal cells, capillary lumina (*asterisk*), and macrophages with complex cytoplasmic content (*circles*); adrenal medulla (M). Bar = 20 μm. (**B**) Ultrastructure of a large ZR macrophage showing the nucleus (N), the complex heterogeneous content of lipofuscin (Lp), and mitochondria of parenchyma cells (m). Bar = 1 μm. (**C**) Ultrastructural acid phosphatase cytochemistry of a macrophage with fine dense precipitate on complex granules (*arrows*), indicating their lysosomal nature, and lipid droplets (l). Bar = 1 μm.

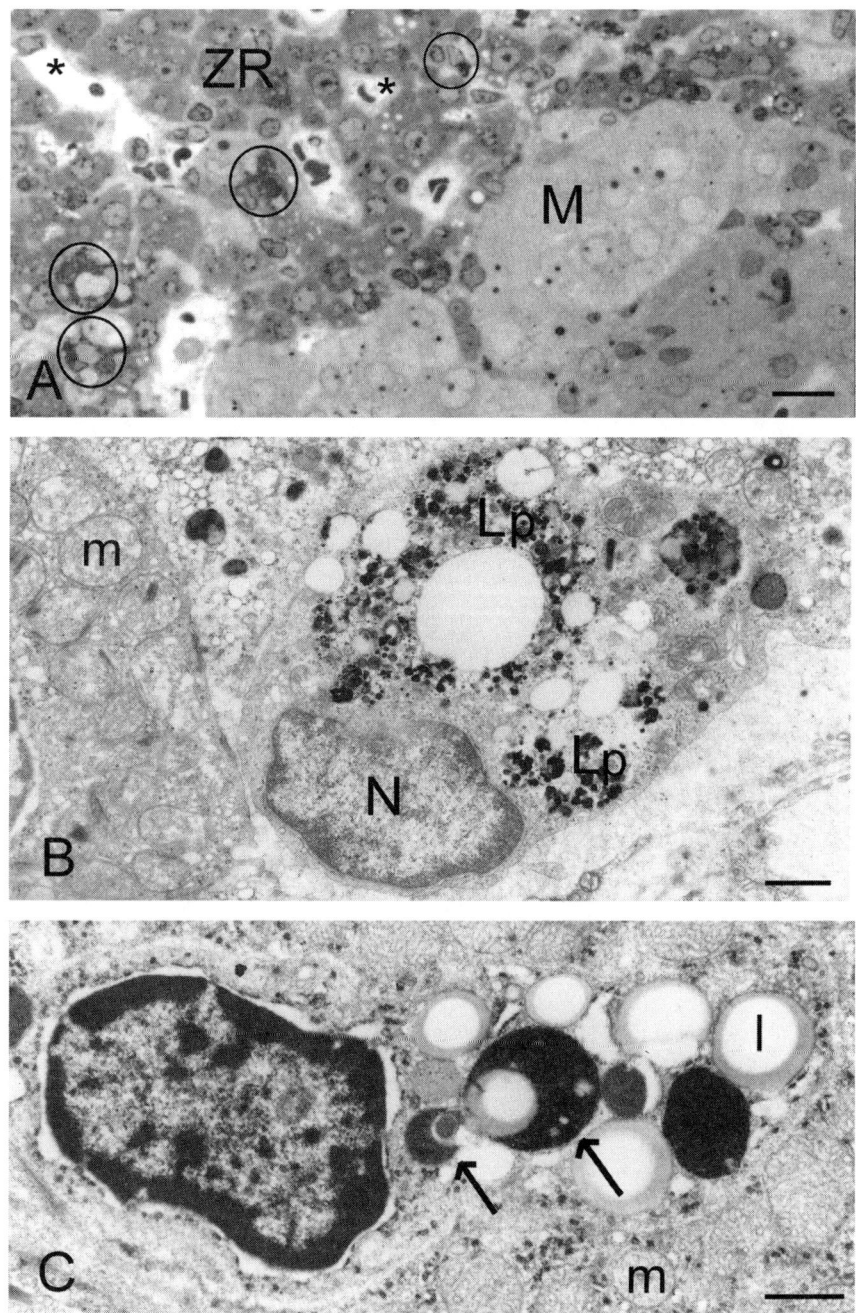

FIGURE 1. *See previous page for legend.*

TABLE 1. Macrophage Vv (%), Nv (× 10³/mm³), and CV (μm³) at different ages[a]

	VvCt	VvDx	NvCt	NvDx	CVCt	CVDx
2m	1.21 ± 0.23	2.04 ± 0.45	1.42 ± 0.15	2.73 ± 0.27	797.4 ± 157.8	730.2 ± 115.2
6m	2.01 ± 0.45	2.27 ± 0.26	2.90 ± 0.17[A]	2.35 ± 0.21	715.9 ± 199.0	826.0 ± 107.2
12m	2.59 ± 0.56	2.90 ± 0.26	3.07 ± 0.35[A]	3.92 ± 0.34	827.0 ± 161.8	749.2 ± 69.2
18m	3.74 ± 0.64[A,B]	4.37 ± 0.55	3.09 ± 020[A]	3.58 ± 0.16	1227.0 ± 203..9	1186.0 ± 149.6[A]
24m	4.99 ± 0.72[A,B,C]	7.90 ± 1.99[A,B,C,d]	3.03 ± 0.25[A]	4.86 ± 1.12[A,B,c,d]	1629.0 ± 160.6[A,B,C]	1437.0 ± 232.5[A,B]
P<	0.01	0.01	0.01	0.01	0.05	0.05

[a] a, b, c, and d refer to comparisons with 2, 6, 12, and 18 months, respectively, for $P<.05$ in LSD procedure of Fisher; A, B, C, and D report comparisons for $P<.01$. Means ± standard error of controls (Ct) and dexamethasone injected (Dx), $n = 4$.

the ultrastructural level, they appeared as lipofuscin granules: clumps of round structures with heterogeneous electronic density interspersed with dense, membrane-like features, all surrounded by a membrane (FIG. 1B). The content of some granules had a positive reaction for acid phosphatase, indicating their lysosomal origin (FIG. 1C).

In dexamethasone-injected animals, the structure of the AC and ZR parenchyma cells was maintained. In some sections, the width of the IZ appeared smaller, whereas in others that was not apparent. Parenchyma cells appeared smaller; in some, the nuclei were irregularly shaped and in others they had shrunk. Some nuclei were observed in an intracapillary location. Cells with ultrastructural features similar to monocytes were seen more frequently; macrophages had a similar location as in controls and appeared to contain a larger amount of the cytoplasmic features described.

Quantitative

The results for Vv (%), Nv ($\times 10^3$/mm^3), and CV (μm^3) are depicted in TABLE 1. There was a statistically significant increase in macrophage Vv and Nv ($P < .01$) and CV ($P < .05$).

DISCUSSION

Macrophages are cells originating from monocytes and may be observed throughout the body. They include the histiocytes of the connective tissue and the various types of macrophages present in different tissues and organs.

Macrophages are widely known for their ability to phagocytose microorganisms, particles, dead cells, or cell debris. However, there is a large body of evidence showing that macrophages also are involved in immunity and inflammatory processes through the secretion of multiple products[6] and therefore are likely to modulate locally the functioning of neighbor cells. This applies, in particular, to macrophages located in the adrenal cortex.[7]

As in other tissues, in the AC they have a subendothelial location, next to the parenchyma cells, and are present in all zones but are more numerous at the IZ.[8] This distribution pattern, which may be related to different functions, agrees with the migration theory. According to it,[9] adrenocortical cells originate at the outer cell layers, differentiate, and move centripetally to die ultimately at the innermost layers (ZR), where they are removed by the macrophages.

In the saline-injected rats in our study, we found an age-related increase in macrophage Vv, Nv, and average cell volume, which suggests a continuous process of phagocytosis, likely of ZR dead cells or their debris. The presence of larger macrophages presenting the cytoplasm filled with apparently undigested debris suggests so.

The ZR, taken as part of the IZ, forms a functionally distinct compartment of the AC, whose main regulator is the ACTH. The administration of ACTH is followed by an enhancement of steroidogenic enzyme activity, enlargement of IZ cell volume, mitochondrial and smooth endoplasmic reticulum compartments, and an increase in steroid output.[2,10] When ACTH is suppressed, after hypophysectomy or corticosteroid administration, these features are reversed[2,10] and apoptosis is seen at the ZR and its transition to ZF.[1]

Macrophages of dexamethasone-injected rats maintained the steady age-related increase in Vv, Nv, and cell volume. However, their Vv and Nv were higher, and average cell volume was lower, when compared with controls. Such a finding, indicating that a higher number of smaller macrophages occupy a larger volume, suggests a recent migration of monocytes into the adrenal and their activation into macrophages.

The age-related increase in macrophages at the ZR also may occur as a result of their secretory role with local modulatory effect. In fact, macrophages secrete interleukin-1, which causes corticosterone release in the rat adrenal, whether directly or indirectly.[7] Taking into account the previous observation of an age-related decrease in secretory ability of IZ cells despite an increase in circulating levels of ACTH,[4] it is likely that macrophages may operate as paracrine regulators in an attempt to enhance corticosterone production and secretion. Additional studies would be necessary to enlighten us regarding the relative contribution of phagocytosis and secretion in this setting.

ACKNOWLEDGMENT

In memory of Prof. Manuel Miranda Magalhães (1935–2002), Full Professor of the Faculty of Medicine of Porto and former member of the New York Academy of Sciences.

REFERENCES

1. WYLLIE, A.H., J.F.R. KERR, I.A.M. MACASKILL, *et al.* 1973. Adrenocortical cell deletion: the role of ACTH. J. Pathol. **111:** 85–94.
2. NUSSDORFER, G.G. 1986. Cytophysiology of the adrenal cortex. Int. Rev. Cytol. **98:** 1–405.
3. SAVILL, J. 1997. Recognition and phagocytosis of cells undergoing apoptosis. Br. Med. Bull. **53:** 491–508.
4. ALMEIDA, H., M.C. MAGALHÃES & M.M. MAGALHÃES. 1998. Age-related changes in the inner zone of the adrenal cortex of the rat—a morphologic and biochemical study. Mech. Ageing Develop. **105:** 1–18.
5. WEIBEL, E.R. & R.P. BOLENDER. 1973. Stereological techniques for electron microscopic morphometry. *In* Principles and Techniques of Electron Microscopy. Vol. 3. M.A. Hayat, Ed.: 237–296. Van Nostrand-Reinhold. New York.
6. NATHAN, C.F. 1987. Secretory products of macrophages. J. Clin. Invest. **79:** 319–326.
7. EHRHART-BORNSTEIN, M., J.P. HINSON, S.R. BORNSTEIN, *et al.* 1998. Intraadrenal interactions in the regulation of adrenocortical steroidogenesis. Endocrinol. Rev. **19:** 101–143.
8. SURLEFF, S.V. & J.M. PAPADIMITRIOU. 1981. The mononuclear phagocytes of the rat adrenal. Am. J. Pathol. **104:** 258–271.
9. LONG, J.A. 1975. Zonation of the mammalian adrenal cortex. *In* Handbook of Physiology. Section 7 (Endocrinology). Vol 6. R.O. Greep & E.B. Astwood, Eds.: 13–24. American Physiological Society. Washington, DC.
10. ESTIVARIZ, F.E., P.J. LOWRY & S. JACKSON. 1992. Control of adrenal growth. *In* The Adrenal Gland. 2nd ed. V.H.T. James, Ed.:1–42. Raven Press. New York.

Looking for Immunological Risk Genotypes

CALOGERO CARUSO, ALESSANDRA AQUINO, GIUSEPPINA CANDORE, LETIZIA SCOLA, GIUSEPPINA COLONNA-ROMANO, AND DOMENICO LIO

Gruppo di Studio sull'Immunosenescenza, Dipartimento di Biopatologia e Metodologie Biomediche, Palermo, Italy

ABSTRACT: Several functional markers of the immune system may be used either as markers of successful aging or conversely as markers of unsuccessful aging. Particularly, a combination of high CD8 and low CD4 and poor T cell proliferation has been associated with a higher two-year mortality in very old subjects. Therefore, genetic determinants of longevity should reside in those polymorphisms for the immune system genes that regulate immune responses. Concerning these changes in T cell subpopulations, how much they depend on the immunogenetic background and how much they depend on individual antigenic load, such as chronic infections, should be assessed. As previously demonstrated in our population, the interleukin (IL)–2 high-producer genotype is less frequent in old men than in young people; conversely, the IL-10 high-producer genotype is increased in old men. In this study, we tried to assess the role of low- and high-producer genotypes for IL-10 and IL-2 in the CD4 and CD8 absolute values, taking into account gender and age. The results suggest that old men carrying an anti-inflammatory IL-10 high-producer genotype or a proinflammatory IL-2 low-producer genotype show the lowest values of CD8 cells. Although in our study we were not able to show any correlation with CD4 values and no functional assessment of T cell was performed, these results suggest that cytokine genotypes may be involved in the subpopulation dynamics in old age.

KEYWORDS: CD4; CD8; IL-2; IL-10; polymorphisms

INTRODUCTION

Some people live in good health to great age while others die relatively young; we do not understand why this is so. However, several studies show that longevity may be correlated with optimal functioning of the immune system. In fact, both longitudinal and cross-sectional studies performed in the last years have indicated that several functional markers of the immune system may be used either as markers of successful aging or conversely as markers of unsuccessful aging. Particularly, several early studies already suggested a positive association between a "good" T cell function and individual longevity. More recently, several studies have focussed on CD4 and CD8 T cell absolute values, being a combination of CD8 and low CD4 and

---

Address for correspondence: Prof. Calogero Caruso, M.D., Gruppo di Studio sull'Immunosenescenza, Dipartimento di Biopatologia e Metodologie Biomediche, Corso Tukory 211, 90134 Palermo, Italy. Voice: +39-09-1655-5911; fax: +39-09-1655-5933.
marcoc@unipa.it

poor T cell proliferation associated with a higher two-year mortality in very old subjects.[1,2]

As discussed by Pawelec et al.,[1] in these kinds of studies the "chicken and egg" question has to be asked: that is, Do people live longer because of "good" immune function, or do they possess good immune function because other factors have enabled them to survive longer? Thus, to better understand the role of immune system in longevity, we have to search for immunogenetic markers of longevity. In other words, whether immune system plays a key role in the attainment of successful aging, then genetic determinants of longevity should reside in those polymorphisms for the immune system genes that regulate immune responses as cytokines.[2]

On the whole, data on cytokine polymorphisms suggest that polymorphic alleles of inflammatory cytokines, involved in high cytokine production, play an important role in age-related inflammatory diseases, that is, in unsuccessful aging. Reciprocally, they suggest that controlling inflammatory status may allow better attainment of successful aging. In fact, the major findings reported in the recent articles on cytokine polymorphisms and longevity suggest that those individuals who are genetically predisposed to produce low levels of inflammatory cytokines or high levels of anti-inflammatory cytokines have an increased capacity to reach the extreme limits of human life span.[1–3]

Concerning the change in T cell subpopulations assessed as markers of unsuccessful aging, the matter should be to assess how much these changes depend on the immunogenetic background and how much depend on the natural history of the individual, that is, on an extra burden of antigenic load such as chronic infections. Further steps should include studies able to relate immunological and immunogenetic markers.[2,4]

As previously demonstrated in our population, the interleukin (IL)–2 (that is a type 1 proinflammatory cytokine) high-producer genotype is less frequent in old men than in young people; conversely, the IL-10 (that is a type 2 anti-inflammatory cytokine) high-producer genotype was increased in old men. These gender-related effects are difficult to explain. However, it is well known that men and women may follow different strategies to reach longevity.[3,5]

In this study, we tried to assess the role of low- and high-producer genotypes for IL-10 and IL-2 in the CD4 and CD8 absolute values, taking into account gender and age. For this purpose, we classified –1082 G/G genotype of IL-10 as high producer and GA or AA as low producer[3] and –330 TG and GG genotype of IL-2 as high producer and TT as low producer.[5]

MATERIALS AND METHODS

Studied subjects were randomly selected from the Sicilian population. None of these was affected by neoplastic, infectious, or autoimmune diseases or was experiencing any drug-influencing immune functions at the time of the study. Informed consent was obtained according to Italian laws. For this study, we selected 80 individuals (age range, 21–101; 20 men and 60 women). Blood samples were collected in tripotassium EDTA sterile tubes and an aliquot was put away for cytometry analysis of subpopulations, and, on the other sample, genomic DNA extraction was performed and DNA was stored at $-20°C$ for the cytokine genotype analysis.

In all the freshly collected blood samples, we identified the lymphocyte population by using forward and side-angle scatter on a FACScan flow cytometer (Becton Dickinson, Mountain View, CA, USA). Samples were treated with fluorochrome-conjugated monoclonal antibodies anti-CD3 (fluoroscein-isothiocyanate), CD4, CD8 (phycoerythrin; Caltag, Burlingame, CA, USA) to identify lymphocyte subpopulations by two-color fluorescence. Forward and side-angle scatter were collected as linear signals, and all fluorescent emissions were collected on a four-decade logarithmic scale. All measurements were made with the same instrument setting, and at least 10^4 cells were analyzed by using Lysis II software (Becton Dickinson).[6]

Complete linkage of allele −819C with allele −592C and of allele −819T with allele −592A and the presence of only three different allele combinations, −1082G, −819C, and −592C GCC, ACC, and ATA, are characteristic of the IL-10 polymorphisms in Caucasoid populations.[7] In the previous study, only −1082 SNP was shown to be associated with longevity; therefore, in this study we limited ourselves to the analysis of the −1082 G→A SNP. This biallelic polymorphism was identified using ARMS-PCR, as previously described.[7] The functional IL-2 polymorphism, known to be involved in different cytokine production, at 330 (T→G) was analyzed by a multiplex SSP based on a set of four primers as described by Reynard et al.[5,8]

Statistical analysis was performed using Statistical Package for Social Sciences for Windows (SPSS). $P < .05$ was considered significant.

RESULTS AND DISCUSSION

FIGURE 1 shows the distribution of subset absolute values according to age, gender, and cytokine producer genotypes. The correlations between absolute values and age, according to gender and genotypes are depicted.

FIGURE 1A, B shows the distribution of CD4 subset absolute values according to age, gender, and IL-10 or, respectively, IL-2 producer genotypes. The correlations between absolute values and age, according to gender and genotypes are depicted. No significant difference in the distribution was observed taking into account gender, age, or genotype.

FIGURE 1C, D shows the distribution of CD8 subset absolute values according to age, gender, and IL-10 or, respectively, IL-2 producer genotypes. The correlations between absolute values and age, according to gender and genotypes are depicted. FIGURE 1C shows that taking into account gender, age, and genotype a significant difference ($P < .05$) was observed, because old men IL-10 high producers showed the lowest values of CD8 (114 vs. 345). Concerning IL-2 genotypes, again taking into account gender, age, and genotype, a significant difference ($P < .05$) was observed because old men IL-2 low producers showed the lowest values of CD8 (174 vs. 426; FIG. 1D).

In this study, we have analyzed in our group of old and old oldest people, typed for IL-10 and IL-2 genotypes, known to be associated to longevity,[3,5,7] the relationship between high- or low-producer genotypes and lymphocyte subpopulations. The results seem to indicate that cytokine genotypes may be involved in the subpopulation dynamics in old age. In particular, our preliminary results suggest that old men carrying an antiinflammatory IL-10 high-producer genotype or a proinflammatory IL-2 low-producer genotype show the lowest values of CD8 cells. It is intriguing that

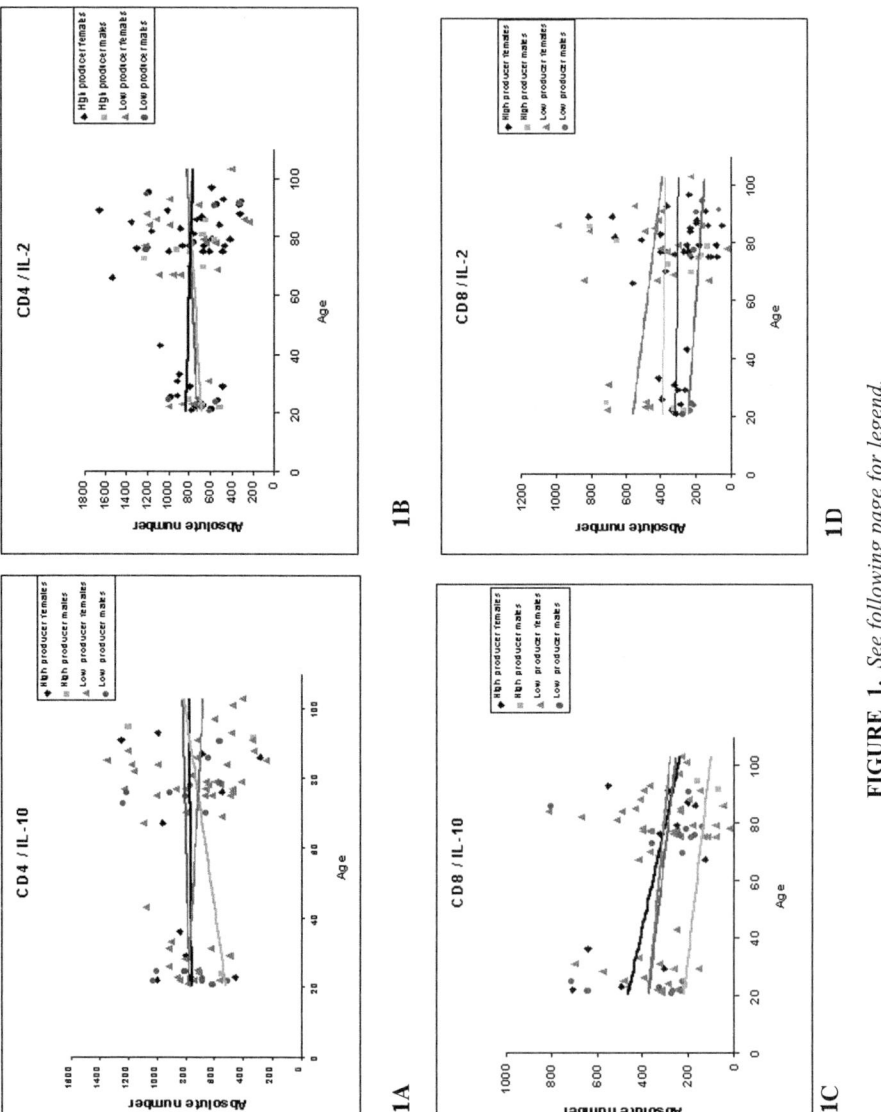

FIGURE 1. See following page for legend.

a combination of high CD8 and low CD4 and poor T cell proliferation has been claimed to be associated with a higher two-year mortality in very old subjects.[1,2,4] However, in our study we were not able to show any correlation with CD4 values, and no functional assessment of T cells was performed.

Thus, concerning the change in T cell subpopulations assessed as markers of unsuccessful aging, our results suggest that T subset changes might depend on the immunogenetic background and not only on the natural history of the individual, that is, on an extra burden of antigenic load such as chronic infections.[2] However, note that an efficient control of chronic infections also depends on the immunogenetic background of the host.[9,10]

ACKNOWLEDGMENTS

The "Gruppo di Studio sull'immunosenescenza" coordinated by Professor C. Caruso is funded by grants from MIUR, Rome (40%, to C.C. and D.L.; 60% to C.C., D.L., G.C., and G.C.-R.), and from Ministery of Health Projects "Immunological parameters age-related" and "Genetic and nongenetic determinants of healthy aging."

REFERENCES

1. PAWELEC, G. et al. 2002. T cells and aging. Front Biosci. **7:** d1056–d1183.
2. CANDORE, G. et al. 2003. Immunological and immunogenetic markers of successful and unsuccessful ageing. Adv. Cell Aging Gerontol. **13:** 29–45.
3. LIO, D. et al. 2003. Inflammation, genetics and longevity: further studies on the protective effects in men of IL-10 –1082 promoter SNP and its interaction with –308 TNF-α promoter SNP. J. Med. Genet. **40:** 296–299.
4. PAWELEC, G. et al. 2002. Is human immunosenescence clinically relevant? Looking for "immunological risk phenotypes." Trends Immunol. **23:** 330–332.
5. CANDORE, G. et al. 2002. Polymorphisms of IL-2, IL-10 and IFN-γ genes in Sicilian elderly: implication for longevity. Biogerontology 3 (Suppl. 1): 36–37.
6. POTESTIO, M. et al. 1999. Age-related changes in the expression of CD95 (Apo1/Fas) on blood lymphocytes. Exp. Gerontol. **34:** 659–673.
7. LIO, D. et al. 2002. Gender specific association between –1082 IL-10 promoter polymorphism and longevity. Genes Immun. **3:** 30–33.
8. REYNARD, M.P. et al. 2000. Allele frequencies of polymorphisms of the tumour necrosis factor-alpha, interleukin-10, interferon-gamma and interleukin-2 genes in a North European Caucasoid group from the UK. Eur. J. Immunogenet. **27:** 241–249.

FIGURE 1. Distribution of subset absolute values according to age, gender, and cytokine producer genotypes. The correlations between absolute values and age, according to gender and genotypes are depicted. (**A**, **B**) Distribution of CD4 subset absolute values according to age, gender, and IL-10 or, respectively, IL-2 producer genotypes. The R values are ◆, .02; ■, .31; ▲, –.13; ●, .06 (**A**) and, respectively, ◆, –.07; ■, .20; ▲, –.06; ●, .13 (**B**). Panels **C** and **D** show the distribution of CD8 subset absolute values according to age, gender and IL-10 or, respectively, IL-2 producer genotypes. The R values are: ◆, –.43; ■, –.77; ▲, –.18; ●, .20 (**C**) and, respectively, ◆, .03; ■, .02; ▲, –.22; ●, –.64 (**D**). Concerning CD8 subset, taking into account gender, age, and genotype, a significant difference ($P < .05$) was observed because old men IL-10 high producers showed the lowest values of CD8 (114 vs. 345) (**C**), and old men IL-2 low producers showed the lowest values of CD8 (174 vs. 426) (**D**).

9. CARUSO, C. et al. 2001. Immunogenetics of longevity. Is major histocompatibility complex polymorphism relevant to the control of human longevity? A review of literature data. Mech. Ageing Dev. **122:** 445–462.
10. SCOLA, L. et al. 2003. IL-10 and TNF-alpha polymorphisms in a sample of Sicilian patients affected by tuberculosis: implication for ageing and life span expectancy. Mech. Ageing Dev. **124:** 569–572.

Total Deletion of *in Vivo* Telomere Elongation Capacity

An Ambitious but Possibly Ultimate Cure for All Age-Related Human Cancers

AUBREY D. N. J. DE GREY,[a] F. CHARLES CAMPBELL,[b] INDERJEET DOKAL,[c] LESLIE J. FAIRBAIRN,[d] GERRY J. GRAHAM,[e] COLIN A. B. JAHODA,[f] AND ANDREW C. G. PORTER[g]

[a]*Department of Genetics, University of Cambridge,* Cambridge CB2 3EH, United Kingdom

[b]*Department of Surgery, Queen's University of Belfast,* Belfast, Ireland

[c]*Department of Haematology, Imperial College, London,* United Kingdom

[d]*Paterson Institute for Cancer Research, Manchester,* United Kingdom

[e]*Cancer Research UK Beatson Laboratories, Glasgow,* Scotland

[f]*School of Biological and Biomedical Sciences, University of Durham,* United Kingdom

[g]*Faculty of Medicine, Imperial College, London,* United Kingdom

ABSTRACT: Despite enormous effort, progress in reducing mortality from cancer remains modest. Can a true cancer "cure" ever be developed, given the vast versatility that tumors derive from their genomic instability? Here we consider the efficacy, feasibility, and safety of a therapy that, unlike any available or in development, could never be escaped by spontaneous changes of gene expression: the total elimination from the body of all genetic potential for telomere elongation, combined with stem cell therapies administered about once a decade to maintain proliferative tissues despite this handicap. We term this therapy WILT, for whole-body interdiction of lengthening of telomeres. We first argue that a whole-body gene-deletion approach, however bizarre it initially seems, is truly the only way to overcome the hypermutation that makes tumors so insidious. We then identify the key obstacles to developing such a therapy and conclude that, while some will probably be insurmountable for at least a decade, none is a clear-cut showstopper. Hence, given the absence of alternatives with comparable anticancer promise, we advocate working toward such a therapy.

KEYWORDS: cancer; telomerase; ALT; stem cell therapy; chemoresistance; gene targeting

Address for correspondence: Dr. Aubrey D.N.J. de Grey, Department of Genetics, University of Cambridge, Downing Street, Cambridge CB2 3EH, UK. Voice: +44-1223-765665; fax: +44-1223- 333992.

ag24@gen.cam.ac.uk

INTRODUCTION

The reason cancer is so hard to combat is depressingly simple; it comes down to just two facts. First, cancer cells are very similar in most respects to the non–cancer cells from which they arose, making selective ablation of cancer cells intrinsically fraught. Second, unlike all other aspects of age-related degeneration, cancer can acquire additional means of survival in response to whatever the body, or the clinician, may throw at it. Each cell in a tumor is a furnace of inventive potential, constantly experimenting with new combinations of gene expression as a result of its profound genomic instability and the availability of 6Gb of DNA to rearrange.

What therapies might, in principle, overcome this versatility? An answer is evident when we consider the mechanisms whereby tumors escape endogenous or medical attack, because those mechanisms have one very tangible thing in common: changes of gene expression. Immune stimulation is often escaped by loss of antigen presentation.[1] Angiogenesis inhibition is escaped by upregulating alternative angiogenic pathways.[2] Chemotherapy may be escaped by numerous mechanisms, including upregulating transporters that keep the cell free of the toxin, or specific DNA repair capacities.[3] Telomerase inhibitors[4] are too new for clinical data to be available, but can, in theory, be escaped by overexpression of telomerase or degradation or export of the inhibitor.

We should therefore seek therapies that make such changes of gene expression impossible or at least highly improbable, even for the ever-inventive cancer cell. In principle, the **deletion** (not merely inhibition) of a gene whose function is essential for cancers to progress would present a major challenge to cancer cells. Creation of a new gene out of nothing does of course occur on evolutionary time scales, but it is many orders of magnitude rarer than mutations causing changes of expression, so tumors would never have enough cells or enough time to achieve it.

Unfortunately, cancer cells have the same genome as non–cancer cells. Selective deletion of a gene from cancer cells, but not others, faces the usual gene-expression problems: cancer cells can readily escape by downregulating the DNA maintenance machinery on which targeted deletion depends, and the need to avoid killing too many non–cancer cells intrinsically limits any such treatment's therapeutic index.

A way around this is to eliminate the gene from **all** cells, and somehow to make it nonessential to the non–cancer cell (or, at least, to the tissue of which that cell is a part) while preserving the cancer cell's absolute requirement for it. This is the approach discussed here. The genes in question are those responsible for maintaining telomere length through large numbers of cell divisions by telomere elongation. Tissue integrity would be preserved by, about every ten years, reseeding the stem cell compartments of all tissues reliant on continuous cell division with stem cells whose telomeres had been lengthened *ex vivo* but whose telomere elongation machinery was deleted (FIG. 1). Transformation of a living organism—ultimately, a human—to a totally telomere elongation–incompetent state would be performed gradually, using a variety of techniques discussed below. We suggest that, if (as we foresee) it could be implemented without serious side effects, this therapy would almost completely eliminate cancer as an age-related cause of death, something which no other present or currently contemplated therapy would do. In fact, one's risk of cancer would actually **decline** with age as telomere elongation–competent cells were progressively depleted.

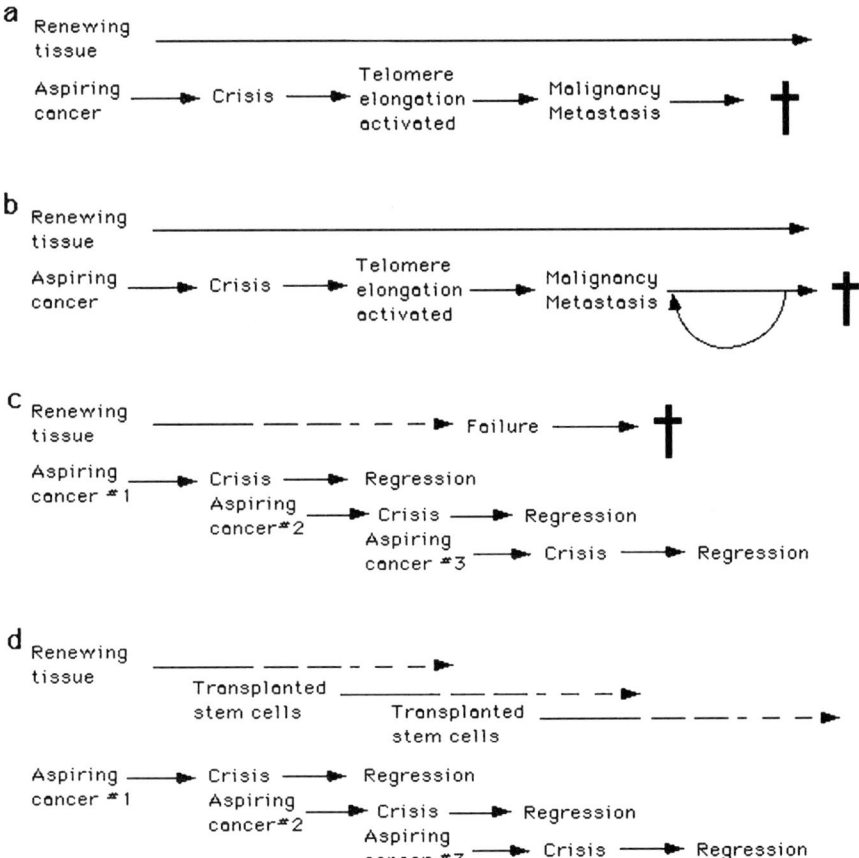

FIGURE 1. The WILT concept. An untreated cancer sufferer (**a**) dies rapidly once the cancer achieves malignancy and metastasis. Conventional treatments (**b**) delay death somewhat, but the cancer typically evolves gene expression changes that outmaneuver the treatment. A hypothetical telomere-elongation-negative human (**c**) could not develop metastatic cancer, but would die relatively young from failure of constantly renewing tissues. A beneficiary of WILT (**d**) would maintain function of such tissues through periodic stem cell transplantation, so would not die of either cause.

Here we discuss the plethora of obstacles to the development (even on a multi-decade time scale) of such therapy, which we term WILT, whole-body interdiction of lengthening of telomeres. We conclude that, while many of those obstacles are daunting, none is so insurmountable as to justify dismissing this approach. We foresee a considerable risk that, as sophisticated cell and gene therapy technologies mature in the next decade or two, progress in reducing age-specific cancer death rates will lag behind that for other major killers,[5] and that the proportion of people dying from cancer will thus rise sharply. It may be that only by developing ambitious but extremely powerful anticancer therapies, such as WILT, can this be prevented.

EFFICACY

Requirement of Telomere Elongation for Human Cancer Progression

A typical clinically relevant cancer contains around 2^{40} (10^{12}) cells. Thus, at least 40 cell generations have occurred in that cancer, starting from the initiating non–cancer cell. In fact, however, this is a gross underestimate: (1) there is abundant cell death in cancer, and (2) the development of cancer is a multistage process. Suppose, for simplicity, that a cancer develops as a result of two mutations—one to escape growth control and, later, one to induce angiogenesis. The former may allow it to grow to, say, 10^6 cells; the second, to 10^{12} cells. That second mutation, however, will have occurred in just one of the 10^6 cells that harbored the first. Thus, starting from the cell in which the first mutation occurred, there will have been not 40 but 60 divisions—even ignoring the contribution of cell death.

In practice, since cancer progression in humans requires many more than two mutations (except some rare childhood cancers), there are probably at least a few hundred cell generations between the originating non–mutant cell and the clinically relevant cancer.[6] It is this that makes prevention of telomere elongation a realistic way to prevent cancers from ever reaching an advanced stage. No human cell has ever been observed to divide more than 100 times without telomere elongation machinery. Moreover, even though the "end-replication problem"[7,8] that originally inspired the telomere-based explanation of this "Hayflick limit"[9] suggests that telomere loss per cell generation could be much slower than is typically seen *in vitro*,[10] only a modest extension of replicative capacity results from growth in low oxygen.[11] Direct evidence for the absolute requirement of telomere elongation for progression of human cancers is widespread.[12–14]

Telomerase

All mammals maintain telomere length in rapidly dividing cells by reverse transcription of a 6-base RNA template, of which the telomere is a many-copy DNA tandem repeat. The RNA including the template (hereafter TERC) and the reverse transcriptase (hereafter TERT) form a heterodimer called telomerase, which adds copies of this sequence to the end of one strand; the other strand is elongated by standard DNA replication machinery.[15] TERC is ubiquitous in human tissues, but TERT is expressed only at trace levels in tissues that require telomere elongation and is undetectable in quiescent and postmitotic cells.[16,17] In about 90% of human cancers, however, TERT is highly expressed and telomere length thereby stabilized.[18] Many human non–cancer cell types that normally senesce (have a finite replicative capacity) in culture have been "immortalized" (given indefinite replicative capacity) by introducing constitutively active TERT.[19–21]

Though telomerase may have cytoprotective properties not directly related to cell division–associated telomere elongation,[22] it seems that neither telomerase subunit has any **essential** physiological function except telomere elongation. For TERT in humans, this is shown by its absence in nearly all cells and very low levels in any cell type. In laboratory mice, which maintain their telomere length several organismal generations "ahead of the game" (allowing serial inbreeding of telomerase knockout mice, in which telomeres in the germ line progressively shorten), knockout of either TERC or TERT confers no detectable phenotype for three generations.[23,24] Thus, these genes are prime targets for WILT.

Alternative Lengthening of Telomeres

However, about 10% of human cancers—predominantly mesenchyme-derived ones, such as sarcomas, in which the proportion approaches 50%—do not express telomerase but nonetheless maintain telomere length indefinitely both *in vivo* and *in vitro*.[25] They do so by a mechanism termed ALT, for alternative lengthening of telomeres. Moreover, cancers of epithelial tissues may express ALT rarely only because they have the easier option to activate telomerase (which may be suppressed less thoroughly in epithelial than in mesenchymal tissues). Hence, epithelial-derived cancers might turn ALT on as easily as sarcomas do if the telomerase route were denied them. A therapy that eliminated the ability of cancer to activate telomerase but left ALT untouched might thus only modestly reduce age-specific cancer mortality rates.

The mechanism of ALT clearly involves a recombination-like process, but the molecular details have not been determined. Short telomeres are the recipients of ALT events (but perhaps not exclusively), but it is unclear whether the telomere repeats added are chromosomal or extrachromosomal in origin. One model proposes that t-loop structures initiate intratelomeric rolling circle replication in ALT cells, though there is currently no supporting evidence for this mechanism in human cells. A second model (which has some supporting evidence[26]) proposes strand invasion and copying of telomere repeats from a donor to a recipient telomere in a BIR (breakage-induced repair)–like process.[27]

Even with our limited current understanding of ALT, however, we can make one observation that gives cause for optimism that, once its underlying genetic etiology is discovered, it will be amenable to the same sort of manipulation as for telomerase. There are formally three types of possible explanation for why ALT is seen in certain cancers but not in normal tissues. One is that, like telomerase, ALT is an activation of a gene or genes that are normally turned off in the cell type in which the cancer arises. (Candidate genes might be ones involved in meiosis or in a form of DNA repair that is only activated under certain circumstances, for example.) The second is that telomere elongation by recombination is a side effect of a constitutive process (a ubiquitous DNA repair process, for example): that is, that it is happening all the time in normal cells but is counterbalanced by a shortening process, and so progressive telomere lengthening is not seen in such cells. Indeed, there seems to be a system for actively shortening telomeres that have been lengthened by ALT.[28] If this second mechanism were the basis of ALT, it would be a blow to the potential efficacy of WILT, because no gene would be available to be deleted without rapidly deleterious effects in normal cells. This seems unlikely, however, because a constitutive system in which telomere elongation by recombination is balanced by shortening of overly long telomeres would maintain telomere length by default in all tumors and there would be no pressure to activate telomerase. Additionally, telomeric recombination has not been detected in normal cells.[26,29] Finally there is the possibility that the active players in ALT are indeed active in normal cells (performing nontelomeric DNA maintenance), but that, rather than being constantly lengthened and reshortened, some system protects telomeres from being adventitiously lengthened by this machinery in the first place, and this is lost in ALT cells. In this scenario, however, since the hypothetical constitutive function of the ALT machinery is certainly not interchromosomal recombination, it seems plausible that (once it had been identified) judicious site-directed mutagenesis could delete its capacity for such recombination while preserving its constitutive function.

Hence, in summary, until the molecular basis of ALT is understood, we cannot state how or whether it can be ablated along with telomerase as part of WILT, but there is reason for optimism.

Chemotherapy and Chemoresistance

The characteristic that most centrally defines a cancer cell is its high division rate. Thus, the cell types that are hardest to distinguish from cancer cells, when designing a therapy, are those that themselves divide fast, such as in the bone marrow, skin, and gut. The blood, in particular, is maintained by the rapid division of transit amplifying cells in bone marrow whose ablation as a result of anticancer therapy is highly prejudicial to the welfare or even survival of the patient.[30]

Conveniently, the tissues most at risk in this regard are just those that would also—again because of their rapid division—be eventually compromised by WILT. Such tissues must be maintained by the periodic introduction of new cells that have been engineered *ex vivo*. This *ex vivo* manipulation can potentially include manipulations to diminish sensitivity to anticancer agents.

In fact, many groups have been exploring such an approach (independently of WILT, of course).[31,32] A prominent stratagem has been to exploit the cell's spectacularly laborious mechanism for reversing a particular type of DNA damage—alkylation of guanine at position 6; this is done by a protein that transfers the alkyl group to itself and is then ubiquitinated and destroyed, rather than acting catalytically. This protein, O^6-alkylguanine-DNA-alkyltransferase (ATase) is a first-class target for chemotherapeutic agents because of two additional features: first, there are small molecules that mimic O^6-alkylation in DNA and act as pseudosubstrates of the protein leading to its inactivation, and second, there are single amino acid changes to the protein that render it almost completely resistant to such inactivation (FIG. 2). Hence, before chemotherapy with a combination of inactivator and O^6-alkylating agent, the patient can be transplanted with hemopoietic stem cells engineered to express inactivator-resistant ATase; then, a dose of the inhibitor/O^6-alkylating agent combination that the cancer cell cannot survive will ablate native bone marrow but leave the transplanted cells (and hence the patient) unscathed.[33]

This approach possesses an inherent shortcoming: engineered marrow—which must necessarily contain hemopoietic stem cells—could give rise to new cancers, which would be resistant to some chemotherapeutic challenges. Since hemopoietic stem cells can repopulate many tissues other than the blood,[34,35] this problem might be severe if the patient lives many years after the treatment. However, when implemented in combination with WILT, no such concern exists: such cancers might arise, but they could not reach a life-threatening stage.

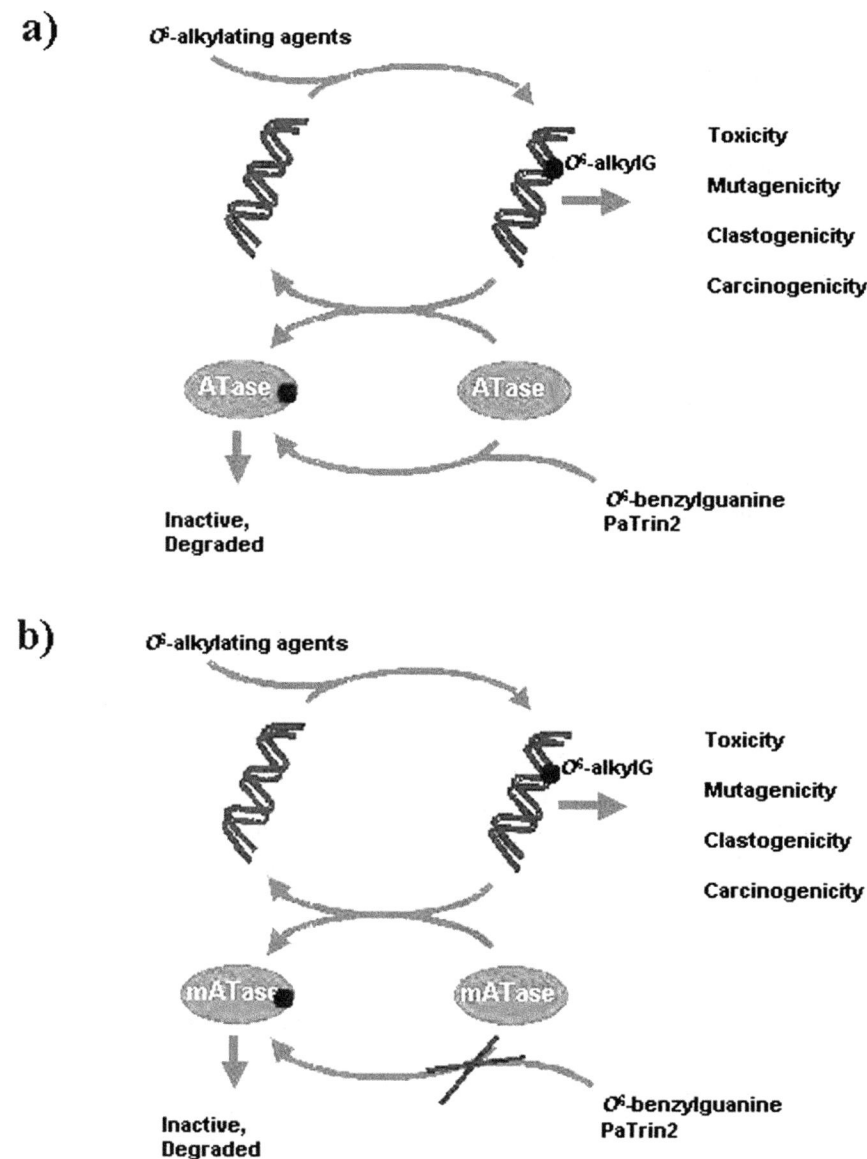

FIGURE 2. Mechanism of ATase activity and inactivation. (**a**) O^6-alkylating agent modification of DNA leads to incorporation of alkyl groups at the O^6 position of guanine and to subsequent genotoxic events. ATase repairs O^6-alkylguanine lesions in a stoichiometric and autoinactivating manner. Small molecule pseuodosubstrates of ATase lead to inactivation and thus to sensitivity of cells to O^6-alkylating agents. (**b**) Certain point-mutated versions of ATase are unable to react with pseudosubstrates, yet retain their DNA-repair capacity.

Telomerase Capture: A Possible Cancer Escape Route from Whole-Body Interdiction of Lengthening of Telomeres?

The WILT concept assumes that creating a new gene is far harder than changing expression patterns. However, genomes can gain genes by lateral gene transfer. Could tumors escape WILT that way?

A formal possibility is that the reverse transcriptase of a retrovirus might be recruited for telomere elongation; these work very differently from TERT, however,[36] so this seems remote. Alternatively, a cell engineered to lack telomerase but to be chemoresistant might fuse, *in vivo*, with one that was present natively and hence retained telomerase genes. Cell fusion (and phagocytosis of apoptotic bodies, which could be equivalent) has been demonstrated *in vitro*,[37–39] but its *in vivo* relevance remains unknown. Such fusion products would, anyway, still be susceptible to chemotherapeutic agents to which resistance had not been transgenically conferred, so this would not seriously subvert WILT.

FEASIBILITY

Stem Cell Technology

We purposely say little here about the prospects for developing the stem cell technology needed for WILT. Clearly WILT could not be implemented until we can transform adult cells into stem cells of all rapidly renewing tissues, expand them very substantially *in vitro* and introduce them into the person from whom they came;[40] these are major advances. Numerous other advances necessary for WILT, however, are also very considerable, so that we do not foresee any prospect of its being developed in under ten years, even in the best case. Progress in stem cell technology is presently so rapid that nothing can meaningfully be predicted about where it will stand in ten years, let alone thereafter. Hence, we merely note that the necessary sophistication of stem cell therapy is likely to exist by then, and focus here on the many other prerequisites for implementing WILT.

Ex Vivo *Genetic Manipulation*

Three genetic alterations are entailed in WILT (plus, perhaps, adding an inducible "suicide gene" for safety): (1) deletion of telomere-elongation genes, (2) introduction of chemoresistance, and (3) elongation of telomeres to the length seen in a typical stem cell.

Of these, the last is probably easiest, because it does not require genomic integration. Expression of telomerase from an extrachromosomal transgene, in a cell that has already undergone the other required genetic changes, would extend telomeres to somewhat more than the desired length. The cells would then be grown for enough generations to allow confirmation of loss of the extrachromosomal transgene. Additionally, by incorporating a suicide gene such as HSVTk into the extrachromosomal construct, it should be possible to selectively eliminate (using ganciclovir) any cells that retain the construct.[41]

Chemoresistance could be conferred by introducing a transgene (e.g., encoding a drug-resistant ATase) at a random position in the genome. This approach, however, in common with most gene addition strategies for gene therapy, faces the severe problems of transgene silencing and instability after transplantation (not to mention potentially deleterious effects on genes close to the integration site), even if pre-transplant selection is used to enrich for transgene-expressing cells. Such problems can be avoided by modification of an endogenous gene; the fact that chemoresistance can sometimes be conferred by one or two amino acid changes[31] to an endogenous gene is particularly valuable in this context. The best-established technique for endogenous gene modification is gene targeting by homologous recombination between a target locus and a plasmid carrying several kbp of homologous dsDNA.[42–45] Other, less developed methods involve triplex-forming oligonucleotides,[46] single-stranded oligonucleotides,[47,48] or RNA/DNA oligonucleotides (RDOs).[49,50] The choice of technique would be driven mainly by the incidence of accompanying random mutations, rather than of the desired alteration, because selection for ATase inhibitor resistance, for example, can be used to enrich for rare events. Although the incidence of accompanying random integrations is easier to assess (by simple Southern analysis) in standard gene targeting methods, oligonucleotides have the attraction that they are relatively easy to prepare and deliver. It is therefore important that oligonucleotide-based methods be thoroughly validated, characterized, and optimized.

A problem with altering endogenous genes is that the target tissues are often sensitive to chemotherapeutic drugs because they naturally express low levels of drug-resistance mechanisms such as ATase. Thus, small changes to endogenous genes might be more appropriate for ubiquitously expressed enzymes such as thymidylate synthetase or dihydrofolate reductase, where specific mutations confer resistance to specific antimetabolites.[51,52] Other alternatives are to combine point mutations in the coding regions with genomic changes to alter expression patterns, or to deliver the drug resistance transgene on a mammalian artificial chromosome.[53,54]

Deletion of telomere-elongation genes is more challenging. First, deletion of both copies of at least two to four genes will be desirable. Second, these deletions will not confer an inherent selectable advantage on the cells (though with gene targeting this might be addressed by replacing the gene by a selectable marker). Third, the alterations must delete large portions of the relevant genes, because less drastic changes (such as single-base-pair changes to introduce a stop codon or frameshift) might be too easily reverted in a cancer. This may constrain the choice of technique: targeted deletions (see FIG. 3) of several kbp (or Mbp if Cre/lox technologies are used) are a well-established capability of standard gene targeting methods,[45,55–57] while oligonucleotide-mediated approaches have so far been limited to base changes or deletions of only one or two base pairs (although multiple modifications could be introduced sequentially). This situation may change, however, as oligonucleotide-based methods are developed in mammalian cells. In *E. coli*, for example, single-stranded oligonucleotides can generate a deletion of 3.3 kb as efficiently as a single base-pair change.[58]

Modification of multiple nonselectable genes is daunting because of the generally very low efficiencies of modification. Gene targeting frequencies of one per million transfected cells are not atypical, for example, and random integration frequencies are often 1–3 logs higher. Furthermore, the initially reported[59] high frequencies of RDO-mediated gene modification have often not been reproduced.[50] The efficiency of standard gene targeting and of oligo-based methods in general will therefore need

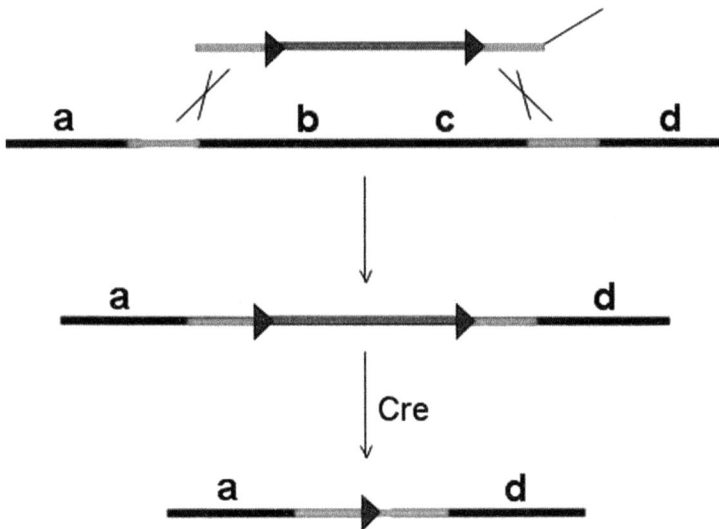

FIGURE 3. Making a genomic deletion by gene targeting. Regions of homology between the targeting construct (*top*) and the target locus are at the ends of the construct. In the first step, homologous recombination between the target gene and target locus deletes a portion of the target gene, replacing it with a drug resistance cassette (*central part of the construct*). If desired, the latter can be removed by the action of a site-specific recombinase (e.g., Cre) on flanking sequences (*triangles*; e.g., LoxP).

to be improved. Numerous approaches are being explored,[45,60,61] many based on promoting and impairing the machinery for homologous recombination and nonhomologous end-joining, respectively, and many improvements have already been reported. Other approaches can be envisaged, however. For example, methods for *in vitro* evolution of target-specific endonucleases may well emerge within the next decade, and these should be powerful tools, as it is known that double-strand breaks in the target gene can improve gene-targeting efficiencies by 2–3 logs.[62] Adeno-associated viruses also seem promising.[63] Aside from WILT, there are already powerful incentives for developing such approaches: as a means of determining gene function and as cures for single-gene disorders, such as cystic fibrosis and thalassemia. Our understanding of the important variables in gene modification should thus continue to grow and lead to better efficiency, and modification of multiple nonselectable target genes should become realistic.

In Vivo *Genetic Manipulation*

Genetic alteration of rapidly dividing cells for WILT will almost certainly always be easiest by an *ex vivo* procedure. Apart from the intrinsic difficulties of somatic gene therapy, the result of deleting telomere elongation function in such cell types would be the long-term inviability of the tissue and the need to replenish it (discussed below), so the cells whose genetic engineering is required will already have to be manipulated in other ways *ex vivo* to give them the desired properties. However, several important cancer types, including sarcomas and gliomas, derive from relatively quiescent cells whose total requirement for cell division in a lifetime is low. Repopulating such tissues with engineered cells appears very challenging.

It may, therefore, be necessary to alter these cell types *in situ*. Unfortunately, this seems unlikely to be achievable soon by gene targeting, given the rate of random integration noted above. However, several groups are working to improve the reproducibility of high-efficiency oligonucleotide-mediated gene targeting, and other approaches are also on the horizon.[61]

Finally, we must remember that a therapy so advanced and technically difficult as WILT is not likely to become an attractive option until considerable progress has been made against all other major causes of death and debilitation—particularly cardiovascular disease, neurodegeneration, and diabetes—because only then will the limitations of more conventional anticancer approaches become apparent as a steep rise in the proportion of people dying of cancer. Such advances will surely also require effective *in vivo* genetic manipulation.[5] Thus, this aspect of WILT is not, in fact, a substantive obstacle to its development by the time it is needed.

SIDE EFFECTS

Cancer Promotion?

Cells with very short telomeres are genetically unstable. Indeed, in humans it is considered likely that an initial phase of inadequate telomere maintenance early in tumorigenesis confers a "mutator" phenotype, accelerating the occurrence of further mutations—including activation of telomerase or ALT—that allow the tumor to progress.[64]

This phenomenon should not affect the efficacy of WILT, however. When telomere elongation cannot be activated, the mutator phenotype will, if anything, hasten the tumor's demise by increasing the accumulation of mutations that prevent cell division.

Telomerase Knockout Mice

The best laboratory models currently available for exploring the WILT concept are mice engineered to lack telomerase. Even though mouse embryonic stem cells lacking telomerase acquire an ALT-like character,[65] this is not seen *in vivo*—perhaps because it is too rare, or perhaps because ALT is incompatible with the normal differentiated state of some mouse tissues. Thus, mice lacking telomerase can be inbred for successive generations to yield mice with telomeres too short to sustain highly proliferative tissues for the animal's normal lifetime.[66] The most prominent phenotypes observed are in the gonads, blood, and skin. Interestingly, mice lacking p53 as well as telomerase show a delay in the major phenotype that can be measured at an early enough age not to be masked by the cancers that result from lack of p53, namely sterility: $TERC^{-/-}$ $p53^{-/-}$ mice can be bred for two generations longer than the simple TERC knockouts.[67]

It is important to understand why p53 ablation accelerates death from cancer even in late-generation telomerase knockout mice.[68] The number of cell divisions needed for a mouse cancer to grow big enough to kill it is considerably fewer than in a human, for several reasons: (1) the cancer need not grow as big; (2) it need not metastasize, whereas most human cancers only become life-threatening after metastasis; and (3) the telomere damage-detection system in mice is simpler—in particular, the Rb pathway does not exert a strong protective effect[69]—so fewer mutations are required. Also, as noted earlier, mouse cells can activate ALT quite easily *in vitro*; it has not been determined whether cancers developed by TERC$^{-/-}$ p53$^{-/-}$ mice (or, indeed, by TERC$^{-/-}$ mice) are phenotypically ALT-like, though they do become ALT-like after serial transplantation.[70] The anticancer effect of short telomeres is therefore challenging to assay in mice. However, when these confounders are minimized, the effect is dramatic: in TERC$^{-/-}$ Apc^{Min} mice, a mild reduction in telomere length increased the incidence of cancer at a given age, but severe telomere shortening reduced that risk to the point where no deaths at all occurred by the age at which all TERC$^{+/+}$ animals had died.[71] Other models of cancer in TERC$^{-/-}$ mice also show resistance to cancer progression.[72]

Dyskeratosis Congenita

Humans have shorter telomeres than most mammals (including nonhuman primates[73]), and their gestation is longer. This is probably why humans lacking telomerase activity are not found: they would not develop to term. However, a disease has been known for nearly 100 years[74] that exhibits symptoms quite like those of late-generation telomerase knockout mice: it is called dyskeratosis congenita (DC). Indeed, the genetic basis for nearly half the known cases of DC is a mutation in one of two genes whose product is telomere associated, and in both cases patients have shorter telomeres than age-matched controls (FIG. 4).

One of these genes is TERC.[75] Several TERC mutations have been identified in different DC families. These mutations are present in only one of the TERC alleles, and families display autosomal dominant transmission of the DC phenotype. Of interest is that many sufferers only acquire symptoms in middle age, and, in particular, are fertile, since pedigrees exist. Moreover, the age of onset of DC in offspring tends (though the small number of sufferers so far identified precludes firm conclusions) to be considerably earlier than in parents, and grandchildren tend to develop symptoms in childhood[75] (also I.D., unpublished data). This suggests cumulative telomere shortening in the germ line.

The other gene is named dyskerin. Unlike TERC, most dyskerin mutations so far seen in humans are missense alterations, presumably hypomorphic. Intriguingly, dyskerin knockout mice die at embryonic day 6.[76] Dyskerin must thus have a non-telomeric function (it seems inconceivable that telomere maintenance defects could be so rapidly lethal); there is suggestive evidence that it is pseudouridylation of ribosomal RNA.[77] Mutations in dyskerin, which on average cause an earlier age of onset of symptoms than those in TERC, cause depletion of TERC to around 20% of normal,[78] so the dominant phenotype of TERC mutations is probably simple haploinsufficiency. DC promotes cancer,[79] but insufficient tissue has been available, thus far, to address key questions, such as whether DC tumors express telomerase or ALT.

DC sufferers are potential beneficiaries of the techniques to prevent side effects of WILT that will be discussed below. One, bone marrow transplantation, is a stan-

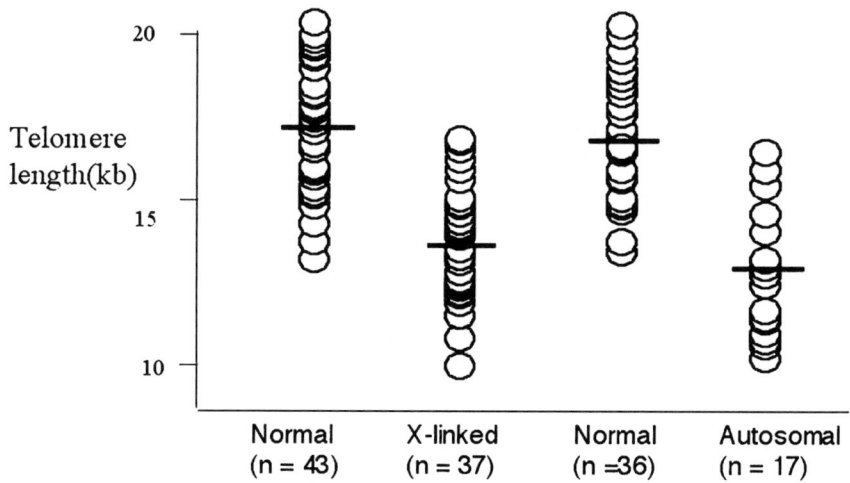

FIGURE 4. Both X-linked (dyskerin) and autosomal (TERC) DC cause shortened telomeres.

dard treatment already. With anticipated advances in stem cell manipulation, such treatments should become more feasible and effective, and DC may become a truly curable disease.

AVOIDANCE OF SIDE EFFECTS

The problems that would certainly arise from ablating telomere elongation can, in principle, be avoided by periodically reseeding all highly proliferative tissues with stem cells whose telomeres have been lengthened *ex vivo* (but whose autonomous telomere elongation competence has not been restored, or has been restored but then removed again). While this is conceptually straightforward, in practice it faces major obstacles, which vary from tissue to tissue. Below we consider three key tissues needing this restoration and the difficulties to be overcome.

Bone Marrow Reseeding

The hemopoietic system is a rapidly renewing tissue for which replenishment techniques already exist: bone marrow transplantation (BMT) has long been routine. New problems would arise, however, in BMT for WILT.

First, for complete reseeding of the hemopoietic system, substantial expansion of the transplantable stem cell population *ex vivo* would be required. Current efforts at expanding stem cell numbers using combinations of cytokines[80] have been limited by several factors. First, the most primitive stem cells, the so-called long-term repopulating stem cells, are typically not expanded and are frequently lost by differentiation following prolonged culture in *ex vivo* expansion conditions. These are the key stem cells for long-term maintenance of a transplant,[81] so this largely explains the failure of transplantability of *ex vivo*–expanded stem cell populations. Thus, there is much current interest in characterizing factors that will allow self-renewal of these cells against a block in differentiation. Recently, many researchers have focused on members of the Notch ligand family in this respect.[82] However, although results are promising, these analyses are at an early stage.

A further complication is that following such culture, these cells will typically be proliferating. Under normal circumstances, most stem cells are not proliferating, and there is abundant evidence for a requirement for a G_0/G_1 state of hemopoietic stem cells for proper homing and engraftment following transplantation.[83] Thus, pre-transplantation resetting of this "quiescent" status will be essential. This may be achieved using combinations of the well-characterized inhibitors of stem cell proliferation appropriate for long-term repopulating stem cells.[84] The same applies to molecules involved in the *in vivo* homing and engraftment of hemopoietic stem cells: expression of these molecules, such as the chemokine receptor CXCR4, may be altered by culture conditions[85] and need to be reset before transplantation.

Third, BMT works best when the stem cell niche has already been denuded of native cells.[86] In certain diseases of the hemopoietic system, however, this is not seen,[87] indicating that functionally compromised stem cells are less resistant to displacement by incoming, more robust ones. For second and subsequent WILT reseedings, it may thus be possible to rely on the fact that many of the previous reseeding's stem cells will be nearing exhaustion in terms of telomere length. The first treatment, however, might need chemotherapeutic or radiation-mediated depletion of the marrow to allow the engineered cells to engraft.

Gut Reseeding

The gut lining consists of a juxtaposition of finger-shaped structures, termed villi, and invaginations, termed crypts. It is maintained by stem cells at or near the crypt base that generate rapidly dividing cells that migrate up out of them and along the villi, eventually being shed at the tip.

Several years ago, one of us (F.C.C.) and his colleagues developed a technique for surgically repopulating the mouse colon with cells extracted from the small intestine. Despite considerable *ex vivo* handling, cell aggregates that had been plated onto freshly denuded colon developed *in vivo* into morphologically normal crypts containing all four of the differentiated cell types normally observed.[88] Clearly this augurs well for maintaining the gut in the context of WILT.

However, daunting problems remain. One is fibrosis. The mouse work involved only a small area of colon; when similar surgery was done on newborn pigs, the resulting fibrosis precluded restoration of functional intestine (F.C.C., unpublished data). Further, for application to humans there would be a requirement to avoid surgery. The gut may, like the bone marrow, resist engraftment of new stem cells in tissue already replete with them, so denudation may be required; this might be possible using endoscopy technology, but that would risk short-term impairment of gut function. Finally, gut stem cells cultured *in vitro* lose proliferative capacity after only a few divisions. This sensitivity may or may not be alleviated by more sophisticated culturing technology (such as low oxygen).

Skin Reseeding

DC sufferers and late-generation TERC$^{-/-}$ mice both show severe epidermal dysfunction, and this will undoubtedly be a tissue needing replenishment in the context of WILT. However, epidermal function depends critically on the underlying tissue—the dermis.[89] The dermis–epidermis interaction seems to be central to epidermal maintenance and regeneration. Also, most of our skin grows hair, and it may be the hair follicles, from which several important types of skin cancer are believed to originate, that hold the key to effective skin regeneration.[90]

As elsewhere, an important requirement for skin reseeding with a frequency of around a decade will be to control the differentiation process so that stem cells divide rarely enough to survive. Several factors have been reported to exert appropriate influences. One is 14-3-3σ, which inhibits differentiation.[91] Reliable identification of stem cells is also important; high levels of β1 integrin expression,[92] high α6 integrin with low CD71 expression,[93] Keratin 19,[94] and p63[95] are among markers championed as being diagnostic of the keratinocyte stem cell state. A definitive marker would permit refinement of techniques already developed for isolating a pure population of these cells for tissue engineering purposes.[96]

A particularly useful tool for studying skin regeneration is the corneal epithelium. Its central region can be removed without removing the stem cells from the surrounding germinal region (the limbus) and grafted onto denuded dorsal dermis; the corneal cells are rapidly reprogrammed to a follicular state, including development of normal hair follicles.[97] Importantly, hair follicle formation actually precedes formation of new epidermis, and epidermal differentiation spreads from the neck of the follicle (FIG. 5), reinforcing the idea that the follicle can be a repository of stem cells for the epidermis.[90] Also, this type of transdifferentiation work illustrates the possibility of using stem cells from an organ like the eye to repopulate another like skin.

Taken together, these and other observations give cause for optimism regarding skin regeneration, whether for WILT or for more traditional applications, such as treatment of burns or DC. Since the dermis is a very slowly renewing tissue, its capacity to orchestrate the behavior of its epidermal coating affords us great flexibility in the introduction of WILT cells. There is still some uncertainty as to the numbers and exact location of stem cells in hair follicles, but the most widely held view is that they undergo bursts of activity corresponding with the periodic initiation of the follicle growth cycle.[98] Certainly a follicle (not to mention its epidermal neighborhood) contains more cells than a villus. Moreover, matrix epithelial cells at the base of actively growing follicles are among the fastest dividing cells in the body: in human scalp the matrix replaces itself every 23 hours, and corresponding mouse cells are thought to divide every 13 hours.[99,100] Since the active growing phase in scalp follicles can last several years, this represents many generations at the transit amplifying stage. Thus, the skin should not only be relatively straightforward to repopulate: it should also not need reseeding very often.

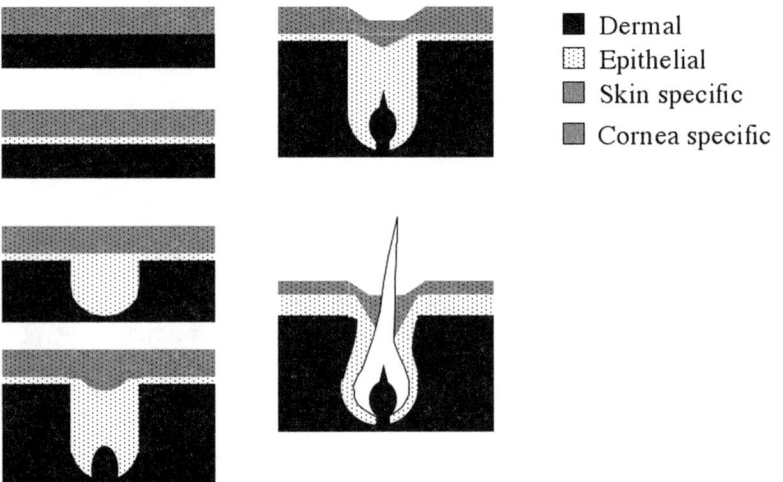

FIGURE 5. Corneal epithelium is reprogrammed by the dermis as hair-forming epidermis, starting with the hair follicle. Epidermis formation after grafting of corneal epithelium proceeds through basal layer formation, placode formation, epidermis formation at the follicle edge, and finally hair growth. *Black*, dermal; *dots*, epithelial; *dark gray*, skin specific; *light gray*, cornea specific.

As a practical consideration and on the question of whether periodic reseeding of skin cells would be an acceptable practice and taken up if available, it is worth noting that many people currently pay for (often very painful) chemical or laser "peels" of skin merely for cosmetic antiaging purposes.

Reseeding of Other Tissues

Similar techniques would presumably have to be developed for many other epithelial tissues in order to make WILT a viable therapy. These include the lung, on which stem cell therapy is already an active area of research, given its potential to treat diseases such as cystic fibrosis.[101] Though several such tissues may present specific difficulties, we feel that the techniques developed for the three tissues discussed above will probably be sufficiently versatile to be relatively easily adapted to these other tissues.

Frequency of Reseeding

The utility of WILT depends on all rapidly renewing tissues surviving for at least several years with stem cells that lack all telomere extension function. This implies stem cell generation times of at least two months. That may be the natural rate in blood;[102] what about other tissues?

The tissue ostensibly of greatest concern here is the gut. In both DC sufferers and TERC$^{-/-}$ mice, gut phenotypes tend to arise contemporaneously with those of other tissues such as the blood. (In DC there is an important exception—certain sufferers of Hoyeraal-Hreidarsson syndrome, a severe allelic variant of DC,[103] show gut abnormalities before other problems.) Yet, mouse hemopoietic stem cells divide only every few weeks,[102] whereas gut stem cells have been calculated to divide once a day.[104] (This calculation depends on how many stem cells are present per crypt, which remains unclear: crypts are monoclonal,[105] but cells at an early stage of differentiation can return to the stem cell niche,[106] so maybe stem cells can also sometimes divide symmetrically to form two stem cells, as in the hemopoietic system.[107]) If blood and gut stem cell division frequencies differ by an order of magnitude, how can the age at which telomere maintenance deficiency affects those two tissues be comparable? In DC there might be tissue-specific factors—for example, the gut might express more TERC—but no such loophole seems available for TERC$^{-/-}$ mice. Resolution of this paradox is of high priority, as it may reveal aspects of stem cell population dynamics that can be exploited for many therapeutic purposes. For WILT, however, the implication is inescapable that the gut should survive as long between transplants as the blood.

Senescent Cell Ablation

Telomere elongation-incompetent stem cells, when compromised by over-short telomeres, may not fall obligingly upon their swords: they may need to be actively eliminated. Cultured cells with over-short telomeres remain alive in a distinctive "senescent" state long after losing the ability to divide; similar cells have been observed *in vivo*.[108,109] They seem to be very rare except in cartilage,[109] but might be deleterious even so;[110] WILT might raise their abundance considerably, with unknown consequences.

Luckily, however, the possibility that even rare senescent cells may do harm *in vivo* has prompted work on their removal.[111] One strategy being pursued is to incorporate into cells a "suicide" gene that induces apoptosis if the cell adopts a senescent gene expression profile. Vaccination against cell surface markers of the senescent state is also a plausible approach. This work is at an early stage, but the fact that it is already being aggressively attempted gives cause for optimism that it will be perfected within the ten-year minimum time frame that we foresee for WILT.

Immune Memory

Unlike the gut lining and epidermis, the blood comprises not only short-lived cells but also a small minority of long-lived ones. The immune system relies on two types of long-term memory, and the possibility and consequences of loss of this memory as a result of WILT must be considered.

One type is the memory of previous infections. While memory cells are undoubtedly good for us, they may be of diminishing importance as we make progress against the many other aspects of aging that make the elderly more susceptible to infection in the first place. The immune system of a young person contains relatively few memory cells, but one would not replace it with that of a centenarian. Additionally, to the extent that it may be desirable to preserve memory cell abundance and function, the same technology proposed here for stem cell renewal may also be applicable to memory cells, which are relatively oligoclonal and could be amplified along with telomere lengthening *ex vivo*.

The other type of memory is self/nonself discrimination. Here we must bear in mind that lymphocytes cannot participate in an immune response until maturation in either the thymus or the bone marrow. One part of this maturation process is the preemption of an autoimmune response, mainly by clonal deletion of cells that could react to self antigens.[112] The memory of which cells to delete is thus not stored in the hemopoietic system itself but in the stromal cells that vet immature lymphocytes. In the thymus, some of these cells are epithelial in origin and are maintained by stem cells,[113] so retention of their self/nonself memory during *ex vivo* manipulation would be needed. Critically, however, these cells—and also those of other provenance, such as bone marrow–derived dentritic cells at the cortex/medulla boundary within the thymus—do not undergo the genomic reorganization that occurs in the lymphocytes themselves. Thus, since the cells to be used for reseeding will be autologous, the selective pattern that their descendents in the thymus and bone marrow subsequently impose on maturing lymphocytes will be the same as that imposed by native cells—that is, a faithful self/nonself divide. Autoimmune consequences of WILT thus seem unlikely.

PUTTING IT ALL TOGETHER: DEVELOPMENT AND IMPLEMENTATION

Developing WILT in Mice

Reseeding of rapidly renewing tissues can be explored not only in normal mice, but also in telomerase-negative ones. Sixth-generation $TERC^{-/-}$ mice have a shortened life span as a result of failure of highly proliferative tissues;[66] successful reseeding of such tissues should, in principle, restore these animals' longevity. Similarly, mice with constitutive p53 activity exhibit shortened life span due to an accelerated decline of function of various tissues, even though they are markedly protected from cancer;[114] such mice, when made $TERC^{-/-}$ in addition, would be ideal subjects for testing the benefit of reseeding relevant tissues.

WILT in Humans: When Should It Be Initiated?

Several issues of clinical judgement would arise when and if WILT became safely and affordably available. The first is whether it would be advisable to use WILT preemptively, on individuals who did not yet have cancer. This may not be generally advisable, as the main motivation would be to use high-dose chemotherapy to deplete "native" (telomere-elongation competent) stem cells, and the side effects of chemotherapy are considerable. However, factors such as a family history of early death from cancer may alter this judgement.

A related issue concerns the frequency of administration of chemotherapy after a patient's first WILT treatment. If the reseeding of all relevant tissues is efficient, it should be possible to raise chemotherapy doses to a point that kills the large majority of "native" stem cells as well as the patient's cancer itself, thus greatly reducing the risk of subsequent cancers. This will ultimately be limited, however, by the toxicity of chemotherapy to cell types that are not replenished from stem cells, as well as by the degree of chemoresistance of the engineered cells. Thus, especially at advanced ages when new tumors may be appearing more often, it may become appropriate to administer chemotherapy at milder doses but higher frequency.

The question of subsequent fertility must also be considered, since the proposed high doses of chemotherapy might well cause permanent sterility, at least in males. This should be surmountable, however, by a variety of assisted reproduction technologies—not least by the option of introducing engineered germ-line stem cells in the same way as is proposed here for other constantly renewing tissues. Germ-line manipulations raise unique ethical and safety issues, of course, but these can only be evaluated when what the therapy might offer is clearly delineated.

CONCLUSION

The idea of eliminating from the body a function known to be essential for survival is a conceptual leap that takes substantial justification even to contemplate, let alone implement. However, here we have examined its ramifications in detail and found that none is so clear-cut as to preclude the possibility that WILT might be feasible. Given (1) the acknowledged inadequacy of present cancer therapies, (2) that no foreseeable therapy that could be escaped by changes of gene expression will do much better, and (3) the likelihood that progress against other aspects of age-related decline will make cancer a progressively bigger menace,[5] we conclude that serious consideration should be given, even at this early stage, to development and refinement of the many techniques that would be necessary to make WILT work.

ACKNOWLEDGMENTS

We are much indebted to Nicola Royle of the Department of Genetics, University of Leicester, who participated (along with all of us) in the round-table meeting at which the WILT concept was first evaluated and also in the preparation of this article. She played as great a role as the other authors, contributing vital specialist expertise about ALT, but withdrew from authorship because of her concerns at the social and environmental consequences of the greatly increased human healthy life expectancy that successful development of WILT would help to bring about. We are equally indebted to Steven Artandi of Stanford University, an equally vital participant in the aforementioned roundtable, who contributed expertise about telomerase knockout mice; he was, however, unable to devote any time to the preparation of this manuscript and therefore felt that he should not be an author.

REFERENCES

1. MULLER, L., R. KIESSLING, R.C. REES & G. PAWELEC. 2002. Escape mechanisms in tumor immunity: an update. J. Environ. Pathol. Toxicol. Oncol. **21:** 277–330.
2. TWOMBLY, R. 2002. First clinical trials of endostatin yield lukewarm results. J. Natl. Cancer Inst. **94:** 1520–1521.
3. SIKIC, B.I. 1999. Modulation of multidrug resistance: a paradigm for translational clinical research. Oncology **13:** 183–187.
4. WHITE, L.K., W.E. WRIGHT & J.W. SHAY. 2001. Telomerase inhibitors. Trends Biotechnol. **19:** 114–120.

5. DE GREY, A., B.N. AMES, J.K. ANDERSEN, *et al.* 2002. Time to talk SENS: critiquing the immutability of human aging. Ann. N.Y. Acad. Sci. **959:** 452–462.
 6. REDDEL, R.R. 2000. The role of senescence and immortalization in carcinogenesis. Carcinogenesis **21:** 477–484.
 7. OLOVNIKOV, A.M. 1971. [Principle of marginotomy in template synthesis of polynucleotides.] Dokl. Akad. Nauk SSSR **201:** 1496–1499.
 8. WATSON, J.D. 1972. Origin of concatemeric T7 DNA. Nat. New Biol. **239:** 197–201.
 9. HAYFLICK, L. & P.S. MOORHEAD. 1961. The limited in vitro lifetime of human diploid cell strains. Exp. Cell Res. **25:** 585–621.
10. VON ZGLINICKI, T. 2002. Oxidative stress shortens telomeres. Trends Biochem. Sci. **27:** 339–344.
11. PACKER, L. & K. FUEHR. 1977. Low oxygen concentration extends the lifespan of cultured human diploid cells. Nature **267:** 423–425.
12. HIYAMA, E., K. HIYAMA, T. YOKOYAMA, *et al.* 1995. Correlating telomerase activity levels with human neuroblastoma outcomes. Nat. Med. **1:** 249–255.
13. HIRANO, Y., K. FUJITA, K. SUZUKI, *et al.* 1998. Telomerase activity as an indicator of potentially malignant adrenal tumors. Cancer **83:** 772–776.
14. LIN, Y., H. MIYAMOTO, K. FUJINAMI, *et al.* 1996. Telomerase activity in human bladder cancer. Clin. Cancer Res. **2:** 929–932.
15. SHIPPEN-LENTZ, D. & E.H. BLACKBURN. 1990. Functional evidence for an RNA template in telomerase. Science **247:** 546–552.
16. RAMIREZ, R.D., W.E. WRIGHT, J.W. SHAY & R.S. TAYLOR. 1997. Telomerase activity concentrates in the mitotically active segments of human hair follicles. J. Invest. Dermatol. **108:** 113–117.
17. HSIAO, R., H.W. SHARMA, S. RAMAKRISHNAN, *et al.* 1997. Telomerase activity in normal human endothelial cells. Anticancer Res. **17:** 827–832.
18. SHAY, J.W. & S. BACCHETTI. 1997. A survey of telomerase activity in human cancer. Eur. J. Cancer **33:** 787–791.
19. BODNAR, A.G., M. OUELLETTE, M. FROLKIS, *et al.* 1998. Extension of life-span by introduction of telomerase into normal human cells. Science **279:** 349–352.
20. RAMIREZ, R.D., C.P. MORALES, B.S. HERBERT, *et al.* 2001. Putative telomere-independent mechanisms of replicative aging reflect inadequate growth conditions. Genes Dev. **15:** 398–403.
21. HERBERT, B.S., W.E. WRIGHT & J.W. SHAY. 2002. p16(INK4a) inactivation is not required to immortalize human mammary epithelial cells. Oncogene **21:** 7897–7900.
22. CHEONG, C., K.U. HONG & H.W. LEE. 2003. Mouse models for telomere and telomerase biology. Exp. Mol. Med. **35:** 141–153.
23. RUDOLPH, K.L., S. CHANG, H.W. LEE, *et al.* 1999. Longevity, stress response, and cancer in aging telomerase-deficient mice. Cell **96:** 701–712.
24. YUAN, X., S. ISHIBASHI, S. HATAKEYAMA, *et al.* 1999. Presence of telomeric G-strand tails in the telomerase catalytic subunit TERT knockout mice. Genes Cells **4:** 563–572.
25. HENSON, J.D., A.A. NEUMANN, T.R. YEAGER & R.R. REDDEL. 2002. Alternative lengthening of telomeres in mammalian cells. Oncogene **21:** 598–601.
26. VARLEY, H., H.A. PICKETT, J.L. FOXON, *et al.* 2002. Molecular characterization of intertelomere and intra-telomere mutations in human ALT cells. Nat. Genet. **30:** 301–305.
27. MALKOVA, A., E.L. IVANOV & J.E. HABER. 1996. Double-strand break repair in the absence of RAD51 in yeast: a possible role for break-induced DNA replication. Proc. Natl. Acad. Sci. USA **93:** 7131–7136.
28. PERREM, K., T.M. BRYAN, A. ENGLEZOU, *et al.* 1999. Repression of an alternative mechanism for lengthening of telomeres in somatic cell hybrids. Oncogene **18:** 3383–3390.
29. BAIRD, D.M., J. COLEMAN, Z.H. ROSSER & N.J. ROYLE. 2000. High levels of sequence polymorphism and linkage disequilibrium at the telomere of 12q: implications for telomere biology and human evolution. Am. J. Hum. Genet. **66:** 235–250.
30. MAUCH, P., L. CONSTINE, J. GREENBERGER, *et al.* 1995. Hematopoietic stem cell compartment: acute and late effects of radiation therapy and chemotherapy. Int. J. Radiat. Oncol. Biol. Phys. **31:** 1319–1339.

31. RAFFERTY, J.A., I. HICKSON, N. CHINNASAMY, et al. 1996. Chemoprotection of normal tissues by transfer of drug resistance genes. Cancer Metastasis Rev. **15:** 365–383.
32. MAZE, R., H. HANENBERG & D.A. WILLIAMS. 1997. Establishing chemoresistance in hematopoietic progenitor cells. Mol. Med. Today **3:** 350–358.
33. HOBIN, D.A. & L.J. FAIRBAIRN. 2002. Genetic chemoprotection with mutant O^6-alkylguanine-DNA-alkyltransferases. Curr. Gene Ther. **2:** 1–8.
34. PROCKOP, D.J. 1997. Marrow stromal cells as stem cells for nonhaematopoietic tissues. Science **276:** 71–74.
35. KRAUSE, D.S. 2002. Plasticity of marrow-derived stem cells. Gene Ther. **9:** 754–758.
36. MILLER, M.C., J.K. LIU & K. COLINS. 2000. Template definition by Tetrahymena telomerase reverse transcriptase. EMBO J. **19:** 4412–4422.
37. TERADA, N., T. HAMAZAKI, M. OKA, et al. 2002. Bone marrow cells adopt the phenotype of other cells by spontaneous cell fusion. Nature **416:** 542–545.
38. YING, Q.L., J. NICHOLS, E.P. EVANS & A.G. SMITH. 2002. Changing potency by spontaneous fusion. Nature **416:** 545–548.
39. BERGSMEDH, A., A. SZELES, M. HENRIKSSON, et al. 2001. Horizontal transfer of oncogenes by uptake of apoptotic bodies. Proc. Natl. Acad. Sci. USA **98:** 6407–6411.
40. GURDON, J.B. & A. COLMAN. 1999. The future of cloning. Nature **402:** 743–746.
41. SPENCER, D.M. 2000. Developments in suicide genes for preclinical and clinical applications. Curr. Opin. Mol. Ther. **2:** 433–440.
42. CAPECCHI, M.R. 1989. Altering the genome by homologous recombination. Science **244:** 1288–1292.
43. KOLLER, B.H. & O. SMITHIES. 1992. Altering genes in animals by gene targeting. Annu. Rev. Immunol. **10:** 705–730.
44. PORTER, A.C. & M.J. DALLMAN. 1997. Gene targeting: techniques and applications to transplantation. Transplantation **64:** 1227–1235.
45. YANEZ, R.J. & A.C. PORTER. 1998. Therapeutic gene targeting. Gene Ther. **5:** 149–159.
46. KNAUERT, M.P. & P.M. GLAZER. 2001. Triplex forming oligonucleotides: sequence-specific tools for gene targeting. Hum. Mol. Genet. **10:** 2243–2245.
47. IGOUCHEVA, O., V. ALEXEEV & K. YOON. 2001. Targeted gene correction by small single-stranded oligonucleotides in mammalian cells. Gene Ther. **8:** 391–399.
48. KENNER, O., A. KNEISEL, J. KLINGLER, et al. 2002. Targeted gene correction of hprt mutations by 45 base single-stranded oligonucleotides. Biochem. Biophys. Res. Commun. **299:** 787–792.
49. BRACHMAN, E.E. & E.B. KMIEC. 2002. The "biased" evolution of targeted gene repair. Curr. Opin. Mol. Ther. **4:** 171–176.
50. TAUBES, G. 2002. Gene therapy. The strange case of chimeraplasty. Science **298:** 2116–2120.
51. LANDIS, D.M., C.C. HEINDEL & L.A. LOEB. 2001. Creation and characterization of 5-fluorodeoxyuridine-resistant Arg50 loop mutants of human thymidylate synthase. Cancer Res. **61:** 666–672.
52. ALLAY, J.A., D.A. PERSONS, J. GALIPEAU, et al. 1998. In vivo selection of retrovirally transduced hematopoietic stem cells. Nat. Med. **10:** 1136–1143.
53. LARIN, Z. & J.E. MEJIA. 2002. Advances in human artificial chromosome technology. Trends Genet. **18:** 313–319.
54. COOKE, H. 2001. Mammalian artificial chromosomes as vectors: progress and prospects. Cloning Stem Cells **3:** 243–249.
55. MOMBAERTS, P., A.R. CLARKE, M.L. HOOPER & S. TONEGAWA. 1991. Creation of a large genomic deletion at the T-cell antigen receptor beta-subunit locus in mouse embryonic stem cells by gene targeting. Proc. Natl. Acad. Sci. USA **88:** 3084–3087.
56. MULLER, U. 1999. Ten years of gene targeting: targeted mouse mutants, from vector design to phenotype analysis. Mech. Dev. **82:** 3–21.
57. MILLS, A.A. & A. BRADLEY. 2001. From mouse to man: generating megabase chromosome rearrangements. Trends Genet. **17:** 331–339.
58. ELLIS, H.M., D. YU, T. DITIZIO & D.L. COURT. 2001. High efficiency mutagenesis, repair, and engineering of chromosomal DNA using single-stranded oligonucleotides. Proc. Natl. Acad. Sci. USA **98:** 6742–6746.

59. KREN, B.T., P. BANDYOPADHYAY & C.J. STEER. 1998. In vivo site-directed mutagenesis of the factor IX gene by chimeric RNA/DNA oligonucleotides. Nat. Med. **4:** 285–290.
60. VASQUEZ, K.M., K. MARBURGER, Z. INTODY & J.H. WILSON. 2001. Manipulating the mammalian genome by homologous recombination. Proc. Natl. Acad. Sci. USA **98:** 8403–8410.
61. WESTPHAL, S.P. 2002. Designer animals made easy. New Scientist **173:** 6.
62. JASIN, M. 1996. Genetic manipulation of genomes with rare-cutting endonucleases. Trends Genet. **12:** 224–228.
63. HIRATA, R., J. CHAMBERLAIN, R. DONG & D.W. RUSSELL. 2002. Targeted transgene insertion into human chromosomes by adeno-associated virus vectors. Nat. Biotechnol. **20:** 735–738.
64. LOEB, L.A. 2001. A mutator phenotype in cancer. Cancer Res. **61:** 3230–3239.
65. NIIDA, H., Y. SHINKAI, M.P. HANDE, *et al.* 2000. Telomere maintenance in telomerase-deficient mouse embryonic stem cells: characterization of an amplified telomeric DNA. Mol. Cell. Biol. **20:** 4115–4127.
66. LEE, H.W., M.A. BLASCO, G.J. GOTTLIEB, *et al.* 1998. Essential role of mouse telomerase in highly proliferative organs. Nature **392:** 569–574.
67. CHIN, L., S.E. ARTANDI, Q. SHEN, *et al.* 1999. p53 deficiency rescues the adverse effects of telomere loss and cooperates with telomere dysfunction to accelerate carcinogenesis. Cell **97:** 527–538.
68. ARTANDI, S.E. & R.A. DEPINHO. 2000. A critical role for telomeres in suppressing and facilitating carcinogenesis. Curr. Opin. Genet. Dev. **10:** 39–46.
69. SMOGORZEWSKA, A. & T. DE LANGE. 2002. Different telomere damage signaling pathways in human and mouse cells. EMBO J. **21:** 4338–4348.
70. CHANG, S., C.M. KHOO, M.L. NAYLOR, *et al.* 2003. Telomere-based crisis: functional differences between telomerase activation and ALT in tumor progression. Genes Dev. **17:** 88–100.
71. RUDOLPH, K.L., M. MILLARD, M.W. BOSENBERG & R.A. DEPINHO. 2001. Telomere dysfunction and evolution of intestinal carcinoma in mice and humans. Nat. Genet. **28:** 155–159.
72. GONZALEZ-SUAREZ, E., E. SAMPER, J.M. FLORES & M.A. BLASCO. 2000. Telomerase-deficient mice with short telomeres are resistant to skin tumorigenesis. Nat. Genet. **26:** 114–117.
73. KAKUO, S., K. ASAOKA & T. IDE. 1999. Human is a unique species among primates in terms of telomere length. Biochem. Biophys. Res. Commun. **263:** 308–314.
74. ZINSSER, F. 1906. Atropha cutis reticularis cum pigmentatione, dystropia ungium et leukoplakia oris. Ikonogr. Dermatol. **5:** 219–223.
75. VULLIAMY, T., A. MARRONE, F. GOLDMAN, *et al.* 2001. The RNA component of telomerase is mutated in autosomal dominant dyskeratosis congenita. Nature **413:** 432–435.
76. HE, J., S. NAVARRETE, M. JASINSKI, *et al.* 2002. Targeted disruption of Dkc1, the gene mutated in X-linked dyskeratosis congenita, causes embryonic lethality in mice. Oncogene **21:** 7740–7744.
77. RUGGERO, D., S. GRISENDI, F. PIAZZA, *et al.* 2003. Dyskeratosis congenita and cancer in mice deficient in ribosomal RNA modification. Science **299:** 259–262.
78. MITCHELL, J.R., E. WOOD & K. COLLINS. 1999. A telomerase component is defective in the human disease dyskeratosis congenita. Nature **402:** 551–555.
79. DOKAL, I. 2000. Dyskeratosis congenita in all its forms. Br. J. Haematol. **110:** 768–779.
80. MCNIECE, I. & R. BRIDDELL. 2001. Ex vivo expansion of hematopoietic progenitor cells and mature cells. Exp. Hematol. **29:** 3–11.
81. GRAHAM, G.J. & E.G. WRIGHT. 1997. Haemopoietic stem cells: their heterogeneity and regulation. Int. J. Exp. Pathol. **78:** 197–218.
82. OHSHI, K., B. VARNUM-FINNEY & I.D. BERNSTEIN. 2002. Delta-1 enhances marrow and thymus repopulating ability of human $CD34^+CD38^-$ cord blood cells. J. Clin. Invest. **110:** 1165–1174.
83. YONG, K.L., A. FAHEY, A. PIZZEY & D.C. LINCH. 2002. Influence of cell cycling and cell division on transendothelial migration of $CD34^{(+)}$ cells. Br. J. Haematol. **119:** 500–509.
84. GRAHAM, G.J. 1997. Growth inhibitors in haemoiesis and leukaemogenesis. Baillieres Clin. Haematol. **10:** 467–483.

85. WHETTON, A.D. & G.J. GRAHAM. 1999. Homing and mobilization in the stem cell niche. Trends Cell Biol **9**: 233–238.
86. STEWART, F.M., S. ZHONG, J. WUU, et al. 1998. Lymphohematopoietic engraftment in minimally myeloablated hosts. Blood **91**: 3681–3687.
87. GEORGES, G.E. & R. STORB. 2002. Stem cell transplantation for aplastic anemia. Int. J. Hematol. **75**: 141–146.
88. TAIT, I.S., N. FLINT, F.C. CAMPBELL & G.S. EVANS. 1994. Generation of neomucosa in vivo by transplantation of dissociated rat postnatal small intestinal epithelium. Differentiation **56**: 91–100.
89. JAHODA, C.A. & A.J. REYNOLDS. 2001. Hair follicle dermal sheath cells: unsung participants in wound healing. Lancet **358**: 1445–1448.
90. TAYLOR, G., M.S. LEHRER, P.J. JENSEN, et al. 2000. Involvement of follicular stem cells in forming not only the follicle but also the epidermis. Cell **102**: 451–461.
91. DELLAMBRA, E., O. GOLISANO, S. BONDANZA, et al. 2000. Downregulation of 14-3-3sigma prevents clonal evolution and leads to immortalization of primary human keratinocytes. J. Cell Biol. **149**: 1117–1130.
92. WATT, F.M. 1998. Epidermal stem cells: markers, patterning and the control of stem cell fate. Phil. Trans. R. Soc. Lond. B **353**: 831–837.
93. TANI, H., R.J. MORRIS & P. KAUR. 2000. Enrichment for murine keratinocyte stem cells based on cell surface phenotype. Proc. Natl. Acad. Sci. USA **97**: 10960–10965.
94. MICHEL, M., N. TOROK, M.J. GODBOUT, et al. 1996. Keratin 19 as a biochemical marker of skin stem cells in vivo and in vitro: keratin 19 expressing cells are differentially localized in function of anatomic sites, and their number varies with donor age and culture stage. J. Cell Sci. **109**: 1017–1028.
95. PELLEGRINI, G., E. DELLAMBRA, O. GOLISANO, et al. 2001. p63 identifies keratinocyte stem cells. Proc. Natl. Acad. Sci. USA **98**: 3156–3161.
96. DUNNWALD, M., A. TOMANEK-CHALKLEY, D. ALEXANDRUNAS, et al. 2001. Isolating a pure population of epidermal stem cells for use in tissue engineering. Exp. Dermatol. **10**: 45–54.
97. FERRARIS, C., G. CHEVALIER, B. FAVIER, et al. 2000. Adult corneal epithelium basal cells possess the capacity to activate epidermal, pilosebaceous and sweat gland genetic programs in response to embryonic dermal stimuli. Development **127**: 5487–5495.
98. COTSARELIS, G., T.T. SUN & R.M. LAVKER. 1990. Label-retaining cells reside in the bulge area of pilosebaceous unit: implications for follicular stem cells, hair cycle, and skin carcinogenesis. Cell **61**: 1329–1337.
99. BULLOUGH, W.S. & E.B. LAURENCE. 1958. The mitotic activity of the follicle. *In* The Biology of Hair Growth. W. Montagna & R.A. Ellis, Eds.: 171–187. Academic Press, Inc. New York.
100. VAN SCOTT, E.J., T.M. EKEL & R. AUERBACH. 1963. Determinants of rate and kinetics of cell division in scalp hair. J. Invest. Dermatol. **4**: 269–273.
101. MASON, R.J., M.C. WILLIAMS, H.L. MOSES, et al. 1997. Stem cells in lung development, disease and therapy. Am. J. Respir. Cell. Mol. Biol. **16**: 355–363.
102. ABKOWITZ, J.L., D. GOLINELLI, D.E. HARRISON & P. GUTTDORP. 2000. In vivo kinetics of murine hemopoietic stem cells. Blood **96**: 3399–3405.
103. KNIGHT, S.W., N.S. HEISS, T.J. VULLIAMY, et al. 1999. Unexplained aplastic anaemia, immunodeficiency, and cerebellar hypoplasia (Hoyeraal-Hreidarsson syndrome) due to mutations in the dyskeratosis congenita gene, DKC1. Br. J. Haematol. **107**: 335–339.
104. MARSHMAN, E., C. BOOTH & C.S. POTTEN. 2002. The intestinal epithelial stem cell. BioEssays **24**: 91–98.
105. SCHMIDT, G.H., D.J. GARBUTT, M.M. WILKINSON & B.A. PONDER. 1985. Clonal analysis of intestinal crypt populations in mouse aggregation chimaeras. J. Embryol. Exp. Morphol. **85**: 121–130.
106. KIM, K.M. & D. SHIBATA. 2002. Methylation reveals a niche: stem cell succession in human colon crypts. Oncogene **21**: 5441–5449.
107. DE HAAN, G. & G. VAN ZANT. 1999. Dynamic changes in mouse hematopoietic stem cell numbers during aging. Blood **93**: 3294–3301.
108. DIMRI, G.P., X. LEE, G. BASILE, et al. 1995. A biomarker that identifies senescent human cells in culture and in aging skin in vivo. Proc. Natl. Acad. Sci. USA **92**: 9363–9367.

109. MARTIN, J.A. & J.A. BUCKWALTER. 2002. Aging, articular cartilage chondrocyte senescence and osteoarthritis. Biogerontology 3: 257–264.
110. CAMPISI, J. 1997. Aging and cancer: the double-edged sword of replicative senescence. J. Am. Geriatr. Soc. 45: 482–488.
111. CAMPISI, J. 2003. Consequences of cellular senescence and prospects for reversal. Biogerontology 4 (Suppl. 1): 13.
112. LO, D., C.R. REILLY, L.C. BURKLY, et al. 1997. Thymic stromal cell specialization and the T-cell receptor repertoire. Immunol. Res. 16: 3–14.
113. BLACKBURN, C.C., N.R. MANLEY, D.B. PALMER, et al. 2002. One for all and all for one: thymic epithelial stem cells and regeneration. Trends Immunol. 23: 391–395.
114. TYNER, S.D., S. VENKATACHALAM, J. CHOI, et al. 2002. p53 mutant mice that display early ageing-associated phenotypes. Nature 415: 45–53.

Insights into Aging Obtained from p53 Mutant Mouse Models

MELISSA DUMBLE,[a] CATHERINE GATZA,[a,b] STUART TYNER,[a] SUNDARESAN VENKATACHALAM,[c] AND LAWRENCE A. DONEHOWER[a,d]

[a]*Department of Molecular Virology and Microbiology, Baylor College of Medicine, Houston, Texas 77030, USA*

[b]*Interdepartmental Graduate Program in Cell and Molecular Biology, Baylor College of Medicine, Houston, Texas 77030, USA*

[c]*Department of Biochemistry and Cell and Molecular Biology, University of Tennessee, Knoxville, Tennessee 37996, USA*

[d]*Department of Molecular and Cellular Biology, Baylor College of Medicine, Houston, Texas 77030, USA*

ABSTRACT: Cancer suppression is an integral component of longevity in organisms with renewable tissues. A number of genes in the mammalian genome function in cancer prevention, and some of these have been directly implicated in longevity assurance. One such longevity assurance gene is the tumor suppressor p53, a transcription factor that is mutated or dysregulated in most human cancers. Early studies have linked p53 to the induction of cellular senescence, whereas recent reports implicate it as a potential regulator of organismal aging. We have shown by gene inactivation studies that loss of p53 function enhances tumor susceptibility and reduces longevity in the mouse. A recent serendipitously generated p53 mutant allele resulted in a hypermorphic version of p53 that displays increased cancer resistance, yet also mediates decreased longevity. The reduced longevity is accompanied by the accelerated onset of a variety of aging phenotypes. These include a 20% decrease in median life span, early osteoporosis, lordokyphosis, organ atrophy, delayed wound healing, and a reduced regenerative response after various stresses. Since the initial characterization of these mutant mice, we have attempted to elucidate the underlying molecular and cellular mechanisms that could be influencing the early aging phenotypes. Molecular studies of the p53 mutant allele product indicate that it induces an increase in p53 activity in both *in vitro* and *in vivo* contexts. The age-associated loss of organ cellularity and reduced tissue regenerative responses in the mutant mice are consistent with an accelerated loss of stem cell functional capacity. Our model is that enhanced growth inhibitory activity of p53 produces an earlier loss of the ability of stem cells to produce adequate numbers of progenitor and mature differentiated cells in each organ. Currently, we are performing stem cell functional assays from p53 mutant and wild-type mice to test this model. One challenge for the future will be to find

Address for correspondence: Lawrence A. Donehower, Department of Molecular Virology and Microbiology, Baylor College of Medicine, Houston, TX 77030. Voice: 713-798-3594; fax: 713-798-3190.
larryd@bcm.tmc.edu

Ann. N.Y. Acad. Sci. 1019: 171–177 (2004). © 2004 New York Academy of Sciences.
doi: 10.1196/annals.1297.027

ways to manipulate p53 function to provide increased cancer resistance, yet still enhance overall organismal longevity.

KEYWORDS: p53; tumor suppressor; mouse; aging model; accelerated aging; stem cells

INTRODUCTION

In humans and laboratory mice, cancer risk increases dramatically with age, making cancer a prominent age-associated disease. Both cancer and aging are associated with the accumulation of cellular DNA damage over time. Cancer-associated DNA damage often is manifested in genetic alterations that affect normal maintenance of genomic integrity and cellular growth and death control. In the aging organism, DNA damage can induce stress responses such as apoptosis that allow the removal of cells that are nonfunctional or potentially cancerous. The regenerative capacity of the adult tissue stem cells allows replacement of the cast off cells through the continual production of progenitor and terminally differentiated cells. Thus, in the normal animal, organ homeostasis is maintained through a balance between proliferation and apoptosis. Disruptions in the homeostatic balance that lead to decreased apoptosis or increased proliferation often are associated with cancer.

One interesting question is whether alterations in organ homeostatic mechanisms (independent of those associated with cancer) also can affect the organismal aging process. It is well established that the progressive loss of organ function in human aging is accompanied by atrophy and loss of cellularity in many tissues. Could this organ atrophy be a result of dysfunctional homeostasis brought on by deficiencies in cell proliferation or increases in cell apoptosis? As hypothesized by Van Zant and Liang,[1] age-related declines in tissue stem cell function could play a key role in altering organ homeostasis. Growing evidence suggests that aging has important qualitative effects on stem cells, including reduction of self-renewal capacity, restriction of the breadth of developmental potency, and response to stress-related demands.[1] Although the precise relationships of stem cell functionality to overall aging phenotypes and longevity remain unclear, it seems likely that stem cell–related declines are an important component affecting the aging process.

It is particularly important that stem cells, because of their developmental potency, remain relatively protected from environmental and endogenous insults. Indeed, there is some evidence that stem cells do have very effective stress response, toxin export, and damage repair systems.[1] One critical integrator of the cellular stress response is the p53 protein. p53 is considered a prototypical tumor suppressor, and its inactivation through either structural mutation or functional dysregulation occurs in most human cancers.[2,3] When the dividing cell is subjected to a variety of stresses, p53 is activated to induce a cell cycle arrest or apoptosis. A p53-induced cell cycle arrest allows time for the stress-induced damage to be repaired before entry into S phase or mitosis, thus preventing deleterious fixation of damage and mutations in the DNA of progeny cells. In other contexts, it may be more advantageous for the organism to eliminate damaged cells, and p53 can efficiently induce apoptosis by transcriptionally activating a battery of proapoptotic genes. Thus, p53 protects the organism from nascent cancer cells, but the ability to arrest or kill cells also raises the possibility that it can affect organ homeostasis through its effects on stem cell growth and death. There is some evidence that reduction in p53 dosage does increase stem cell proliferative capacity in experimental contexts.[4–6]

The primary approach of our laboratory has been to understand p53 function through the generation of mouse models with mutant versions of p53. We showed that inactivation of p53 in the germ line of mice resulted in drastically increased tumor susceptibility.[7] More recently, we have generated a p53 mutant mouse that appears to display hypermorphic p53 activity. This mutant mouse, the p53$^{+/m}$ mouse, exhibits enhanced cancer resistance but shows reduced longevity and the accelerated onset of an array of aging-associated phenotypes.[8] The nature of the early aging phenotypes in the p53$^{+/m}$ mouse suggested the possibility of p53 effects on stem cell phenotypes. The interrelationship of p53, stem cells, and aging thus is the focus of this article.

RESULTS AND DISCUSSION

The p53 mutation in the p53$^{+/m}$ mouse was the result of an aberrant gene targeting event in embryonic stem cells. Along with the intended single inactivating point mutation in exon 7, we obtained a deletion of the first 6 exons of the 11-exon p53 gene. This resulted in expression of a chimeric transcript initiated at a gene upstream of p53 and then spliced into exon 7 sequences of the p53 gene. This transcript resulted in translation of a 24 kDa C-terminal p53 peptide (the m protein) that was missing the transactivation and DNA binding domains that are critical for the transcriptional activity of the protein. The truncated m protein was expressed, albeit at low levels, in several tissues of the p53$^{+/m}$ mouse (S. Venkatachalam, unpublished data). Our initial hypothesis was that this deleted allele of p53 would behave essentially as a null allele and that p53$^{+/m}$ mice would develop tumors with a similar incidence and spectrum as that observed for the original p53$^{+/-}$ mice that we had engineered.[9] In fact, p53$^{+/m}$ mice were surprisingly resistant to spontaneous cancers. Only 2 of 35 p53$^{+/m}$ mice (~6%) exhibited tumors over their life span (FIG. 1). This compared with an almost 100% cancer development in p53$^{+/-}$ mice and a 45% cancer incidence in wild-type (p53$^{+/+}$) mice of the same predominantly C57BL/6 background.

Despite being almost cancer-free, the p53$^{+/m}$ mice had a median longevity that was significantly less than that of their more cancer-prone p53$^{+/+}$ counterparts (96 weeks vs. 118 weeks; FIG. 1). The decreased p53$^{+/m}$ longevity could be caused in part by some of the early aging–associated phenotypes observed in them. Alternatively, the decrease in longevity could be associated with some subtle pathology unrelated to aging. However, most of the phenotypes observed in the older p53$^{+/m}$ mice could legitimately be considered markers of early aging (TABLE 1). They appeared completely normal in appearance up to the age of ~14 months, but between 14 and 20 months of age (middle age for this strain of laboratory mouse) they began to show reductions in body mass, lordokyphosis (hunchbacked spine), lethargy, and ruffled fur. Timed deaths and necropsies of older p53$^{+/m}$ and p53$^{+/+}$ mice revealed atrophy in many of the organs of the p53$^{+/m}$ mice. The spleen, thymus, liver, kidney, and testes of the p53$^{+/m}$ mice showed a marked loss of mass and organ cellularity compared with age- and sex-matched organs from wild-type mice. Whole-body radiographs of the p53$^{+/m}$ mice showed global osteoporosis beginning at ~12 months of age, and

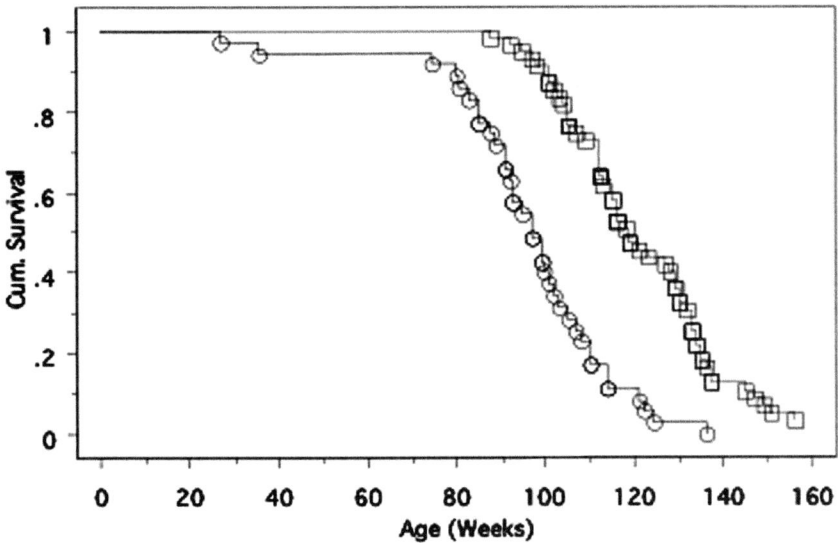

FIGURE 1. Longevity of $p53^{+/+}$ and $p53^{+/m}$ mice. Kaplan–Meier survival plots for 35 $p53^{+/m}$ mice (*circles*) and 56 $p53^{+/+}$ mice (*squares*) of similar C57BL/6 × 129/Sv genetic background are shown. The reduced $p53^{+/m}$ longevity is highly significant by log-rank analysis ($P < .00001$). Only 2 of 35 $p53^{+/m}$ mice exhibited tumors during their life span, whereas 27 of 56 $p53^{+/+}$ mice succumbed to tumors.

loss of bone density was particularly substantial by 18–24 months of age. Histopathology on bone cross-sections from aged $p53^{+/+}$ and $p53^{+/m}$ mice confirmed the osteoporotic diagnosis. Skin sections from the $p53^{+/m}$ mice also showed a pronounced thinning of the dermis and subcutaneous adipose layer in the $p53^{+/m}$ mice, another aging marker in both mice and humans. Skeletal muscle atrophy in a variety of muscle groups in the $p53^{+/m}$ mice was marked. Other aging markers noted in the aged $p53^{+/m}$ mice were loss of hair regeneration capacity, diminished wound healing, reduced anesthetic tolerance, and decreased ability to produce mature white blood cells after hematopoietic progenitor ablation (TABLE 1). Note that not all aging-associated markers or pathologies were accelerated in the $p53^{+/m}$ mice, so that this model can best be described as exhibiting segmental features of accelerated aging.

In addition to characterization of the biological markers for aging, we are examining molecular markers in tissues of the $p53^{+/m}$ mice that could provide further evidence that they are undergoing accelerated aging. One aging marker used with preliminary success is the senescence-associated beta-galactosidase assay. First described by Campisi and colleagues,[10] this assay appears to be quite specific for senescent, but not prescenescent or quiescent cells. Senescent cells express a beta-galactosidase, histochemically detectable by blue staining at pH 6.0, upon incubation in X-gal. We found that liver and spleen tissue sections from young 3-month $p53^{+/+}$ and $p53^{+/m}$ mice displayed very few X-gal–positive senescent cells. However,

TABLE 1. Aging-related phenotypes in p53$^{+/+}$ and p53$^{+/m}$ mice

Phenotype	p53$^{+/+}$	p53$^{+/m}$
Median life span	118 weeks	96 weeks
Maximum life span	164 weeks	136 weeks
Cancer incidence	>45%	<6%
Body weight	reduced at 30 months	reduced at 18 months
Liver, spleen, kidney weights	minimal loss of mass	25–40% reduction in mass at 24 months
Lymphoid atrophy	moderate	pronounced
Lordokyphosis	modest	pronounced
Osteoporosis	minimal	pronounced
Blood chemistry	normal	normal
Urinalysis	normal	normal
Peripheral WBC, RBC counts	normal	normal
Male fecundity	normal	normal
Hair graying and alopecia	minimal	minimal
Hair regrowth	modestly reduced	greatly reduced
Dermal thickness	moderately reduced	greatly reduced
Subcutaneous adipose	moderately reduced	greatly reduced
Wound healing	normal re-epithelialization	reduced epithelialization
Muscle atrophy	minimal	pronounced
Tolerance of anesthetic stress	well tolerated	poorly tolerated
5-FU myeloablation	robust WBC replenishment	reduced WBC replenishment
Tissue SA-beta-gal staining	moderate increase with age	pronounced increase with age

18–21-month-old p53$^{+/m}$ and p53$^{+/+}$ tissues showed more than a 10-fold increase in senescent cell counts over their younger counterparts, as might be expected for a bona fide aging marker. Moreover, the average percentage of senescent cells in each old p53$^{+/m}$ tissue section was over twice that observed in the old p53$^{+/+}$ section, consistent with the earlier appearance of aging phenotypes in the p53$^{+/m}$ mice (C. Gatza, unpublished data). We are currently in the process of assessing the status of other molecular aging markers in the p53$^{+/m}$ mice that are based on cDNA array analysis of young versus aged tissues.

Our preliminary assumption was that the early aging phenotypes observed in the p53$^{+/m}$ mice were a result of a hyperactive p53 state. The increased cancer resistance was certainly consistent with this. However, given that there was only one intact wild-type p53 allele in the p53$^{+/m}$ mice and thus 50% of the normal level of p53, how could the p53 state be hyperactive? Our current favored hypothesis, with some evidence to support it,[8] is that the truncated p53 m protein can interact with wild-type p53 to increase its activity. Since p53 in unstressed cells is primarily in a latent inactive state, perhaps the interaction of the truncated m with wild-type p53 could convert some of the latent wild-type p53 into a more active conformation. There is evidence for this type of activity from literature reports indicating that C-terminal p53 fragments and peptides can increase wild-type p53 transcriptional activation and DNA binding activity.[11,12] *In vitro*, we showed that the m allele–generated protein of 24 kDa could directly interact with wild-type forms of p53 and could enhance wild-type p53 transcriptional activation activity on a p53 reporter construct[8] (S. Venkatachalam, unpublished data). *In vivo*, the $p53^{+/m}$ cells showed an enhanced p53 response to ionizing radiation, as measured by wild-type p53 protein levels and p53 target gene RNA expression.[8]

The reduced longevity of the $p53^{+/m}$ mice associated with the pronounced age-associated organ atrophies and reduced regenerative responses suggested to us that stem cell function could be an important component of these phenotypes. We hypothesize that increased p53 activity in the $p53^{+/m}$ stem cells could inhibit stem cell and/or progenitor cell proliferation and/or differentiation. Early in their life span, the $p53^{+/m}$ mice have ample stem cell functional reserves to maintain organ homeostasis, but with age this stem reserve declines more precipitously compared with wild-type mice. Eventually, the loss of stem cell function may manifest itself as classic aging phenotypes (e.g., osteoporosis, muscle atrophy, organ atrophy). We are currently examining the $p53^{+/m}$, $p53^{+/+}$, $p53^{+/-}$, and $p53^{-/-}$ mice to determine how p53 dosage may affect stem cell/progenitor cell proliferation, numbers, and overall functionality. Preliminary data from our laboratory indicate that reduction of p53 dosage in $p53^{+/-}$ and $p53^{-/-}$ hematopoietic stem cells augments their proliferative capacity and ability to reconstitute mature tissues (M. Dumble, unpublished data). Interestingly, the $p53^{+/m}$ hematopoietic stem cells exhibit reduced numbers and similar proliferative activities compared with their $p53^{+/+}$ counterparts, despite the fact that the $p53^{+/m}$ mice have only one intact wild-type p53 allele. These stem cell studies were performed on young mice, indicating that the decreased $p53^{+/m}$ stem cell numbers preceded the appearance of their subsequent aging phenotypes. Initial assays on older $p53^{+/m}$ mice confirmed a reduced number of hematopoietic stem cells compared with their older $p53^{+/+}$ counterparts (M. Dumble, unpublished data). These preliminary results suggest the possibility that the $p53^{+/m}$ mice do have reduced stem cell functional activity and that this reduction could be at least partially responsible for the early aging phenotypes in these mice.

If decreases in stem cell functionality in the $p53^{+/m}$ mice are responsible for some of their early aging phenotypes, does this mean that reduction of p53 activity could delay aging phenotypes and prolong life? Because virtually all of the $p53^{+/-}$ mice develop early tumors, this seems unlikely on the surface. However, interestingly, two $p53^{+/-}$ mice in our colony that avoided tumors lived significantly longer than the longest lived $p53^{+/+}$ mouse in our colony (L. A. Donehower, unpublished observations). This result suggests that perhaps the $p53^{+/-}$ animals would have increased longevity if tumors somehow could be prevented. We currently are initiating experimental protocols to reduce tumorigenesis in the $p53^{+/-}$ mice in an attempt to obtain significant numbers of these tumor-free animals to test their longevity phenotypes. Another challenge is the manipulation of the structure of p53 to obtain a version that retains or enhances its tumor-fighting functions while somehow increasing stem cell functionality and prolonging longevity. Such approaches potentially could convert p53 from a longevity assurance gene to a longevity enhancement gene.

REFERENCES

1. VAN ZANT, G. & Y. LIANG. 2003. The role of stem cells in aging. Exp. Hematol. **31:** 659–672.
2. LEVINE, A.J. 1997. p53, the cellular gatekeeper for growth and division. Cell **88:** 323–331.
3. VOGELSTEIN, B., D. LANE & A.J. LEVINE. 2000. Surfing the p53 network. Nature **408:** 307–310.
4. DONEHOWER, L.A. 2002. Does p53 affect organismal aging? J. Cell. Physiol. **192:** 23–33.
5. PALACIOS, R., C. BUCANA & X. XIE. 1996. Long-term culture of lymphohematopoietic stem cells. Proc. Natl. Acad. Sci. USA **93:** 5247–5252.
6. SHOUNAN, Y., A. DOLNIKOV, K.L. MACKENZIE, et al. 1996. Retroviral transduction of hematopoietic progenitor cells with mutant p53 promotes survival and proliferation, modifies differentiation potential and inhibits apoptosis. Leukemia **10:** 1619–1628.
7. DONEHOWER, L.A., M. HARVEY, B.L. SLAGLE, et al. 1992. Mice deficient for p53 are developmentally normal but susceptible to spontaneous tumours. Nature **356:** 215–221.
8. TYNER, S.D., S. VENKATACHALAM, J. CHOI, et al. 2002. p53 mutant mice that display early ageing-associated phenotypes. Nature **415:** 45–53.
9. DONEHOWER, L.A. 1996. The p53-deficient mouse: a model for basic and applied cancer studies. Semin. Cancer Biol. **7:** 269–278.
10. DIMRI, G.P., X. LEE, G. BASILE, et al. 1995. A biomarker that identifies senescent human cells in culture and in aging skin in vivo. Proc. Natl. Acad. Sci. USA **92:** 9363–9367.
11. SELIVANOVA, G., V. IOTSOVA, I. OKAN, et al. 1997. Restoration of the growth suppression function of mutant p53 by a synthetic peptide derived from the p53 C-terminal domain. Nat. Med. **3:** 632–638.
12. SELIVANOVA, G., L. RYABCHENKO, E. JANSSON, et al. 1999. Reactivation of mutant p53 through interaction of a C-terminal peptide with the core domain. Mol. Cell. Biol. **19:** 3395–3402.

Engineering Anticancer T Cells for Extended Functional Longevity

GRAHAM PAWELEC,[a] ERMINIA MARIANI,[b] JULIE McLEOD,[c] ARIE BEN-YEHUDA,[d] TAMAS FÜLÖP,[e] MARTIN ARINGER,[f] AND YVONNE BARNETT[g]

[a]*Center for Medical Research, ZMF, University of Tübingen Medical School, D-72072 Tübingen, Germany*

[b]*University of Bologna, I-40136 Bologna, Italy*

[c]*University of the West of England, Bristol BS16 1QY, England*

[d]*Hadassah University Hospital, IL-91120 Jerusalem, Israel*

[e]*Université de Franche-Comté, F-25030 Besançon, France*

[f]*University of Vienna, A-1090 Vienna, Austria*

[g]*University of Ulster, Coleraine BT52 1SA, Northern Ireland*

ABSTRACT: Like other somatic cells, human T lymphocytes have a finite replicative capacity *in vitro*, and, by implication and consistent with the limited data available, *in vivo* as well. An accumulation of dysfunctional T cells may be detrimental under conditions of chronic antigenic stress (chronic infection, cancer, autoimmunity). Using T cells from young donors to model the process of T cell clonal expansion *in vitro* under these conditions reveals age-associated increasing levels of oxidative DNA damage and microsatellite instability (MSI), coupled with decreasing DNA repair capacity, telomerase induction and telomere length, decreased levels of expression of the T cell costimulator CD28 and consequently reduced secretion of the T cell growth factor interleukin-2 (IL-2). However, data from similar experiments using T cell clones (TCCs) derived from extremely healthy very elderly donors ("successfully aged") indicate that DNA repair is better maintained, MSI less prevalent, and (already short) telomere lengths are maintained. Nonetheless, oxidative DNA damage is seen to the same extent, and clonal longevity is also similar in these clones. DNA damage levels are reduced by culture in 5% oxygen, but longevity is not improved. This may be because of the requirement for intermittent reactivation via receptor pathways dependent on free radical production in T cells. These recent findings from our international immunosenescence research consortium suggest that strategies other than telomere maintenance, better protection against free radicals, or improved DNA repair will be required for functional longevity extension of human TCCs. To obtain sufficient cells for adoptive immunotherapy of cancer, alternative avenues need exploration; currently, these include enforced expression of certain heat shock proteins and proteasome compo-

Address for correspondence: Graham Pawelec, Center for Medical Research, ZMF, University of Tübingen Medical School, Waldhörnlestrasse 22, D-72072 Tübingen, Germany. Voice: +49-7071-298-2805; fax: +49-7071-294467.
graham.pawelec@uni-tuebingen.de

nents, and interference with the expression of negative regulatory receptors expressed by T cells.

KEYWORDS: T cell clones; cell culture longevity; DNA damage; DNA repair; telomere length; costimulation; antigenic stress; oxidative stress

INTRODUCTION

Tumor cells are at least initially immunogenic and can be recognized and destroyed by T lymphocytes. Tumors escape this immune destruction by a wide variety of strategies including T cell suppression. Many of the characteristics of the dysfunctional T cells found associated with tumors are shared with those found in aging. These include shortened telomeres, increased levels of oxidative DNA damage, decreased DNA repair, decreased expression of positive and increased expression of negative costimulatory receptors, curtailed proliferative capacity, altered cytokine secretion patterns, and changes in apoptosis induction (increased resistance of CD8 and increased susceptibility of CD4 T cells). We suggest that many of these changes are caused by chronic antigenic stress (stimulation by tumor antigens in cancer patients and by persistent viruses in the elderly). This results in anergy and replicative senescence, which compromise the immune status of the host. These processes can be modeled *in vitro* in long-term clonal cultures and interventions for their prevention screened with a view to application *in vivo*. Additionally, extending the life span of tumor-specific T cells *in vitro* is a useful aim in itself, because these cells could be more effectively exploited for the adoptive immunotherapy of cancer if their functional integrity could be maintained over many more population doublings than currently possible. Currently, promising approaches to achieve these aims include gene transfer (hTERT, proteasome ß1 or ß5 chains, HSP70 or 90, and possibly DNA repair enzymes, etc.), manipulation of the cytokine environment, or intervening in apoptosis control pathways. Some of these interventions may find application in both aging and cancer therapy. The following summarizes some of the first results from an international research consortium seeking to characterize biomarkers of aging specifically in the human clonal T lymphocyte longitudinal model, to compare these parameters for TCCs derived from "successfully aged" extremely healthy ("senior European" [SENIEUR]-selected) donors or normal young donors, and to develop interventions for extending functional TCC longevity in a safe manner.

CHRONIC ANTIGENIC STRESS

Numerous tumor-specific antigens have been described, mostly MHC class I–restricted and targeted by CD8 T cells, but also increasing numbers of MHC class II–restricted antigens targeted by CD4 T cells.[1] Naive T cells require activation via their highly polymorphic receptor for antigen (TCR) together with stimulation via monomorphic costimulatory receptors such as CD28. Contact with antigens under appropriate conditions, such as presentation by activated dendritic cells, commits the T cells to a certain number of cell divisions (clonal expansion), the purpose of which is to generate sufficiently high numbers of antigen-specific cells to mediate a successful immune response. Such clonal expansion is closely regulated by mechanisms which are just beginning to be understood. In the face of chronic antigenic stimulation, that is, when the source of antigen cannot be cleared, the immune response may become dysregulated. In the elderly, persistent herpes viruses, especially cytomegalovirus (CMV), provide a reservoir of antigen and a constant stimulus to T cell–mediated immunity. It is paramount that an effective immune response to CMV is maintained because reactivation of this virus (which does not normally occur in a clinically noticeable manner in the elderly) would be fatal (as can be seen in the major clinical problem that CMV still represents for severely immunosuppressed hematopoietic stem cell transplant recipients). We have documented the presence of many dysfunctional CMV-specific T cells in some elderly people and suggest that this is an important contributor to the immune risk phenotype (IRP) that we are developing to predict incipient mortality based on longitudinal aging studies currently being performed in Sweden.[2,3] The majority of such CMV-specific cells in the elderly express little costimulatory receptor CD28, but instead a very high level of a negative receptor, KLRG1,[4] which prevents them from proliferating.[5] Thus, these T cells, which are likely to be apoptosis resistant and anergic, accumulate but fail to function properly, for example, in terms of their production of antiviral cytokines such as interferon-γ.[4]

In the case of CD4 T cells, on the other hand, the problem may be that clonal exhaustion manifests as clonal deletion rather than accumulation. Thus, cultured CD4 TCCs become more rather than less susceptible to apoptosis triggered via stimulation through the receptor for antigen[6] so that such antigen-specific cells eventually would be lost to the organism under conditions of chronic antigenic stress. Indeed, as well as accumulation of CMV-specific CD8 cells in the elderly, which contribute to the IRP, decreased numbers of CD4 cells and an inverted CD4:8 ratio (as in AIDS patients) also seem to be an important component of the IRP.[7] Therefore, we suggest that chronic antigenic stress results in an accumulation of dysfunctional CD8 cells, selective clonal deletion of CD4 cells, and consequently decreased immune responses to the target. For the cancer patient, this is disastrous. We further hypothesize that dysfunctional CD8 cells accumulate *because* of selective loss of the CD4 helper cells. We therefore suggest that replacing the lost CD4 cells will "rejuvenate" the response. This could be approached by generating such CD4 cells *in vitro* and infusing them into the patient ("adoptive immunotherapy") or intervening *in vivo* to achieve this aim ("active immunotherapy"). As a prelude to the first approach, we have been studying the characteristics of human CD4 TCCs *in vitro* as they progress through their finite life spans, and we have sought differences between TCCs derived from the very old, successfully aged and the normal young in this respect.

STUDIES ON CD4 T CELL CLONES

As part of a pan-European immunosenescence research program (Immunology and Ageing in Europe, ImAginE, www.medizin.uni-tuebingen.de/imagine/) we have generated and distributed TCCs to several centers. Preliminary data from the initial concerted investigation on the same set of TCCs are summarized here. The study materials consisted of three TCCs derived from a very healthy SENIEUR donor, and four TCCs derived from two normal young healthy controls. These cells were cultured under standard conditions using the same medium, feeder cells, and cytokines and tested by different members of the consortium from the earliest time point possible (~26 population doublings [PDs]) up to the end of their life span (~80 PDs for the longest lived). The first point to emerge from these studies was that, unexpectedly, TCC longevities did not differ regardless of the source of cells to be cloned (for recent review, see Pawelec et al.[8]). This may seem a minor point, but probably because of the laborious nature of this type of work, such data were essentially lacking in the literature. Several immunological and cell biological parameters have now been studied using some of these clones. The formation of "immunological synapses" by stimulated old cells was altered compared with the young in that certain signaling molecules such as p56lck were not equally well recruited, whereas other parameters, such as exclusion of CD45, were not affected. It was confirmed that, as expected, the density of expression of the costimulatory receptor CD28 decreased with increasing numbers of PD, coupled with a decreased level of IL-2 production, as previously observed by ourselves and others.[9] Perhaps because of decreased levels of CD28 costimulation and IL-2 production, autocrine proliferative capacity decreased, and levels of induced telomerase declined. Concordantly, the density of CD25 and CD122 expression (α and β chains of the IL-2 receptor) also decreased, as did the common γ chain (CD132). The previously observed increased susceptibility of these TCCs to CD3 antibody–mediated activation-induced cell death[6] was extended to include apoptosis induced by more physiological fas ligand signaling. Here, we observed the first difference between TCCs derived from SENIEUR donors and those derived from young donors; namely, the former showed greater resistance to apoptosis than the latter. These results need to be confirmed with larger numbers of clones; if true, they may provide an interesting clue to differential regulation of apoptosis in the successfully aged. The second difference between SENIEUR-derived and young donor-derived TCCs was observed for their capacity to repair DNA damage: this was maintained over the entire life span of the former but decreased with increasing PD of the latter. These findings are perhaps reflected in the observed differences in microsatellite instability (MSI) in these clones: when tested over six loci at three different culture ages, it was found that SENIEUR-derived clones acquired MSI in a total of 5 of 15 assessments, whereas this figure was 13 of 22 for the other clones (33% vs. 59%). This suggests that mismatch repair capacity was better maintained in the SENIEUR donor-derived clones. Nonetheless, application of a Comet assay modified to detect oxidative DNA damage revealed similar age-associated increased levels of such damage in all clones, regardless of donor source. This apparent paradox requires further exploration.

Intriguingly, although telomerase induction also decreased with increasing PD in all clones, telomere dynamics in SENIEUR-derived cells were different. Telomere lengths in TCCs from young individuals decreased with increasing PD, as expected, but the lengths of the already-short telomeres in SENIEUR-derived clones were maintained. Nonetheless, the TCCs were no longer-lived from SENIEUR than younger donors. Therefore, the alternative telomere maintenance mechanism in SENIEUR-derived clones does not seem to prevent their clonal deletion. It could be that the amount of telomere DNA damage, rather then length *per se*, is the critical factor here, as reported for other cell types. Therefore, despite better maintenance of telomere length and DNA repair capacity, SENIEUR-derived clones are not longer-lived than others. Use of lowered oxygen tension culture conditions also provided data consistent with the interpretation that overall DNA damage and repair were not directly associated with increased longevity. Thus, culture in 5% rather than 20% oxygen resulted in a clear reduction in oxidative DNA damage but failed to increase the life span of the clones. In fact, if anything, the life span was reduced (but this may be because TCCs require intermittent restimulation via the TCR for continued proliferation, and signaling therefrom requires free radical production). Nonetheless, addition of the antioxidant N-tert-butyl-a-phenylnitrone (PBN) did slightly increase rather than decrease the life span of the clones and had a similar effect on both SENIEUR (average 10.6% increase) and non-SENIEUR–derived clones (average 11.2% increase). This apparent paradox is also not yet resolved but could be related to reducing the levels of free radicals from damage-causing to less damage-causing but still sufficient for signaling.

REMEDIATION

To recap, cultured human CD4 TCCs accumulate oxidative DNA damage during culture; reducing this with PBN slightly extends life span, but reducing it with low oxygen decreases life span. Better maintenance of DNA repair, less MSI, and maintenance of telomere length, however, are not associated with increased longevity. The fact that TCCs exhibiting these differences have similar longevities obviously suggests that these factors are, somewhat counterintuitively, not critical. Therefore, age-associated changes shared between the SENIEUR and non-SENIEUR clones may be more important. Thus, the decreased levels of expression of CD28, probably resulting in decreased costimulation and contributing to the observed declining IL-2 secretion and levels of all three IL-2 receptor chains, as well as most likely the decreased telomerase induction seen,[10] may be an important factor. Knowledge of CD28 expression regulation then would be crucial for manipulating TCC longevity. Little is known of this, but some data on regulation of CD28 expression in senescent cells are available.[11] Moreover, not only has it been reported that the cytokine TNF-α can downregulate CD28,[12] but recent findings suggest that IL-12 may be able to upregulate CD28 expression at least on certain freshly isolated CD28-negative CD4 T cells, although this has not yet been demonstrated for CD28$^+$ cells which have become CD28-negative in culture.[13] We have observed that a minority of clones reexpresses CD28 during progression through their life span, and that this may correlate with their loss of ability to secrete TNF-α.[14] Moreover, the reexpressed CD28 appears to be functional in that autocrine proliferative capacity is also reacquired (FIG. 1). However, despite upregulation of functional CD28, these clones *still* manifest a finite life span, and the inclusion of neutralizing antisera to TNF-α extends longevity only to a certain extent, in fact, about the same as PBN (~10–15%; FIG. 2).

The effect of supplementation with the cytokine IL-12 and other cocktails of cytokines including IL-7 and IL-15 remains to be explored. Note also that it is not only the CD28 costimulatory receptor on T cells that influences the outcome of activation via the TCR, but a whole host of receptors, delivering negative as well as positive signals on ligation. This is a very complicated system, probably not even all the members of which have yet been identified, because new molecules are still being reported.[15] TABLE 1 summarizes current awareness of the T cell costimulatory receptor family.

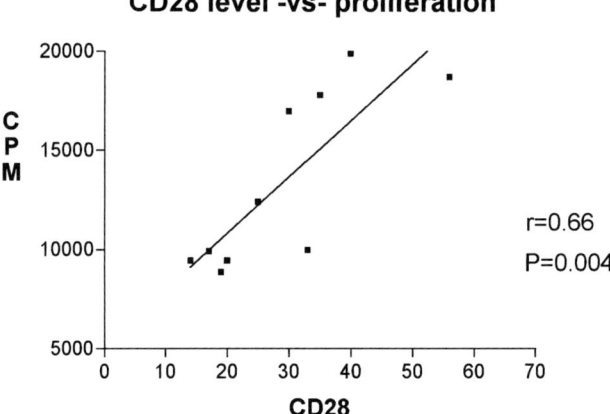

FIGURE 1. CD28 expression level, measured by FACS as median fluorescence intensity, plotted against autocrine proliferative capacity (CPM) assessed by tritiated thymidine incorporation 2 days after restimulation of TCCs at different ages and during CD28 expression loss and re-acquisition.

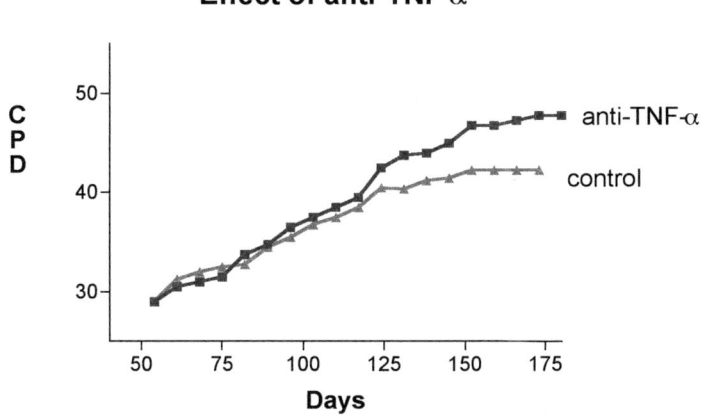

FIGURE 2. Effect of blocking the action of autocrine TNF-α production using neutralizing antiserum supplementation. CPD, cumulative population doublings. Symbols show growth in the presence of TNF-α antiserum (*squares*) and in the presence of control antiserum (*triangles*).

TABLE 1. T cell costimulation

Receptor	Ligand	Main effect
CD 28	CD80, 86	Strong positive constimulation
CD 152	CD80, 86	Dominant negative constimulation
ICOS	B7RP-1	Accessory positive constimulation
PD-1	PD-L1, L2	Weak negative constimulation when IL-2 limiting (blocks ICOS, not CD28)
BTLA	B7x	Similar to PD-1? What differences?

OTHER APPROACHES

Other approaches to longevity extension may include enforced expression of heat shock proteins (because there is an age-associated decrease in expression of various stress response proteins with age in humans[16]) or proteasome ß1 or ß5 chains (because age-associated impaired proteasome function is associated with decreased stress resistance which can be reversed by gene transfection[17]). Whether a more differentiated approach to manipulating DNA repair pathways in mammalian cells, as in yeast,[18] will offer any benefit remains to be tested. Clearly, the use of hTERT and the mechanisms of its action, particularly in the light of our findings on telomere length above, and the still unresolved issue of why hTERT "immortalization" does[19] or does not[20] work (in human CD8 clones), also require further investigation. Finally, blockade of negative receptors such as KLRG-1 and CD152 also may be beneficial.

ACKNOWLEDGMENTS

The experimental work performed under the aegis of "Immunology and Ageing in Europe" was supported by each participating laboratory; funding for coordination was supplied by EU contract no. QLK6-CT-1999-02031. G.P.'s work was supported by the Deutsche Forschungsgemeinschaft (DGF Pa 361-7/1).

REFERENCES

1. HALDER, T., G. PAWELEC, A.F. KIRKIN, et al. 1997. Novel class II-restricted melanoma antigens. Cancer Res. **57:** 3238–3244.
2. PAWELEC, G., Q. OUYANG, G. COLONNA-ROMANA, et al. 2002. Is human immunosenescence clinically relevant? Looking for "immunological risk phenotypes." Trends Immunol. **23:** 330–332.
3. PAWELEC, G., Q. OUYANG, W. WAGNER & A. WIKBY. 2003. Pathways to a robust immune response in the elderly. In Impact of Immune Senescence on Human Aging. J.D. Mountz, H.-C. Hsu, Eds.: 1–13. Immunol Allergy Clin N America Series. Vol 23, WB Saunders. Philadelphia.
4. OUYANG, Q., W.M. WAGNER, D. VOEHRINGER, et al. 2003. Age-associated accumulation of CMV-specific CD8(+) T cells expressing the inhibitory killer cell lectin-like receptor G1 (KLRG1). Exp. Gerontol. **38:** 911–920.
5. VOEHRINGER, D., M. KOSCHELLA & H. PIRCHER. 2003. Lack of proliferative capacity of human effector and memory T cells expressing killer cell lectin-like receptor G1 (KLRG1). Blood **100:** 3698–3702.

6. PAWELEC, G., D. SANSOM, A. REHBEIN, et al. 1996. Decreased proliferative capacity and increased susceptibility to activation-induced cell death in late-passage human CD4+ TCR2+ cultured T cell clones. Exp. Gerontol. **31:** 655–668.
7. WIKBY, A., B. JOHANSSON, J. OLSSON, et al. 2002. Expansions of peripheral blood CD8 T-lymphocyte subpopulations and an association with cytomegalovirus seropositivity in the elderly: the Swedish NONA immune study. Exp. Gerontol. **37:** 445–453.
8. PAWELEC, G., Y. BARNETT, E. MARIANI & R. SOLANA. 2002. Human CD4+ T cell clone longevity in tissue culture: lack of influence of donor age or cell origin. Exp. Gerontol. **37:** 265–269.
9. PAWELEC, G., A. REHBEIN, H. HAEHNEL, et al. 1997. Human T-cell clones in long-term culture as a model of immunosenescence. Immunol. Rev. **160:** 31–42.
10. VALENZUELA, H.F. & R.B. EFFROS. 2002. Divergent telomerase and CD28 expression patterns in human CD4 and CD8 T cells following repeated encounters with the same antigenic stimulus. Clin. Immunol. **105:** 117–125.
11. VALLEJO, A.N., E. BRYL, K. KLARSKOV, et al. 2002. Molecular basis for the loss of CD28 expression in senescent T cells. J. Biol. Chem. **277:** 46940–46949.
12. BRYL, E., A.N. VALLEJO, C.M. WEYAND & J.J. GORONZY. 2001. Down-regulation of CD28 expression by TNF-alpha. J. Immunol. **167:** 3231–3238.
13. WARRINGTON, K.J., A.N. VALLEJO, C.M. WEYAND & J.J. GORONZY. 2003. CD28 loss in senescent CD4+ T cells: reversal by interleukin-12 stimulation. Blood **101:** 3543–3549.
14. PAWELEC, G. 2003. Cultured T cell clones as models for immunosenescence. *In* Basic Biology and Clinical Impact of Immunosenescence. G. Pawelec, Ed.: 295–307. Advances in Cell Aging and Gerontology series. Vol 13. Elsevier. Amsterdam.
15. WATANABE, N., M. GAVRIELI, J.R. SEDY, et al. 2003. BTLA is a lymphocyte inhibitory receptor with similarities to CTLA-4 and PD-1. Nat. Immunol. **4:** 670–679.
16. RAO, D.V., K. WATSON & G.L. JONES. 1999. Age-related attenuation in the expression of the major heat shock proteins in human peripheral lymphocytes. Mech. Age. Dev. **107:** 105–118.
17. CHONDROGIANNI, N., L.L. STRATFORD, I.P. TROUGAKOS, et al. 2003. Central role of the proteasome in senescence and survival of human fibroblasts: induction of a senescence-like phenotype upon its inhibition and resistance to stress upon its activation. J. Biol. Chem. **278:** 28026–28037
18. LIU, L., S. CHENG, A.J. VAN BRABANT & E.B. KMIEC. 2002. Rad51p and Rad54p, but not Rad52p, elevate gene repair in *Saccharomyces cerevisiae* directed by modified single-stranded oligonucleotide vectors. Nucleic Acids Res. **30:** 2742–2750.
19. HOOIJBERG, E., J.J. RUIZENDAAL, P.J. SNIJDERS, et al. 2000. Immortalization of human CD8+ T cell clones by ectopic expression of telomerase reverse transcriptase. J. Immunol. **165:** 4239–4245.
20. MIGLIACCIO, M., M. AMACKER, T. JUST, et al. 2000. Ectopic human telomerase catalytic subunit expression maintains telomere length but is not sufficient for CD8+ T lymphocyte immortalization. J. Immunol. **165:** 4978–4984.

Telomerase Expression Is Differentially Regulated in Birds of Differing Life Span

MARK F. HAUSSMANN,[a] DAVID W. WINKLER,[b] CHARLES E. HUNTINGTON,[c] IAN C. T. NISBET,[d] AND CAROL M. VLECK[a]

[a]*Department of Ecology, Evolution and Organismal Biology, Iowa State University, Ames, Iowa, 50011, USA*

[b]*Department of Ecology and Evolutionary Biology, Cornell University, Ithaca, New York 14853, USA*

[c]*Bowdoin College, Harpswell, Maine, 04079, USA*

[d]*I. C. T. Nisbet & Company, North Falmouth, Massachusetts 02556, USA*

ABSTRACT: Cellular senescence caused by telomere shortening has been suggested as one potential causal agent of aging. In some tissues, telomeres are maintained by telomerase; however, telomerase promotes tumor formation, suggesting a trade-off between aging and cancer. We predicted that telomerase activity should vary directly with life span. We determined telomerase activity in bone marrow in cross-sectional samples from two short-lived bird species and two long-lived bird species. The two short-lived species had high telomerase activity as hatchlings but showed a sharp downregulation in both the young and old adults, whereas the two long-lived species had relatively high telomerase activity in bone marrow that did not decrease with age. In zebra finches, the age-related change in telomerase activity varied in different tissues. Telomerase activity increased late in life in skeletal muscle, liver, and gonad, but not in blood or bone marrow.

KEYWORDS: telomerase; life span; bird; aging; telomere

One cannot consider the wide variation in life spans of different species without reflecting on the underlying physiological and molecular mechanisms. One potential mechanism is telomere regulation. Cellular replicative senescence caused by the shortening of telomeres has been suggested as a causal agent of aging and age-related diseases.[1] Organismal aging is normally accompanied by telomere shortening, which has been shown in several species including birds and mammals.[2] In some tissues, telomeric repeats are maintained by telomerase, a ribonucleoprotein capable of maintaining telomeres.[3] Expressing telomerase is associated with a cost, however, because its presence promotes tumor formation.[4] The association between aging and cancer suggests a trade-off. Downregulation of telomerase and the subsequent ero-

---

Address for correspondence: Mark F. Haussmann, Department of Ecology, Evolution and Organismal Biology, Iowa State University, Ames, IA 50011. Voice: 515-294-2759; fax: 515-294-8457.
hauss@iastate.edu

Ann. N.Y. Acad. Sci. 1019: 186–190 (2004). © 2004 New York Academy of Sciences.
doi: 10.1196/annals.1297.029

sion of telomeres with age protects organisms by decreasing the possibility of runaway proliferation and tumor formation. This mechanism acts as an antagonistic pleiotropy, affording beneficial effects early in life, but eventually contributing to senescence.[5]

We have shown that birds and mammals with longer life spans lose telomeric repeats slower than species with shorter life spans.[2] This suggests that telomerase expression has been adjusted through natural selection to alter the rate at which telomeres shorten and thereby contribute to life span modification. We predict that evolutionary strategies in telomerase activity may vary with life span. Species with a short life span and rapid rate of telomere shortening due to lack of telomerase expression should be protected from tumor formation until the end of life. At this point, critically short telomeres may be rescued by forced telomerase expression, which leads to an increased incidence of cancer. Species with long life span and a slow rate of telomere shortening due to tightly regulated expression of telomerase should be at risk for tumor formation throughout life but have delayed cellular replicative senescence compared with short-lived species.

To initiate a test of these predictions, we determined telomerase activity in cross-sectional samples from zebra finches (*Taeniopygia guttata*), tree swallows (*Tachycineta bicolor*), common terns (*Sterna hirundo*), and Leach's storm-petrels (*Oceanodroma leucorhoa*). The reported maximum life spans in the wild for these species range from 5 to 36 years and includes two relatively short-lived species, zebra finch (5 years) and tree swallow (11 years), and two relatively long-lived species common tern (27 years) and Leach's storm petrel (36 years). Within each species, telomerase activity was measured in the bone marrow of hatchlings, young adults at first breeding (at ~10% of maximum life span), and old adults (at ~ 60% of maximum life span). In zebra finches, telomerase activity also was measured in blood, muscle, liver, and gonadal tissue to determine if telomerase expression was variable between tissues and at different ages.

Birds were euthanized and tissues were immediately snap-frozen in liquid nitrogen. Tissues were ground into cell lysates and their protein concentrations were determined by Bradford assay. Telomerase activity was detected using the PCR-based TRAPeze XL Telomerase Detection Kit (Intergen Company, Norcross, GA). The yield of the PCR was determined by measuring the fluorescence of the reaction in a spectrofluorometer.

Telomerase profiles in bone marrow varied with life span. The two short-lived species had high telomerase activity as hatchlings but showed a sharp downregulation in both the young and old adults (zebra finches $F_{2,9} = 23.80$, $P = .0003$; tree swallows $F_{2,7} = 6.89$, $P = .02$). The two long-lived species had relatively high telomerase activity in bone marrow that did not decrease with age (common terns $F_{2,7} = 0.40$, $P = .69$; Leach's storm-petrels $F_{2,9} = 1.97$, $P = .20$). In the various zebra finch tissues, telomerase activity varied with age ($F_{2,56} = 8.1056$, $P = .0008$). Telomerase activity in blood and bone marrow was relatively high in hatchling birds and then decreased in young and old adults (FIG. 1). In contrast, whereas telomerase activity in muscle, liver, and gonadal tissue was relatively low in young adults, it increased in old birds (FIG. 1).

These results are in agreement with our predictions for short- and long-lived organisms outlined above. In the long-lived common tern and Leach's storm-petrel, telomerase is expressed in bone marrow throughout life and telomeres of blood cells

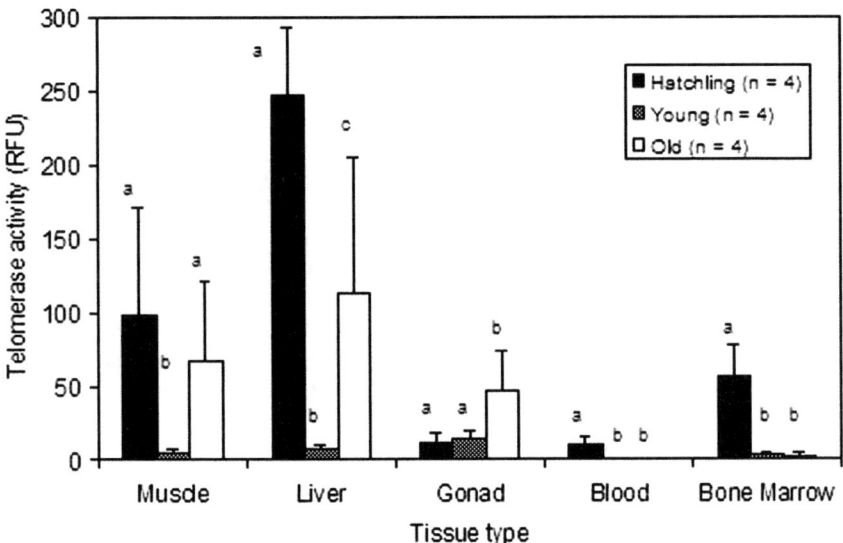

FIGURE 1. Telomerase activity in muscle, liver, gonad, blood, and bone marrow of hatchling, mature, and old zebra finches measured in relative fluorescence units (RFU). Telomerase activity within each tissue varied with age (ANOVA, $P < .0001$). Superscripts that differ denote significant differences within a tissue type (Student's t test, $P < .05$).

shorten very slowly or not at all.[2] How these birds express telomerase throughout life and appear to avoid its tumor-promoting tendencies is of great interest. In contrast, in the short-lived zebra finch and tree swallow, telomerase expression in bone marrow is reduced after fledging, possibly to deter tumor production and blood cell telomeres shorten relatively quickly.[2] In young adult zebra finch, there was a sharp downregulation of telomerase activity in all tissues except gonad, but in old birds, telomerase expression increased in muscle, liver, and gonad. This upregulation may serve to rescue tissues with critically short telomeres, although it is also possible that this activity may indicate neoplastic tissue. It is interesting that telomerase activity does not increase in the bone marrow of old birds, and this may be caused by high tumor susceptibility in this tissue.

The pattern of telomerase expression is variable among species, in different tissues and at different developmental time points. In the chicken, telomerase activity was detected in early embryos and in all tissues throughout organogenesis. Subsequently, telomerase was downregulated in the majority of somatic tissues.[6] Chickens are a short-lived species that also display our short life span strategy in telomere expression.

Some of the finding in this study challenge current opinion.[7] Telomerase is thought to be highly expressed in almost all stem cells but was low in bone marrow of adult zebra finches and tree swallows. Telomerase should be very low or absent in normal differentiated tissues, but increased in zebra finch muscle, liver, and gonad late in life. Telomerase also should gradually decrease with age, but its activity in bone marrow remained constant at all age classes in common terns and Leach's storm-petrels.

Long-lived bird species lose telomeres at a slower rate than short-lived birds,[2] and this may be caused by increased telomerase expression throughout life. Telomerase's ability to reduce telomere loss by elongating telomeres *de novo* is thought to extend the proliferative life span of cells,[8] and forced telomerase expression in normal human cells extends their proliferative life span.[9] Whether extended proliferative life span of cells translates into extended organismal life span is unknown at this time, and a link between cellular telomere length and organismal health has been proposed only recently.[10]

The major finding of this study is that telomerase profiles in bone marrow differ in short- and long-lived bird species. Whereas two short-lived species downregulated telomerase activity after neonatal life, two very long-lived species express telomerase at the same level throughout life. These results raise other interesting questions. Are these telomerase–life span relationships found in other taxa? How does increased telomerase activity throughout life influence life span, and how do the bird species that express telomerase throughout life avoid its oncogenic costs? These natural animal models for longevity deserve greater study for strategies and mechanisms that have evolved to delay the effects of aging.

ACKNOWLEDGMENTS

David Vleck, Carrie Sanneman, Daniel Hanley, Alexis Blackmer, and Nat Wheelwright assisted in the field. This work was supported in part by a Glenn/American Federation of Aging Research scholarship to M.F.H., a Sigma Xi Grant-in Aid of Research to M.F.H, and a National Institute of Health Grant, RO3 AG022207 to C.M.V. Further support was generously given by Gary Hudson. This manuscript represents contribution no. 164 from the Bowdoin Scientific Station.

REFERENCES

1. VAZIRI, H., I. SCHACHTER, L. UCHIDA, *et al.* 1993. Loss of telomeric DNA during aging of normal and trisomy 21 human lymphocytes. Am. J. Hum. Genet. **52:** 661–667.
2. HAUSSMANN, M.F., D.W. WINKLER, K.M. O'REILLY, *et al.* 2003. Telomeres shorten more slowly in long-lived birds and mammals than in short-lived ones. Proc. R. Soc. Lond. [Biol.] **270:** 1387–1392.
3. GREIDER, C.W. & E. BLACKBURN. 1985. Identification of a specific telomere terminal transferase activity in *Tertahymena* extracts. Cell **43:** 405–413.
4. HARLEY, C.B., N.W. KIM, K.R. PROWSE, *et al.* 1994. Telomerase, cell immortality, and cancer. Cold Spring Harb. Symp. Quant. Biol. **59:** 307–315.
5. WEINSTEIN, B.S. & D. CISZEK. 2002. The reserve-capacity hypothesis: evolutionary origins and modern implications of the trade-off between tumor-suppression and tissue-repair. Exp. Gerontol. **37:** 615–627.
6. TAYLOR, H.A. & M.E. DELANY. 2000. Ontogeny of telomerase in chicken: impact of downregulation on pre- and postnatal telomere length *in vivo*. Dev. Growth Differ. **42:** 613–621.

7. ARAGONA,M., R. MAISANO, S. PANETTA, *et al.* 2000. Telomere length maintenance in aging and carcinogenesis (review). Int. J. Oncol. **17:** 981–989.
8. ENGELHARDT, M., R. KUMAR, J. ALBANELL, *et al.* 1997. Telomerase regulation, cell cycle, and telomere stability in primitive hematopoietic cells. Blood **90:** 182–193.
9. BODNAR, A.G., M. OUELLETTE, M. FROLKIS, *et al.* 1998. Extension of life-span by introduction of telomerase into normal human cells. Science **279:** 349–352.
10. CAWTHON, R.M., K.R. SMITH, E. O'BRIEN, *et al.* 2003. Association between telomere length in blood and mortality in people aged 60 years or older. Lancet **361:** 393–395.

The Role of Cellular Senescence May Be to Prevent Proliferation of Neighboring Cells within Stem Cell Niches

M. D. LYNCH

Addenbrookes Hospital, Cambridge, England

ABSTRACT: It has long been suspected that cellular senescence is an anticancer mechanism; however, it has been difficult to understand the advantage for the organism of retaining mutant cells in a postmitotic state rather than simply deleting them by apoptosis. It is proposed that in certain circumstances apoptosis promotes neoplasia by causing cells adjacent to the deleted cell to divide and that the role of cellular senescence is to prevent this. This may be particularly important in mammalian stem cell niches. After loss of a stem cell from a niche, another stem cell within the same niche divides symmetrically to restore the original number. The most important human malignancies arise from tissues maintained by stem cells, and there is increasing evidence that stem cells are the targets for at least the initial genetic changes that occur during carcinogenesis. If a subset of stem cells within a niche arises containing an oncogenic mutation, then tumor suppressor mechanisms promote apoptosis of these cells, and the niche restores the original number of stem cells by replication of both normal and mutated stem cells. Thus, paradoxically apoptosis increases turnover of mutant cells with associated risk of further genetic changes. However, if in addition mutant cells can become senescent, then the niche is progressively filled by senescent cells until either the mutant cells are eliminated or the niche is completely occupied by postmitotic cells, thereby preventing further evolution of the neoplastic clone. The consequences of this hypothesis are explored by computer modeling.

KEYWORDS: cellular senescence; apoptosis; cancer; stem cells

INTRODUCTION

It has long been suspected that cellular senescence is an anticancer mechanism; however, it has been difficult to understand the advantage for the organism of retaining mutant cells in a postmitotic state rather than simply deleting them by apoptosis.

In any mitotic compartment maintaining a constant number of cells, cells deleted by apoptosis must be replaced by replication of other cells within the compartment. If the compartment contains predominantly or exclusively mutant cells, then death of one mutant cell by apoptosis is likely to trigger the replication of another; thus, paradoxically apoptosis can promote the proliferation of mutant cells thereby accel-

Address for correspondence: M.D. Lynch, Burnside, School Lane, Nutbourne, Chichester, West Sussex PO18 8RZ, England. Voice: +44-01243-373577; fax: +44-01243-373877.
magnuslynch@hotmail.com

erating the acquisition of the multiple genetic changes required for malignancy. It is proposed that this mechanism is of particular importance in stem cell niches.

There is increasing evidence that many mammalian tissues contain stem cells and that these are organized into niches.[1] Each niche contains a small number of stem cells,[1,2] and if a stem cell is deleted by apoptosis, then it is replaced by replication of another stem cell within the same niche.[1,3] The most important malignancies of old age arise from epithelial tissues, and it is likely that at least the initial genetic changes occur in stem cells.

Stem cells in which a genetic alteration has occurred are eliminated by apoptosis;[4,5] however, if a stem cell niche contains predominantly or exclusively mutant stem cells, then apoptosis alone will promote their proliferation. It is proposed that the role of cellular senescence is to prevent this increased turnover. Specifically it is suggested that mutant stem cells can become senescent and persist long term within the stem cell niche so blocking a location that otherwise would be occupied by a dividing stem cell. A computer model was developed to explore the consequences of this hypothesis.

DETAILS OF COMPUTER MODEL

The model was loosely based on the intestinal crypt[2] but was intended to capture the important features of mammalian stem cell niches in general. Although there is no direct evidence for the persistence of senescent stem cells within stem cell niches, senescent keratinocytes are found in the basal layer of the epidermis,[6] which is the location of the stem cells.

Each niche in the model contained six stem cells that were arranged in a circle. "Unit time" was defined as a period of chronological time equal to the time taken for symmetrical stem cell division once G1 transition has occurred. For each stem cell P_{del} and P_{sen} are the probabilities of that cell respectively being deleted or becoming senescent during unit time. Every iteration represented a period equal to unit time and the fate of each stem cell in the niche was determined independently. For normal cells, P_{del} was set at a low level (.05) so that in accord with the situation *in vivo*[2] most iterations did not delete any stem cells with deletion of one or more stem cells progressively less common. P_{sen} was zero for normal cells. Locations vacated by apoptosis were filled by replication of a nondeleted, nonsenescent stem cell two positions on either side within the same niche. The stem cell to be replicated was chosen according to relative probabilities of G1 transition of each of the four candidates, and this probability was three times greater for mutant cells than for normal cells. For each scenario, 1,000 niches were simulated for 1,000 iterations.

RESULTS AND DISCUSSION

To verify the model, we assigned all stem cells in the niche equal properties. After 300 iterations, it was found that all cells within the niche were derived from one of the original stem cells. A similar bottleneck occurs with intestinal stem cells niches *in vivo*.[7] To investigate the capacity of apoptosis alone to eliminate mutant stem cells, we populated all niches with five normal and one mutant stem cell. It was

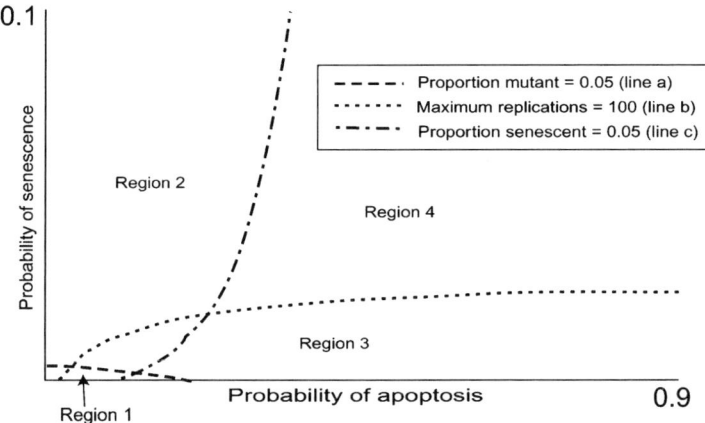

FIGURE 1. A schematic representation of the interaction between apoptosis and cellular senescence in the elimination of mutant stem cells from stem cell niches.

found that as P_{del} for mutant cells increased, the number of mutant cells remaining decreased exponentially, but the maximum replications achieved by a mutant stem cell increased steeply in a linear manner. The factor responsible for the increase in stem cell turnover was niches containing exclusively mutant stem cells, which cannot be eliminated by apoptosis alone. Although the proportion of niches affected is low, the increased turnover is a risk for malignancy because new mutations occur throughout the life span; the absolute number of niches is very high, and mutant stem cells can spread to adjacent niches.[8]

To investigate the interaction between apoptosis and cellular senescence in the elimination of mutant cells, we varied P_{del} and P_{sen} systematically. The results are illustrated schematically in FIGURE 1. At low values of P_{del} and P_{sen} (region 1), there is insufficient elimination of mutant cells; at high values of P_{del}, there is excessive turnover of mutant cells (region 3), and at high values of P_{sen} there is excessive accumulation of senescent cells (region 2). However, in region 4 (bounded lines b and c) apoptosis in combination with senescence achieves efficient elimination of mutant cells without excessive turnover of mutant cells or excessive accumulation of senescent cells. Thus, cellular senescence combined with apoptosis is more efficient than either mechanism alone.

If all mutant stem cells are deleted before they have replicated, then there is no need for senescence; indeed, this appears to be the strategy used by the small intestine where there is a correspondingly low incidence of neoplasia. However, in other mammalian stem cell niches, in particular, the large intestine, the sensitivity to genetic alterations is much lower.[3]

The model presented in this article may clarify several other areas. It is not clear how following an oncogenic stimulus a cell "decides" whether to undergo senescence or apoptosis.[9] This model is consistent with an entirely stochastic decision, although it is likely that the *in vivo* situation is more complex. If a senescent cell is present within a niche, then it is more likely that other malignant stem cells are present within the same niche and this could explain the senescent phenotype,[9] for example, inflammatory cytokines may recruit immune effector cells or directly promote senescence of other stem cells.

Stem cells in the small intestine divide several thousand times during the normal life span,[2] so it is likely that potentially oncogenic stimuli[9] rather than replications *per se* are the most important triggers of stem cell senescence *in vivo*. Furthermore, in this model the rate of self-renewal stem cell replication is determined entirely by the rate of stem cell apoptosis, and this may explain the seemingly paradoxical finding that in some tumor models overexpression of antiapoptotic genes decreases tumor incidence.[10]

In the epidermis, senescent keratinocytes are localized to the basal layer that contains the stem cells.[6] It is predicted that costaining for senescent cells and markers of stem cells such as beta-1-integrin will confirm localization of senescent cells within stem cell niches. A further prediction is that interventions that eliminate senescence in favor of apoptosis will promote neoplasia; however, "one off" removal of senescent cells should not.

In summary, based on several biologically plausible assumptions, this article proposes a candidate mechanism for the anticancer action of cellular senescence; however, whether this is the mechanism that has been chosen by evolution can be determined only by experiment.

ACKNOWLEDGMENTS

I thank Aubrey de Grey for encouraging me to develop the concept that the role of cellular senescence may be to prevent proliferation of neighboring cells.

REFERENCES

1. SPRADLING, A., D. DRUMMOND-BARBOSA & T. KAI. 2001. Stem cells find their niche. Nature **414:** 98–104.
2. POTTEN, C.S. & M. LOEFFLER. 1990. Stem cells: attributes, cycles, spirals, pitfalls, and uncertainties: lessons for and from the crypt. Development **110:** 1001–1020.
3. POTTEN, C.S. 1977. Extreme sensitivity of some intestinal crypt cells to X and gamma irradiation. Nature **269:** 518–521.
4. EVAN, G.I., A.H. WYLLIE, C.S. GILBERT, *et al.* 1992. Induction of apoptosis in fibroblasts by c-myc protein. Cell **69:** 119–128.
5. ZORNIG, M., A. HUEBER, W. BAUM, *et al.* 2001. Apoptosis regulators and their role in tumorigenesis. Biochim. Biophys. Acta. **1551:** F1–F37.
6. DIMRI, G.P., X. LEE, G. BASILE, *et al.* 1995. A biomarker that identifies senescent human cells in culture and in aging skin in vivo. Proc. Natl. Acad. Sci. USA **92:** 9363–9367.
7. WILLIAMS, E.D., A.P. LOWES, D. WILLIAMS, *et al.* 1992. A stem cell niche theory of intestinal crypt maintenance based on a study of somatic mutation in colonic mucosa. Am. J. Pathol. **141:** 773–776.
8. BRAAKHUIS, B.J., M.P. TABOR, J.A. KUMMER, *et al.* 2003. A genetic explanation of Slaughter's concept of field cancerization: evidence and clinical implications. Cancer Res. **63:** 1727–1730.
9. CAMPISI, J. 2001. Cellular senescence as a tumor-suppressor mechanism. Trends Cell. Biol. **11:** S27–S31.
10. DE LA COSTE, A., A. MIGNON, M. FABRE, *et al.* 1999. Paradoxical inhibition of c-myc-induced carcinogenesis by Bcl-2 in transgenic mice. Cancer Res. **59:** 5017–5022.

The Aging/Precancerous Gastric Mucosa
A Pilot Nutraceutical Trial

F. MAROTTA,[a] R. BARRETO,[b] H. TAJIRI,[c] J. BERTUCCELLI,[d] P. SAFRAN,[d] C. YOSHIDA,[d] AND E. FESCE[a]

[a]*Hepato-Gastroenterology Unit, S. Giuseppe Hospital, Milano, Italy*

[b]*Department of Gastroenterology, Instituto Nacional de la Nutrition S. Zubiran, Mexico City, Mexico*

[c]*Endoscopy Unit, Internal Medicine Department, Jikei University Medical School, Tokyo, Japan*

[d]*Osato Research Institute, Bioscience Laboratory, Gifu, Japan*

ABSTRACT: The aim of this study was to test the effect of antioxidant supplementation on enzymatic abnormalities and free radical–modified DNA adducts associated with premalignant changes in the gastric mucosa of elderly patients with HP-negative atrophic gastritis (CAG). Sixty patients with atrophic gastritis and intestinal metaplasia underwent a nutritional interview and a gastroscopy with multiple biopsy samples in the antrum that were processed for histology and for assaying: alpha-tocopherol, MDA, xanthine oxidase (XO), ornithine decarboxylase (ODC), and 8-OHdG. Patients were randomly allocated into three matched groups and supplemented for 6 months with (1) vitamin E, 300 mg/day; (2) multivitamin, two tablets t.i.d.; and (3) Immun-Age 6 g/day nocte (ORI, Gifu, Japan), a certified fermented papaya preparation with basic science-validated antioxidant/immunomodulant properties. Ten dyspeptic patients served as controls. Histology and biochemistry were blindly repeated at 3 and 6 months. CAG patients showed a significantly ($P < .05$) increased level of mucosal MDA and XO concentration that were reverted to normal by each supplementation ($P < .05$). All supplements caused a significant decrease of ODC ($P < .01$), but Immun-Age yielded the most effective ($P < 0.05$) and was the only one significantly decreasing 8-OhdG ($P < 0.05$). These data suggest that antioxidant supplementation, and, namely, Immun-Age, might be potential chemopreventive agents in HP-eradicated CAG patients and especially in the elderly population.

KEYWORDS: oxidative stress; atrophic gastritis; ODC activity; 8-OhdG; antioxidants

INTRODUCTION

Atrophic gastritis changes are commonly found to be increased with age and with an annual incidence of 1–3%. Although the prevalence of this condition often

Address for correspondence: Prof. Francesco Marotta, M.D., Ph.D., via Pisanello, 4, 20146 Milano, Italy. Voice/fax: +39-024077243.
fmarchimede@libero.it

parallels the one of *Helicobacter pylori*, such association does not follow a strictly direct correlation as seen in some long-term studies.[1] Indeed, several other causative factors have been involved such as alcohol, nonsteroidal anti-inflammatory drugs, smoking, biliary reflux, and thermal injury. Moreover, genetic variables in the host may contribute to the susceptibility or resistance to the progression of chronic gastritis to gastric atrophy and, finally, to intestinal-type gastric cancer. Indeed, adenocarcinoma of the stomach is the second most common malignancy in the world, and the principal cause of mortality from cancer in the developing regions of Asia, Africa, and South America. There has been an increasing interest on abnormality in ornithine decarboxilase (ODC) activity in association with clinical premalignant and malignant lesions of the gastrointestinal tract. Evidence for involvement of active oxygen species in the promotion stage of carcinogenesis has been repeatedly reported.[2] Indeed, one of these free radical–modified DNA adducts, 8-hydroxydeoxyguanosine (8-OhdG), has recently received a great deal of attention as a potential biomarker.[3] Indeed, 8-hydroxyguanine is one of the major products of base damage when DNA is exposed to physiologically relevant systems producing OH and $^1O_2$. The purpose of the current investigation was to test the effect of oral supplementation of a certified papaya-fermented product (Immune-Age FPP; Osato Research Institute, Gifu, Japan), which is endowed by an effective acid- and heat-resistant antioxidant property,[4] on enzymatic abnormalities and free radical–damaged DNA parameters associated with premalignant changes in the upper gastrointestinal mucosa.

MATERIALS AND METHODS

Sixty patients with known atrophic gastritis and intestinal metaplasia and with a recent negative result of urea breath test were selected as our population study group. Each of these patients was carefully interviewed for dietary habit with particular attention to an estimated vitamin intake, alcohol, smoking, and drugs or nutraceutical consumption. In particular, patients were instructed not to consume any vitamin or "health supplement" during the study period. All subjects underwent a routine upper gastrointestinal endoscopy during which multiple biopsy samples were taken in the antrum. Biopsy samples were processed for routine histology with particular attention to intestinal metaplasia and *H. pylori* presence. The other samples were processed to test alpha-tocopherol, malonyldialdehyde, xanthine oxidase, ODC activity, 8OHdG, and for mRNA expression for ODC, COX-2, and gastrin by reverse transcription polymerase chain reaction (RT-PCR).

An overall plasma antioxidant status also was assessed at entry. Patients were divided in three groups comparable for age, gender, drinking, and smoking habit. After overnight fasting, all patients underwent baseline blood chemical evaluation as described below. All subjects were randomly allocated into one of the following 6-month supplementation trial: (1) Immun-Age FPP 6 g/day nocte (FPP, obtained from biofermentation of carica papaya, pennisetum purpureum, and sechium edule; Osato Research Institute, Gifu, Japan); (2) vitamin E 300 IU/day nocte; (3) multivitamin preparation (Supradyn, Roche, Switzerland) two tablets t.i.d. All the above histological and biochemical parameters were repeated at 3 and 6 months. Histological assessment was conducted in a blind fashion and reviewed by one experienced investigator (R.B.).

RESULTS

There was no statistical difference among the groups for dietary composition during the study period. Routine blood chemistry were within the reference range at entry and did not change during the study period, irrespective of the treatment used.

Plasma Oxidant/Antioxidant Status

The baseline oxidant/antioxidant assessment at entry, as measured by the serum level of α-tocopherol, malonyldialdehyde, superoxide dismutase, hydroperoxide, and glutathione peroxidase, was within normal limits, and it did not change irrespective of any of the antioxidant treatments used.

Gastric Mucosal Oxidant/Antioxidant Assessment

As compared with controls, mucosal concentration of MDA and XO in patients with atrophic/metaplastic changes were significantly higher ($P<.05$). Each of the three antioxidant treatments used brought about a normalization of this parameter ($P<.05$) without any significant difference among them.

ODC Activity in Gastric Mucosa

As compared with control dyspeptic subjects, patients with CAG showed a significant increased concentration of ODC in gastric mucosa ($P<.05$). All three supplementations caused a significant improvement of this parameter. However, at 6-month observation, Immune-Age FPP yielded the most significant improvement ($P<.05$ vs. the two other supplements).

8-OhdG Concentration in Gastric Mucosa

Patients with CAG showed a significant increase of 8-0hdG ($P<.05$) which was unrelated to other tested parameters. Such abnormality was not affected either by vitamin E or by multivitamin supplement throughout the study period. However, Immune-Age FPP brought about a significant, although partial, decrease at the end of the study period ($P<.05$).

Gene Expression Study

The expression of COX-2 and ODC was significantly upregulated in the gastric mucosa of patients with atrophic gastritis and, in particular, in 18%, 26%, and 22% in groups treated with Immun-Age FPP, vitamin E, and multivitamin preparation, respectively. However, only the former treatment yielded a significantly reduced expression ($P<.05$ vs. baseline value).

CONCLUSION

Although the incidence of gastric cancer is declining, it remains a common cause of death from malignancy worldwide. Strong epidemiological evidence supports the correlation of age and markers of poverty with both *H. pylori* prevalence and

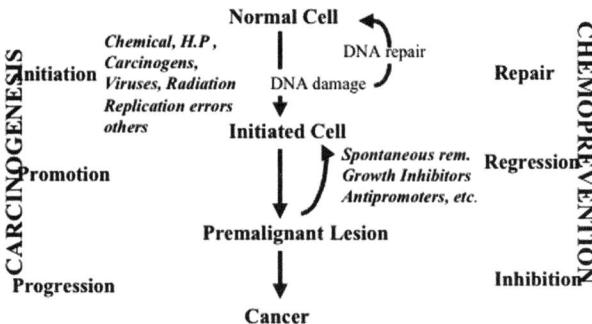

FIGURE 1. An overview on the multistep theory of carcinogenesis. H.P., *H. pylori*.

stomach cancer. There is substantial evidence to support a sequence of histological changes in the mucosa before the development of intestinal-type gastric carcinoma. The development of inflammatory gastritis progresses to gastric atrophy, to intestinal metaplasia, to dysplasia, and finally to intestinal type carcinoma. On the other hand, increased concentrations of lipid peroxidation products have been found in the serum of gastric cancer patients. Oxidative damage to DNA may result in base modification, sugar damage, stand break, and DNA–protein cross-links. Of these, modification of guanine by hydroxyl radicals at the C-8 site, frequently estimated as 8-OhdG, is the most commonly studied lesion. Albeit there have been scanty reports tackling the issue of vitamin/antioxidant supplementation in patients with premalignant gastrointestinal lesions in view of reducing ODC activity,[5] although a lack of a more comprehensive study of the issue still remains. From this study, it appears that patients with CAG, although maintaining a normal plasmatic redox status, show a significant impairment of it at a mucosal level. Virtually any antioxidant supplement[7] seems to improve such an abnormality to a certain extent. However, this is the first study showing that a nutritional intervention with a product endowed with immunomodulator and NO modulator[8] properties associated with lipid[4] and protein[9] antioxidant effect can significantly improve oncological biomarker in the gastric mucosa, something which poses some hopes, given the multistep characteristic of gastric carcinogenesis (FIG. 1). The positive preliminary data thus obtained are all the more encouraging when considering the rather inconclusive results coming from survey trials[6] which are likely to have been biased by the intrinsic limitations involved in any large-scale epidemiological study. This holds particular interest when considering that, although *H. pylori* is now recognized as one of the most widespread human pathogens in the world, it is difficult to eradicate by antibiotic therapy in 15–20% of individuals. Ongoing *in vitro* studies by a French group seem to suggest that a 500-dalton fraction of Immun-Age FPP has the best antioxidant/immunomodulator properties (unpublished data).

REFERENCES

1. VALLE, J., M. KEKKI, P. SIPPONEN, et al. 1996. Long term course and consequences of Helicobacter pylori gastritis. Scand. J. Gastroenterol. **31:** 546–550.
2. KENSLER, T.W. & B.G. TAFFE. 1986. Free radicals in tumor promotion. Adv. Free Radic. Biol. Med. **2:** 347–387.
3. SHIGENAGA, M.K. et al. 1989. Urinary 8-hydroxy-2′-deoxyguanosine as a biomarker of in vivo oxidative DNA damage. Proc. Natl. Acad. Sci. USA **86:** 9697–9701.
4. MAROTTA, F., H. TAJIRI, P. SAFRAN, et al. 1999. Ethanol-related gastric mucosal damage: evidence of a free radical-mediated mechanism and beneficial effect of oral supplementation with Bionormalizer, a novel natural antioxidant. Digestion **60:** 538–543.
5. BUKIN, Y.V., V.A. DRAUDIN-KRYLENKO, E.N. ORLOV, et al. 1995. Effect of prolonged beta-carotene or DL-alpha-tocopheryl acetate supplementation on ornithine decarboxylase activity in human atrophic stomach mucosa. Cancer Epidemiol. Biomarkers Prev. **4:** 865–870.
6. DAWSEY, S.M., G.Q. WANG, P.R. TAILOR, et al. 1994. Effects of vitamin/mineral supplementation on the prevalence of histological dysplasia and early cancer of the esophagus and stomach: results from the Dysplasia Trial in Linxian, China. Cancer Epidemiol. Biomarkers Prev. **3:** 167–172.
7. XU, G.P., P.J. SONG & P.I. REED. 1993. Effects of fruit juices, processed vegetable juice, orange peel and green tea on endogenous formation of N-nitrosoproline in subjects from a high-risk area for gastric cancer in Moping County, China. Eur. J. Cancer Prev. **2:** 327–335.
8. RIMBACH, G., Y.C. PARK, Q. GUO, et al. 2000. Nitric oxide synthesis and TNF-α secretion in RAW 264.7 macrophages. Mode of action of a fermented papaya preparation. Life Sci. **67:** 679–694.
9. RIMBACH, G., Q. GUO, T. AKIYAMA, et al. 2000. Ferric nitrilotriacetate-induced DNA and protein damage: inhibitory effect of a fermented papaya preparation. Anticancer Res. **20:** 2907–2914.

Cancer as "Rejuvenescence"

SVETLANA V. UKRAINTSEVA[a] AND ANATOLY I. YASHIN[a,b]

[a]*Max Planck Institute for Demographic Research, Rostock, Germany*
[b]*Center for Demographic Studies, Duke University, Durham, North Carolina 27708, USA*

ABSTRACT: Comparative analysis of malignant and senescent cells shows that their phenotypic features are in many instances contrary. Cancer cells do not "age"; their metabolic and growth characteristics are opposite to those observed with cellular aging (both replicative and functional). In many such characteristics, cancer cells resemble embryonic cells. One can say that cancer manifests itself as a local uncontrolled "rejuvenation" in an organism. Available evidence from human and animal studies suggests that the opposite phenotypic features of aging and cancer arise from the opposite regulation of common genes, such as those participating in apoptosis/growth arrest or in growth signal transduction pathways in the cell. For instance, in aging cells and organisms, proto-oncogenes are often downregulated, while tumor suppressors are permanently expressed. In cancer cells the situation is just the opposite: the proto-oncogenes are commonly overexpressed, while tumor suppressors are downregulated. This fact may have various applications for the development of new antiaging and anticancer treatments. First, genes that are oppositely regulated in cancer and aging could be candidate targets for antiaging interventions. Their "cancerlike" regulation, if strictly controlled, might help to rejuvenate the aging organism. Recent evidence from human and animal studies in support of this view is discussed. Second, the fact that cancer cells do not "age" implies that these cells may have a survival advantage in the surrounding of senescent cells. This could be a partial reason for an increase in the risk of cancer with age, because the proportion of senescent cells increases in an organism with age, too. In such a situation, the rejuvenation of normal cells surrounding the tumor might be a perspective anticancer treatment. For instance, a controlled activation of oncogenes in normal host cells or the grafting of young proliferating cells (such as embryonic stem cells) in the area near a malignant tumor might help to supplant cancer cells rather than to kill them.

KEYWORDS: cancer; aging; apoptosis; signal transduction; oncogenes; tumor suppressors; growth arrest

OPPOSITE PHENOTYPES OF CANCER AND AGING

A comparison between malignant and aging cells shows that cancer cells do not "age"; their metabolic, proliferative, and growth characteristics are the opposite of those observed in cellular aging (both replicative and functional).[1,2] Indeed, cancer cells are potentially immortal (due to avoiding apoptosis), while aging cells (both proliferating and postmitotic) normally die via apoptosis. Cancer cells can proliferate to an unlimited extent. Aging proliferating cells, however, exhibit a decline in proliferative ability with each cell division and finally suffer irreversible growth arrest (also called replicative senescence). Whereas cancer cells are de-differentiating, the final stage of normal cellular development is terminal differentiation. Cancer cells often have an increased metabolism, while functionally aging cells (e.g., postmitotic neurons) decline in metabolic activity. Cancer cells may secrete factors that increase blood supply, and produce embryonic proteins, such as α-fetoprotein, while aging cells do not. Many of these cancer features are inherent to most "young" cells in an organism, that is, embryonic cells. Embryonic cells proliferate vigorously, are capable of extensive migration, secrete factors that increase the local supply of blood, and produce enzymes capable of degrading basement membranes.[1] Thus, cancer and aging are in many instances opposite phenotypic conditions. One might even say that cancer manifests itself as local and uncontrolled "rejuvenescence" in an organism. Understanding the mechanisms creating such "antiaging" condition in an aging organism may help in developing both antiaging and anticancer interventions.

Recent evidence suggests that cancer and aging share common genes, which are oppositely expressed, however. These are proto-oncogenes and tumor suppressors. They normally contribute to apoptosis/growth arrest and growth signal transduction pathways in the cell. The proto-oncogenes are downregulated in aging cells, while in cancer cells they are overexpressed. Tumor suppressors are permanently expressed in aging cells, while in cancer cells they are downregulated. We propose that controlled "cancerlike" expression of some of these genes may have an antiaging effect on cells and organisms.

OPPOSITE PHENOTYPES OF CANCER AND AGING ARISE FROM THE OPPOSITE REGULATION OF COMMON SIGNALING PATHWAYS

Apoptosis/Growth Arrest

P53. The potential immortality of cancer cells results from their ability to avoid apoptosis. The unlimited growth and proliferation of cancer cells are linked to their ability to avoid irreversible growth arrest.[2] Both these qualities require the suppression of the *p53* tumor suppressor gene.[3] The latter is a transcription factor that induces apoptosis or cell circle arrest at the G1-S phase. It is downregulated in most human cancers.[3,4] As for aging, the *p53* is permanently expressed in senescent and postmitotic cells.[5] Mice carrying the *p53* mutation with a phenotypic effect analogous to the upregulation of this gene display an early aging phenotype along with a lower risk of cancer development.[6] On the other hand, long-living mutant mice, $p66^{Shc-/-}$, have shown an impaired *p53* apoptotic response. The introduction of the null *p53* allele has protected $Ku80^{-/-}$ and $mTR^{-/-}$ mice from premature aging typical of these mutants, indicating that the senescence phenotypes were *p53*-dependent.[6] During the IABG 10th Congress, Van Heemst demonstrated that individuals with Pro/Pro genotype of *p53* (corresponding to reduced apoptosis in cell) have significantly increased both the survival rates and the proportion of deaths from cancer at the oldest ages (85+).

Thus, it follows that the upregulation of the *p53* tumor suppressor gene is required for both cellular and an organism's aging, while its downregulation may have an antiaging effect on cells and (at least in some cases) on organisms.

Fas. One apoptotic pathway involves the transduction of a signal from outside the Fas-ligand to the "death" receptor, CD95 (or Fas), on the cellular membrane. This signal activates a cascade of caspases, which are intracellular enzymes destroying cell proteins. The expression of CD95 is weaker on cancer cells. As regards aging, the proportion of $CD4^+$ and $CD8^+$ lymphocytes expressing the Fas receptor is significantly higher in serum taken from old compared to young individuals (45% vs. 29%).[7] It is possible to induce an *in vitro* apoptosis in 55% of the CD4+ cells of old (65–95) donors, but only in 26% of the cells of young (20–29) donors.[7] Other studies show that the Fas receptor is weakly expressed on the lymphocytes of newborns; however, its expression progressively increases in adulthood.

Bcl-2. Another apoptotic way involves the release of cytochrome *C* from mitochondria and the following activation of effector caspases. The expression of *Bcl-2* blocks this apoptotic activity of mitochondria. The *Bcl-2* is known as a proto-oncogene overexpressed in some cancers. As for aging, the density of this protein is lower in lymphocytes taken from old individuals compared to young ones.

Thus, available evidence suggests that key genes contributing to apoptosis/growth arrest are oppositely expressed in cancer and aging cells (TABLE 1). There is also evidence—although limited—that the downregulation of the *p53* tumor suppressor gene has an antiaging effect on cells and organisms. The latter, however, needs further investigation.

The Growth Signal Transduction Pathway

The proliferation, the growth signal autonomy, and the de-differentiation of cancer cells are all associated with the upregulation of the growth signal transduction pathway. This typical pathway involves the transmission of a signal from an external growth factor to the growth factor receptor on a cellular membrane (such as tyrosine kinase receptor), and then to cytoplasmic proteins (e.g., GSP and RAS), passing the signal to a nucleus transcription factor such as *myc*. The latter has the ability to induce cell division and suppress cell differentiation.[4] The majority of known proto-oncogenes normally participate in the growth signal transduction pathway. Among these, *ras*, *myc*, and tyrosine kinase receptors are particularly involved in both aging and cancer.

Myc. Elevated *myc* transcription is found in many human cancers. However, it is expressed at much higher levels not only in cancer but also in normal young proliferating cells when compared to terminally differentiated nondividing ones.[4] The sustained expression of the *myc* rescued rat embryo cells from senescence. On the other hand, significantly decreased levels of *c-myc* transcription have been found in late-passage human fibroblasts compared to earlypassage cells.

Ras. It is also proto-oncogene activated in many cancers. As for aging, RAS activity has been found to be lower in cells isolated from old rats compared to young ones. The *ras* expression weakened during *in vitro* senescence of human fibroblasts.

TABLE 1. Signaling pathways oppositely manifested in cancer and aging

Gene	Function	Apoptosis/growth arrest		
		In cancer cells	In aging cells	In aging organism
p53	Induces apoptosis/growth arrest Tumor suppressor	Downregulated in most human cancers (Soussi, 2000; Hickman, 2002)	Elevated expression (Kulju and Lehman;[5] Antropova et al., 2002)	Upregulating mutation is associated with early aging phenotype and lower cancer risk in mice (Donehower[6])
CD95	"Death" receptor of apoptotic signal	Decreased expression (Pinkoski and Green, 2000)	Higher expression on cells from adults compared with newborns (Miyawaki et al., 1992)	Proportion of cells expressing CD95 is higher in older individuals (Aggarwal and Gupta[7])
Bcl-2	Antiapoptotic protein Proto-oncogene	Overexpressed in some cancers (Ross, 1997)	Decreased levels (Miyashita et al., 1994; Peters and Vousden[4])	Decreased expression in lymphocytes from older individuals (Aggarwal and Gupta[7])

Gene	Function	Growth signal transduction		
		In cancer cells	In aging cells	In aging organism
myc	Transcription factor Proto-oncogene	Overexpressed in many cancers (Peters and Vousden[4])	Decreased expression in senescent cells (Dean et al., 1986; Peters and Vousden[4])	Sustained expression of the myc rescued rat embryo cells from senescence (Schwab and Bishop, 1988)
ras	Signal transducer Proto-oncogene	Activated in some cancers (Frame and Balmain, 2000)	Decreased expression in senescent cells (Delgado et al., 1986)	Activity is lower in old rats (Pahlavani and Vargas, 2000). Controlled expression extends the reproductive life span in yeast (Jazwinski et al.[8])
Tyrosine kinase receptors	Growth factor receptors (e.g., erb-B, TRK) Proto-oncogenes	Overexpressed in some cancers (Peters and Vousden[4])	Receptor density and mitogenic response decrease with donor age (Reenstra et al., 1996; DeKeyser et al., 1994; Hou et al., 2002)	Overexpression of tkr-1 increases longevity and stress-resistance in nematodes (Murakami and Johnson[9])

Interestingly, the controlled expression of the v-Ha-ras in yeast has extended their reproductive life span nearly twofold.[8]

Tyrosine kinase receptors. These receptors are overexpressed in some human cancers.[4] As for aging, human fibroblasts express fewer epidermal growth factor receptors and display a weaker mitogenic response to the growth factor with increasing donor age. It has been demonstrated that upregulation of a tyrosine kinase receptor may increase both longevity and stress resistance in nematodes. The overexpression of *tkr-1* has improved their survival (average 65%) and resistance to heat and ultraviolet irradiation.[9]

Thus, there is strong evidence that proto-oncogenes participating in growth signal transduction are oppositely expressed in cancer and aging cells. There is also some evidence that controlled activation of the proto-oncogenes may have an antiaging effect on cells and organisms. One should notice that recently it has been proposed that the signal transduction pathway (regardless of the role it plays in human cancer) is a conserved regulator of aging in different species.[10] Mutations of many relevant genes (e.g., *daf-2* and *age-1* in *C. elegans*) have been found to increase longevity in experimental animals. However, only a few such mutations resulted in the *activation* of a known proto-oncogene.[9] Thus, additional studies are needed to explore the effect of the controlled "cancerlike" regulation of genes involved in growth signaling pathways on aging and longevity.

CONCLUDING REMARKS AND DISCUSSION

The comparative analysis shows that phenotypes of cancer and aging are in many instances contrary. Cancer cells do not "age"; their metabolic, proliferative, and growth characteristics are opposite to those observed in cellular aging (both replicative and functional). That is, cancer manifests itself as local uncontrolled "rejuvenation" in an organism. Available data suggest that the opposite phenotypic features of aging and cancer arise from the opposite regulation of common signaling pathways such as apoptosis/growth arrest and growth signal transduction pathways. Genes normally managing cellular aging promote cancer when contrarily expressed (TABLE 1).

This finding may help to developing new antiaging and anticancer interventions. First, the controlled activation of oncogenes or the downregulation of tumor suppressors might produce an antiaging effect on cells and (possibly) on an organism. The latter, however, needs careful investigation.

Second, the fact that cancer cells do not "age" suggests that these cells may have a survival advantage in the surrounding senescent cells. Cancer risk could increase with age, partly because the proportion of the senescent cells increases in the aging organism. In this situation, the rejuvenation of normal host cells surrounding the tumor could be a perspective anticancer treatment. For instance, grafting young proliferating cells (such as embryonic/stem cells) in the area of a malignant tumor might help to supplant cancer cells rather than to kill them.

REFERENCES

1. BAST, R.C. *et al.*, Eds. 2000. Holland-Frei Cancer Medicine. Fifth edition. Decker. Hamilton, Ontario, Canada.

2. HANAHAN, D. & R.A. WEINBERG. 2000. The hallmarks of cancer. Cell **100:** 57–70.
3. HICKMAN, J.A. 2002. Apoptosis and tumourigenesis. Curr. Opin. Genet. Dev. **12:** 67–72.
4. PETERS, G. & K.H. VOUSDEN, Eds. 1997. Oncogenes and Tumour Suppressors. Oxford University Press. New York.
5. KULJU, K.S. & J.M. LEHMAN. 1995. Increased p53 protein associated with aging in human diploid fibroblasts. Exp. Cell Res. **217:** 336–345.
6. DONEHOWER, L. 2002. Does p53 affect organismal aging? J. Cell. Physiol. **192:** 23–33.
7. AGGARWAL, S. & S. GUPTA. 1998. Increased apoptosis of T cell subsets in aging humans: altered expression of Fas (CD95), Fas ligand, Bcl-2, and Bax. J. Immunol. **160:** 1627–1637.
8. JAZWINSKI, S.M., J.B. CHEN & J. SUN. 1993. A single gene change can extend yeast life span: the role of Ras in cellular senescence. Adv. Exp. Med. Biol. **330:** 45–53.
9. MURAKAMI, S. & T.E. JOHNSON. 1998. Life extension and stress resistance in *Caenorhabditis elegans* modulated by the tkr-1 gene. Curr. Biol. **8:** 1091–1094.
10. KENYON, C. 2001. A conserved regulatory system for aging. Cell **105:** 165–168.

Functional Analysis of Clusterin/Apolipoprotein J in Cellular Death Induced by Severe Genotoxic Stress

IOANNIS P. TROUGAKOS AND EFSTATHIOS S. GONOS

Laboratory of Molecular and Cellular Aging, Institute of Biological Research and Biotechnology, National Hellenic Research Foundation, Athens 11635, Greece

ABSTRACT: Clusterin/apolipoprotein J (CLU) is a secreted heterodimeric glycoprotein that is reportedly upregulated during tumorigenesis, as well as during cell injury or death. Despite extensive efforts, CLU function during cellular death remains largely elusive. We are using as a model system to study CLU function three human osteosarcoma (OS) cell lines, namely, Sa OS, KH OS, and U-2 OS cells, induced to die after exposure to severe genotoxic stress mediated by the chemotherapeutic drug doxorubicin (DXR). We initially applied small interfering RNA (siRNA)–mediated specific knockdown of the CLU protein in OS cells. In all three cell lines, CLU knockdown resulted in increased sensitization to DXR-induced apoptosis. Supportively, moderate levels of forced transgene-mediated CLU stable overexpression in KH OS cells could rescue them from DXR-mediated apoptosis. In contrast, stable overexpression of high CLU levels in Sa OS and U-2 OS cells augmented apoptosis induced by cell exposure to severe DXR-mediated genotoxic stress. In summary, our data provide evidence that, although CLU is essential for cellular homeostasis, it may become highly cytotoxic in certain cellular contexts when it accumulates in high amounts intracellularly either by direct synthesis or by uptake from the extracellular milieu.

KEYWORDS: apoptosis; clusterin/apolipoprotein J; doxorubicin

INTRODUCTION

Clusterin/apolipoprotein J (CLU) is a secreted glycoprotein that is translated from a single mRNA as a preprotein that matures by limited proteolysis and glycosylation to form a disulfide-linked heterodimeric glycoprotein of ~70–80 kDa.[1] CLU has been implicated in a variety of physiological processes and is overexpressed in many severe physiological disturbances, such as carcinogenesis and various neurological diseases including Scrapie, Alzheimer's disease, and AIDS encephalitis.[2,3] We cloned CLU as a gene overexpressed during cellular senescence[4] and showed

---

Address for correspondence: Efstathios S. Gonos, Laboratory of Molecular and Cellular Aging, Institute of Biological Research and Biotechnology, National Hellenic Research Foundation, 48 Vas. Constantinou Ave., Athens 11635, Greece. Voice: +30-210-7273756; fax: +30-210-7273677.

sgonos@eie.gr

Ann. N.Y. Acad. Sci. 1019: 206–210 (2004). © 2004 New York Academy of Sciences.
doi: 10.1196/annals.1297.033

that it is induced in normal human cells exposed to various types of stress[4,5] and accumulates in the human serum during aging and at several age-related diseases.[6] Another defining prominent and intriguing CLU feature is its upregulation during cell injury and apoptosis.[3] Nevertheless, despite extensive efforts CLU function and precise involvement in all these disorders and cell death remains puzzling.

We are using as a model system to study CLU function during cell death the Sa OS, KH OS, and U-2 OS osteosarcoma (OS) cell lines. By using specific small interfering RNA (siRNA)–mediated CLU knockdown, we demonstrated that CLU knockdown sensitizes OS cells to genotoxic stress and consequent apoptosis induced by doxorubicin (DXR). In contrast, transgene-mediated CLU protein overexpression could rescue only KH OS cells from high doses of DXR, whereas in U-2 OS and Sa OS cells CLU significantly augmented cell death. Thus, CLU may either function cytoprotectively or may promote cell death after severe genotoxic stress, thereby providing a balance between cellular survival and death.

MATERIALS AND METHODS

Identification of the appropriate CLU cDNA sequence to be targeted, synthesis of the required RNA oligonucleotides, and cell treatment with the RNA duplexes was done essentially as described.[7] The siRNA Cl-I oligonucleotide targets the sequence 5′ AAccagagctcgcccttctacTT 3′ of the human CLU mRNA.

The human CLU full-length cDNA was directly subcloned into the pcDNA3.1/Myc-His(+) mammalian expression vector (Invitrogen; cat. no. V800-20) as described.[5] OS cells were transfected with either the pcDNA3.1 empty vector or the pcDNA3.1^{CLU} construct by using the Lipofectamine 2000 reagent (Invitrogen, cat. no. 11668-027) as per the manufacturer's instructions. To avoid clonal variability, we isolated pools of stable transfectants from the selection medium three weeks later and propagated them accordingly.

Ongoing apoptosis of CLU knockdown or CLU transgenic OS cells treated for 24 h with low to relatively high DXR concentrations was determined by measuring the cytoplasmic histone-associated DNA fragments with a Cell Death Detection ELISA^{PLUS} photometric enzyme-immunoassay method (Roche), as suggested by the manufacturer.

RESULTS AND DISCUSSION

SiRNA-mediated CLU knockdown at the three OS cell lines appeared quite effective and resulted in a significant growth retardation and higher rates of spontaneous endogenous apoptosis (data to be reported elsewhere). When these cells were exposed to a gradually increasing concentration of DXR, it became apparent that CLU knockdown resulted in a significant cell sensitization to genotoxic stress and consequent apoptosis induced by DXR even at low doses (FIG. 1a). These results are in agreement with previous studies demonstrating that treatment of prostate cancer cells with CLU-specific antisense oligonucleotides resulted in increased cellular chemosensitivity.[8]

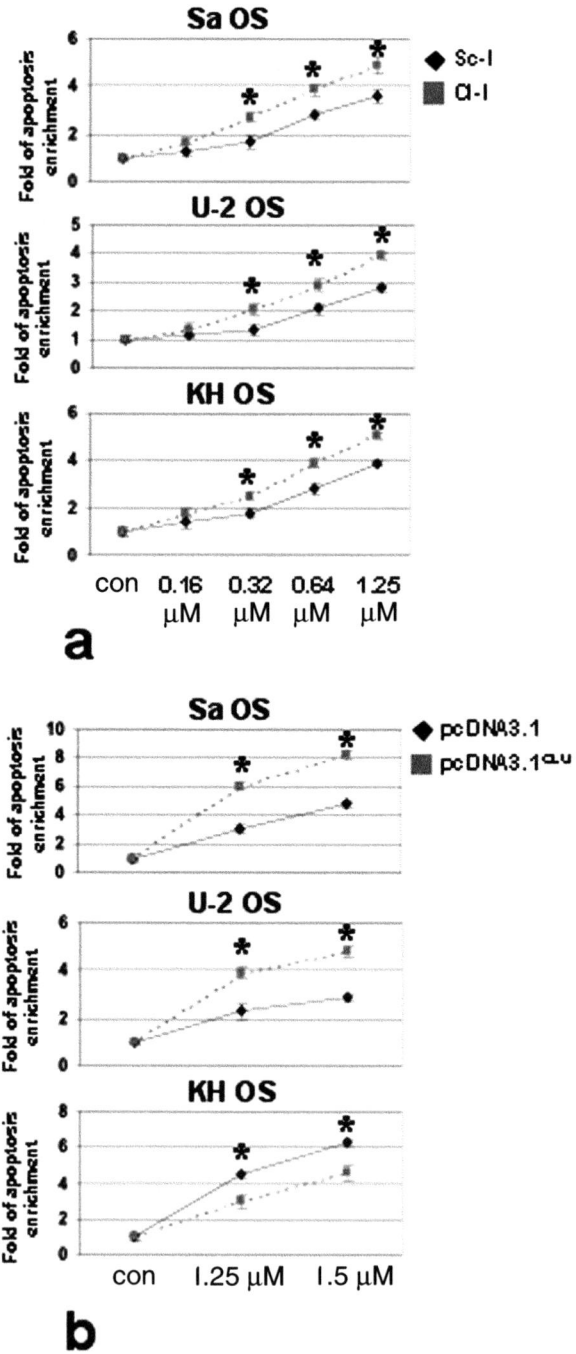

FIGURE 1. *See following page for legend.*

In an attempt to verify these data, we artificially overexpressed CLU in the three OS cell lines (not shown) and assayed apoptosis after cell exposure to relatively high doses of DXR. As shown in FIGURE 1b, only at KH OS cells (where only a moderate CLU overexpression could be achieved [not shown]) did CLU accumulation effectively inhibit apoptosis induction. Surprisingly, at Sa OS and U-2 OS transgenic cells that stably overexpress high amounts of the CLU protein, it was found that CLU augmented apoptosis (FIG. 1b). These results resemble the intriguingly distinct and usually opposing functions proposed for CLU during apoptosis because, although CLU overexpression reportedly promotes cytoprotection in prostate cancer cells,[8] its accumulation correlates with cellular death in mouse skin tumor cells[9] and in neurons.[10] Our data are also in line with recent evidence suggesting that forced expression of intracellular CLU fragments may initiate the formation of protein aggregates and cell death.[11] We conclude that, as shown after CLU knockdown in OS cells, CLU is an essential molecule in cellular homeostasis whose primary function is cytoprotective. On the other hand, CLU also may become deleterious in certain cell types if it accumulates in high amounts either by direct synthesis or by uptake from the extracellular milieu.

ACKNOWLEDGMENTS

This work was supported by the following European Union full-cost grants to E.S.G.: "Cellage" (QLK6-CT-2001-00616) and "Functionage" (QLK6-CT-2001-00310).

REFERENCES

1. WILSON, M.R. & S.B. EASTERBROOK-SMITH. 2000. Clusterin is a secreted mammalian chaperone. Trends Biochem. Sci. **25:** 95–98.
2. CALERO, M., A. ROSTAGNO, E. MATSUBARA, et al. 2000. Apolipoprotein J (clusterin) and Alzheimer's disease. Microsc. Res. Tech. **50:** 305–315.
3. TROUGAKOS, I.P. & E.S. GONOS. 2002. Clusterin/apolipoprotein J in human aging and cancer. Int. J. Biochem. Cell. Biol. **34:** 1430–1448.
4. GONOS, E.S., A. DERVENTZI, M. KVEIBORG, et al. 1998. Cloning and identification of genes that associate with mammalian senescence. Exp. Cell Res. **240:** 66–74.

FIGURE 1. (a) siRNA-mediated CLU knockdown in OS cells induces cell sensitization to DXR-mediated genotoxic stress and subsequent apoptosis. Cells were exposed to gradually increasing concentrations of DXR (0.16–1.25 μM), and apoptosis was assayed by a cell death detection ELISA photometric enzyme-immunoassay method. Sc-I, scrambled siRNA oligonucleotide; Cl-I, the CLU-specific siRNA oligonucleotide. (b) Stable overexpression of the CLU protein in low levels at KH OS cells inhibits apoptosis (*bottom panel*), whereas stable CLU overexpression at high amounts in U-2 OS and Sa OS cells augments apoptosis induced by cell exposure to relatively high doses of DXR (1.25 or 1.5 μM) that result to a severe genotoxic stress. pcDNA3.1, pool of cells transfected with the empty vector; pcDNA3.1^{CLU}, pool of cells transfected with the full-length CLU cDNA. Data points represent the mean of three **a** or two **b** independent experiments; *bars* denote SD; *asterisks* indicate differences from control at $P < .01$.

5. PETROPOULOU, C., I.P. TROUGAKOS, E. KOLETTAS, et al. 2001. Clusterin/apolipoprotein J is a novel biomarker of cellular senescence, that does not affect the proliferative capacity of human diploid fibroblasts. FEBS Lett. **509:** 287–297.
6. TROUGAKOS, I.P., M. POULAKOU, M. STATHATOS, et al. 2002. Serum levels of the senescence biomarker clusterin/apolipoprotein J increase significantly in diabetes type II and during development of coronary heart disease or at myocardial infarction. Exp. Gerontol. **37:** 1175–1187.
7. ELBASHIR, S.M., J. HARBORTH, W. LENDECKEL, et al. 2001. Duplexes of 21-nucleotide RNAs mediate RNA interference in cultured mammalian cells. Nature **411:** 494–498.
8. GLEAVE, M.E., H. MIYAKE, T. ZELLWEGER, et al. 2001. Use of antisense oligonucleotides targeting the antiapoptotic gene, clusterin/testosterone-repressed prostate message 2, to enhance androgen sensitivity and chemosensitivity in prostate cancer. Urology **58:** 39–49.
9. KALKA, K., N. AHMAD, T. CRISWELL, et al. 2000. Up-regulation of clusterin during phthalocyanine 4 photodynamic therapy-mediated apoptosis of tumor cells and ablation of mouse skin tumors. Cancer Res. **60:** 5984–5987.
10. WALTON, M., D. YOUNG, E. SIRIMANNE, et al. 1996. Induction of clusterin in the immature brain following a hypoxic-ischemic injury. Brain Res. Mol. Brain Res. **39:** 137–152.
11. DEBURE, L., J.L. VAYSSIERE, V. RINCHEVAL, et al. 2003. Intracellular clusterin causes juxtanuclear aggregate formation and mitochondrial alteration. J. Cell Sci. **116:** 3109–3121.

Evidence of Preferential Protein Targets for Age-Related Modifications in Peripheral Blood Lymphocytes

SYLVIE POGGIOLI, JEAN MARY, HILAIRE BAKALA, AND BERTRAND FRIGUET

Laboratoire de Biologie et Biochimie Cellulaire du Vieillissement, IFR 117, Université Paris 7-Denis Diderot, Paris, France

ABSTRACT: Oxidatively modified proteins have been analyzed in aging human peripheral blood lymphocytes since protein modification by oxidation and other related pathways are believed to contribute to the intracellular age-related accumulation of damaged proteins, a process that has been associated with the cellular functional deficits that occur with age. Advanced glycation end products (AGE) were quantified and the pattern of glycated proteins analyzed by two-dimensional gel electrophoresis followed by Western blotting using an anti-AGE antibody raised against glycated RNAse. The protein silver stain and the immunoblot patterns were not superimposable, indicating that glycoxidative modifications are targeting only a restricted set of proteins. Modification of proteins with the lipid peroxidation product 4-hydroxy-2-nonenal has also been studied. The patterns of modified proteins have been analyzed using two-dimensional gel electrophoresis followed by Western blotting with an antibody recognizing 4-hydroxy-2-nonenal protein adducts using the same proteomic approach as for glycoxidative modifications. Specific protein targets for these modifications, that might serve as biomarkers of aging lymphocytes, are currently characterized and identified by mass spectrometry.

KEYWORDS: Keywords: protein glycation; protein oxidative modifications; human lymphocytes; aging biomarkers; proteomics

INTRODUCTION

Human aging is characterized by the alteration of physiological functions and especially by the decline of the immune system, referred to as immunosenescence.[1,2] Aging is also characterized by the intracellular accumulation of damaged macromolecules, including nucleic acids, lipids, and proteins. Indeed, protein carbonyl content, taken as a signature of protein oxidative damage, has been reported to increase in such proportion that old individuals would have one third of their proteins carrying the modification.[3] Because protein modification by oxidation and

---

Address for correspondence: Bertrand Friguet, Laboratoire de Biologie et Biochimie Cellulaire du Vieillissement, IFR 117, Université Paris 7-Denis Diderot, Paris, France. Voice/fax: +33-1-44-27-82-34.

bfriguet@paris7.jussieu.fr

other related pathways are believed to contribute to the intracellular age-related accumulation of damaged proteins, oxidatively modified proteins have been analyzed in aging human peripheral blood lymphocytes (PBLs). In lymphocytes, increased levels of both lipofuscin and the advanced glycation end product (AGE) pentosidine with age already have been reported.[4,5] Therefore, we have investigated the appearance of both AGE-modified proteins[6] and proteins modified by the lipid peroxidation product 4-hydroxy-2-nonenal (HNE). In fact, both modifications of the model protein glucose-6-phosphate dehydrogenase have been shown to induce resistance to degradation by the proteasome.[7,8] Therefore, these modifications appear to be good candidates for the generation of modified proteins that would be poor substrates for degradation by the proteasome and then would accumulate and alter lymphocyte cellular function with aging. AGE-modified proteins and HNE-modified proteins were characterized using an anti-AGE antibody raised against glycated RNAse and an antibody raised against HNE-modified KLH, respectively. The patterns of both glycated proteins and HNE-modified proteins were analyzed by two-dimensional gel electrophoresis followed by Western blotting with either anti-AGE or anti-KLH-HNE antibody. In both cases, the protein silver stain and the immunoblot patterns were not superimposable, indicating that the modifications are targeting only a restricted set of proteins. The corresponding modified proteins, whose identification is currently achieved by mass spectrometry (LC/MS/MS) might serve as biomarkers of aging lymphocytes.

MATERIALS AND METHODS

PBL Purification and Protein Samples Preparation

PBLs were prepared from human blood samples from healthy young (20–25 years old) and old donors (86–91 years old). Blood was diluted in PBS, pH 7.2, and centrifuged on a Ficoll gradient. The buffy coat was collected, washed in PBS, and pelleted by centrifugation at 400g for 45 min at room temperature. The cytosolic extracts were obtained after sonication of the cells in a lysis buffer containing 10 mM Tris HCl, pH 7.6, supplemented with 1 mM EDTA and 1 mM DTT followed by centrifugation at 10,000g for 30 min at 4°C. The soluble cytosolic extracts then were aliquoted and stored at −80°C.

Two-Dimensional Gel Electrophoresis, Western Blotting, and Image Analysis

Cytosolic proteins (150 µg) were precipitated by cold ethanol and suspended in 370 µL of two-dimensional sample buffer (7 M urea, 2 M thiourea, 4% [w/v] CHAPS, 1% [w/v] DTT, 2% [v/v] Pharmalytes, pH 3.0–10.0). Then, the cytosolic proteins were separated by two-dimensional gel electrophoresis. The first dimension isoelectric focusing was performed on Immobiline Drystrips (pH 3.0–10.0, 18 cm) in the Multiphor II device (Amersham Biosciences) for 27,000 Vh. After electrofocusing, the immobilines were prepared for SDS-PAGE, and the second dimension SDS-PAGE was run vertically on a 12% (w/v) polyacrylamide gel using the cooling Protean II system (Bio-Rad). The gels were fixed and silver stained as previously described[6] or electroblotted on a nitrocellulose membrane overnight at 30 V. The blots then were incubated for 2 h in 20 mM Tris-HCl, pH 7.6, supplemented with 137 mM NaCl, 0.01% (v/v) Tween-20, 3% (w/v) BSA (buffer B) at room temperature, and the specific detection of modified proteins was achieved after incubation for 1 h at room temperature with the rabbit polyclonal antibody raised against either AGE-modified RNAse or KLH-HNE. The membrane then was washed three times in buffer B and incubated with the horseradish peroxidase (HRP)-linked secondary antibody (NA 934 Amersham Biosciences) for 1 h at room temperature. After three washes, the modified proteins were finally revealed by ECL (Amersham Pharmacia Biotech) upon 5-min exposure of the films. The silver-stained gels and the films were digitized with a JX-330 scanner (Sharp). The spot detection and quantification were done with the Imagemaster 2D Elite software (Amersham Biosciences), and the data were expressed as spot volumes in pixels.

RESULTS AND DISCUSSION

Advanced glycation end products were characterized using the polyclonal anti-AGE antibody, and a small but significant (40%) increase of protein glycation in cytosolic extracts from old donors versus young donors was observed by enzyme-linked immunosorbent assay. To further analyze the pattern of glycated proteins, we performed two-dimensional gel electrophoresis followed by Western blotting with the same anti-AGE antibody. The protein silver stain and the immunoblot patterns were not superimposable indicating that glycation is targeting only a restricted set of proteins. Among these preferential protein targets, seven of them exhibited a significant age-related increased immunoreactivity with the anti-AGE antibody suggesting that the corresponding modified proteins might serve as biomarkers of aging lymphocytes. Identification of several target proteins has been achieved by mass spectrometry (LC/MS/MS). Protein modification with the lipid peroxidation product 4-hydroxy-2-nonenal also has been studied. Using the same proteomic approach as for AGE-modifications, we analyzed the patterns of HNE-modified proteins in cytosolic extracts from old donors and young donors by using two-dimensional gel electrophoresis followed by Western blotting with an antibody recognizing HNE-protein adducts. As observed for protein glycation, the protein silver stain and the immunoblot patterns were also not superimposable, indicating that the modifications are targeting only a restricted set of proteins. Among these preferential protein targets, six of them exhibited an age-related increased immunoreactivity with the polyclonal anti-HNE antibody, suggesting that these specific protein targets might also serve as biomarkers of aging lymphocytes. Interestingly, the protein targets for modification by HNE were different from those modified by AGE. Further identification of these proteins, assessment of the precise nature of the modification(s) and modification site(s), and the study of the impact of such modification(s) on the function of the protein may provide insight on the effects of protein glycation, glycoxidation, and other oxidative modifications in the aging process. Finally, proteomic approaches (reviewed in Dierick et al.[9] and Schoneich[10]) aimed at identifying either protein expression or posttranslational modification profiles appear to have great potential for addressing new issues for molecular studies of biological aging.

ACKNOWLEDGMENTS

The support of our laboratory is by a European Union "Protage" grant (QLK6-CT-1999-02193).

REFERENCES

1. ASPINALL, R. & D. ANDREW. 2000. Immunosenescence: potential causes and strategies for reversal. Biochem. Soc. Trans. **28:** 250–254.
2. PAWELEC, T., Y. BARNETT, R. FORSEY, et al. 2002. T cells and aging. Front. Biosci. **7:** D1056–D1183.
3. STADTMAN, E.R. & R.L. LEVINE. 2000. Protein oxidation. Ann. N.Y. Acad. Sci. **899:** 191–208.
4. BEREGI, E., O. REGIUS & K. RAJCZY. 1991. Comparative study of the morphological changes in lymphocytes of elderly individuals and centenarians. Age Ageing **20:** 55–59.
5. SELL, D.R., M. PRIMC, I.A. SCHAFER, et al. 1998. Cell-associated pentosidine as a marker of aging in human diploid cells in vitro and in vivo. Mech. Ageing Dev. **105:** 221–240.
6. POGGIOLI, S., H. BAKALA & B. FRIGUET. 2002. Age-related increase of protein glycation in peripheral blood lymphocytes is restricted to preferential target proteins. Exp. Gerontol. **37:** 1207–1215.
7. FRIGUET, B. & L.I. SZWEDA. 1997. Inhibition of the multicatalytic proteinase (proteasome) by 4-hydroxy-2-nonenal cross-linked protein. FEBS Lett. **405:** 21–25.
8. BULTEAU, A.L., P. VERBEKE, I. PETROPOULOS, et al. 2001. Proteasome inhibition in glyoxal-treated fibroblasts and resistance of glycated glucose-6-phosphate dehydrogenase to 20 S proteasome degradation in vitro. J. Biol. Chem. **276:** 45662–45668.
9. DIERICK, J.F., M. DIEU, J. REMACLE, et al. 2002. Proteomics in experimental gerontology. Exp. Gerontol. **37:** 721–734.
10. SCHONEICH, C. Proteomics in gerontological research. 2003. Exp. Gerontol. **38:** 473–481.

Protective Effects of Mutant Ubiquitin in Transgenic Mice

D. A. GRAY, M. TSIRIGOTIS, J. BRUN, M. TANG, M. ZHANG, M. BEYERS, AND J. WOULFE

Ottawa Health Research Institute, Ottawa, Ontario K1H 8L6, Canada

ABSTRACT: The K48R mutant ubiquitin can exert profound *in vivo* protective effects against a variety of insults, including agents of direct clinical relevance. The manipulation of the ubiquitin/proteasome pathway has enormous potential for clinical benefit, and it is not unreasonable to expect that such benefits will include diseases of aging.

KEYWORDS: ubiquitin; mutant; transgenic; mice; life span; K48R

The ubiquitin/proteasome pathway (UPP) is responsible for elimination of damaged and misfolded proteins, and there is reason to believe that a decline in the efficiency of the UPP accompanies and may contribute to human aging.[1] For many of its functions, ubiquitin must be assembled into chains, and it is the varying topology of these chains that allows ubiquitin to serve apparently separate functions in distinct cellular pathways. In yeast, it has been established that mutant isoforms of ubiquitin unable to participate in ubiquitin chain assembly through lysine 48 (K48) linkages exert a dominant negative effect on proteolysis.[2] In contrast, mutant ubiquitin engineered to interfere with K63-linked chain assembly imparts a DNA repair deficit in yeast.[3] To explore the consequences of analogous mutations in the context of mammalian cells *in vivo*, we have created transgenic mouse strains in which wild-type or mutant ubiquitin is expressed at high levels from the human UbC promoter. The rationale and details of transgene construction have been described previously.[4,5]

All the ubiquitin lines we have created to date are viable and fertile. Homozygous individuals from all strains have reached three years of age, arguing against any dramatic reduction in life span; with current data, we can draw no conclusions about the potential extension of life span in these strains. In order to determine if alterations in ubiquitin might predispose to protein or DNA damaging agents as has been observed in yeast, we have subjected the mice to various biological and chemical insults. Contrary to our initial expectations, mice expressing K48R mutant ubiquitin insults were remarkably resistant to various stressors that would be expected to provide a burden of misfolded or aberrant protein. A classic yeast methodology for delivering such a burden is to grow cells in the presence of canavanine, a naturally occurring arginine analogue whose incorporation during translation generates struc-

---

Address for correspondence: D.A. Gray, Ottawa Health Research Institute, 501 Smyth Road, Ottawa, Ontario K1H 8L6, Canada. Voice: 613-737-7700, ext. 6896; fax: 613-247-3524.
dgray@ohri.ca

turally aberrant proteins. Yeast cells expressing K48R mutant ubiquitin are sensitive to canavanine,[2] as are mammalian neuroblastoma cells.[5] When mouse pups were injected intraperitoneally with canavanine, we observed a marked failure to thrive in nontransgenic animals. Expression of K48R mutant ubiquitin resulted in considerable protection against canavanine toxicity, as evidenced by weight gain in the neonatal pups.

$ts1$ is a neuropathogenic retrovirus encoding an envelope protein that misfolds at the body temperature of an adult mouse (the neonatal body temperature is permissive for replication of the virus, allowing systemic infection). Mice infected with $ts1$ as neonates invariably succumb to spongiform degeneration of the spinal cord and hindbrain at approximately one month postinfection. Whereas transgenic mice expressing wild-type ubiquitin or K63R mutant ubiquitin developed disease with latency similar to that of nontransgenic control animals, the latency period was doubled in mice expressing K48R mutant ubiquitin. These animals were partially resistant to the $ts1$ virus replication, generating viral titers roughly a log lower at equivalent time points.[6]

Bacterial lipopolysaccharide (LPS) injection is a potent means of inducing endotoxic shock, an NF-κB-dependent activation of innate immunity in mice. Transgenic lines and nontransgenic control mice of the same genetic background (FVB-N) were injected intraperitoneally with LPS at various dosages. Animals were monitored at frequent intervals for a variety of physiological parameters including body weight, body temperature, and blood pressure. Animals found to be outside humane end points (e.g., having sustained more than 10% loss of body weight) were euthanized. Whereas LPS given at 40 mg/kg produced profound illness in nontransgenic mice as well as the transgenic animals expressing wild-type or K63R mutant ubiquitin, the K48R mutant transgenics were much healthier both by appearance and by the physiological parameters measured.

Finally, cohorts of mice were treated with an intraperitoneal dosage of cisplatin, a cancer chemotherapeutic agent, at 15 mg/kg body weight. At this dosage, cisplatin not only induces DNA damage (the activity thought to be of primary therapeutic importance), but also induces a stress response involving NF-κB and other mediators. Once again, mice expressing K48R mutant ubiquitin fared significantly better than animals expressing the wild-type or K63R mutant isoforms of ubiquitin, as evidenced by loss of body weight (FIG. 1).

The apparent paradox presented by our *in vivo* results clearly arises from an unexpected consequence of an altered UPP in the mice expressing K48R mutant ubiquitin. These results are also at odds with our previous observations in stable cell lines expressing identical ubiquitin transgenes.[5] It is likely that elements of organismal biology are at play in the current series of experiments that are not well modeled by cell culture experiments. For example, all of the current experiments feature a direct or indirect NF-κB response, and NF-κB activation is regulated by the UPP at various levels.[7,8] The modulation of NF-κB activation in K48R mice (the sequelae of which would include, for example, dampening of cytokine release) might explain a great deal of what we have observed in our *in vivo* experiments, and we are actively investigating this possibility. The related issue of nitric oxide and its downstream effects is another common thread in our experiments worthy of further investigation. Altered ubiquitin metabolism can be expected to impinge on the regulation of transcription, and using microarray analyses we are investigating the extent to which

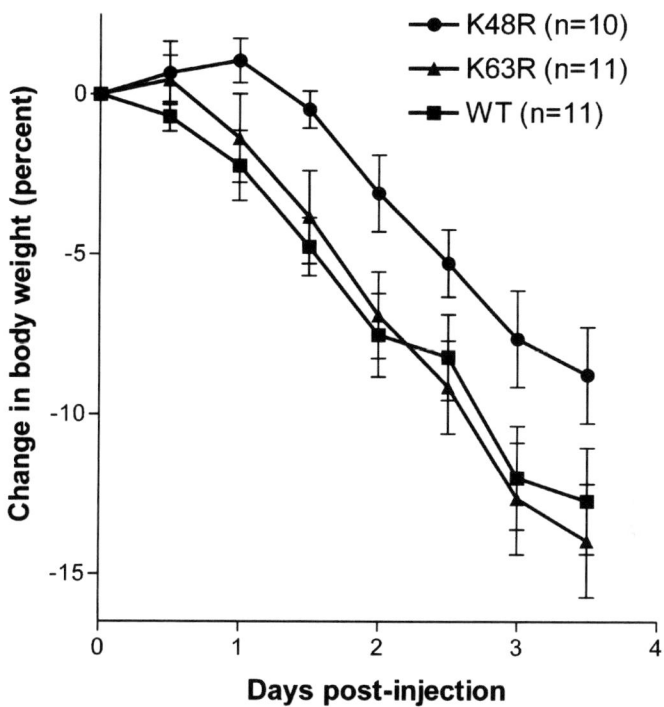

FIGURE 1. Loss of body weight in various cohorts of mice. Mice expressing K48R mutant ubiquitin fared significantly better than animals expressing the wild-type or K63R mutant isoforms of ubiquitin. See text.

transcription is reprogrammed in our ubiquitin transgenics. Ubiquitin also plays an important role in directing trafficking of proteins internalized by endocytosis and is required for ERAD (endoplasmic reticulum associated degradation), the degradative pathway charged with elimination of misfolded proteins extracted from the ER. There may be important alterations in vesicle trafficking in K48R mice, and these must also be investigated further.

In summary, we have discovered that K48R mutant ubiquitin can exert profound *in vivo* protective effects against a variety of insults, including agents of direct clinical relevance. The manipulation of the UPP has enormous potential for clinical benefit[9] and it is not unreasonable to expect that such benefits will include diseases of aging. In the coming months, we hope to determine if the general robustness of our K48R mice not only protects them against toxic insults, but also extends their life span in the absence of such stressors. There is evidence in at least one tissue that aging is delayed in these mice.[10]

REFERENCES

1. GRAY, D.A., M. TSIRIGOTIS & J. WOULFE. 2003. Ubiquitin, proteasomes, and the aging brain. Sci. Aging Knowl. Environ. **2003:** RE6.
2. FINLEY, D. *et al.* 1994. Inhibition of proteolysis and cell cycle progression in a multi-ubiquitination-deficient yeast mutant. Mol. Cell. Biol. **14:** 5501–5509.
3. SPENCE, J. *et al.* 1995. A ubiquitin mutant with specific defects in DNA repair and multi-ubiquitination. Mol. Cell. Biol. **15:** 1265–1273.
4. TSIRIGOTIS, M. *et al.* 2001. Analysis of ubiquitination *in vivo* using a transgenic mouse model. Biotechniques **31:** 120–126, 128, 130.
5. TSIRIGOTIS, M. *et al.* 2001. Sensitivity of mammalian cells expressing mutant ubiquitin to protein-damaging agents. J. Biol. Chem. **276:** 46073–46078.
6. ZHANG, M. *et al.* 2003. Effects of mutant ubiquitin on *ts*1 retrovirus–mediated neuropathology. J. Virol. **77:** 7193–7201.
7. SEARS, C. *et al.* 1998. NF-kappa B p105 processing via the ubiquitin-proteasome pathway. J. Biol. Chem. **273:** 1409–1419.
8. DENG, L. *et al.* 2000. Activation of the IkappaB kinase complex by TRAF6 requires a dimeric ubiquitin-conjugating enzyme complex and a unique polyubiquitin chain. Cell **103:** 351–361.
9. ADAMS, J. 2001. Proteasome inhibition in cancer: development of PS-341. Semin. Oncol. **28:** 613–619.
10. RASOULPOUR, R.J. *et al.* 2003. Altered ubiquitination protects the testis from cryptorchid injury and aging. Am. J. Pathol. In press.

Algae Extract Protection Effect on Oxidized Protein Level in Human *Stratum Corneum*

CARINE NIZARD,[a] SYLVIE POGGIOLI,[b] CATHERINE HEUSÈLE,[a] ANNE-LAURE BULTEAU,[b] MARIELLE MOREAU,[a] ALEX SAUNOIS,[a] SYLVIANNE SCHNEBERT,[a] CHRISTIAN MAHÉ,[a] AND BERTRAND FRIGUET[b]

[a]*LVMH Branche Parfums et Cosmetiques, 45804, Saint Jean de Braye, Cedex, France*
[b]*EA 1306 Université Paris 7-Denis Diderot, Paris, France*

ABSTRACT: Modification of proteins by reactive oxygen species is implicated in different disorders. The proteasome is a multicatalytic proteinase in charge of intracellular protein turnover and of oxidized proteins degradation. Consequently, proteasome function is very important in controlling the level of altered proteins in eukaryotic cells. Evidence for a decline in proteasome activity during skin photo-aging has been provided in Bulteau *et al.* in 2002. The ability of a lipid algae extract (*Phaeodactylum tricornutum*) to stimulate 20S proteasome peptidase activities was described by Nizard *et al.* in 2001. Furthermore, keratinocytes treated with *Phaeodactylum tricornutum* extract and then UVA and UVB irradiated, exhibited a sustained level of proteasome activitiy comparable to the one of nonirradiated cells. The level of modified proteins can be quantified by measurement of protein carbonyl content (Oxyblot technique), which has been shown to increase with aging and other disorders. In this paper, it is described that, in the presence of this lipid algae extract, the level of oxidized proteins is reduced, as assessed by the Oxyblot technique. These results are obtained both with culture of human keratinocytes and *stratum corneum* skin cells (obtained by stripping) from human volunteers. Altogether, these results argue for the presence of compounds in this algae extract that have a stimulating and/or protective effect on proteasome activity, resulting in a decreased level of protein oxidation.

KEYWORDS: *stratum corneum*; carbonyls; oxidized proteins; aging

INTRODUCTION

The epidermis is a dynamic system whose metabolic activity is regulated in large part by the integrity of the permeability barrier. This barrier resides in the *stratum corneum* and comprises a unique two-compartment system of structural protein-enriched corneocytes embedded in a lipid-enriched intercellular matrix. Premature aging of the skin results from a decrease in its capacity to resist the attacks made upon it by environmental factors, for example, sources of oxydative stress. The deleterious cellular effects of these agents are partially mediated by the formation of

Address for correspondence: Carine Nizard, LVMH Branche Parfums et Cosmetiques, 45804, Saint Jean de Braye, Cedex, France. Voice: +33-1-43-25-67-14; fax: +33-1-43-25-16-15.
carine.nizard-u505@bhdc.jussieu.fr

reactive oxygen species (ROS) that alter genomic integrity and can lead to skin carcinogenesis. ROS cause cellular damage by direct reaction with DNA, proteins, and lipids. Protein carbonyls may be formed either by oxidative cleavage of proteins or by direct oxidation of lysine, arginine, proline, and threonine residues.[1] Furthermore, carbonyl groups may derive from reactions of proteins with aldehydes (4-hydroxy-2-nonenal, malonaldehyde) produced during lipid peroxidation or with reactive carbonyl species (RCS) generated as a consequence of the reaction of reducing sugars or their oxidation products with lysine residues of proteins.

The proteasome is a multicatalytic proteinase in charge of intracellular protein turnover and of oxidized protein degradation. Consequently, proteasome function is very important in controlling the level of altered proteins in eukaryotic cells. We provided evidence for a decline in proteasome activity during skin photoaging.[2] In this study, measurement of protein carbonyl content (Oxyblot technique), which has been shown to increase with aging and other disorders, is assessed in *stratum corneum* skin cells (obtained by stripping) from human volunteers, treated or not with *Phaeodactylum tricornutum* lipid-rich algae extract.

MATERIAL AND METHODS

Humans

Seventeen healthy subjects (Caucasian; from 19 to 69 years old). Each person received placebo and 0.0003% *P. tricornutum* extract on each forearm, twice a day for 21 days.

Isolation of Human Stratum Corneum Proteins

The forearms of each subject were cleaned with ethanol and the first tape stripping was discarded to avoid contamination with surface lipids. Three strippings were performed sequentially and pooled. Proteins were obtained after tape stripping of skin with D-Squame tape adhesive disks (CuDerm Corporation, Dallas, Texas) and extraction using 2% SDS, 0.5 mM tris-HCl pH 7; 10 % glycerol; 5% 2-mercaptoethanol, lysis buffer. Disks were subjected to agitation for 3 hours at 4°C. Protein extracts were analyzed for protein content (DC protein assay, Bio-RAD, Hercules, California), and stored at −80°C until used.

Protein Carbonyl Detection

The derivatization of carbonyl groups of proteins by dinitrophenyl hydrazine (DNPH) was performed on 5 µg of epidermal proteins diluted in 6% SDS by adding 10% DNPH for 15 minutes at room temperature. The reaction was stopped with 25% tris-2M. This mix was diluted by water/glycerol (v/v) and sample buffer 11X (687 mM tris-HCl, pH 6.8, 22% SDS, 1.1 M 2-mercaptoethanol, bromophenol blue) and then a fraction containing 0.2 µg of proteins was electrophoresed on a 12% polyacrylamide gel and transferred onto a nitrocellulose membrane. The membrane was blocked 1 hour at room temperature with 1% BSA in TBS, Tween 20 0.01% (T-TBS), incubated with an anti-DNP antibody (1/100) in 1% BSA, T-TBS for 1 hour at room temperature, rinsed three times for 5 minutes and one time for 15 minutes in T-TBS.

After incubating 1 hour at room temperature with the secondary antibody (HRP-conjugated), the oxidized proteins were detected by chemoluminescence (ECL, Amersham Biosciences, Buckinghamshire, UK). The films were scanned and then analyzed with the Image Master 1D Elite software (Amersham Biosciences). The total amount of protein was controlled by SDS PAGE: 2 µg of each sample was separated on 12% polyacrylamide gel and stained by Coomassie blue. The gels were scanned and the signal in each lane was quantified with Image Master 1D Elite software.

RESULTS AND DISCUSSION

In this study, we have analyzed the level of protein carbonyls in human *stratum corneum* using an immunoblotting technique (Oxyblot). To investigate the level of oxidized proteins in the *stratum corneum*, we examined the first three layers of the skin. Indeed, we previously examined as far as the tenth layer (data not shown) and observed a protein oxidation gradient with increased levels toward outer *stratum corneum* layers. Therefore, in order to optimize our ability to observe differences between extracts from placebo- and *P. tricornutum*-treated donors, we decided to work only with the first three layers. We observed that application of 0.0003%

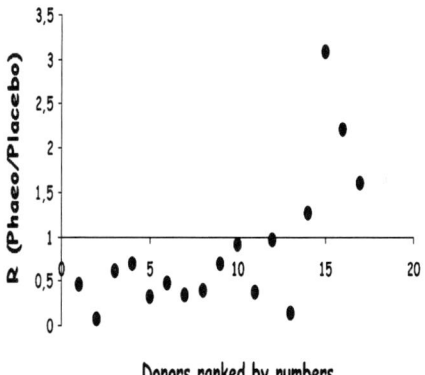

FIGURE 1. Effect of *Phaeodactylum tricornutum* extract on the level of oxidized proteins. Extracts from human stratum corneum were electrophoresed by SDS-PAGE and visualized using anti-DNP-antibody. The same extracts were electrophoresed by SDS-PAGE and stained by Coomassie blue. For oxyblots, results (total value of the spot volumes) are expressed as OXY(Phaeo) for extracts from 0.0003% *Phaeodactylum*-treated arm or OXY(Placebo) for extracts from placebo-treated arm. The total value of spot volumes from Coomassie blue gels is expressed as COM(Phaeo) or COM(Placebo). The effect of *Phaeodactylum* is expressed as R(PHAEO) and calculated as the ratio between OXY(Phaeo)J21/COM(Phaeo)J21 and OXY(Phaeo)J1/COM(Phaeo)J1. The effect of placebo is expressed as R(PLACEBO) and calculated as the ratio between OXY(Placebo)J21/COM(Placebo)J21 and OXY(Placebo)J1/COM(Placebo)J1. The final ratio, R(PHAEO/PLACEBO), presented in the figure, is calculated as R(PHAEO)/R(PLACEBO) and represents the effect of *Phaeodactylum* compared to placebo. The further R is below 1, the greater is the effect of *Phaeodactylum*, in terms of decreasing oxidized protein level.

P. tricornutum algae extract twice a day for three weeks is able to decrease the amount of oxidized proteins in thirteen out of seventeen people. Donors who have $R \geq 1$ (see FIG. 1 legend for the definition of R) are from 22 to 53 years old and no evidence for relationship between age and R levels was demonstrated.

The skin epidermis diplays a highly active metabolism of polyunsaturated fatty acids (PUFA). *P. tricornutum* algae extract contains about 95% of fatty acids (mostly composed of ecosapentanoic acid (EPA) which is a PUFA) and about 1% of xanthopylls (which are a group of oxygenated carotenoids). Dietary EPA has been shown to maintain an adequate antioxydant level after UVB irradiation of mouse skin.[3] Furthermore, it has been shown that xantophylls can interact with $^1O_2$, proffering a defense against oxidative damage.[4] We previously described the ability of a lipid algae extract (*P. tricornutum*) to stimulate 20S proteasome peptidase activities. Furthermore, keratinocytes treated with *P. tricornutum* extract and then UVA- and UVB-irradiated, exhibited a sustained level of proteasome activitiy compared to that of nonirradiated cells.[5] In conclusion, these data are consistent with our results, providing evidence that *P. tricornutum* algae extract could be of great dermatologic and cosmetic interest by virtue of its antioxidant properties and its ability to decrease protein oxidation.

REFERENCES

1. BERLETT, B.S. & E.R. STADTMAN. 1997. Protein oxidation in aging, disease, and oxidative stress. J. Biol. Chem. **272:** 20313–20316.
2. BULTEAU, A.L., M. MOREAU, C. NIZARD, *et al.* 2002. Impairment of proteasome function upon UVA- and UVB irradiation of human keratinocytes. Free Radical Biol. Med. **11:** 1157–1170.
3. MOISON, R.M. & G.M. BEIJERSBERGEN VAN HENEGOUWEN. 2001. Dietary eicosapentaenoic acid prevents systemic immunosuppression in mice induced by UVB radiation. Radiat. Res. **156:** 36–44.
4. NIYOGI, K., K.O. BJORKMAN & A.R. GROSSMAN. 1997. The roles of specific xanthophylls in photoprotection. Proc. Natl. Acad. Sci. USA **94:** 14162–14167.
5. NIZARD, C., B. FRIGUET, M. MOREAU, *et al.*2001. Inventors; LVMH-Recherche, assignee. PCT Application WO 02/080876. Use of *Phaeodactylum* algae extract as cosmetic agent promoting the proteasome activity of skin cells and cosmetic composition comprising same. Date of application: April 3.

Heat Shock Protein 47 Expression in Aged Normal Human Fibroblasts

Modulation by *Salix alba* Extract

CARINE NIZARD,[a] EMMANUELLE NOBLESSE,[a] CÉCILLE BOISDÉ,[a] MARIELLE MOREAU,[a] ANNE-MARIE FAUSSAT,[b] SYLVIANNE SCHNEBERT,[a] AND CHRISTIAN MAHÉ[a]

[a]*LVMH Branche Parfums et Cosmétiques, 45804, Saint Jean de Braye, Cedex, France*

[b]*IFR 58, Institut des Cordeliers, Paris, France*

ABSTRACT: Heat shock protein (HSP) 47 is a specific chaperone of procollagen. This heat shock protein is responsible for the correct three-dimentional organization of procollagen and its control-quality prior secretion. The aim of the study is to evaluate the level of HSP 47 in aged, photoaged, and senescent fibroblasts and its modulation by a plant extract (*Salix alba*). The level of HSP 47 and/or procollagen expression in fibroblasts was measured by real-time RT-PCR (mRNA transcripts) and by flow cytometry (immunochemistry technique for measurement of arbitrary fluorescence intensity). Immunochemistry techniques and confocal microscopy were used to vizualize the cellular localization of HSP 47 and procollagen. These parameters were compared with different age donors, nonsenescent, and senescent fibroblasts. Fibroblasts were irradiated by a noncytotoxic dose of UVA (6 J/cm^2), and HSP 47 level was evaluated. *S. alba* extract was tested for its capacity to modulate HSP 47 expression. Colocalization of HSP 47 and procollagen was shown by confocal microscopy, indicating that HSP 47 could play a role of procollagen molecular chaperone in the cellular model. It was also shown that the HSP 47 level is decreased in old-donor cells, senescent, and irradiated cells. This decrease can be modulated by a *S. alba* extract (polyphenols rich) in a dose-dependent manner. The evaluation of HSP 47 expression in the experimental conditions can lead to a new approach of aging and photoaging, pointing out the implication of this chaperone in these pathophysiologic phenomena. Modulation of HSP 47 expression by this family of molecules could be of cosmetic and/or dermatologic interest.

KEYWORDS: HSP 47; fibroblasts; aging; polyphenols; *Salix alba*

INTRODUCTION

Nature has evolved antistress mechanisms, many of which involve proteins. Some of these proteins are molecular chaperones. Integrity and functionality of antistress mechanisms, including the molecular chaperones and their coding genes, are key

Address for correspondence: Carine Nizard, LVMH Branche Parfums et Cosmétiques, 45804, Saint Jean de Braye, Cedex, France. Voice: +33-1-43-25-67-14; fax: +33-1-43-25-16-15.
carine.nizard-u505@bhdc.jussieu.fr

elements in the maintenance of all cellular proteins within functional, efficient ranges of concentration and configuration.

Heat shock protein (HSP) 47, derived from the serpin family of proteins, interacts transiently with procollagen during its folding, assembly, and transport from the endoplasmic reticulum (ER) of mammalian cells. It has been suggested that it carries out a diverse range of functions, such as acting as a molecular chaperone, facilitating the folding and assembly of procollagen molecules, retaining unfolded molecules within ER, and assisting the transport of correctly folded molecules from the ER to the golgi apparatus.[1]

As individuals age, their skin undergoes marked structural changes. In habitually exposed areas, cumulative solar-induced cutaneous changes are superimposed on these intrinsic age-associated structural associations. As regards the dermis, the dermal thickness decreases progressively with age. In aged skin, there is an apparent increase of the collagen network. This probably results from compression of collagen bundles, giving a more compact appearance due to age-related loss of the ground substance that normally occupies the spaces between individual bundles. In addition, aged skin shows marked architectural alterations. The collagen fibers are arranged in disarray in thick, coarse, tangled bundles, and/or aggregates of loosely woven, straight fibers.[2]

Is collagen and its assembly and transport affected by a defective HSP 47 molecule enhancing senescence? Given the collagen deterioration characterisic of senescence, it is tempting to speculate that a sick HSP 47 would considerably enhance this manifestation of aging.

In this paper we have assessed the effect of a polyphenol-rich plant extract (*Salix alba* or willow commercially named Astressyl®) on old- and young-donor normal human fibroblasts, on HSP 47 expression.

MATERIAL AND METHODS

Antibodies and Probes

Monoclonal mouse anti-HSP 47 (colligin) antibody (StressGen Biotechnologies Corp., Victoria, BC, Canada); IgG goat antimouse Alexafluor 488 (Molecular Probes, Eugene, Oregon).

Cell Culture

All cell culture media and chemicals were purchased from Gibco Life Technologies (Cergy Pontoise, France) and Sigma (St. Louis, Missouri). Dermal cells were prepared by means of plastic surgery (facial liftings) from 20- and 70-year-old healthy female donors.

Fibroblasts are grown as monolayers in Dubelco's modified Eagle's medium (DMEM) containing 1 g/L glucose, supplemented by 10% SVF. *S. alba* extract named, Astressyl (SILAB, Brive, France), is an aqueous solution. Cells were treated 6 hours with 2% (v/v) Astressyl.

Flow Cytometry

Cells were trypsinated and then fixed in 3.7% formaldehyde. Each pellet (10^6 cells) was incubated 1 hour at room temperature with 1/500 anti-HSP 47 antibody diluted in PBS-BSA (1%, w/v) and 30 minutes at room temperature with 1/100 secondary antibody diluted in PBS-BSA (1%, w/v). Analysis was performed on an ALTRA cell sorter (Beckmann Coulter) and with Expo32 software.

RESULTS AND DISCUSSION

Before examining the expression of HSP 47 in normal fibroblasts, we assessed the cellular viability and dose-effect of Astressyl (data not shown). A 6-hour cell treatment with 2% Astressyl induces optimal results with no cellular mortality.

FIGURE 1 shows a difference between the level of HSP 47 in older donor (70 years) compared to younger donor (20 years). The decrease is significant in old-donor cells according to the Kolmogorov-Smirnov test ($S = 0.2657$), which is adapted to cytometry results analysis.

Treatment with 2% Astressyl of young-donor cells, induces no clear increase of HSP 47 level. A significant increase ($S = 0.2856$) is observed when treatment is performed on 70-year-old donor cells. This level is approximately similar to the level of control young-donor cells.

Evidence from several lines of investigation has indicated that photoaging, when superimposed on the intrinsic aging process, plays a major role in age-associated degenerative changes of the skin. Our face-skin biopsy samples provided cells in

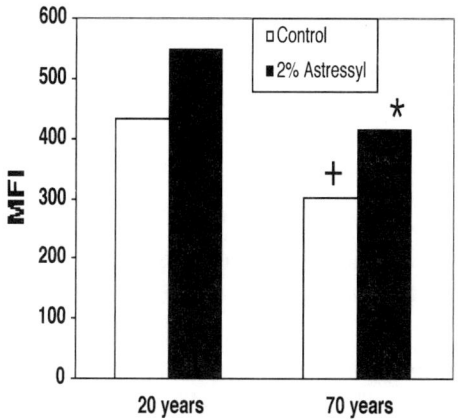

FIGURE 1. Astressyl® induction of HSP 47. Cells are treated by 2% (v/v) Astressyl for 6 hours. HSP 47 expression is presented as mean fluorescence intensity (MFI) of 10,000 normal human fibroblasts of 20- and 70-year-old donors determined by flow cytometry. Statistical analysis is performed by Expo 2 software (Beckmann Coulter) using the Kolmogorov-Smirnov statistical test, which is significant when $S > 0.2$. (∗ means significant compared to 20-year-old control cells; + means significant compared to 70-year-old control cells.)

which aging and photo-aging are evidently overlaping. These two processes have in common a free-radical component. As expected from the "free-radical theory of aging," there is an accumulation of oxidation products such as oxidized proteins and lipid metabolites during the aging process. HSP 47 protein could be a possible target for free-radical attack that could be translated in terms of a defect in its synthesis and its expression. We could hypothesize that the HSP 47 level is not only lowered, but that its function could be altered (collagen processing alteration). An accumulation of damaged HSP 47 protein may be the result of an increase in the rate of protein oxidation and/or decrease in the rate of degradation of oxidized protein. It has been well demonstrated that the multicatalytic proteasome is the major proteolytic system involved in the removal of oxidized protein. Aging and photoaging are also described as factors implicated in proteasome inhibition.[3] Although the link between HSP 47 degradation and proteasome is not yet described, we could hypothesize that, like some HSP, age-damaged HSP 47 could be much less degraded by age-altered proteasome.

Our results are consistent with studies that described age-related attenuation of some HSP in primary cultured fibroblasts.[4] Furthermore, an altered expression of HSP 47 in high population doubling level (PDL) has been described.[5]

S. alba extract, commercially named Astressyl, is rich in tannins, which are phenolic compounds characterized by their ability to bind N-containing organic structures such as amino acids and proteins. However, little is known about the mechanisms involved in the formation of tannin–protein complexes. It was suggested that hydrophobic interactions play an important role during tannin complexation. It has been showed that *S. alba* extract contains mainly procyanidins.[6] Recent studies have shown that procyanidins in grape seeds possess anti-inflammatory, antiarthritic, and antiallergic properties and prevent heart disease and skin aging. In other studies, polyphenols have been shown to exert a much stronger oxygen free-radical scavenging effect than vitamins C and E.

HSP 47 could be protected (like many other proteins not studied here) by *S. alba* extract from free radicals implicated in the aging phenomenon. An explanation of the maintenance of HSP 47 level with age could be the high radical-scavenging capacity of tannins. The nonsignificant effect of Astressyl on young-donor cells could be explained by the already high level of HSP 47, which could not be further enhanced.

Taken together, these results could be of great cosmetic or dematologic interest by virtue of *S. alba* extract's ability to induce HSP 47 expression.

REFERENCES

1. TASAB, M., M.R. BATTEN & N.J. BULLEID. 2000. Hsp47: a molecular chaperone that interacts with and stabilizes correctly-folded procollagen. EMBO J. **19:** 2204–2211.
2. LAVKER, R.M., P.S. ZHENG & G. DONG. 1987. Aged skin: a study by light, transmission electron, and scanning electron microscopy. J. Invest. Dermatol. **88:** 44s–51s.
3. BULTEAU, A.L., M. MOREAU., C. NIZARD, *et al.* 2002. Impairment of proteasome function upon UVA- and UVB irradiation of human keratinocytes. Free Radical Biol. Med. **11:** 1157–1170.
4. DEGUCHI, Y., S. NEGORO & S. KISHIMOTO. 1988. Age-related changes of heat shock protein gene transcription in human peripheral blood mononuclear cells. Biochem. Biophys. Res. Commun. **157:** 580–584.

5. MIYAISHI O., Y. ITO, K. KOZAKI, et al. 1995. Age-related attenuation of HSP47 heat response in fibroblasts. Mech. Ageing Dev. **77:** 213–226.
6. BEHRENS, A., N. MAIE, H. KNICKER & I. KOGEL-KNABNER. 2003. MALDI-TOF mass spectrometry and PSD fragmentation as means for the analysis of condensed tannins in plant leaves and needles. Phytochemistry **62:** 1159–1170.

RAGE: A New Pleiotropic Antagonistic Gene?

A. SIMM, B. BARTLING, AND R-E. SILBER

Department of Cardio-Thoracic Surgery, University of Halle-Wittenberg, Ernst-Grube Str. 40, D-06120 Halle, Germany

ABSTRACT: Advanced glycation end products (AGEs) are the result of a nonenzymatic reaction of reducing sugars with primary amino groups of proteins (Maillard reaction). They accumulate in various tissues in the course of aging. Because AGEs induce protein cross-links and oxidative stress (radicals) within cells and tissues, they have been implicated in the development of many degenerative diseases. Binding of AGEs to receptors like RAGE induces the release of profibrotic cytokines, such as TGF-β or proinflammatory cytokines, such as TNF-α or IL-6. AGE inhibitors or breakers, such as aminoguanidine or ALT-711, inhibit the age-induced heart hypertrophy or stiffness of the large arteries. On the other hand, little is known about the physiological role of RAGE as the receptor of AGEs. Investigations about the expression of RAGE in lung tissue and lung tumors may give a hint for such a role.

KEYWORDS: receptor; advanced glycation end products; aging; human; heart

Cardiovascular diseases are the leading cause of death in the Western World. The cardiovascular risk is greatly increased in elder humans, and especially in those with type 1 or type 2 diabetes. This can be explained, in part, by the association of diabetes with hypertension and arteriosclerosis. On the other hand, the underlying molecular mechanisms are not yet completely known. Posttranslational modification of proteins via nonenzymatic glycation are directly associated with high glucose and oxidative stress. This reaction starts with the formation of a Schiff base from the carbonyl group of a reducing sugar, such as glucose, and a primary amino group. The Schiff base rearranges to the Amadori product. Over time, in a series of reactions including dehydrations and especially oxidation reaction, a heterogeneous group of compounds is formed, the advanced glycation end products (AGEs), which exhibit characteristic absorbance and fluorescence properties.[1]

AGE cross-linking of peptides and proteins is protease-resistant and causes irreversible damage to tissues and activation of different cell types, such as macrophages/monocytes, cardiac fibroblasts, and vascular smooth muscle cells. Activation of these cells leads to the generation of reactive oxygen species (ROS), which induce the oxidation of DNA and the peroxidation of membrane lipids. Increasing evidence

Address for correspondence: PD Dr. Andreas Simm, Department of Cardio-Thoracic Surgery, University of Halle-Wittenberg, Ernst-Grube Str. 40, D-06120 Halle, Germany. Voice: +49-345-557-2647; fax: +49-345-557-2782.
andreas.simm@medizin.uni-halle.de

Ann. N.Y. Acad. Sci. 1019: 228–231 (2004). © 2004 New York Academy of Sciences.
doi: 10.1196/annals.1297.038

suggests a role for AGE-induced oxidative stress in the pathogenesis of normal aging and age-related chronic diseases, including diabetes.[2] Accumulation of AGEs during normal aging occurs in long-lived proteins, such as collagens, lens crystalline, and cartilage. AGE deposits have been immunolocalized in the skin, lung, kidney, intestine, intervertebral disks, as well as in the heart and arteries (especially in atherosclerotic plaques) of aged and diabetic patients.[3] Furthermore, the pathophysiological significance of AGE-induced oxidative stress is supported by animal and clinical studies showing an improvement in arterial and cardiac compliance after treatment with ALT-711, an inhibitor of AGE–cross-linking.[4]

In the last decade, a number of receptors have been identified that bind AGEs, including AGE-R1, AGE-R2, AGE-R3, the scavenger receptor II, and the receptor for AGEs (RAGE).[5] Among them, RAGE seems to be the most important, as it is responsible for the activation of intracellular signal transduction pathways, such as the ERK kinases, the p38^{MAPK}, the JNK kinases, and the NF-κB pathway. The receptor RAGE, primarily identified as a 35-kD protein and predominantly expressed in lung, recognizes families of ligands such as S100/calgranulins, β-sheet fibrils, and amphoterin, which is important for neurite outgrowth. RAGE has been shown to be implicated in inflammation; for example, binding of S100A12 of the S100/calganuulin family to RAGE in murine macrophages resulted in the elaboration of interleukin-1β and tumor necrosis factor-α.[6] An elevated expression of RAGE has been demonstrated in cardiovascular tissue in diabetic rats.[7] Furthermore, the involvement of AGE–RAGE interaction in the pathogenesis of accelerated arteriosclerosis in diabetes has been shown in diabetic Apo-E-knock-out mice. Treatment of these mice with soluble RAGE (the extra cellular domain of RAGE) leads to a complete reduction of diabetes-induced arteriosclerotic plaques.[8] These and other results clearly demonstrate that RAGE plays an important pathophysiological role during aging and age-related degenerative diseases. As no gene exists without any physiological function, RAGE may fit the concept of the pleiotropic antagonism. This concept of an evolutionary basis for the development of age-related diseases postulates that genes that are beneficial during the reproductive phase of life may become deleterious in the elderly.

First results in the field of oncology may suggest a positive physiological function of RAGE. Growth of neuroblastoma cells on an amphoterin-coated surface leads to neurite outgrowth and differentiation of these cells. Application of amphoterin inhibits transendothelial migration of tumor cells as well as the formation of pulmonary metastasis.[9] Nevertheless, there is still contradictory data. Some groups found an upregulation of RAGE in gastric and pancreatic tumors, while, in contrast, we and others found a downregulation of RAGE in lung cancer. It has been suggested that first amphoterin, which is highly expressed in the lung, mediates cell differentiation via RAGE, and second, that a downregulation of the receptor may be considered to be a critical step in lung tumor formation.[10] These data indicate that RAGE may be involved in the regulation of the cell differentiation, while it is still unclear if RAGE indeed promotes or inhibits tumor growth.

In summary, a great deal of information about the pathophysiological role of RAGE during aging is available. In contrast, there is little data to indicate a physiological role of this receptor. As an example of a pleiotropic antagonistic gene, RAGE may interfere with differentiation processes that are needed during youth, but it is known as an important trigger for degenerative diseases during aging (FIG. 1).

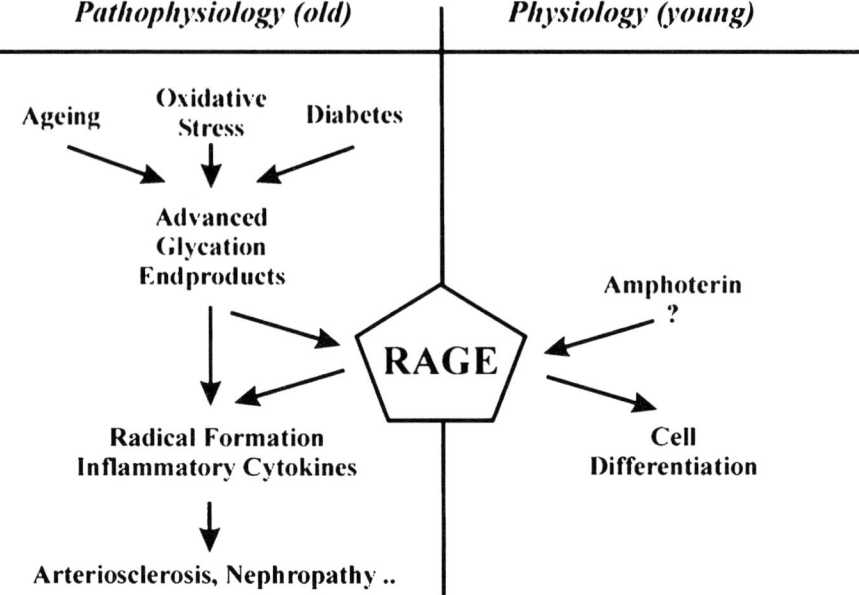

FIGURE 1. RAGE as a pleiotropic antagonistic gene.

ACKNOWLEDGMENT

This work was supported by the DFG SFB-598 Herzversagen im Alter, TPA5.

REFERENCES

1. WESTWOOD, M.E. & P.J. THORNALLEY. 1997. Glycation and advanced glycation endproducts. *In* The Glycation Hypthesis. C. Colacao, Ed.: 59–87. Landes Bioscience. Georgetown, Texas.
2. VLASSARA, H. & M.R. PALACE. 2002. Diabetes and advanced glycation endproducts. J. Intern. Med. **251:** 87–101.
3. SCHLEICHER, E.D., E. WAGNER & A.G. NERLICH. 1997. Increased accumulation of the glycoxidation product N(epsilon)-(carboxymethyl)lysine in human tissues in diabetes and aging. J. Clin. Invest. **99:** 457–468.
4. ASIF, M., J. EGAN, S. VASAN, *et al.* 2000. An advanced glycation endproduct cross-link breaker can reverse age-related increases in myocardial stiffness, Proc. Natl. Acad. Sci. USA **97:** 2809–2813.
5. THORNALLEY, P.J. 1998. Cell activation by glycated proteins. AGE receptors, receptor recognition factors and functional classification of AGEs. Cell. Mol. Biol. (Noisy-le-grand) **44:** 1013–1023.
6. SCHMIDT, A.M., S.D. YAN, S.F. YAN & D.M. STERN. 2000. The biology of the receptor for advanced glycation end products and its ligands. Biochim. Biophys. Acta **1498:** 99–111.

7. SCHMIDT, A.M. & V.D. D'AGATI. 2000. Expression of advanced glycation end products and their cellular receptor RAGE in diabetic nephropathy and nondiabetic renal disease, J. Am. Soc. Nephrol. **11:** 1656–1666.
8. PARK, L., K.G. RAMAN, K.J. LEE, *et al.* 1998. Suppression of accelerated diabetic atherosclerosis by the soluble receptor for advanced glycation endproducts. Nat. Med. **4:** 1025–1031.
9. HUTTUNEN, H.J., C. FAGES, J. KUJA-PANULA, *et al.* 2002. Receptor for advanced glycation end products-binding COOH-terminal motif of amphoterin inhibits invasive migration and metastasis. Cancer Res. **62:** 4805–4811.
10. SCHRAML, P., I. BENDIK & C.U. LUDWIG. 1997. Differential messenger RNA and protein expression of the receptor for advanced glycosylated end products in normal lung and non-small cell lung carcinoma. Cancer Res. **57:** 3669–3671.

Genetic Correction of Mitochondrial Diseases

Using the Natural Migration of Mitochondrial Genes to the Nucleus in Chlorophyte Algae as a Model System

DIEGO GONZÁLEZ-HALPHEN,[a] SOLEDAD FUNES,[b] XOCHITL PÉREZ-MARTÍNEZ,[c] ADRIÁN REYES-PRIETO,[d] M. GONZALO CLAROS,[e] EDGAR DAVIDSON,[f] AND MICHAEL P. KING[f]

[a]*Departamento de Genética Molecular, Instituto de Fisiología Celular, Universidad Nacional Autónoma de México, 04510 México D.F., Mexico*

[b]*Institut fur Physiologische Chemie, Ludwig-Maximilians-Universität München, Butenandtstrasse 5, München 81377, Germany*

[c]*Department of Molecular Biology and Genetics, Cornell University, Ithaca, New York 14853, USA*

[d]*Departamento de Botánica, Instituto de Biología, Universidad Nacional Autónoma de México, Mexico City, Mexico*

[e]*Departamento de Biología Molecular y Bioquímica, Facultad de Ciencias, Universidad de Málaga, Málaga E-29071, Spain*

[f]*Department of Biochemistry and Molecular Pharmacology, Thomas Jefferson University, Philadelphia, Pennsylvania 19107-5541, USA*

ABSTRACT: Mitochondrial diseases display great diversity in clinical symptoms and biochemical characteristics. Although mtDNA mutations have been identified in many patients, there are currently no effective treatments. A number of human diseases result from mutations in mtDNA-encoded proteins, a group of proteins that are hydrophobic and have multiple membrane-spanning regions. One method that has great potential for overcoming the pathogenic consequences of these mutations is to place a wild-type copy of the affected gene in the nucleus, and target the expressed protein to the mitochondrion to function in place of the defective protein. Several respiratory chain subunit genes, which are typically mtDNA encoded, are nucleus encoded in the chlorophyte algae *Chlamydomonas reinhardtii* and *Polytomella* sp. Analysis of these genes has revealed adaptations that facilitated their expression from the nucleus. The nucleus-encoded proteins exhibited diminished physical constraints for import as compared to their mtDNA-encoded homologues. The hydrophobicity of the nucleus-encoded proteins is diminished in those regions that are not involved in subunit–subunit interactions or that contain amino acids critical for enzymatic reactions of the proteins. In addition, these proteins have unusually large mitochondrial targeting sequences. Information derived from these studies should be applicable toward the development of genetic therapies for human diseases resulting from mutations in mtDNA-encoded polypeptides.

Address for correspondence: Michael P. King, Thomas Jefferson University, 233 S. 10th Street, BLSB 308, Philadelphia, PA 19107-5541. Voice: 215-503-4845; fax: 215-503-5393.
Michael.King@jefferson.edu

Ann. N.Y. Acad. Sci. 1019: 232–239 (2004). © 2004 New York Academy of Sciences.
doi: 10.1196/annals.1297.039

KEYWORDS: mitochondrial diseases; mitochondrial genomes; gene therapy; chlorophyte algae; allotopic expression; gene migration

INTRODUCTION

Since pathogenic mutations in the human mitochondrial genome (mtDNA) were first described,[1,2] more than 100 point mutations and numerous mtDNA rearrangements associated with mitochondrial diseases have been reported.[3] Despite the molecular genetic characterization of these mutations, no effective therapies exist for mitochondrial diseases. Allotopic expression is one potential approach to gene therapy for human diseases resulting from mutations in mtDNA-encoded protein genes. This entails the functional expression of a mitochondrial gene that has been relocated in the nucleus.[4,5] This strategy would allow the expression of a mitochondrial protein from the nucleus of cells harboring an mtDNA-encoded mutant form of the protein. The allotopic expression of a mitochondrial gene was pioneered with the *atp8* gene of yeast.[4] Some eukaryotes contain nucleus-encoded genes that are normally found in the mtDNA in the vast majority of organisms. The characteristics of these relocated genes are discussed here. These characteristics suggest genetic modifications that may facilitate allotopic expression of a mitochondrial gene.

MITOCHONDRIAL GENOMES AND MITOCHONDRIAL GENE MIGRATION

The endosymbiotic event that gave rise to mitochondria was followed by a massive migration of genes to the nucleus,[6] a process that continues to this day, as exemplified by organisms that contain the same protein encoded in both the mitochondrial and the nuclear genomes, such as, subunit ATP9 of *Neurospora crassa*,[7] and the COX II subunit of legumes.[8] Most nucleus-encoded proteins destined for the mitochondrial matrix or inner membrane, the innermost mitochondrial compartments, require a mitochondrial targeting sequence (MTS). This is generally a small, N-terminal cleavable presequence of 20 to 40 residues, capable of forming an amphiphilic alpha-helix that is recognized by the mitochondrial import apparatus. After import, the MTS is usually removed by a mitochondrial processing peptidase.

The migration of mitochondrial genes to the nucleus gave rise to the present highly reduced mtDNAs that encode a limited set of protein and RNA components.[6] Mitochondria that possess a complete set of oxidative phosphorylation (OX-PHOS) complexes— I, II, III, IV, and ATP synthase—usually contain the genes *nad1, nad2, nad3, nad4, nad4L, nad5, nad6, cox1, cox2, cox3, cob, atp6,* and *atp8* that encode highly hydrophobic membrane proteins with two to seventeen transmembrane stretches.[6] In the mtDNA of green algae *Chlamydomonas reinhardtii, Chlamydomonas eugametos,* and *Polytomella parva,* members of the "Reinhardtii" clade,[9] there is a conspicuous absence of the *nad3, nad4L, cox2, cox3, atp6,* and *atp8* genes encoding essential membrane proteins that participate in OX-PHOS.[10–12]

Several hypotheses have been proposed to explain why mitochondrial genomes preserve a limited set of genes encoding OX-PHOS components (reviewed in Ref. 13). These include (1) the presence of some organellar proteins in the cytoplasm may have detrimental effects on the cell; (2) highly hydrophobic cytoplasm-synthesized organellar proteins could be misrouted to other cell compartments, such as the endoplasmic reticulum; (3) the retention of genes in the mitochondrial genome may allow them to be rapidly regulated by the organelle redox state; and (4) highly hydrophobic proteins may not be readily imported into mitochondria, and must be synthesized *in situ* to be properly inserted into the inner mitochondrial membrane. Additionally, in some organisms the evolution of a mitochondrial genetic code different from the nuclear code may inhibit the functional expression of mitochondrial genes relocated in the nucleus. Also, mitochondrial genes in some organisms have acquired complex processing requirements, such as mRNA editing, that would prevent their expression from the nucleus. As outlined below, we favor the hypothesis that hydrophobicity[14] is the ultimate limiting step for the functional relocation to the nucleus of mitochondrial genes encoding polytopic membrane proteins.

MIGRATION OF MITOCHONDRIAL GENES TO THE NUCLEUS IN *CHLOROPHYTE ALGAE*

In members of the genera *Chlamydomonas* and *Polytomella*, some mitochondrial genes that are retained in the mtDNA of the vast majority of eukaryotes have migrated to the nucleus. Among these are *cox2*, encoding subunit II of cytochrome *c* oxidase (COX II);[15] *cox3*, encoding subunit III of cytochrome *c* oxidase (COX III);[16] *atp6* encoding subunit ATP6 of F_1F_0-ATP synthase;[17] and *nad4L*, encoding subunit NAD4L of the NADH-ubiquinone oxidoreductase [GenBank accession number AY216718]. These four subunits are essential components of their corresponding enzyme complexes.

Mitochondrial genes adapted for expression in the nucleus exhibit several distinct features that facilitate nuclear expression.[18] A number of modifications that occur in the chlorophyte algal genes *cox2a*, *cox2b*, *cox3*, *atp6*, and *nad4L* contribute to their ability to be expressed from the nucleus and are described below:

(1) *Acquisition of promoters.* Relocated genes must acquire promoters and other regulatory elements to be expressed in the nucleus. The chlorophyte algal promoters that regulate the expression of the relocated mitochondrial genes have yet to be characterized.

(2) *Acquisition of polyadenylation signals.* The polyadenylation signal of *C. reinhardtii* nuclear genes is present in the relocalized mitochondrial genes.

(3) *Acquisition of introns.* Several introns with orthodox splicing sites are present in some of the relocalized chlorophyte mitochondrial genes. The *cox2a* and *cox3* genes of both algae, and *cox2b* and *atp6* of *C. reinhardtii* contain introns, while *nad4L* of *C. reinhardtii* and *cox2b* of *Polytomella* sp. lack introns.

(4) *Change in codon usage.* The chlorophyte algae of the "Reinhardtii" clade exhibit a biased codon usage in their nuclear genes. The relocated mitochondrial genes of *C. reinhardtii* and *Polytomella* sp. exhibit codon usage patterns similar to other nuclear genes and that are distinct from mtDNA-encoded genes.

(5) *Acquisition of a region encoding a MTS. C. reinhardtii* MTSs vary in size. COX IIA, COX III, ATP6, and NAD4L exhibit unusually large MTSs of 143, 119, 107, and 133 residues, respectively. Shorter MTSs of 30 to 70 residues are associ-

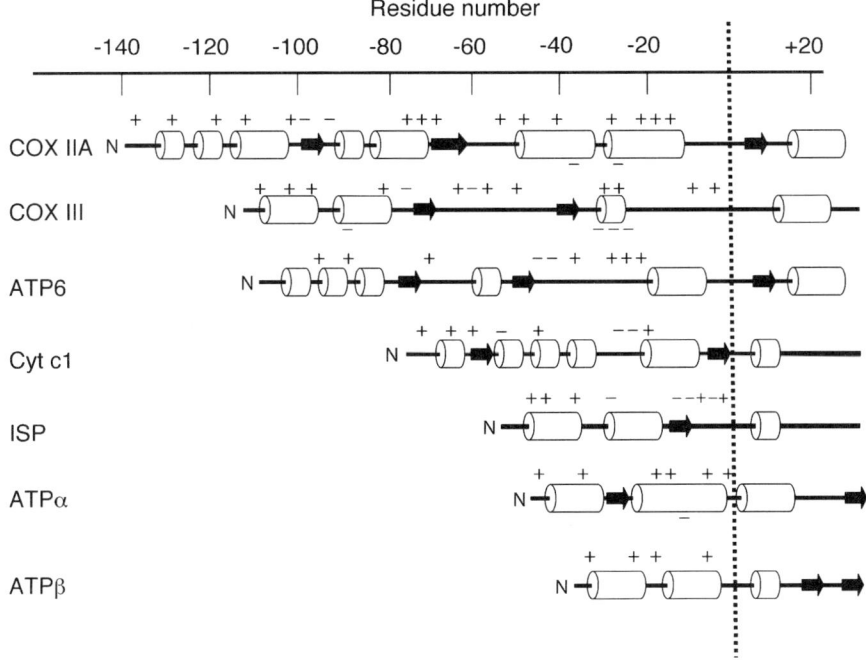

FIGURE 1. Secondary structure analysis of different *C. reinhardtii* mitochondrial targeting sequences. Predicted alpha helices are depicted as *cylinders*, beta sheets as *bold arrows*, and random coils as *straight lines*. The *vertical dashed line* separates the MTSs from the mature portions of the proteins. Residues are indicated as *negative numbers* for MTSs and as *positive numbers* for the N-terminal regions of the mature proteins. The *C. reinhardtii* nucleus-encoded mitochondrial proteins analyzed were COX IIA of cytochrome *c* oxidase [GenBank AF305080]; COX III of cytochrome *c* oxidase [AF233515]; ATP6 of the F_0 sector of F_1F_0-ATP synthase [AF411119]; cytochrome c_1 (Cyt c_1)[AF245393]; the Rieske-type iron-sulfur protein (ISP) [X91795]; ATPalpha, the alpha subunit of F_1F_0-ATP synthase [X94149]; and ATPbeta, the beta subunit of F_1F_0-ATP synthase [X61624].

ated with proteins targeted to the mitochondrial matrix. As with other MTSs, it is predicted that these long MTSs form amphiphilic α-helices (FIG. 1) that are important for binding with the mitochondrial outer membrane receptors (reviewed in Ref. 19). Long presequences may improve the efficiency of import of nucleus-encoded, highly hydrophobic proteins into mitochondria.[20–22]

(6) *Diminished hydrophobicity.* The membrane domains of nucleus-encoded mitochondrial proteins are less hydrophobic and are spaced further apart than their mtDNA-encoded counterparts. Both mesohydrophobicity (*meso*H), a measure of the distance between hydrophobic domains, and the maximum hydrophobicity of the putative transmembrane segments (<H>) are predictors of the likelihood that a protein could be imported into the mitochondrion.[21,23,24] The nucleus-encoded COX IIA, COX IIB, COX III, ATP6, and NAD4L of chlamydomonad algae exhibit reduced *meso*H and <H> compared to their mtDNA-encoded counterparts, which

presumably facilitates their import into mitochondria.[24] In particular, hydropathy analysis of the algal COX III and ATP6 sequences showed that the decrease of mean hydrophobicity occurs mostly in those transmembrane regions of the protein that are not involved in subunit–subunit interactions or in the function of the subunit.[16,17] A similar phenomenon is observed for the relocated mitochondrial *sdh3* gene of angiosperms.[25]

In leguminous species that express both mitochondrial and nuclear *cox2* genes, the nucleus-encoded COX II proteins have a lower hydrophobicity than the mtDNA-encoded COX II. A chimeric protein, consisting of mitochondrial COX II with the MTS of the nuclear COX II subunit, was not imported into mitochondria.[26] However, this protein could be imported after the introduction of two amino acid substitutions in the first transmembrane alpha-helix, which introduced fewer hydrophobic residues in the nucleus-encoded COX II.[26] Therefore, structural changes that diminish hydrophobicity can allow import into mitochondria of a nucleus-encoded protein that is normally mtDNA encoded. These results support the hypothesis[14,16,21] that hydrophobicity limits the functional relocalization of mitochondrial genes to the nucleus.

(7) *Fragmentation of genes*. The splitting of mitochondrial genes may be another mechanism that can facilitate their migration to the nucleus. In both *Polytomella* sp. and *C. reinhardtii*, the *cox2* gene encoding COX II of cytochrome *c* oxi-

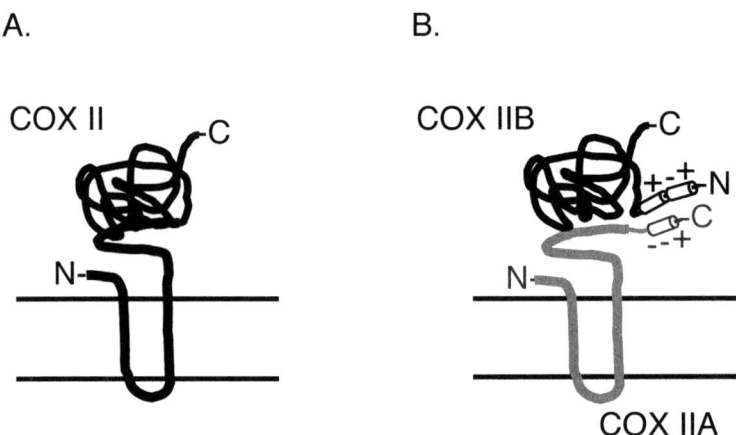

FIGURE 2. Cytochrome *c* oxidase subunit II from *Chlamydomonas* and *Polytomella* is a heterodimer. Most COX II subunits are single polypeptides encoded by single mitochondrial genes (**A**). In Chlamydomonad algae (**B**), COX IIA (*gray*) is encoded by the nuclear gene *cox2a* and corresponds to the N-terminal, hydrophobic half of a canonical COX II protein. COX IIB (*black*) is encoded by the nuclear *cox2b* gene and corresponds to the soluble C-terminal half of a conventional COX II protein.[15] The chlorophyte COX IIA and COX IIB subunits contain unique C- and N-terminal extensions, respectively, not present in orthodox COX II subunits, that may interact through their highly charged α-helices (represented as *cylinders*), to assemble and stabilize the two COX II proteins in the mature cytochrome *c* oxidase complex. N represents the N-terminus of the protein; C represents the C-terminus.

dase has not only relocated to the nucleus but has been split into two separate nuclear genes, *cox2a* and *cox2b*.[15] *cox2a* encodes COX IIA, corresponding to the N-terminal half of a typical single-polypeptide COX II, including the two transmembrane regions. *cox2b* encodes COX IIB, equivalent to the C-terminal domain of an orthodox COX II, which is located in the intermembrane space. COX IIA and COX IIB assemble noncovalently to give a heterodimeric COX II in the mature cytochrome *c* oxidase complex (FIG. 2). *cox2a* and *cox2b* genes are also present in the chlorophyte alga *Scenedesmus obliquus*, but in this alga *cox2b* has migrated to the nucleus, while *cox2a* was retained in the mtDNA. This indicates that the division of *cox2* into two genes occurred in the mtDNA of an ancestral chlorophyte.[27] The fragmentation of a highly hydrophobic protein containing two or more putative transmembrane stretches into simpler protein modules may facilitate their import into mitochondria.[15,21] Proper assembly of the protein modules may be mediated by interactions between charged N- and C-terminal extensions (FIG. 2).

(8) In conclusion, structural modifications have occurred during the relocation of mitochondrial genes to the nucleus. The diminished mesohydrophobicity seems to be of particular importance for hydrophobic mitochondrial OX-PHOS proteins whose genes are localized in the nucleus.

ALLOTOPIC EXPRESSION OF MITOCHONDRIAL GENES AND ITS APPLICATIONS TO HUMAN MITOCHONDRIAL GENE THERAPY

Human mitochondrial and *C. reinhardtii* ATP6 subunits have been allotopically expressed in human cells with mutations in the mtDNA-encoded *atp6* gene.[28,29] Remarkably, expression of *C. reinhardtii* ATP6 improved ATP synthesis in human cells, despite the evolutionary distance between green algae and vertebrates. A similar approach was used in cells harboring a mutation in the *nad4* gene using a nucleus-encoded human NAD4 subunit of complex I.[30] However, these investigations revealed that the allotopic expression of highly hydrophobic human mitochondrial OX-PHOS subunits is inefficient and still must be optimized. Some features of the *cox2*, *cox3*, *atp6*, and *nad4L* genes that are naturally nucleus-localized in some organisms could be used to enhance the efficiency of allotopic expression of mitochondrial genes in humans with mitochondrial diseases.[31,32] The hydrophobicity of the human proteins could be diminished in the same regions where hydrophobicity has been reduced by evolution in chlamydomonad algae. Site-directed mutagenesis that diminishes hydrophobicity of some residues in certain transmembrane stretches, and the addition of appropriate MTSs, might prove sufficient to improve the efficiency of allotopic expression. For hydrophobic proteins with multiple membrane helices, nuclear expression of mitochondrial genes could be accomplished as two or more nuclear genes with each gene encoding a subset of the membrane-spanning domains of the protein. N-Terminal and C-terminal extensions could be added to facilitate functional assembly of split proteins in the mitochondrial inner membrane. Alternatively, insertion of inteins, self-splicing intervening protein sequences, in the allotopically expressed proteins may facilitate their association in the mitochondrial inner membrane.[33]

ACKNOWLEDGMENTS

Work in our groups is supported by Grants TW01176 from NIH/Fogarty, USA; 27754N from CONACyT, Mexico; and IN202598 from DGAPA, UNAM, Mexico. The authors acknowledge the technical assistance of Miriam Vázquez-Acevedo.

REFERENCES

1. HOLT, I.J., A.E. HARDING & J.A. MORGAN HUGHES. 1988. Deletions of muscle mitochondrial DNA in patients with mitochondrial myopathies. Nature **331:** 717–719.
2. WALLACE, D.C., G. SINGH, M.T. LOTT, et al. 1988. Mitochondrial DNA mutation associated with Leber's hereditary optic neuropathy. Science **242:** 1427–1430.
3. DIMAURO, S. & A.L. ANDREU. 2000. Mutations in mtDNA: Are we scraping the bottom of the barrel? Brain Pathol. **10:** 431–441.
4. GEARING, D.P. & P. NAGLEY. 1986. Yeast mitochondrial ATPase subunit 8, normally a mitochondrial gene product, expressed in vitro and imported back into the organelle. EMBO J. **5:** 3651–3655.
5. ZULLO, S.J. 2001. Gene therapy of mitochondrial DNA mutations: a brief, biased history of allotopic expression in mammalian cells. Semin. Neurol. **21:** 327–335.
6. GRAY, M.W., G. BURGER & B.F. LANG. 1999. Mitochondrial evolution. Science **283:** 1476–1481.
7. BITTNER-EDDY, P., A.F. MONROY & R. BRAMBL. 1994. Expression of mitochondrial genes in the germinating conidia of *Neurospora crassa*. J. Mol. Biol. **235:** 881–897.
8. ADAMS, K.L., D.O. DALEY, Y.-L. QIU, et al. 2000. Repeated, recent and diverse transfers of a mitochondrial gene to the nucleus in flowering plants. Nature **408:** 354–357.
9. PRÖSCHOLD, T., B. MARIN, U.G. SCHLOSSER & M. MELKONIAN. 2001. Molecular phylogeny and taxonomic revision of *Chlamydomonas* (Chlorophyta). I. Emendation of *Chlamydomonas* Ehrenberg and *Chloromonas* Gobi, and description of Oogamochlamys gen. nov. and Lobochlamys gen. nov. Protist **152:** 265–300.
10. VAHRENHOLZ, C., G. RIEMEN, E. PRATJE, et al. 1993. Mitochondrial DNA of *Chlamydomonas reinhardtii*: the structure of the ends of the linear 15.8-kb genome suggests mechanisms for DNA replication. Curr. Genet. **24:** 241–247.
11. DENOVAN-WRIGHT, E.M., A.M. NEDELCU & R.W. LEE. 1998. Complete sequence of the mitochondrial DNA of *Chlamydomonas eugametos*. Plant Mol. Biol. **36:** 285–295.
12. FAN, J. & R.W. LEE. 2002. Mitochondrial genome of the colorless green alga *Polytomella parva*: two linear DNA molecules with homologous inverted repeat termini. Mol. Biol. Evol. **19:** 999–1007.
13. ALLEN, J.F. 2003. The function of genomes in bioenergetic organelles. Philos. Trans. R. Soc. Lond. B Biol. Sci. **358:** 19–37.
14. POPOT, J.-L., & C. DE VITRY. 1990. On the microassembly of integral membrane proteins. Annu. Res. Biophys. Chem. **19:** 369–403.
15. PÉREZ-MARTÍNEZ, X., A. ANTARAMIAN, M. VÁZQUEZ-ACEVEDO, et al. 2001. Subunit II of cytochrome *c* oxidase in Chlamydomonad algae is a heterodimer encoded by two independent nuclear genes. J. Biol. Chem. **276:** 11302–11309.
16. PÉREZ-MARTÍNEZ, X., M. VÁZQUEZ-ACEVEDO, E. TOLKUNOVA, et al. 2000. Unusual location of a mitochondrial gene. Subunit III of cytochrome *c* oxidase is encoded in the nucleus of Chlamydomonad algae. J. Biol. Chem. **275:** 30144–30152.
17. FUNES, S., E. DAVIDSON, M.G. CLAROS, et al. 2002. The typically mitochondrial DNA-encoded ATP6 subunit of the F1F0-ATPase is encoded by a nuclear gene in *Chlamydomonas reinhardtii*. J. Biol. Chem. **277:** 6051–6058.
18. BRENNICKE, A., L. GROHMANN, R. HIESEL, et al. 1993. The mitochondrial genome on its way to the nucleus: different stages of gene transfer in higher plants. FEBS Lett. **325:** 140–145.
19. EMANUELSSON, O. & G. VON HEIJNE. 2001. Prediction of organellar targeting signals. Biochim. Biophys. Acta **1541:** 114–119.

20. GALANIS, M., R.J. DEVENISH & P. NAGLEY. 1991. Duplication of leader sequence for protein targeting to mitochondria leads to increased import efficiency. FEBS Lett. **282:** 425–430.
21. CLAROS, M.G., J. PEREA, Y. SHU, *et al.* 1995. Limitations to *in vivo* import of hydrophobic proteins into yeast mitochondria. The case of a cytoplasmically synthesized apocytochrome *b*. Eur. J. Biochem. **228:** 762–771.
22. CLAROS, M.G., J. PEREA & C. JACQ. 1996. Allotopic expresion of a yeast mitochondrial maturase to study mitochondrial import of hydrophobic proteins. Methods Enzymol. **264:** 389–403.
23. CLAROS, M.G. 1995. MitoProt, a Macintosh application for studying mitochondrial proteins. Comput. Appl. Biosci. **11:** 441–447.
24. CLAROS, M.G. & P. VINCENS. 1996. Computational method to predict mitochondrially imported proteins and their transit peptides. Eur. J. Biochem. **241:** 779–786.
25. ADAMS, K.L., M. ROSENBLUETH, Y.-L. QIU & J.D. PALMER. 2001. Multiple losses and transfers to the nucleus of two mitochondrial succinate dehydrogenase genes during angiosperm evolution. Genetics **158:** 1289–1300.
26. DALEY, D.O., R. CLIFTON, & J. WHELAN. 2002. Intracellular gene transfer: reduced hydrophobicity facilitates gene transfer for subunit 2 of cytochrome *c* oxidase. Proc. Natl. Acad. Sci. USA **99:** 10510–10515.
27. FUNES, S., E. DAVIDSON, A. REYES-PRIETO, *et al.* 2002. A green algal apicoplast ancestor. Science **298:** 2155.
28. MANFREDI, G., J. FU, J.E. SADLOCK, *et al.* 2001. Allotopic expression of human ATPase6 in NARP mutated cells. Mitochondrion **1**(Suppl.1): S24.
29. OJAIMI, J., J. PAN, S. SANTRA, *et al.* 2002. An algal nucleus-encoded subunit of mitochondrial ATP synthase rescues a defect in the analogous human mitochondrial-encoded subunit. Mol. Biol. Cell **13:** 3836–3844.
30. GUY, J., X. QI, F. PALLOTTI, *et al.* 2002. Rescue of a mitochondrial deficiency causing Leber Hereditary Optic Neuropathy. Ann. Neurol. **52:** 534–542.
31. DAVIDSON, E. & M.P. KING. 1997. Advances in human mitochondrial diseases. Trends Cardiovasc. Med. **7:** 16–24.
32. SCHON, E.A. 2000. Mitochondrial genetics and disease. Trends Biochem. Sci. **25:** 555–560.
33. DE GREY, A.D. 2000. Mitochondrial gene therapy: an arena for the biomedical use of inteins. Trends Biotechnol. **18:** 394–399.

Where and When Do Somatic mtDNA Mutations Occur?

KONSTANTIN KHRAPKO, KONSTANTIN EBRALIDSE, AND YEVGENYA KRAYTSBERG

Beth Israel Deaconess Medical Center and Harvard Medical School, Gerontology Division, Boston, Massachusetts 02215, USA

ABSTRACT: It is generally assumed that somatic mtDNA mutations are originally created in the cells where these mutations are currently found. Accumulating data indicate, however, that cells with a particular mtDNA mutation tend to "cluster," that is, occur repeatedly within a given sample, but not in the others. Clusters likely are clonal, which implies that mtDNA mutations do not originate in the cells that currently carry them, but rather in those cells' progenitors, such as stem or satellite cells, or even earlier in the development. Importantly, a majority of mtDNA mutations appear to belong to such clusters, and thus mutational events in progenitor cells may be one of the major sources of mtDNA mutations in healthy aging tissue. More research including the analysis of multiple samples per individual is needed to confirm the existence of clustering and to distinguish between the possible clustering mechanisms.

KEYWORDS: mtDNA mutations; muscle fibers; clusters; somatic; aging

INTRODUCTION

The mitochondrial theory of aging[1,2] postulates that somatic mutations in mitochondrial DNA accumulate with age and cause various intracellular adverse effects that ultimately contribute to some age-related degenerative changes. An interesting question is where and when the actual mutational events take place. Intuitively, it seems reasonable to assume that most mutations originate in the old damaged cells with high ROS levels and poor repair capabilities. However plausible, this hypothesis is not necessarily correct. For example, somatic mtDNA mutations are subject to clonal expansion within various types of cells.[3,4] A founder mutation of a clone should have arisen in the cell in advance to give the expansion process enough time to proceed. Although the rates of expansion are unknown, expansion may take as long as many years, an estimation based on the time necessary for certain diseases caused by mtDNA mutations to develop. In other words, the founder mutations of clonal expansions currently observed in a tissue might have arisen years earlier in cells that had been much younger at that time.

Address for correspondence: Konstantin Khrapko, Gerontology Division, Beth Israel Deaconess Medical Center and Harvard Medical School, Burlington Ave. 21–27, Room 554E, Boston, MA 02215. Voice: 617-632-0334; fax: 509-693-7397.
khrapko@hms.harvard.edu

We hypothesized elsewhere[5] that a large proportion of somatic mtDNA mutations in nonpathological aging tissue may belong to clonal expansions that are not limited to individual cells, but rather span different scales from small clusters of mutant cells to the whole organism depending on how early the founder mutation arises. For example, a mutation in the oocyte has a chance to be seeded throughout different tissues, while a mutation in a stem cell will result in a fully mutant turnover unit based on such a stem cell. Interestingly, a few recent reports appear to require such a hypothesis to explain the observed distributions of mutations.

CELLS WITH mtDNA MUTATIONS ARE CLUSTERED BY THE KIND OF MUTATION

Two groups have recently reported that muscle fibers carrying mtDNA individually rare mutations appear to "cluster" in different individuals by the kind of mutation.[6,7] In other words, a sample from one individual may contain multiple fibers containing a particular mutation, while samples from many other individuals do not contain such a mutation at all. In one study,[6] a total of 218 muscle fibers collected from biopsy samples of 14 different individuals were screened for mutations in selected coding regions of the mitochondrial genome: 17 mutant fibers were found, with 1 clonally expanded mutation per fiber, as expected. Some fibers contained the same type of mutation; interestingly, in all but 1 case, fibers sharing the same mutation originated from the same sample. Specifically, of 17 mutant fibers, a group of 4, a group of 3, and two pairs of fibers each shared the sample of origin as well as a mutation in common (both point mutations and large deletions were involved). One more mutation was a part of 10% heteroplasmy. Another paper[7] reports a study of only 24 fibers from 4 people; however, about 30 individual mtDNA molecules per fiber were sequenced within a portion of the control region. Similarly, 42 different mutations were observed in more than one fiber, but in all cases the fibers carrying the same mutation were from the same individual (with the exception of a few high-incidence mutations, which apparently are also subject to clustering, as discussed below).

It is worth emphasizing that clustered mutant cells not only exist, but they are apparently responsible for a majority of mtDNA mutations in a tissue. In the first report,[6] 12 of 17 mutant fibers belong to clusters. It seems most likely that clustered mutations described in the second report[7] also represent a majority of mutations in the tissue, although primary data are not available. The two studies deal with two different classes of mutations. Fayet et al.[6] scored mutations in the coding regions, which most likely caused mitochondrial function defects in the fibers where they were clonally expanded. Mutations scored by Del Bo et al.[7] are located in the control region and are unlikely to be directly related to mitochondrial function. Thus, clustering of mutant cells is independent of the functional relevance of the mutation.

A few other studies, of human brain,[8] heart,[9,10] and murine liver,[11] also hint that cells with mtDNA mutations may be clustered. In these studies, individually rare mutations appear multiple times in particular individuals, although lack of cell-by-cell analysis or insufficient number of cases/mutations makes them less convincing than the two above referenced recent papers. Another group of studies concerned with high-incidence mutations (which thus are found in many individuals) demonstrate significant variation of the fraction of these mutations from individual to individual,[12–15] which may represent a phenomenon closely related to clustering of the low-frequency mutations.

MECHANISMS OF CLUSTERING

One possible explanation of the person-specific clustering could be that every person with a "cluster" of cells with identical mutations has a genetic predisposition for generating or selecting mutations of that particular kind, or has been exposed to a very specific external mutagen. However, in this case, every kind of clustered mutation would require a specific defective biochemical pathway (responsible either for creating or for failing to repair the particular mutation) or a specific environmental mutagen as an explanation. However, the number of different kinds of mutations that happen to be in the clusters is quite large. In other words, one would need to assume that people commonly carry "mutator" genotypes of one of many types or are often significantly exposed to one of many environmental mutagens. Linkage analysis of multiple mutations also argues against this mechanism at least in one case.[5]

An alternative hypothesis that clusters are clones seems more plausible. In this interpretation, the mutations in a cluster are assumed to originate from a single mutational event, which therefore should have happened in a precursor cell that gave rise to all the mutant cells in the cluster. Apparently, precursor cells may be of the "early" or "late" type. Tissues other than muscle provide ample examples of what could be called late precursors, that is, those that arise after development is largely completed. Solid tumors frequently contain almost homoplasmic somatic mtDNA mutations.[16,17] Such tumors are essentially huge clusters of cells with an mtDNA mutation that they inherited from the tumor precursor cell that was homoplasmic for the mtDNA mutation.[18] Similarly, a relatively high proportion of crypts in the aged human colon will be entirely composed of cells with mtDNA mutations, apparently because stem cells feeding these crypts carry homoplasmic mtDNA mutations.[19] Sporadic mitochondrial disease is an example of "early" precursors carrying mtDNA mutations, which apparently are cells involved in forming of multiple organs or at least the whole organs.[20,21]

It would be interesting to determine which type of precursor is responsible for clusters of mutant fibers observed in muscle. The expected difference between the late and the early precursors is the size of the clusters they produce. Late precursors, that is, resident satellite cells, are expected to produce local clusters. The expected size of such clusters is on the order of a millimeter, as suggested by recent muscle grafting experiments.[22] Apparently, satellite cells are capable of migrating over millimeter distances, leaving a patchy pattern of daughter fiber segments on their way. The clusters of mutant fibers created in this way could look like low-density distributions, potentially not inconsistent with the observed distribution of mutant fibers in real tissue. In contrast, early mutant precursors should seed mutant cells throughout a tissue or the whole organism (also at low density) since the development of muscle involves significant intermingling of the progeny of muscle precursor cells.[23]

To distinguish between the late and the early origin of clusters, it is necessary to explore the distribution of mutant cells at distances exceeding the expected size of local clusters in muscle. Unfortunately, most studies include only a single biopsy per person, and a series of sequential sections is analyzed, which does not permit distinguishing between the two types of mechanisms. Even probing different portions of the same biopsy sample might be helpful in this respect, as well as information regarding spatial distribution of mutant fibers.

CONCLUDING REMARKS

An idea that mtDNA mutations originate mostly in the precursors of the cells that carry the mutations currently appears to explain the clustered distribution of cells with mtDNA mutations in muscle, although it remains no more than a testable hypothesis. It is not clear how early most of the mutations are normally acquired. If mutations had arisen in recent precursors, the clusters of mutant fibers are expected to be local, although not necessarily compact. If mutations had arisen in early precursors, mutant fibers should be distributed throughout muscle tissue. This latter possibility deserves a few additional comments.

First, it appears that the border between the origin and distribution of mtDNA mutations in case of sporadic mtDNA disease and normal aging becomes blurred. One may expect every shade of gray, from dense distribution of cells with high percentage of pathogenic mutation to a loose distribution of cells with low fraction of benign mutation. There thus should exist borderline cases (apparently much more frequent that mtDNA disease) where phenotype is subclinical. Such cases have a potential to explain subtle age-related phenomena like frailty. Second, the ideas of early origin of mtDNA mutations find an analogy in recent hypotheses regarding early origin of somatic mutations in nuclear DNA,[24] as well as the high initial damage load hypothesis advocated by the Gavrilovs,[25] which is featured elsewhere in this volume. Finally, clonality of mtDNA mutations implies that it may be difficult to find correlation between mtDNA mutational load and certain end points (like post-ischemic recovery) unless one knows which mutations should be sought for in a particular individual. A blind approach involving the use of standard marker mutations, for example, common deletion, may be inefficient. This potentially may help to explain the poor correlation between the abundance common deletion and post-ischemic recovery reported elsewhere in this issue (see Gavrilov & Gavrilova[25] and Rosenfeldt et al.[26]).

ACKNOWLEDGMENTS

We are grateful to Aubrey de Grey for stimulating discussions. This work was supported in part by NIH Grant Nos. ES 11343 and AG 19787.

REFERENCES

1. HARMAN, D. 1972. The biologic clock: the mitochondria? J. Am. Geriatr. Soc. **20**(4): 145–147.
2. LINNANE, A.W. et al. 1989. Mitochondrial DNA mutations as an important contributor to ageing and degenerative diseases. Lancet **1**(8639): 642–645.

3. MULLER-HOCKER, J. *et al.* 1993. Different *in situ* hybridization patterns of mitochondrial DNA in cytochrome *c* oxidase–deficient extraocular muscle fibres in the elderly. Virchows Arch. A Pathol. Anat. Histopathol. **422:** 7–15.
4. NEKHAEVA, E. *et al.* 2002. Clonally expanded mtDNA point mutations are abundant in individual cells of human tissues. Proc. Natl. Acad. Sci. USA **99**(8): 5521–5526.
5. KHRAPKO, K. *et al.* 2003. Clonal expansions of mitochondrial genomes: implications for *in vivo* mutational spectra. Mutat. Res. **522**(1–2): 13–19.
6. FAYET, G. *et al.* 2002. Ageing muscle: clonal expansions of mitochondrial DNA point mutations and deletions cause focal impairment of mitochondrial function. Neuromuscul. Disord. **12**(5): 484–493.
7. DEL BO, R. *et al.* 2003. High mutational burden in the mtDNA control region from aged muscles: a single-fiber study. Neurobiol. Aging **24**(6): 829–838.
8. JAZIN, E.E. *et al.* 1996. Human brain contains high levels of heteroplasmy in the noncoding regions of mitochondrial DNA. Proc. Natl. Acad. Sci. USA **93**(22): 12382–12387.
9. KAJANDER, O.A. *et al.* 2000. Human mtDNA sublimons resemble rearranged mitochondrial genomes found in pathological states. Hum. Mol. Genet. **9**(19): 2821–2835.
10. BODYAK, N.D. *et al.* 2001. Quantification and sequencing of somatic deleted mtDNA in single cells: evidence for partially duplicated mtDNA in aged human tissues. Hum. Mol. Genet. **10**(1): 17–24.
11. KHAIDAKOV, M. *et al.* 2003. Accumulation of point mutations in mitochondrial DNA of aging mice. Mutat. Res. **526**(1–2): 1–7.
12. MICHIKAWA, Y. *et al.* 1999. Aging-dependent large accumulation of point mutations in the human mtDNA control region for replication [see comments]. Science **286**(5440): 774–779.
13. CALLOWAY, C.D. *et al.* 2000. The frequency of heteroplasmy in the HVII region of mtDNA differs across tissue types and increases with age. Am. J. Hum. Genet. **66**(4): 1384–1397.
14. WANG, Y. *et al.* 2001. Muscle-specific mutations accumulate with aging in critical human mtDNA control sites for replication. Proc. Natl. Acad. Sci. USA **98**(7): 4022–4027.
15. ZHANG, J. *et al.* 2003. Strikingly higher frequency in centenarians and twins of mtDNA mutation causing remodeling of replication origin in leukocytes. Proc. Natl. Acad. Sci. USA **100**(3): 1116–1121.
16. POLYAK, K. *et al.* 1998. Somatic mutations of the mitochondrial genome in human colorectal tumors. Nat. Genet. **20**(3): 291–293.
17. HABANO, W., S. NAKAMURA & T. SUGAI. 1998. Microsatellite instability in the mitochondrial DNA of colorectal carcinomas: evidence for mismatch repair systems in mitochondrial genome. Oncogene **17**(15): 1931–1937.
18. COLLER, H.A. *et al.* 2001. High frequency of homoplasmic mitochondrial DNA mutations in human tumors can be explained without selection. Nat. Genet. **28**(2): 147–150.
19. TAYLOR, R.W. *et al.* 2003. Mitochondrial DNA mutations in human colonic crypt stem cells. J. Clin. Invest. **112**(9): 1351–1360.
20. ZEVIANI, M. *et al.* 1990. Tissue distribution and transmission of mitochondrial DNA deletions in mitochondrial myopathies. Ann. Neurol. **28**(1): 94–97.
21. MARZUKI, S. *et al.* 1997. Developmental genetics of deleted mtDNA in mitochondrial oculomyopathy. J. Neurol. Sci. **145**(2): 155–162.
22. JOCKUSCH, H. & S. VOIGT. 2003. Migration of adult myogenic precursor cells as revealed by GFP/nLacZ labelling of mouse transplantation chimeras. J. Cell Sci. **116**(part 8): 1611–1616.
23. TAJBAKHSH, S. 2003. Stem cells to tissue: molecular, cellular, and anatomical heterogeneity in skeletal muscle. Curr. Opin. Genet. Dev. **13**(4): 413–422.
24. FRANK, S.A. & M.A. NOWAK. 2003. Cell biology: developmental predisposition to cancer. Nature **422**(6931): 494.
25. GAVRILOV, L.A. & N.S. GAVRILOVA. 2004. Early-life programming of aging and longevity: The idea of high initial damage load (the HIDL hypothesis). Ann N.Y. Acad. Sci. **1019:** 496–501.
26. ROSENFELDT, F., F. MILLER, P. NAGLEY, *et al.* 2004. Response of the senescent heart to stress: Clinical therapeutic strategies and quest for mitochondrial predictors of biological age. Ann. N.Y. Acad. Sci. **1019:** 78–84.

Genomic Instability, Aging, and Cellular Senescence

RITA A. BUSUTTIL,[a] MARTIJN DOLLÉ,[a] JUDITH CAMPISI,[b] AND JAN VIJG[a,c]

[a]*Sam and Ann Barshop Center for Longevity and Aging Studies, University of Texas Health Science Center, San Antonio, Texas 78245, USA*

[b]*Life Sciences Division, Lawrence Berkeley National Laboratory, Berkeley, California 94720, USA, and Buck Institute for Age Research, Novato, California 94945, USA*

[c]*Geriatric Research Education and Clinical Center, South Texas Veterans Health Care System, San Antonio, Texas 78229, USA*

> ABSTRACT: Aging can be defined in practical terms as a series of time-related processes that ultimately bring life to a close. Genomic instability has been implicated as a major causal factor in aging. Here, we describe the use of a transgenic mouse model, harboring lacZ reporter genes as part of a plasmid construct integrated at one or more chromosomal locations, to study genomic instability during aging of different mouse organs and tissues as well as in mouse embryonic fibroblasts during primary culture.
>
> KEYWORDS: aging; cancer; oxidative damage; DNA damage; genomic integrity

INTRODUCTION

Aging is a multifactorial process that results in a decline in the fitness of adult organisms, ultimately leading to death. The free radical theory of aging, first proposed by Harman,[1] suggests that aging may be due to the accumulation of macromolecular damage in somatic cells as a result of free radical attack. Reactive oxygen species (ROS) are primarily formed in the mitochondria as a by-product of oxidative phosphorylation. To neutralize the potentially harmful effects of ROS to DNA, virtually all cells possess antioxidant defense mechanisms. However, when ROS production exceeds the capabilities of the antioxidant defenses, cells experience oxidative stress.[2] Oxidative stress results in deleteriously high free radical levels. One consequence of oxidative stress is DNA damage, which, through erroneous repair or replication, can be converted into mutations. Loss of genomic integrity as a consequence of the continuous induction of mutations in the nuclear genome has been considered as a major causal factor in cancer and other forms of age-related cellular degeneration and death.[3,4]

Address for correspondence: Jan Vijg, Sam and Ann Barshop Center for Longevity and Aging Studies, University of Texas Health Science Center, San Antonio, TX 78245. Voice: 210-562-5027; fax: 210-562-5028.
   vijg@uthscsa.edu

AGING *IN VIVO* AND IN CULTURE

Aging has been described as primarily due to cellular functional decline, structural deterioration, and ultimately death. In this respect, it is reasonable to use cell culture models to study basic mechanisms of age-related cellular degeneration. Indeed, Hayflick and Moorhead proposed that aging of an organism could be mimicked to some extent by passaging normal animal cells in culture. They were the first to describe the phenomenon that is now widely termed replicative senescence whereby normal human somatic cells, most notably fibroblasts, can be shown to have only a limited proliferative capacity in culture.[5] Rather than a gradual process of cellular degeneration, it is now clear that senescence is a programmed response to cellular distress and, similar to the apoptosis response, a major defense mechanism against cancer.[6]

In the absence of telomerase, an enzyme that can add telomeric repeats to the telomere ends, telomere shortening has been implicated as the primary cause of replicative senescence in human cells.[6] However, telomere shortening leads to genomic instability and the possibility cannot be ruled out that the senescence response is induced simply by a general loss of genome integrity. Indeed, in the presence of long telomeres, clastogenic agents, such as ionizing radiation, hydrogen peroxide, and mitomycin C, readily induce senescence.[6] Such agents predominantly induce genome rearrangements, which may be the signal that causes the senescence response. The involvement of genomic instability in senescence is supported by the observation that cells of individuals who suffer from Werner syndrome, a premature aging syndrome caused by a heritable mutation in the WRN gene, accumulate chromosomal translocations and large deletions at an extremely high frequency and also undergo senescence earlier than normal adult human fibroblast cells.[7]

Irrespective of its mechanism(s) of induction, it is conceivable that senescence-associated irreversible cell cycle arrest is a major component of the aging process as this occurs *in vivo*.[6]

In contrast to senescence of human cells in culture, senescence of mouse cells takes place independently of telomere shortening. Mouse cells have considerably longer telomeres than human cells and they also constitutively express telomerase. Replicative senescence in mouse cells occurs due to the oxidative stress of standard culture conditions, to which mouse cells appear much more sensitive than human cells.[8] Oxidative stress has also been associated with telomere shortening and human cells undergo senescence more quickly in the presence of oxidative stress.[9] This is in keeping with the observation that human cells cultured in 2–3% O_2, rather than the 20% O_2 of most normal culture conditions, undergo 20–50% more population doublings before exhibiting senescence.[10–14] Mouse cells do not undergo senescence at all in 3% O_2,[8] but readily undergo senescence and subsequent immortalization at 20% O_2.

MODELS FOR STUDYING GENOMIC INSTABILITY *IN VIVO* AND *IN VITRO*

Testing the hypothesis that aging is associated with a general loss of genome integrity has been severely hampered by the lack of methods to quantify and characterize mutations in various organs and tissues of humans or experimental animals. In contrast to DNA damage, DNA mutations are irreversible and cannot be repaired in any other way than through the elimination of the cell. Initially, only large chromosomal changes could be demonstrated by cytogenetic means in peripheral blood lymphocytes or other actively proliferating cells. After the introduction of the HPRT method and several other methods based on selectable target genes, an accumulation of a wider range of mutations was demonstrated, but still mainly in peripheral blood lymphocytes. Interesting exceptions are the early work of Curtis and co-workers, who demonstrated an age-related increase of chromosomal mutations in mouse liver hepatocytes,[15] and Martin and co-workers, who showed an age-related increase of mutations at the HPRT locus in human kidney cells.[16] For both mouse liver and human kidney, the reported mutation frequencies were far higher than generally reported for peripheral blood lymphocytes or splenocytes. This can be explained by a relatively high level of apoptosis in actively proliferating lymphocytes and/or an age-related decrease in apoptosis in liver, evidence for which has been obtained.[17] Interestingly, in human and mouse lymphocytes, the frequency of chromosomal aberrations,[18,19] as well as mutations at the HPRT locus,[20,21] increases with age at about the same rate, as a function of their life span rather than chronological time. This suggests that the accumulation of mutations with age is related to the rate of aging and could be a function of the repair phenotype of the species, as originally predicted by work from Hart and Setlow.[22] Indeed, mutation accumulation at HPRT has been found to accelerate in a mouse model of premature aging[23] and decelerate in calorically restricted mice.[21]

The results described above on genomic instability and aging have been interpreted with caution in view of the fact that the assays used could only be applied to actively proliferating cells. This offers a poor reflection of the *in vivo* system where the majority of adult human and animal cells only rarely undergo cell division. In order to extend these studies to the *in vivo* situation, we have developed transgenic mouse models harboring chromosomally integrated bacterial mutation reporter genes, which can be recovered from their integrated state, transferred to *E. coli*, and then analyzed for mutations.[24] One of these models, based on plasmids containing the lacZ reporter gene, has made it possible to quantify and characterize a wide range of somatic mutations (including large genome rearrangements) in a neutral gene as the animals age and/or develop cancer (see FIG. 1).[24–26] Using these mice, we have demonstrated that mutation frequencies at the lacZ locus accumulate with age in most organs and tissues, albeit at greatly different rates (see FIG. 2A).[26–28] Other investigators have now confirmed these results.[29]

Mutations in the lacZ reporter mouse model can be characterized by restriction digestion and/or sequencing of the positively selected lacZ-mutant plasmids recovered from a mouse tissue.[30] Mutations that do not alter the restriction pattern are considered to be point mutations. Mutations that cause changes in the restriction pattern appeared to be mostly genome rearrangements, that is, deletion, inversion, or translocation events with one breakpoint in a lacZ gene of the plasmid cluster and one breakpoint elsewhere in the mouse genome. Only few mutations were found to be internal deletions, and a transposition of a mouse sequence in a lacZ gene has never been observed.[31] Physical characterization of 49 genome rearrangement mutations, mainly from heart and liver of young and old mice, indicated intrachromosomal deletions or inversions, varying from smaller than 100 kb to 66 Mb, as well as translocation events.[32]

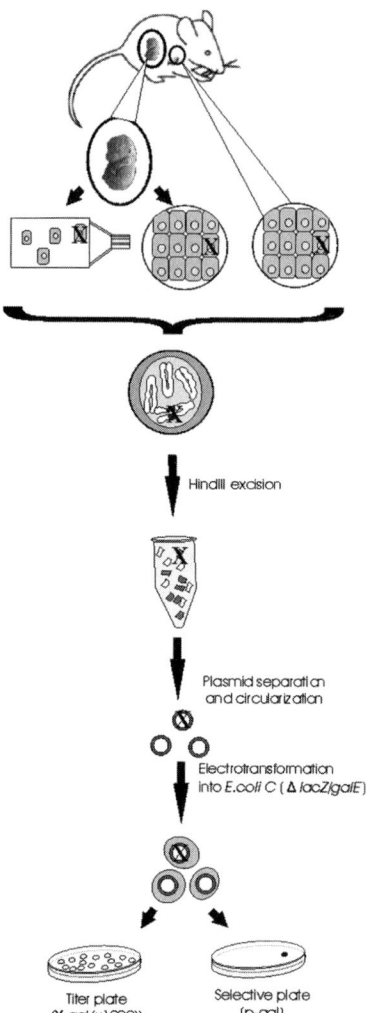

FIGURE 1. Strategy for determining mutation frequency and spectra using transgenic mice carrying integrated lacZ mutation reporter plasmids. A threefold comparison was made, that is, among young adult tissue, embryonic tissue, and first-passage cells isolated from the embryo. After DNA extraction, plasmids (*dark gray areas*), both wild-type and those containing a mutation (X), were excised from genomic DNA with HindIII, followed by their separation from the mouse genomic DNA using magnetic beads, precoated with a lacI repressor protein.[27] The plasmids were then ligated and transferred into *E. coli* C (ΔlacZ, galE$^-$) using electrotransformation. A small amount of transformants were plated on X-gal to determine the total number of recovered plasmids. The remainder was plated on medium containing the lactose analogue, p-gal, to select only those cells harboring a mutation in the lacZ gene. The mutation frequency is the ratio of the colonies on the selective plates versus the colonies on the titer plate (times the dilution factor).

Striking organ specificity with respect to the mutational spectra in aged animals has been observed. In the liver and heart, a considerable fraction of mutations that accumulated with age were the result of large genome rearrangements, including deletions of up to 66 Mb, whereby point mutations in the small intestine and brain were a prominent part of the spectrum.[26,28] Such large chromosomal mutations are likely to adversely affect cell functioning, for example, through partial haploidization or position effects.[31] By extrapolation from the lacZ-plasmid cluster to the entire diploid genome, we have estimated the total load of genome rearrangement mutations in several organs at young and old age. TABLE 1 shows the total mutation frequencies, the frequencies of genome rearrangements, and the load of genome rearrangements per diploid genome for heart and liver.

TABLE 1. Load of genome rearrangements (rearr.) per diploid genome

Organ	Age (months)	LacZ mutant frequency ($\times 10^{-5}$)		Genome rearr. per cell	P
		Total	Genome rearr.		
Liver	4	3.1 ± 0.3	0.9 ± 0.2	9	.014
	32	10.5 ± 2.4	2.7 ± 1.0	27	
Heart	4	4.1 ± 1.4	1.9 ± 0.8	19	.0262
	32	10.1 ± 2.7	3.7 ± 2.0	37	

While the origin of age-related mutations has not yet been determined, it is tempting to speculate that they result from the accumulated effects of endogenous oxidative stress to which these and all aerobic organisms are subject. Indeed, when fibroblasts were isolated from a 14-day-old embryo derived from a mouse harboring the lacZ transgene and brought into culture (FIG. 1), these cells displayed a 3-fold increase in mutation frequency over the embryo tissue from which they were derived (FIG. 2B). Such high spontaneous mutation frequencies are typically only found at old age (FIG. 2B). Most of these mutations were genomic rearrangements and it is reasonable to assume that the rapid mutation accumulation observed during transfer into primary culture is the result of high oxygen tension (typically 20%) associated with standard culture conditions.[33] Oxygen has been demonstrated to induce chromosomal instability.[34] Mammalian tissues generally exist in oxygen (O_2) concentrations ranging from 2% to 8%,[35] well below the atmospheric oxygen level of 20%. However, a similar increase in mutation frequency upon transfer of MEFs in primary culture was found when immediately upon isolation the cells were placed at low oxygen, that is, 3%. In this respect, it is possible that oxygenation during the cell isolation procedure already introduced enough oxidative DNA damage to reach the highest possible level of genome rearrangements compatible with survival.[33]

Also during aging *in vivo*, some tissues showed a significant accumulation of large genome rearrangements,[27] while others predominantly accumulated point mutations. With respect to the latter, it occurred to us that the lacZ point mutational spectra of tissues at old age might reveal signature mutations of oxidative DNA damage, most notably the GC to TA transversion mutation characteristic of 8-oxoguanine, a most frequent form of oxidative DNA damage.[36] While initially, at young age, the types of point mutations were more or less the same, during aging they started to diverge significantly. For example, while in the heart only GC to AT base-pair substitutions at CpG sites were found to accumulate, liver and small intestine showed a more varied pattern (FIG. 2C).[27,28] However, GC to TA transversions, the signature mutation of 8-oxoguanine, were not found to accumulate in heart and only marginally in liver or small intestine.

We then investigated a possible parallel between aging *in vivo* and *in vitro*. Parrinello *et al.* recently showed that primary mouse fibroblasts cultured in 20% O_2 accumulate oxidative DNA damage and undergo senescence owing to severe oxidative stress, and that spontaneous immortalization (which rarely, if ever, occurs in human cells) permits the cells to proliferate despite the damage.[8]

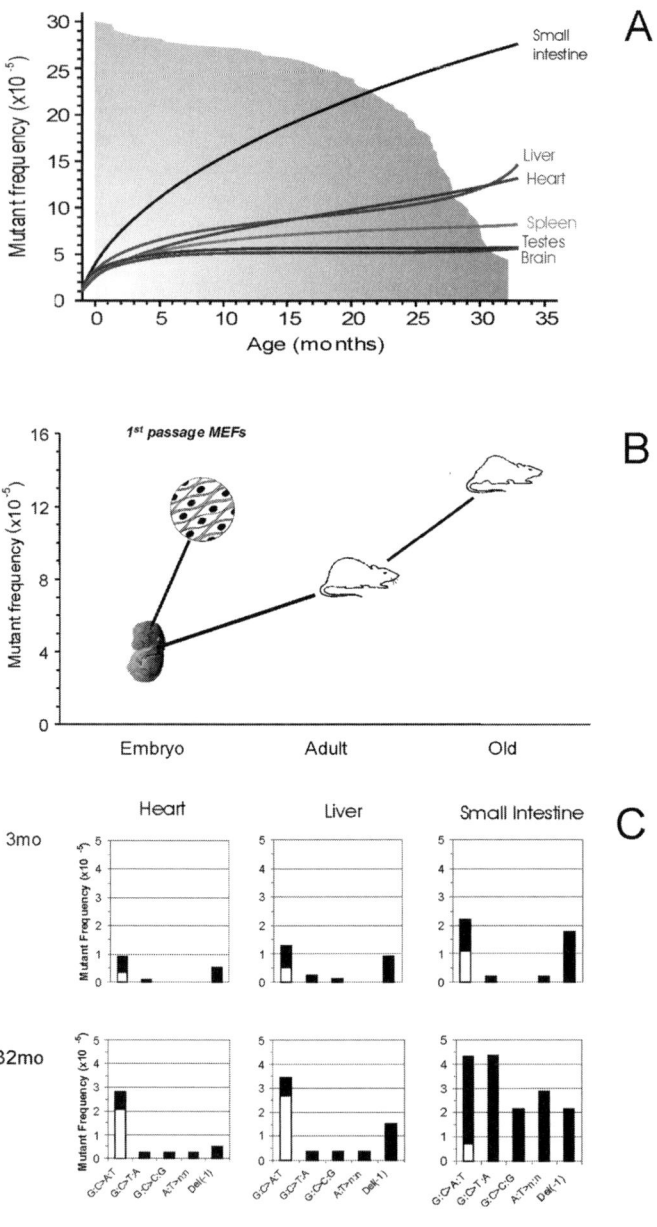

FIGURE 2. *See following page for legend.*

To investigate the possibility of further mutation accumulation at the lacZ locus in the mouse embryonic fibroblasts after their first passage in culture, we studied these cells under ambient (20%) or *in vivo* (3%) oxygen tensions over a series of population doublings. The results indicated a striking further increase in the mutation frequency (on top of the increase in mutation frequency associated with the transfer of cells into primary culture as discussed above) during continued passaging, but only at 20% oxygen (FIG. 3A). This time, the increase was almost entirely due to point mutations, which may be easier to tolerate by the cells than additional genome rearrangements.[33] Sequence characterization of the point mutations that accumulated in MEFs at 20% oxygen demonstrated that they were due to GC to TA transversions (FIG. 3B), the signature mutation of 8-oxoguanine.[37] This demonstrates that GC to TA transversions as a most likely consequence of 8-oxoguanine lesions can be readily detected by the lacZ reporter gene system, but require high levels of oxygen to be induced in substantial numbers.

DISCUSSION

Using a lacZ mutation reporter gene present as a transgenic construct in the mouse genome, we have monitored levels of genomic instability during aging of different organs and tissues *in vivo* and during transfer of mouse embryonic fibroblasts into primary culture followed by continuous passaging at high and low oxygen tension. The results indicate that both *in vivo* aging and *in vitro* aging are associated with increased mutation frequencies, likely as a consequence of oxidative stress. At the high oxygen tension of 20%, which is standard for most culture conditions, mutations were found to accumulate in late-passage cells, most of which could be identified as the GC to TA signature mutation of 8-oxoguanine. At the more physiological level of 3% oxygen, this mutation was almost completely lacking (FIG. 3B), which confirms the results with *in vivo* aged tissues in which this mutation was also absent. Nevertheless, immediately upon transfer into culture, mouse embryonic fibroblasts showed a 2- to 3-fold increase in mutation frequency, which was observed at both 3% and 20% oxygen. Since cells were isolated under atmospheric oxygen, the possibility cannot be ruled out that this temporary exposure was wholly responsible for the observed mutation accumulation. Nevertheless, it is striking that mostly genome rearrangements, not GC to TA transversions, were found to accumulate, which is similar to the results observed for the aging heart and liver *in vivo*. Hence, it is possible that oxidative stress, even at physiological levels, primarily induces genome rearrangement type of events and that GC to TA transversion mutations are strictly associated with very high oxygen tensions.

FIGURE 2. (A) Spontaneous lacZ mutant frequencies with age in various tissues of lacZ line 60 transgenic mice. The *gray faded area* represents the survival curve of the mice (see also Ref. 31). **(B)** Schematic representation of the possible parallels between aging in culture versus aging *in vivo*. The average increase in mutation frequencies of mouse tissues with age is compared to the increase in mutation frequency of mouse embryonic fibroblasts (MEFs) placed immediately into culture. **(C)** Point mutational spectra of heart, liver, and small intestine of young (3 months) and old (32 months) line 60 mice. The *white areas* in the GC to AT bars indicate the fraction of these mutations that occurred at CpG sites.

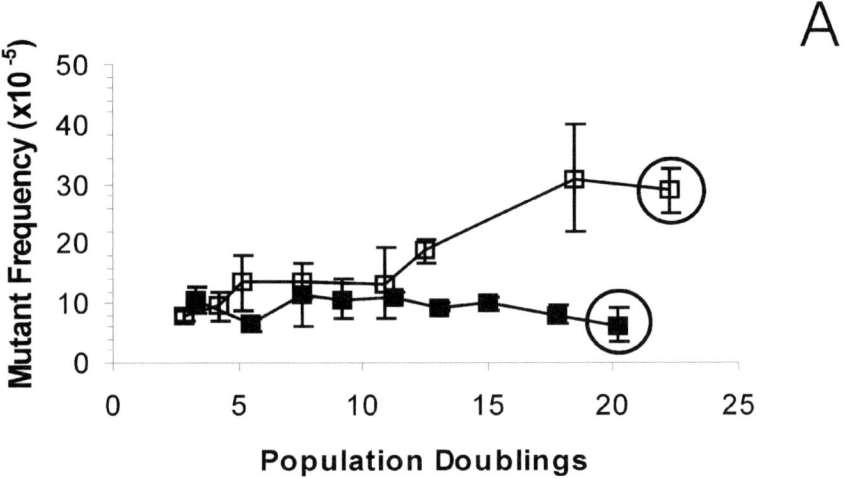

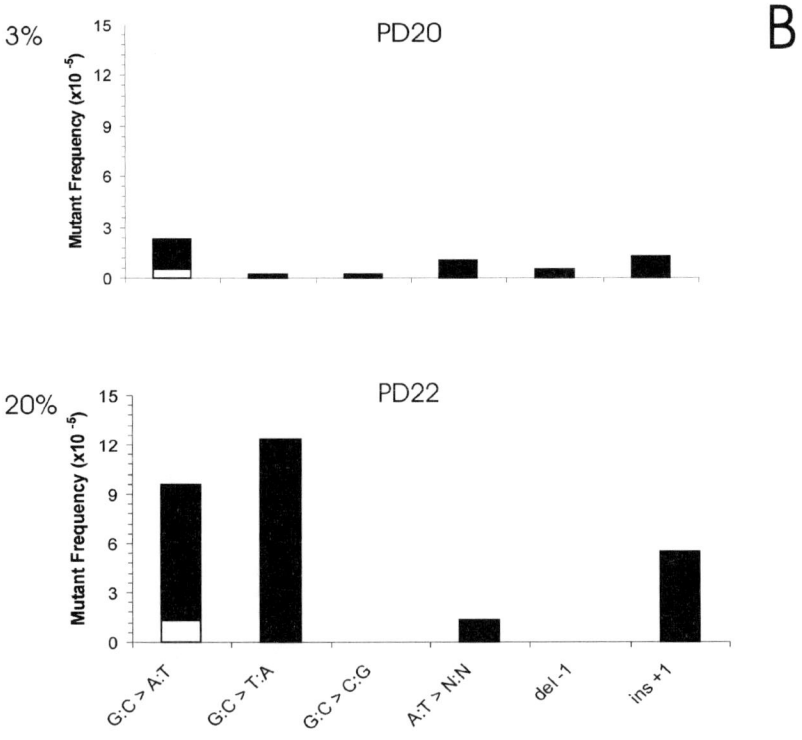

FIGURE 3. *See following page for legend.*

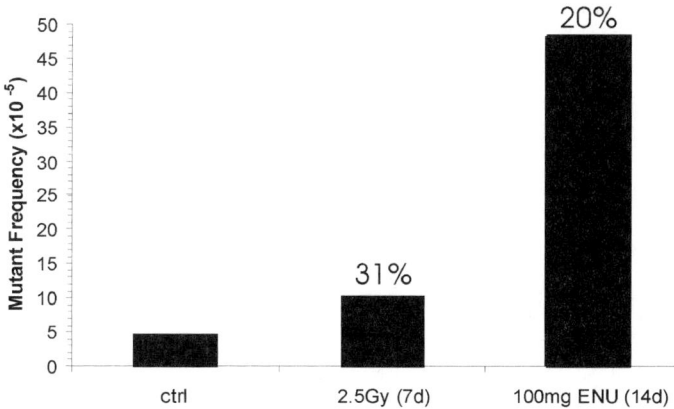

FIGURE 4. Mutation induction in spleen of lacZ-plasmid transgenic mice by about equally toxic doses of ionizing radiation or ethyl nitrosourea (ENU). The percentage of the LD_{50} is indicated above each mutation induction column.

Genome rearrangements are more toxic than point mutations. This is indicated, for example, by the much lower number of mutations induced by clastogens, such as ionizing radiation, than agents such as ENU, at doses of similar toxicity (FIG. 4). Hence, in actively proliferating cells, it is possible that only a limited number of such mutations can be tolerated, which could explain our observation that, during further passaging, eventually only point mutations, that is, GC to TA transversions, accumulate. The effect of genome rearrangements *in vivo* in postmitotic tissues such as heart could also have serious adverse effects. Indeed, the large deletions, involving millions of base pairs, that we found to accumulate in the aging heart could cause partial haploinsufficiency of large numbers of genes. Such gene dose effects could directly affect cellular functions, as well as indirectly, through transcription factors failing to activate target genes at insufficient levels of expression. Chromosomal translocations could adversely affect cell function by causing gene regulatory changes due to position effects.

Based on these results, it is conceivable that cellular degeneration as a consequence of the accumulation of large genome rearrangements is a major component of the aging process. In a cell culture model at 20% oxygen, this would readily induce senescence and/or apoptosis responses, with mouse cells more vulnerable than human cells, possibly as a consequence of inferior genome maintenance systems. At low oxygen, such acute responses may not readily occur and, instead, a more gradual accumulation of mutations might ensue. In the *in vivo* situation, in postmitotic tissues,

FIGURE 3. The effects of oxygen tension on proliferating MEFs. (**A**) LacZ mutation frequencies at 3% and 20% oxygen as a function of population doubling level. (**B**) Point mutational spectra of MEFs cultured in 20% or 3% oxygen. MEFs at the population doubling levels indicated by circles in **A** were harvested, and recovered plasmids were sequenced. The white areas in the GC to AT bars indicate the fraction of these mutations that occurred at CpG sites.

this may lead to diminished cell functioning due to adverse effects of the randomly induced large genome rearrangements on normal patterns of gene expression. In the cell culture model or in actively proliferating tissues *in vivo*, the gradual accumulation of such events may increase susceptibility to immortalization and transformation.

REFERENCES

1. HARMAN, D. 1956. Aging: a theory based on free radical and radiation chemistry. J. Gerontol. **11**: 298–300.
2. CADENAS, E. *et al.* 1982. Active oxygen metabolites and their action in the hepatocyte: studies on chemiluminescence responses and alkane production. Agents Actions Suppl. **11**: 203–216.
3. FAILLA, G. 1958. The aging process and cancerogenesis. Ann. N.Y. Acad. Sci. **71**: 1124–1140.
4. SZILARD, L. 1959. On the nature of the aging process. Proc. Natl. Acad. Sci. USA **45**: 30–45.
5. HAYFLICK, L. & P.S. MOORHEAD. 1961. The serial cultivation of human diploid cell strains. Exp. Cell Res. **25**: 585–621.
6. CAMPISI, J. 2003. Cancer and ageing: rival demons? Nat. Rev. Cancer **3**: 339–349.
7. KASHINO, G. *et al.* 2003. Relief of oxidative stress by ascorbic acid delays cellular senescence of normal human and Werner syndrome fibroblast cells. Free Radical Biol. Med. **35**: 438–443.
8. PARRINELLO, S. *et al.* 2003. Oxygen sensitivity severely limits the replicative life span of murine fibroblasts. Nat. Cell. Biol. **5**: 741–747.
9. VON ZGLINICKI, T. *et al.* 1995. Mild hyperoxia shortens telomeres and inhibits proliferation of fibroblasts: a model for senescence? Exp. Cell Res. **220**: 186–193.
10. CHEN, Q. *et al.* 1995. Oxidative DNA damage and senescence of human diploid fibroblast cells. Proc. Natl. Acad. Sci. USA **92**: 4337–4341.
11. BALIN, A.K., A.J. FISHER & D.M. CARTER. 1984. Oxygen modulates growth of human cells at physiologic partial pressures. J. Exp. Med. **160**: 152–166.
12. SAITO, H., A.T. HAMMOND & R.E. MOSES. 1995. The effect of low oxygen tension on the *in vitro*–replicative life span of human diploid fibroblast cells and their transformed derivatives. Exp. Cell Res. **217**: 272–279.
13. PACKER, L. & K. FUEHR. 1977. Low oxygen concentration extends the life span of cultured human diploid cells. Nature **267**: 423–425.
14. SHIGENAGA, M.K. & B.N. AMES. 1991. Assays for 8-hydroxy-2′-deoxyguanosine: a biomarker of *in vivo* oxidative DNA damage. Free Radical Biol. Med. **10**: 211–216.
15. CURTIS, H. & C. CROWLEY. 1963. Chromosome aberrations in liver cells in relation to the somatic theory of aging. Radiat. Res. **19**: 337–344.
16. MARTIN, G.M. *et al.* 1996. Somatic mutations are frequent and increase with age in human kidney epithelial cells. Hum. Mol. Genet. **5**: 215–221.
17. SUH, Y. *et al.* 2002. Aging alters the apoptotic response to genotoxic stress. Nat. Med. **8**: 3–4.
18. RAMSEY, M.J. *et al.* 1995. The effects of age and lifestyle factors on the accumulation of cytogenetic damage as measured by chromosome painting. Mutat. Res. **338**: 95–106.
19. TUCKER, J.D. *et al.* 1999. Frequency of spontaneous chromosome aberrations in mice: effects of age. Mutat. Res. **425**: 135–141.
20. JONES, I.M. *et al.* 1995. Impact of age and environment on somatic mutation at the hprt gene of T lymphocytes in humans. Mutat. Res. **338**: 129–139.
21. DEMPSEY, J.L., M. PFEIFFER & A.A. MORLEY. 1993. Effect of dietary restriction on *in vivo* somatic mutation in mice. Mutat. Res. **291**: 141–145.
22. HART, R.W. & R.B. SETLOW. 1974. Correlation between deoxyribonucleic acid excision-repair and life-span in a number of mammalian species. Proc. Natl. Acad. Sci. USA **71**: 2169–2173.
23. ODAGIRI, Y. *et al.* 1998. Accelerated accumulation of somatic mutations in the senescence-accelerated mouse. Nat. Genet. **19**: 116–117.

24. BOERRIGTER, M.E. *et al.* 1995. Plasmid-based transgenic mouse model for studying *in vivo* mutations. Nature **377:** 657–659.
25. GOSSEN, J.A. *et al.* 1989. Efficient rescue of integrated shuttle vectors from transgenic mice: a model for studying mutations *in vivo*. Proc. Natl. Acad. Sci. USA **86:** 7971–7975.
26. VIJG, J. *et al.* 1997. Transgenic mouse models for studying mutations *in vivo*: applications in aging research. Mech. Ageing Dev. **99:** 257–271.
27. DOLLÉ, M.E. *et al.* 1997. Rapid accumulation of genome rearrangements in liver, but not in brain of old mice. Nat. Genet. **17:** 431–434.
28. DOLLÉ, M.E. *et al.* 2000. Distinct spectra of somatic mutations accumulated with age in mouse heart and small intestine. Proc. Natl. Acad. Sci. USA **97:** 8403–8408.
29. ONO, T. *et al.* 2000. Age-associated increase of spontaneous mutant frequency and molecular nature of mutation in newborn and old lacZ-transgenic mouse. Mutat. Res. **447:** 165–177.
30. DOLLÉ, M.E. *et al.* 1996. Evaluation of a plasmid-based transgenic mouse model for detecting *in vivo* mutations. Mutagenesis **11:** 111–118.
31. VIJG, J. & M.E. DOLLÉ. 2002. Large genome rearrangements as a primary cause of aging. Mech. Ageing Dev. **123:** 907–915.
32. DOLLÉ, M.E. & J. VIJG. 2002. Genome dynamics in aging mice. Genome Res. **12:** 1732–1738.
33. BUSUTTIL, R.A. *et al.* 2003. Oxygen accelerates the accumulation of mutations during the senescence and immortalization of murine cells in culture. Aging Cell **2:** 287–294.
34. GILLE, J.J., C.G. VAN BERKEL & H. JOENJE. 1994. Mutagenicity of metabolic oxygen radicals in mammalian cell cultures. Carcinogenesis **15:** 2695–2699.
35. VAUPEL, P., F. KALLINOWSKI & P. OKUNIEFF. 1989. Blood flow, oxygen and nutrient supply, and metabolic microenvironment of human tumors: a review. Cancer Res. **49:** 6449–6465.
36. SEKIGUCHI, M. & T. TSUZUKI. 2002. Oxidative nucleotide damage: consequences and prevention. Oncogene **21:** 8895–8904.
37. CUNNINGHAM, R.P. 1997. DNA repair: caretakers of the genome? Curr. Biol. **7:** R576–R579.

Camptothecin Sensitivity in Werner Syndrome Fibroblasts as Assessed by the COMET Technique

J. LOWE, A. SHEERIN, K. JENNERT-BURSTON, D. BURTON, E. L. OSTLER, J. BIRD, M. H. L. GREEN, AND R. G. A. FARAGHER

School of Pharmacy and Biomolecular Science, University of Brighton, Cockcroft Building, Brighton, BN2 4GJ, United Kingdom

ABSTRACT: Werner syndrome (WS) is an inherited genetic disease in which individuals display the premature aging of a selected subset of tissues. The disorder results from the loss of function mutations in the *wrn* gene. *Wrn* codes for a member of the RecQ helicase family with a unique nuclease domain. There is significant evidence that the role of wrn is to assist in the repair and reinitiation of DNA replication forks that have stalled. Loss of the wrn helicase imposes a distinct set of phenotypes at the cellular level. These include premature replicative senescence (in a subset of cell types), chromosomal instability, a distinct mutator phenotype, and hypersensitivity to a limited number of DNA damaging agents. Unfortunately, most of these phenotypes are not suitable for the rapid assessment of loss of function of the wrn gene product. However, WS cells have been reported to show abnormal sensitivity to the drug camptothecin (an inhibitor of topoisomerase type I). A rapid assay for this sensitivity would be a useful marker of loss of wrn function. The COMET (single-cell gel electrophoresis) assay is a rapid, sensitive, versatile, and robust technique for the quantitative assessment of DNA damage in eukaryotic cells. Using this assay, we have found that a significantly increased level of strand breaks can be demonstrated in WS cells treated with camptothecin compared with normal controls.

KEYWORDS: replicative senescence; Werner syndrome; COMET assay; camptothecin

The limited replicative capacity and resulting senescence of somatic cells has been studied *in vitro* since the phenomenon was first observed in the 1960s.[1] Senescence is a cyclin-dependent kinase inhibitor-mediated permanent block to cell cycle progression coupled with a wide range of alterations in the transcriptome. The loss of divisional capacity coupled with the accumulation of senescence cells has been suggested as one of several complimentary causal mechanisms by which mitotic tissue ages.[2] Although a significant amount of circumstantial evidence has been

---

Address for correspondence: R.G.A. Faragher, School of Pharmacy and Biomolecular Science, University of Brighton, Cockcroft Building, Brighton, BN2 4GJ, UK. Voice: +44-1273-642124; fax: +44-1273-679333.
rgaf@brighton.ac.uk

published that is consistent with this hypothesis, few instances of direct experimental support for this theory have emerged to date.[3,4] Perhaps the strongest evidence for a link between replicative senescence and organismal aging is provided by the progeroid syndrome Werner syndrome (WS, MCK227700). WS is an autosomal recessive disorder characterized by accelerated fibroblast senescence and the premature aging of selected tissue lineages within the body.[5,6] WS results from loss of function mutations in the *wrn* gene.[7] This codes for a member of the RecQ family of helicases. The most likely role for this molecule appears to be repair of DNA replication forks that have stalled as a result of base adducts or similar damage. In the absence of wrn, such stalled forks are resolved by a complicated process of recombination and deletion producing an observable "mutator phenotype" characterized by large deletions.[8] Although this process is associated with the production of a significant fraction of intra–S phase arrested cells, we have demonstrated that the accelerated senescence seen in WS fibroblast cultures results principally from telomeric attrition (because it is correctable through the ectopic expression of telomerase).[9] Thus, WS appears to represent a true acceleration of the telomere base divisional counting system that operates in many normal human cell types. On this basis, a plausible hypothesis for the premature dermal aging seen in WS is that it results from the premature accumulation of senescent fibroblasts.

We recently have published two models that seek to explain why some mitotic tissues are very severely affected in WS, whereas others show little or no apparent phenotype. The first of these considers the effect on replicative life span if it is assumed that loss of *wrn* results in an intrinsically increased rate of telomeric deletion.[10] The second assumes that the intrinsic rate of deletion is normal but that removal of cells from the mitotic pool as a consequence of intra–S phase arrest requires additional proliferation from the residual members of that pool.[11] Both models predict that certain mitotic cell types should be essentially unaffected by loss of *wrn*.

Distinguishing between these two models requires a ready supply of different WS cell types. Unfortunately, the disease is relatively rare, deaths are relatively infrequent, and thus the opportunities to acquire patient material are restricted. The new technology of small interfering RNA (shRNA) has the potential to overcome these difficulties and permit the evaluation of the replicative life span of isogenic material with and without functional levels of the *wrn* helicase.[12] An essential prerequisite for the validation of siRNAs (or ribozymes) designed to produce "knockdown" of *wrn* is the existence of a robust and rapid assay for functional loss of the helicase. Of the reported *in vitro* phenotypes displayed by WS cells, only camptothecin sensitivity appears to display the necessary combination of rapidity and sensitivity. An additional complication when seeking to evaluate the effectiveness of shRNA hairpins introduced using retroviral vectors is the need to conduct assays on a clonal basis to control for differing levels of shRNA expression arising from variations in transgene number.

The COMET (single-cell gel electrophoresis) assay is a rapid and sensitive technique for the demonstration of a range of damaged to DNA.[13] In the assay, a single cell suspension is embedded in low melting point agarose on a frosted microscope slide. The embedded cells then are treated with a high salt lysis mixture that removes essentially all proteins leaving supercoiled DNA embedded in the gel. If placed in alkaline buffer and subjected to electrophoresis, DNA containing strand breaks migrates through the agarose toward the anode to form a comet "tail;" undamaged

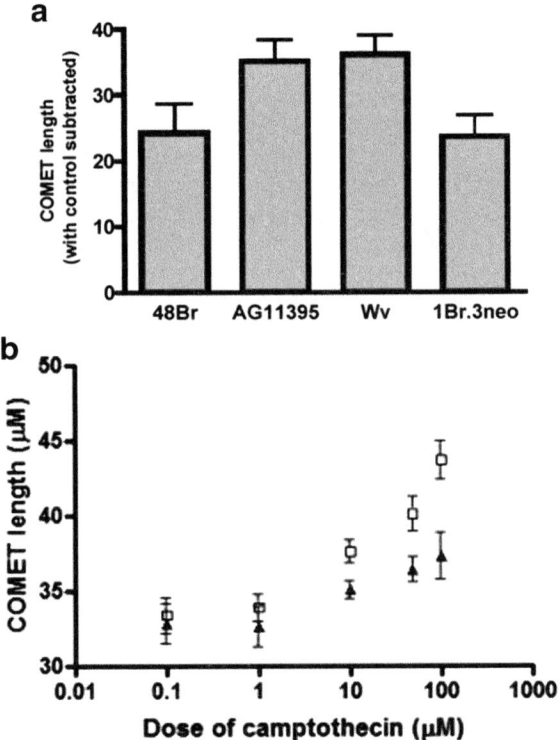

FIGURE 1. (a) A comparison of Comet length in SV40 T antigen immortalized WS and normal fibroblast cell lines after treatment for 1 hour with 10 mm camptothecin ($n = 5$). (b) A comparison of COMET length between hTERT immortalized WS (AGO3141a) and normal (1Br.3) human fibroblasts after treatment for 1 h with variable concentrations of camptothecin ($n \geq 5$, ±SEM). This difference is highly significant ($P < .0001$, two-way ANOVA). (*squares*) AGO3141ahTERT; (*triangles*) 1Br.3hTERT.

DNA remains trapped within the gel. Staining with ethidium bromide combined with image analysis permits the detection and quantitation of tail number and length.

In our initial studies, we sought to determine if a statistically significant difference in the dose-response curve to camptothecin could be demonstrated between T antigen immortalized WS and normal fibroblasts over a dose range of 0.1–10 mm camptothecin.

No statistically significant difference could be shown in COMET length between normal (1Br.3*neo* and 48BR) T antigen immortalized normal fibroblasts ($P = .17$, $n = 5$) or between WS (AG11395 & WV) T antigen immortalized WS fibroblasts ($P = .22$, $n = 5$). However, as can be seen from the sample data in FIGURE 1a, highly significant differences could be demonstrated between either control and either WS cell line ($P < .032$ to $P < .006$). This analysis was subsequently extended to hTERT immortalized WS and normal fibroblasts. At doses above 1 mm, highly significant statistical differences could be shown in the response to camptothecin by WS and normal fibroblasts (see FIG. 1b). From this analysis, we provisionally conclude that detection of camptothecin-induced damage by the COMET assay has the potential to form a rapid and effective screening method for loss of *wrn* induced by shRNA. The technique also may prove of value for other analyses in which the amount of material available for study is limited.

REFERENCES

1. HAYFLICK, L. & P.S. MOORHEAD. 1961. The serial cultivation of human diploid fibroblast cell strains. Exp. Cell Res. **25:** 585–621.
2. FARAGHER, R.G. & D. KIPLING. 1998. How might replicative senescence contribute to human ageing? Bioessays **20:** 985–991.
3. FUNK, W.D., C.K. WANG, D.N. SHELTON, et al. 2000. Telomerase expression restores dermal integrity to in vitro-aged fibroblasts in a reconstituted skin model. Exp. Cell Res. **258:** 270–278.
4. LI, Y., Q. YAN & N.S. WOLF. 1997. Long-term calorie restriction delays age-related decline in proliferation capacity of murine lens epithelial cells in vitro and in vivo. Invest. Ophthmol. Vis. Sci. **38:** 100–108.
5. JAMES, S.E., R.G. FARAGHER, J.L. BURKE, et al. 2000. Werner's syndrome T lymphocytes display a normal in vitro life-span. Mech. Ageing Dev. **121:** 139–149.
6. GOTO, M. 2001. Clinical characteristics of Werner syndrome and other premature ageing syndromes: pattern of ageing in progeroid syndromes. Monogr. Cancer Res. **49:** 27–39.
7. YU, C.E., J. OSHIMA, F. YING-HUI, et al. 1996. Positional cloning of the Werner's syndrome gene. Science **272:** 258–262.
8. FUKUCHI, K., G.M. MARTIN & R.J. MONNAT, JR. 1989. Mutator phenotype of Werner syndrome is characterized by extensive deletions. Proc. Natl. Acad. Sci. USA **86:** 5893–5897.
9. WYLLIE, F.S., C.J. JONES, J.W. SKINNER, et al. 2000. Telomerase prevents the accelerated cell ageing of Werner syndrome fibroblasts. Nat. Genet. **24:** 16–17.
10. OSTLER, E.L., C.V. WALLIS, A.N. SHEERIN & R.G. FARAGHER. 2002. A model for the phenotypic presentation of Werner's syndrome. Exp. Gerontol. **37:** 285–292.
11. BIRD, J., E.L. OSTLER & R.G.A. FARAGHER. 2003. Can we say that senescent cells cause ageing? Exp. Gerontol. **38:** 1319–1326.
12. BRUMMELKAMP, T.R., R. BERNARDS & R. AGAMI. 2002. Stable suppression of tumorigenicity by virus-mediated RNA interference. Cancer Cell **2:** 243–247.
13. CLINGEN, P.H., J.E. LOWE & M.H.L. GREEN. 2000. Measurement of DNA damage and repair capacity as a function of age using the Comet assay. *In* Methods in Molecular Medicine 38: Ageing Methods and Protocols. Y.A. Barnett & C.R. Barnett, Eds.: 143–157. Human Press. Totowa, NJ.

Mitochondrial Dysfunction Is a Common Phenotype in Aging and Cancer

KESHAV K. SINGH

Department of Cancer Genetics, Roswell Park Cancer Institute, Buffalo, New York 14263, USA

ABSTRACT: An interesting clue with regard to molecular mechanisms underlying age-associated cancers is the apparent defect in mitochondrial function. Recent studies demonstrate a progressive decline in mitochondrial function during aging. Studies have established that the decline in mitochondrial function is due to the accumulation of mutations in mitochondrial DNA. These observations suggest that the mitochondrial dysfunction that accompanies aging may exert a major influence on carcinogenesis.

KEYWORDS: aging; cancer; mitochondrial DNA (mtDNA); mitochondrial dysfunction; mutation; oxidative stress

Cancer is a disease associated with aging. In the United States, 60% of all cancer occurs in the age group of 65 years and older, and 70% of all cancer deaths are in this age group. As the U.S. population ages, we anticipate a parallel increase in cancer incidence, with estimates suggesting that a 12% population increase in the age group over the next 20 years will be accompanied by a 60% increase in cancer.[1]

The age-adjusted cancer incidence rate for persons who are 65 years and older is 10 times greater (22,208.1 per 100,000 population) than the rate for persons under 65 years (229.2 per 100,000 population).[1] Unfortunately, we have little understanding about the molecular mechanisms underlying age-associated cancers. However, an interesting clue in this regard is the apparent defect in mitochondrial function associated with both aging and cancer. Recent studies demonstrate a progressive decline in mitochondrial function during aging. Studies have established that the decline in mitochondrial function is due to the accumulation of mutations in mitochondrial DNA (mtDNA). Strikingly, mitochondrial dysfunction is also one of the most common and profound phenotypes of cancer cells, and the mitochondrial dysfunction appears to be associated with accumulation of mitochondrial mutations in all human cancers examined.[2] These observations suggest that the mitochondrial dysfunction that accompanies aging may exert a major influence on carcinogenesis.

Address for correspondence: Keshav K. Singh, Ph.D., Department of Cancer Genetics, Cell and Virus Building, Room 247, Roswell Park Cancer Institute, Elm and Carlton Streets, Buffalo, NY 14263. Voice: 716-845-8017; fax: 716-845-1047.
keshav.singh@roswellpark.org

MITOCHONDRIA PERFORM ESSENTIAL CELLULAR FUNCTIONS

Mitochondria are considered the powerhouse of a cell because they produce more than 80% of the energy (ATP). Indeed, mitochondria perform multiple cellular functions. These include heme synthesis, respiration, and synthesis of lipids, amino acids, and nucleotides. Mitochondria also maintain the intracellular homeostasis of inorganic ions, cell motility, and cell proliferation. Mitochondria are intimately involved in executing programmed cell death (apoptosis). They contain ~1000 proteins that are encoded by the nuclear genome. Only 13 proteins are encoded by the mtDNA. The mitochondrial genome–encoded proteins constitute the essential subunits of the electron transport system. The mitochondrial genome also encodes 2 ribosomal RNAs and 22 transfer RNAs.[2]

MITOCHONDRIAL GENOME IS EXTREMELY SUSCEPTIBLE TO MUTATIONS

Mitochondria are the major source of endogenous reactive oxygen species (ROS) in the cell because they carry the electron transport chain that during oxidative phosphorylation reduces oxygen to water by the addition of electrons.[2] It has been estimated that the endogenous production of ROS within human mitochondria is about 10^7 molecules/mitochondrion/day during normal oxidative phosphorylation.[2,3] Unlike nuclear DNA, mtDNA has no protective histones, so it is relentlessly exposed to ROS generated during oxidative phosphorylation (it is estimated that more than 1% of the oxygen consumed by cells is converted to ROS under physiological conditions).[2] ROS induce more extensive and more persistent damage to mtDNA than to nuclear DNA.[4] ROS also produce more than 20 types of mutagenic base modifications in DNA.[5] These DNA lesions cause mutations in mtDNA that can lead to impairment of mitochondrial function. Taken together, mtDNA is extremely susceptible to mutation by ROS-induced damage.

MITOCHONDRIAL GENETIC DEFECT ASSOCIATED WITH AGING

Human aging is characterized by the progressive decline in function at all levels, including cells, tissues, and organs. Various mechanisms have been proposed, including programmed senescence, molecular cross-linking, increased oxidative stress, and mtDNA mutation, leading to mitochondrial dysfunction.[6] Among these mechanisms, mtDNA mutation has received wide attention. A large number of mtDNA mutations have been reported in human somatic tissues during aging. These mutations include large deletions, point mutations, and small duplication. Among these mutations, a particular deletion of 5 kb has been reported to be common in many tissues and the abundance of this deletion increases with advancing age. It is important to note that mtDNA mutations reported during aging are mosaic, that is, there is uneven distribution of particular mutant mtDNA molecules among the cells of a given tissue. This is because of the intrinsic heteroplasmic nature of the mtDNA population in cells.[6] Unfortunately, the mechanisms underlying mutations in mtDNA are unclear. However, it is likely that increased susceptibility of mtDNA to oxidative damage and limited DNA repair capacity of the proteins involved in mitochondrial repair play a significant role in mutagenesis in aging.[2]

MITOCHONDRIAL GENOTYPE ASSOCIATED WITH LONGEVITY

Several studies have reported an association between the mitochondrial genotype and longevity.[7–9] It is likely that the mitochondrial genotype in the reported cases affects the functioning of the electron transport chain and free radical production that are critical components of the aging process. Indeed, a mutation in the *Caenorhabditis elegans* iron sulfur protein (isp-1) of mitochondrial complex III results in a decreased sensitivity to ROS and an increased life span.[10] A systematic RNA interference (RNAi) screen identified a critical role for the mitochondrial leucyl-tRNA synthetase gene in *C. elegans* longevity.[11] In addition, Tanaka *et al.*[8] recently identified a longevity-associated mitochondrial genotype Mt5178 in Japanese centenarians. This genotype is demonstrated to suppress the occurrence of mtDNA mutations in somatic cells known to increase with age.[6] It also is likely to confer resistance to cancer and mitochondrial diseases in centenarians.

MITOCHONDRIAL GENETIC DEFECT LEADS TO NUCLEAR GENOMIC INSTABILITY

A hallmark of cancer cells is the generation of a mutator phenotype, which results in rapid accumulation of mutations that drive tumor development. To date, it is not clear how mitochondrial dysfunction has an impact on the genetic stability of the nuclear genome. We used *Saccharomyces cerevisiae* as a model organism to analyze the consequences of disrupting mitochondrial function on genetic stability of the nuclear genome. The *CAN1* nuclear gene of *S. cerevisiae* encodes a transmembrane amino acid transporter that renders yeast cells sensitive to the lethal arginine analogue, canavanine. Any inactivating mutation in this gene results in a canavanine-resistant phenotype (CAN^R). We tested the stability of the nuclear genome by measuring the frequency of canavanine-resistant colonies after exposing the wild-type yeast to mitochondrial respiratory chain inhibitors. We compared these results to mutant yeast lacking the entire mitochondrial genome (rho^0) and to yeast with a mitochondrial mutation (rho^-). Our study demonstrates that mitochondrial dysfunction induces mutations in the nuclear genome. Our study also demonstrates that *REV1*, *REV3*, or *REV7* gene products, implicated in error-prone translesion DNA synthesis, mediate the genetic instability of the nuclear genome arising as a result of mitochondrial dysfunction.[12] Our studies conducted in a mammalian cell line also suggest that impaired mitochondrial function leads to increased oxidative stress, reduced DNA repair, and genetic instability.[13] Impaired mitochondrial function can also lead to activation of oncogenes, inhibition of apoptosis, and inactivation of tumor suppressor genes. Of interest here, we have found that mitochondrial dysfunction causes a lack of expression of tumor suppressor genes encoding a family of Claudin proteins (unpublished data). Claudins are tight junction proteins recently reported to be involved in carcinogenesis.[14] As accumulation of mitochondrial mutations is a consistent phenotype of aging and cancer cells, our results in both yeast and mammalian cell models provide a direct link between mitochondrial dysfunction and genomic instability, which have important implications in human aging and cancer.

MITOCHONDRIAL OXIDATIVE STRESS LINKS AGING AND CARCINOGENESIS

Mitochondria are the most important subcellular sites of ROS production in mammalian organs, and the steady state concentration of the ROS in the mitochondria is about 5- to 10-fold higher in mitochondria than in the cytosol or the nucleus.[3] The mtDNA, due to its close proximity to the sites of ROS production and because it is unprotected by histones, is a sensitive target for ROS damage. As a result, mtDNA accumulates mutation ~10 times more than the nuclear DNA. Mutations in mtDNA are reported during both aging and carcinogenesis.[2] Interestingly, mutations in mtDNA lead to oxidative stress.[7] When mitochondria become dysfunctional due to mutation in the mtDNA, they cannot oxidize NADH produced by the catabolism of nutrients. When NADH is accumulated in the cell, the plasma membrane NADH oxidase oxidizes cytosolic NADH to NAD and transfers electrons to oxygen, resulting in increased production of ROS and increased oxidative stress. Increased oxidative stress is involved in carcinogenesis. Oxidative stress accelerates mutagenesis and chromosomal abnormalities.[2] Mitochondria-derived oxidative stress (mDOS) can

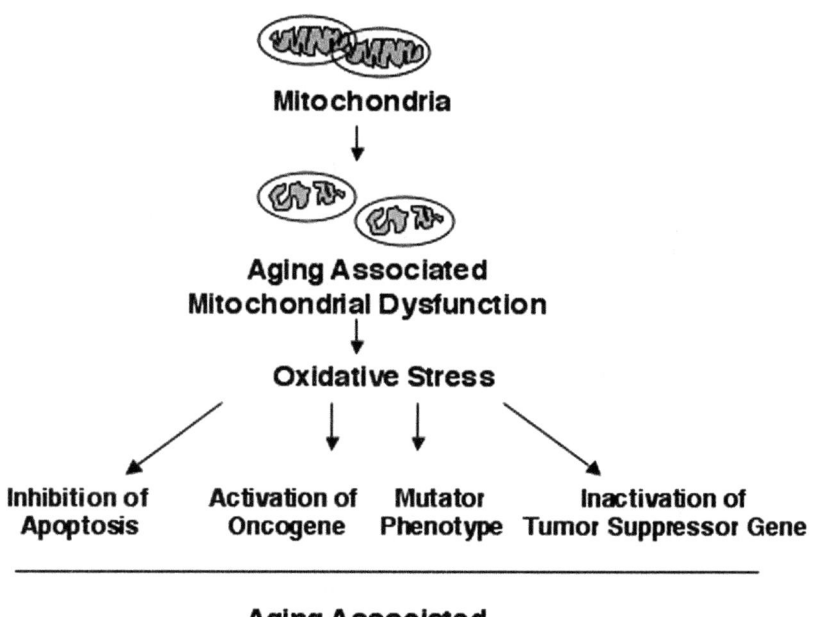

FIGURE 1. Involvement of mitochondria-derived oxidative stress in carcinogenesis. See text for details.

activate the mitogenic signal, inactivate tumor suppressors (such as the Claudins described above), inhibit apoptosis, and activate oncogenes.[2] Inhibition of apoptosis due to mutations in nuclear genes or activation of oncogenes can result in the removal of protective mechanisms against survival of aberrant cells that may instead progress to the tumorigenic state. The involvement of mDOS in carcinogenesis offers a number of intriguing genetic targets for further research in aging and cancer as well as in cancer therapy (see FIG. 1).[14–16]

ACKNOWLEDGMENTS

Research in my laboratory was supported by Grant No. RO1 009714 from the National Institutes of Health.

REFERENCES

1. NIH. 2002. Integrating aging and cancer [http://grants1.nih.gov/grants/guide/pa-files/PA-02-169.html].
2. SINGH, K.K., Ed. 1998. Mitochondrial DNA Mutations in Aging, Disease, and Cancer. Springer Pub. New York.
3. RICHTER, C. 1988. Do mitochondrial DNA fragments promote cancer and aging? FEBS Lett. 241(1–2): 1–5.
4. YAKES, F.M. & B. VAN HOUTEN. 1997. Mitochondrial DNA damage is more extensive and persists longer than nuclear DNA damage in human cells following oxidative stress. Proc. Natl. Acad. Sci. USA 94: 514–519.
5. JARUGA, P. & M. DIZDAROGLU. 1996. Repair of products of oxidative DNA base damage in human cells. Nucleic Acids Res. 24: 1389–1394.
6. NAGLEY, P. & C. ZHANG. 1998. Mitochondrial DNA mutations in aging. In Mitochondrial DNA Mutations in Aging, Disease, and Cancer, pp. 205–238. Springer Pub. New York.
7. TANAKA, M. 2002. Mitochondrial genotypes and cytochrome b variants associated with longevity or Parkinson's disease. J. Neurol. 249(suppl. 2): II11–II18.
8. TANAKA, M., J. GONG, J. ZHANG et al. 2000. Mitochondrial genotype associated with longevity and its inhibitory effect on mutagenesis. Mech. Ageing Dev. 116: 65–76.
9. NIEMI, A.K., A. HERVONEN, M. HURME et al. 2003. Mitochondrial DNA polymorphisms associated with longevity in a Finnish population. Hum. Genet. 112: 29–33.
10. FENG, J., F. BUSSIERE & S. HEKIMI. 2001. Mitochondrial electron transport is a key determinant of life span in Caenorhabditis elegans. Dev. Cell 1: 633–644.
11. LEE, S.S., R.Y. LEE, A.G. FRASER et al. 2003. A systematic RNAi screen identifies a critical role for mitochondria in C. elegans longevity. Nat. Genet. 33: 40–48.
12. RASMUSSEN, A.K., A. CHATTERJEE, L.J. RASMUSSEN & K.K. SINGH. 2003. Mitochondria-mediated nuclear mutator phenotype in Saccharomyces cerevisiae. Nucleic Acids Res. 31: 3909–3917.
13. DELSITE, R., S. KACHHAP, R. ANBAZHAGAN et al. 2002. Nuclear genes involved in mitochondria-to-nucleus communication in breast cancer cells. Mol. Cancer 1(1): 6.
14. KOMINSKY, S.L., P. ARGANI, D. KORZ et al. 2003. Loss of the tight junction protein claudin-7 correlates with histological grade in both ductal carcinoma in situ and invasive ductal carcinoma of the breast. Oncogene 22: 2021–2033.
15. MODICA-NAPOLITANO, J. & K.K. SINGH. 2002. Mitochondria as targets for detection and treatment of cancer [http://www-ermm.cbcu.cam.ac.uk/02004453h.htm].
16. SINGH, K.K., J. RUSSELL, B. SIGALA et al. 1999. Mitochondrial DNA determines the cellular response to cancer therapeutic agents. Oncogene 18: 6641–6646.

The Extent and Significance of Telomere Loss with Age

DUNCAN M. BAIRD AND DAVID KIPLING

Department of Pathology, University of Wales College of Medicine, Heath Park, Cardiff CF14 4XN, United Kingdom

ABSTRACT: By imposing a limit on the proliferative life span of some human cell types, telomere loss and the subsequent onset of replicative senescence have been proposed to contribute to age-related disease. Although there is a large body of *in vitro* data to reveal the mechanisms by which telomere erosion triggers senescence, technical limitations have hampered our ability to understand the full extent of telomere erosion *in vivo*. Thus far, we have evidence of age-related telomere loss; however, the lack of resolution of existing technologies does not allow us to determine if telomere erosion is extensive enough to trigger replicative senescence *in vivo*. This coupled with the considerable interindividual heterogeneity, and the overlap in telomere lengths between young and elder individuals, render any correlation weak and the significance unclear. However, recent technical developments, including adaptations of quantitative telomere fluorescence, *in situ* hybridization (Q-FISH), and the PCR-based single telomere length analysis (STELA), have increased the resolution of telomere length analysis. These technologies promise to provide the evidence required to address the full extent and significance of telomere loss in the human aging process. Here, we review published data on the dynamics of telomere erosion with age in the human body.

KEYWORDS: telomere; aging; senescence

The inability of the DNA replication machinery to completely replicate linear chromosomes results in the loss of telomeric sequences with ongoing cell division.[1] The loss of telomeric DNA, and the subsequent loss of telomere function, is a signal for a cessation of cell division known as replicative senescence. The number of cell divisions before the onset of replicative senescence is proportional to the length of telomeric DNA in the starting cell population; hence, cells with longer telomeres are capable of more cell divisions than those with shorter telomeres. Each cell division results in a loss of ~50–100 bp of DNA; the loss of telomere function, and the onset of replicative senescence, occurs when virtually all telomeric DNA has been lost from an as yet undefined number of individual chromosome ends. The enzyme telomerase, which synthesizes telomere repeats *de novo* and thus maintains telomere length, can facilitate ongoing cell division. However, telomerase is stringently repressed in the majority of human somatic tissues, thereby imposing a limit to the

Address for correspondence: Duncan M. Baird, Department of Pathology, University of Wales College of Medicine, Heath Park, Cardiff CF14 4XN, UK.
bairddm@cardiff.ac.uk

proliferative capacity of cells within those tissues, which when coupled with species specific telomere lengths, is considered to have evolved as a tumor-suppressive mechanism for long-lived species. However, the corollary of this may be that tumor protection results in a loss of proliferative capacity in later life. Hence, many have hypothesized that telomere loss in somatic tissues, as a consequence of ongoing cell division, may result in an age-related accumulation of senescent cells. The presence of senescent cells in somatic tissues may compromise tissue function in various ways, for example, by the simple loss of replicative capacity in actively regenerating tissues. Alternatively, and perhaps more realistically, tissue function could be affected by the characteristic changes in the gene expression profile of senescent cells, for example, the secretion of extracellular matrix-degrading enzymes by senescent fibroblasts. In this situation, a small fraction of senescent cells within a tissue could compromise tissue function, in an age-dependent manner.[2]

There is a considerable interest in understanding the dynamics of telomere erosion in the aging human body. However, we have been limited in our ability to determine telomere length directly from human tissues. The most widely used methodology is terminal restriction fragment (TRF) analysis. This suffers several limitations; it requires at least 100,000 cells, determines TRF length from all chromosome ends simultaneously, and is at best an estimate of mean telomere length. Furthermore, each TRF contains both subtelomeric and telomere repeat variants which can vary by up to 3 kb, which renders comparisons of TRF lengths between individuals difficult. Most crucially, because TRF analysis is a hybridization-based approach, the shortest and thus potentially most interesting telomeres from the perspective of triggering replicative senescence are by their very nature undetectable. Therefore, tissue analysis would not reveal the existence of a small proportion of senescent cells (with short telomeres) that might be compromising tissue function. Furthermore, mixtures of telomerase-positive and negative cell types, with differing replicative histories, will result in extremely heterogeneous TRF smears, making an estimation of mean TRF less informative. Some studies have used cells isolated and grown in culture until sufficient cell numbers were available for analysis. Although this results in less heterogeneous cell populations, the data are confounded by differences in the number of divisions (and therefore telomere loss) before TRF analysis. Most crucially, *in vitro* culture is, by its very nature, selective for the cells that are capable of significant cell division, that is, those with long telomere lengths.

Despite this, several cross-sectional surveys have compared TRF lengths from neonates with elder individuals. Small, but apparently significant, negative correlations of telomere length with age were observed in many different tissue types (summarized in Takubo *et al.*[3]). The majority of tissues analyzed were subjected to telomere degradation of the order of 15–150 bp per year. Telomere loss rates appeared to be related to predicted levels of cell turnover. A good example of this was the difference in telomere erosion rates of endothelial cells between iliac arteries (102 bp/year) and iliac veins (47 bp/year), which was consistent with differential cell turnover in these tissues as a consequence of differing levels of hemodynamic stress.[4] In contrast, relatively static cell populations such as neurons and myocardium displayed no detectable telomere loss.[3] Telomere erosion appears to be ubiquitous in human somatic tissues that are subject to cell turnover during life.

Given the limitations of TRF analysis, it is remarkable that these correlations, although often very weak, have been detected at all. However, most of these studies show considerable overlap in mean TRF lengths between very young and elder individuals. For example, despite an apparent telomere erosion rate of 46 bp/year observed in the renal cortex, more than 25% of individuals older than 60 years had mean TRF lengths within the size range of neonates, with one elderly individual having the largest renal TRF lengths of all.[3] Furthermore, the quoted mean TRF lengths in the elder individuals, usually greater than 7 kb, are significantly longer than those of senescent cell populations (generally of ~4 kb). Consistent with this, fibroblasts derived from elder individuals are capable of long *in vitro* replicative life spans, which do not decline as a function of age.[5] Closer inspection of TRF data from cross-sectional studies reveals that often most detectable telomere erosion appears to occur in the first few years of life, with a reduction in erosion rates in adulthood. This may be a consequence of an increase in cellularity early in life. However, in tissues, such as the immune system, skin, and gastrointestinal mucosa, whose function is underlied by significant cellular turnover, telomere lengths may be stabilized by telomerase activity in stem cells.[6] This was observed by Frenck *et al.*[7] who undertook TRF analysis on peripheral blood leukocytes from individuals within the same families, thereby reducing the intrinsic viability of TRFs. They observed reductions in length of over 1 kb per year in the first 4 years of life, after which telomere erosion leveled out, becoming very gradual for the rest of life.[7] A similar situation was observed in an analysis of hepatic tissue, where it was clear that most erosion occurred in early life, with no apparent loss over the age of 40 years.[8] Therefore, the overall significance of telomere erosion with age is not obvious; this may be because of the limitations in the technologies available to determine telomere length. If more detailed and accurate methods were available, the full extent and consequences of telomere erosion with age may become apparent.

Two technologies recently have emerged that promise to provide the resolution required to address these issues. Telomere quantitative fluorescence *in situ* hybridization has been adapted for use directly in histological sections using confocal microscopy.[9] Telomere length is expressed as a ratio of the telomere fluorescence of cells, within the same tissue section, that are considered to have undergone telomere erosion to that of cells that are considered to have not. When combined with chromosome specific or centromeric probes, telomere length can be compared with the occurrence of genomic rearrangements. This technology is likely to be extremely powerful, particularly when used to examine telomere dynamics in specific disease situations. However, the assumptions that have to be made for the relative telomere dynamics of specific cell types and the inability to determine actual functional telomere length may limit the power of this technology to elucidate telomere dynamics for aging in normal somatic tissues. Another technology that has been described recently, single telomere length analysis (STELA), uses single-molecule PCR to determine telomere length at specific chromosome ends to a high degree of accuracy.[10] Unlike the hybridization-based approaches, it is capable of detecting the full spectrum of telomere lengths, most notably the very short telomeres that are believed to trigger the onset of replicative senescence. Because it is a DNA-based technique, most tissues can be analyzed. The lack of histological information may be overcome, to some extent, by the use of microdissection.

The considerable resolution that these two technologies provide will help us to understand the full extent and significance, in terms of age-related disease and tissue deterioration, of telomere erosion.

REFERENCES

1. HARLEY, C.B., A.B. FUTCHER & C.W. GREIDER. 1990. Telomeres shorten during ageing of human fibroblasts. Nature **345**: 458–460.
2. FARAGHER, R.G. & D. KIPLING. 1998. How might replicative senescence contribute to human ageing? Bioessays **20**: 985–991.
3. TAKUBO, K., N. IZUMIYAMA-SHIMOMURA, N. HONMA, et al. 2002. Telomere lengths are characteristic in each human individual. Exp. Gerontol. **37**: 523–531.
4. CHANG, E. & C.B. HARLEY. 1995. Telomere length and replicative aging in human vascular tissues. Proc. Natl. Acad. Sci. USA **92**: 11190–11194.
5. CRISTOFALO, V.J., R.G. ALLEN, R.J. PIGNOLO, et al. 1998. Relationship between donor age and the replicative lifespan of human cells in culture: a reevaluation. Proc. Natl. Acad. Sci. USA **95**: 10614–10619.
6. KOLQUIST, K.A., L.W. ELLISEN, C.M. COUNTER, et al. 1998. Expression of TERT in early premalignant lesions and a subset of cells in normal tissues. Nat. Genet. **19**: 182–186.
7. FRENCK, R.W., JR., E.H. BLACKBURN & K.M. SHANNON. 1998. The rate of telomere sequence loss in human leukocytes varies with age. Proc. Natl. Acad. Sci. USA **95**: 5607–5510.
8. TAKUBO, K., K. NAKAMURA, N. IZUMIYAMA, et al. 2000. Telomere shortening with aging in human liver. J. Gerontol. A Biol. Sci. Med. Sci. **55**: B533–B536.
9. O'SULLIVAN, J.N., M.P. BRONNER, T.A. BRENTNALL, et al. 2002. Chromosomal instability in ulcerative colitis is related to telomere shortening. Nat. Genet. **32**: 280–284.
10. BAIRD, D.M., J. ROWSON, D. WYNFORD-THOMAS, et al. 2003. Extensive allelic variation and ultrashort telomeres in senescent human cells. Nat. Genet. **33**: 203–207.

Measurement of the 4,834-bp Mitochondrial DNA Deletion Level in Aging Rat Liver and Brain Subjected or Not to Caloric Restriction Diet

P. CASSANO,[a] A. M. S. LEZZA,[a] C. LEEUWENBURGH,[b] P. CANTATORE,[a,c] AND M. N. GADALETA[a,c]

[a]*Department of Biochemistry and Molecular Biology, University of Bari, Bari, Italy*

[b]*University of Florida, Biochemistry of Aging Laboratory, College of Health and Human Performance, Center for Exercise Science, Gainesville, Florida, USA*

[c]*Institute of Biomembrane and Bioenergetics, CNR, Bari, Italy*

ABSTRACT: Several studies have demonstrated an age-related accumulation of the amount of a specific 4834-bp mitochondrial DNA (mtDNA) deletion in different tissues of rat (liver, brain, and skeletal muscle). We investigated the influence of a caloric restriction diet (CR) on a selected age-associated marker of mtDNA damage, as the 4834-bp deletion, using quantitative real-time PCR. The mtDNA deleted level has been determined with respect to the mitochondrial D-loop level, using specific primers and TaqMan probes for each target. In liver we found an age-related increase of the deletion level (twofold) that was reversed and brought back to the adult level by a CR diet. On the contrary, in the brain the age-related increase of the deletion level (eightfold) was not affected by CR at all. The different effect of the CR on the deletion level in liver and brain might be a further element supporting the tissue-specificity of the aging process.

KEYWORDS: caloric restriction; rat liver; rat brain; skeletal muscle; mitochondrial DNA

INTRODUCTION

Aging is a fascinating and highly important topic because of its great social relevance and scientific complexity. One of the most important theories to explain this multifactorial process is the free radicals theory. Such theory involves the damaging role of reactive oxygen species (ROS) on mitochondrial molecular components as lipids, proteins, and DNA. In particular, mitochondrial DNA (mtDNA) damage can include formation of modified bases (adducts) along the molecule as well as of point mutations (single nucleotide substitutions) and of large size rearrangements (dele-

Address for correspondence: P. Cassano, Department of Biochemistry and Molecular Biology, University of Bari, Bari, Italy.
cspr01b1@uniba.it

tions, insertions). Several studies have demonstrated an age-related accumulation of the number of deleted species of mtDNA as well as of the amount of a specific 4,834-bp mtDNA deletion, homologue of the human mtDNA "common deletion," in different tissues of rat.[1–4] However, the different levels of the 4.8-kb deletion measured in mitotic (liver and kidney) versus postmitotic tissues (brain) suggest the possibility of tissue-specific processes in aging rat.[4] The tissue-specificity of age-related mechanisms is supported by the different extent of efficacy of the so far only known treatment able to delay the aging degeneration, namely caloric restriction (CR). CR retards aging in rodents and other animals, including nonhuman primates, by means of various molecular mechanisms, among which the reduction of oxidative stress appears very relevant. Therefore, mitochondria and their function represent a primary target of studies with CR. CR treatment has been reported to decrease the number of mtDNA deleted species in rat skeletal muscle,[1] but very little has been found about other tissues with recent techniques.[5]

RESULTS AND DISCUSSION

We decided to evaluate by quantitative real-time PCR the level of the 4,834-bp mtDNA deletion in tissues of aging rats treated and not with CR. The CR was life-long and kept at 40% compared with *ad libitum* (L) feeding. Assayed animals were adult (12 months) and old (28 months) Fischer rats. The chosen tissues include one mitotic, clearly sensitive to the effect of CR in reducing mitochondrial oxidative stress, that is liver,[6] and one postmitotic, shown sensitive to CR by microarray approach, namely, brain.[7] Data concerning the level of the 4,834-bp mtDNA deletion in liver and brain from adult fed *ad libitum* (AL), old fed *ad libitum* (OL), and old calories-restricted (OR) animals are presented. The level of the 4,834-bp mtDNA deletion has been determined with respect to total mtDNA represented by a PCR product deriving from the mitochondrial D-loop, using specific primers and TaqMan probes (Applied Biosystems) for each target, accurately designed using Primer Express software (Applied Biosystems). The method has been validated by primer limiting experiments to determine the proper primer concentrations, by measurements in previously assayed samples and by evaluating the equal reaction efficiency of the two amplicons. The specificity of the amplification products was checked by 2% agarose gel electrophoresis that showed unique PCR fragments of the expected size. The mitochondrial deletion content was quantified using a 5′-VIC reporter and a 3′-TAMRA quencher dye, and the D-loop quantity with a 5′-6FAM reporter and a 3′-TAMRA quencher dye. Each sample was analyzed in triplicate and fluorescence spectra were monitored by the ABI PRISM 7000 Sequence Detection System (Applied Biosystems). The threshold cycle number (C_t), that is the cycle at which a statistically significant increase in normalized fluorescence is first detected, was used as a measure of input target DNA and to quantify the relative amount of deleted mtDNA to total mtDNA with the following equation: $R = 2^{-\Delta C_t}$, where R is the calculated ratio and ΔC_t is the $C_{t\ deleted\ mtDNA} - C_{t\ D\text{-loop}}$ value. Statistical analysis was conducted with the SSPS Base 11.5 software.

We found in liver an age-related increase of the deletion level in OL animals (the mean value is a twofold increase) that was reversed and brought back to the adult level by lifelong CR. As for brain, we found an age-related increase of the deletion

A. Liver

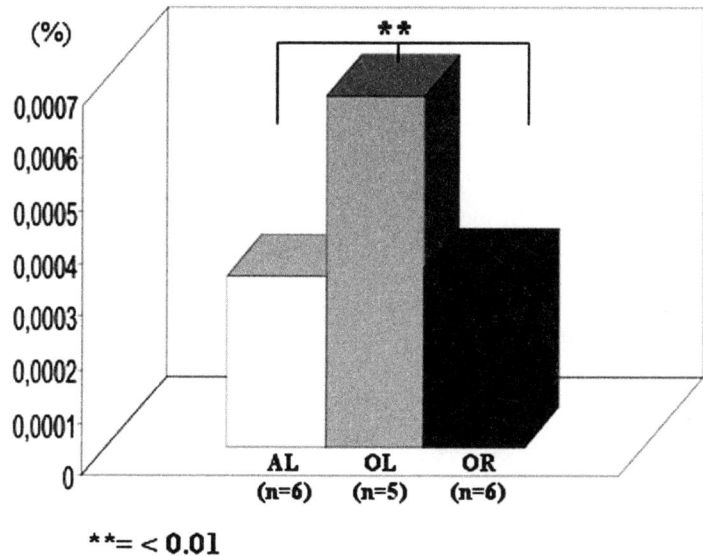

** = < 0.01

B. Brain

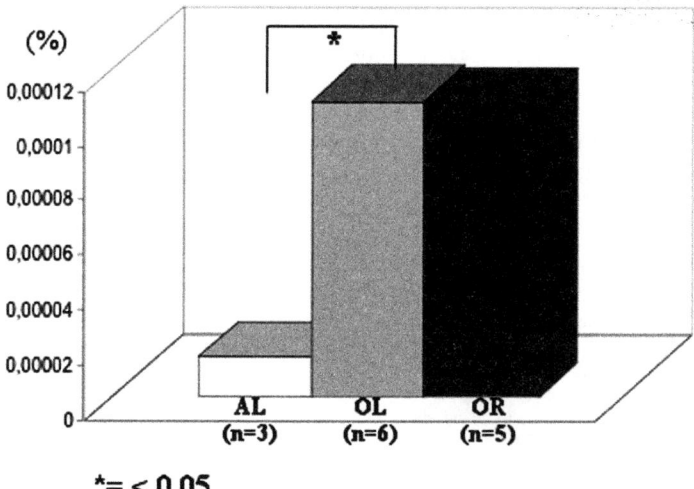

* = < 0.05

FIGURE 1. Quantification of the 4,834-bp mtDNA deletion in adult fed *ad libitum* (AL), old fed *ad libitum* (OL), and old calories-restricted (OR) rat tissues. (**A**) Liver. Statistics, age-related effect: AL vs. OL: $P < .01$ by ANOVA test. Diet-related effect: OR vs. OL: $P < .01$ by ANOVA test. (**B**) Brain. Statistics, age-related effect: AL vs. OL: $P < .05$ by ANOVA test.

level in OL animals (on average an eightfold increase) that was not affected by CR at all (FIG. 1). In particular, the current results show that in liver the deletion was already detectable in all adult animals and homogenously increased by twofold with aging. In brain, vice versa, the deletion level of those adult rats harboring it was much lower than in the liver of the same animals and often was even below the sensitivity of our assay. The different effect of CR on the deletion level in liver and brain might be a further element supporting the tissue-specificity of the aging process. In fact, the mechanism by which fewer ROS are produced in liver of CR rats, that is, the decrease of ROS generation at complex I, should explain the decreased amount of 8-oxo-7,8-dihydro-2-deoxyguanosine (8-oxodG), the most frequent oxidative adduct in DNA, in the mtDNA of restricted rats[6] with respect to the age-increased content of *ad libitum*–fed animals.[8] Because the increase of the 8-oxodG level with age has been correlated in various situations to the increase of the "common" mtDNA deletion,[9] our findings about age and CR effects on deletion level in liver can be easily explained. Liver mitochondria metabolism appears sensitive to changes in the diet that eventually might act through an improved glucoregulation. In brain, aging should be effective on the amount of ROS by-produced by the oxidative phosphorylation leading to an increased content of 8-oxodG in mtDNA. From such age-related change might originate the increase of the deletion level here reported in OL rats. The brain, vice versa, is practically not affected by CR likely because of its different metabolism that does not seem to respond to diet changes with a decreased production of mitochondrial ROS[10] and a lowered level of deletion.

ACKNOWLEDGMENTS

This work has been done with funds from Sigma Tau–Industrie Farmaceutiche Riunite S.p.A., Contract D.S./2000/C.R./no. 20, Italian Space Agency (ASI), Contracts no. I/R/064/01 and I/R/322/02, and Progetto di Ateneo "Biogenesi mitocondriale ed invecchiamento: alterazioni genotipiche e fenotipiche mitocondriali in vari tessuti di ratto." P. Cassano was supported by fellowship from ESF (P.O.P. 2000-2006). The authors thank Ms. R. Longo for word processing.

REFERENCES

1. ASPNES, L., C.M. LEE, R. WEINDRUCH, *et al.* 1997. Caloric restriction reduces fiber loss and mitochondrial abnormalities in aged rat muscle. FASEB J. **11:** 573–581.
2. GADALETA, M.N., G. RAINALDI, A.M.S. LEZZA, *et al.* 1992. Mitochondrial DNA copy number and mitochondrial DNA deletion in adult and senescent rat. Mutat. Res. **275:** 181–193.
3. GADALETA, M.N., G. RAINALDI, A.M.S. LEZZA, *et al.* 1995. Structure and expression of mitochondrial DNA in aging rat: DNA deletions and protein synthesis. *In* Progress in Cell Research. Vol. 5. F. Palmieri *et al.*, Eds.: 231–235. Elsevier Science. Amsterdam.
4. YOWE, D.L. & B.N. AMES. 1998. Quantitation of age-related mitochondrial DNA deletions in rat tissues shows that their pattern of accumulation differs from that of humans. Gene **209:** 23–30.
5. KANG, C.M., B.S. KRISTAL & B.P. YU. 1998. Age-related mitochondrial DNA deletions: effect of dietary restriction. Free Radic. Biol. Med. **24:** 148–154.
6. GREDILLA, R., G. BARJA & M. LOPEZ-TORRES. 2001. Effect of short-term caloric restriction on H_2O_2 production and oxidative DNA damage in rat liver mitochondria and location of the free radical source. J. Bioenerg. Biomembr. **33:** 279–287.

7. LEE, C.-K., R. WEINDRUCH & T.A. PROLLA. 2000. Gene-expression profile of the ageing brain in mice. Nat. Genet. **25:** 294–297.
8. RICHTER, C., J.W. PARK & B.N. AMES. 1988. Normal oxidative damage to mitochondrial and nuclear DNA is extensive. Proc. Natl. Acad. Sci. USA **85:** 6465–6467.
9. LEZZA, A.M.S., P. MECOCCI, A. CORMIO, et al. 1999. Mitochondrial DNA 4,977-bp deletion and OH^8dG levels correlate in old subjects but not in Alzheimer's disease patients brain. FASEB J. **13:** 1083–1088.
10. DREW, B.R. & C. LEEUWENBURGH. 2003. Method for measuring ATP production in isolated mitochondria: ATP production in brain and liver mitochondria of Fischer-344 rats with age and caloric restriction. Am. J. Physiol. Regul. Integr. Comp. Physiol. **285:** R1259–R1267 (July 10 [Epub ahead of print]).

Investigation of the Signaling Pathways Involved in the Proliferative Life Span Barriers in Werner Syndrome Fibroblasts

TERENCE DAVIS,[a] RICHARD G. A. FARAGHER,[b] CHRISTOPHER J. JONES,[a] AND DAVID KIPLING[a]

[a]*Department of Pathology, University of Wales College of Medicine, Heath Park, Cardiff CF14 4XN, Wales*

[b]*School of Pharmacy and Biomolecular Sciences, University of Brighton, Lewes Road, Brighton BN2 4GJ, England*

ABSTRACT: Werner syndrome (WS) fibroblasts enter replicative senescence after a reduced *in vitro* life span. Although this has been postulated as causal in the accelerated aging seen in this disease, controversy remains as to whether WS is showing the acceleration of a normal cellular aging mechanism or, instead, the occurrence of a novel WS-specific process. To address this, we analyzed the signaling pathways involved in senescence in WS fibroblasts. Cultured WS fibroblasts underwent senescence after ~20 population doublings, with the majority of the cells having a 2N DNA content. This was associated with high levels of the CdkIs p16 and p21. Senescent WS cells reentered the cell cycle after microinjection of a p53-neutralizing antibody. Similarly, presenescent WS fibroblasts expressing the E6 and/or E7 oncoproteins bypassed M1 and ultimately reached a second proliferative life span barrier, which strongly resembled the second life span barriers found in normal cells for growth dynamics, cellular morphology, and expression of p16 and p21. The strong similarity between the signaling pathways triggering cell cycle arrest in WS and normal fibroblasts provides support for the defect in WS causing the acceleration of a normal aging mechanism and validates the use of WS as a model for some aspects of human aging.

KEYWORDS: aging; cyclin-dependent kinases; oncoproteins; p53; p21^{WAF1}; p16^{INK4a}; replicative senescence; telomerase; telomeres

Werner syndrome (WS) is a heavily studied human premature aging disorder that, with the exception of central nervous system degeneration, provides a convincing mimic of the normal aging phenotype[1] and is thus an important model disease.

Normal human fibroblasts have a finite capacity to divide after which they enter replicative senescence (M1). Cultures of cells cease to expand as a result of a progressive decline in the growth fraction, consistent with the operation of one or more

Address for correspondence: Terence Davis, Department of Pathology, University of Wales College of Medicine, Heath Park, Cardiff CF14 4XN, Wales. Voice: +44-29-20745575; fax: +44-29-20744276.
davist2@cardiff.ac.uk

mechanisms capable of acting as a cell division "counting" system. This counting mechanism is based on the activation of p53 as a result of the progressive erosion of chromosomal telomeres.[3]

WS fibroblast cultures display a drastic reduction in replicative life span[4] because of an increased rate of decline in the growth fraction compared with normal controls.[5] Loss of the Werner helicase has the potential to produce many abortive DNA replication events that could trigger premature cell cycle exit without involving telomeric loss. Thus, an important question is the extent to which the rapid replicative senescence seen in WS fibroblasts results from an acceleration of normal senescence mechanisms.

Telomere shortening acts as a primary driver of senescence in WS fibroblasts;[6] however, details of the signaling pathway downstream of telomere erosion in WS cells are not fully studied. Here, we have analyzed the signaling pathways involved in cell cycle arrest in WS fibroblasts by the use of HPV E6 and E7 oncoproteins to abrogate components involved in cell cycle control. All methods used in this work were as described.[7]

WS fibroblasts (AG05229) had a replicative life span of 20.5 PDs and thus showed the reduced life span reported for these cells. At M1, the cells had increased in size with increased expression of $p21^{WAF1}$ and SAβ-gal activity compared with growing cells (FIG. 1I). Most of the cells at M1 (>77%) were arrested with a 2N DNA content,[8] consistent with G_1 arrest, with ~20% having higher levels, reflecting G_2 arrest, and/or G_1 tetraploid cells. Thus, although WS cells have a shorter proliferative life span, at senescence their phenotype strongly resembles senescent HCA2 cells.[7,8]

Expression of the HPV16 E6 and/or E7 oncoproteins in presenescent WS cells resulted in evasion of senescence and generated rapidly growing cultures (FIG. 1A). In all cases, the growing cells were small, with a high BrdU labeling index (LI) and low SAβ-gal activity (FIG. 1I). These cultures did not proliferate indefinitely but arrived after variable lengths of time at a second proliferative barrier.

Control cultures (WS.neo) managed three PDs before reaching M1 (FIG. 1A). The E6-expressing cultures (WS.E6) ceased net growth ~20 PDs beyond M1 (FIG. 1A) and entered M^{int}.[7] The cells at M^{int} were large and highly irregular in morphology (FIG. 1D), with a low BrdU LI and high SAβ-gal activity (FIG 1I). TdT analysis showed ~5% positive nuclei, suggestive of apoptosis. The E7-expressing cells (WS.E7) grew rapidly but entered M^{int} after 28 days (six PDs beyond M1), and there were no WS.E7 cells remaining after 56 days (FIG. 1A). The cells were enlarged at M^{int} (FIG. 1E), but were smaller and more regular in morphology than WS cells at M1 or at M2 (FIG. 1C, F), with a moderate BrdU LI, high SAβ-gal activity, and an apoptotic index of 65% (FIG. 1I). E6- and E7-expressing cells (WS.E6E7) avoided M1 and continued growth until the cultures reached crisis (M2) 30 PDs beyond M1 (FIG. 1A). At M2, the cell number declined rapidly, with the cells having an apoptotic index of 67% (FIG. 1I). No WS.E6E7 cells remained after 273 days.

Cycling WS cells showed moderate levels of the CdkI $p21^{WAF1}$ in the nuclei (FIG. 1I). This increased to >90% of the nuclei at M1 (FIG. 1G, I). Expression of E6 caused a decrease in the proportion of nuclei positive for $p21^{WAF1}$, with few nuclei showing staining (FIG. 1I). This was followed by a slow increase in the number of positive nuclei, reaching 15% by M^{int}. Expression of E7 resulted in an increase in the number of positive cells compared with M1 (FIG. 1I), with the level of $p21^{WAF1}$

increasing markedly and being detectable in the cytoplasm of the M^{int} cells (FIG. 1H). Expression of the E6 and E7 proteins together resulted in a decrease in the proportion of nuclei positive for $p21^{WAF1}$ (FIG. 1I), followed by a slow increase in the number of positive nuclei, reaching 11% at M2. The $p21^{WAF1}$ levels were confirmed by immunoblot (FIG. 1J). The low levels of $p21^{WAF1}$ in the E6-expressing cells are presumably caused by abrogation of p53 by the E6 oncoprotein.[8]

The level of the CdkI $p16^{INK4A}$ is very low in cycling WS cells and increases substantially at M1 (FIG. 1J). The level of $p16^{INK4A}$ decreased in E6-infected cells,

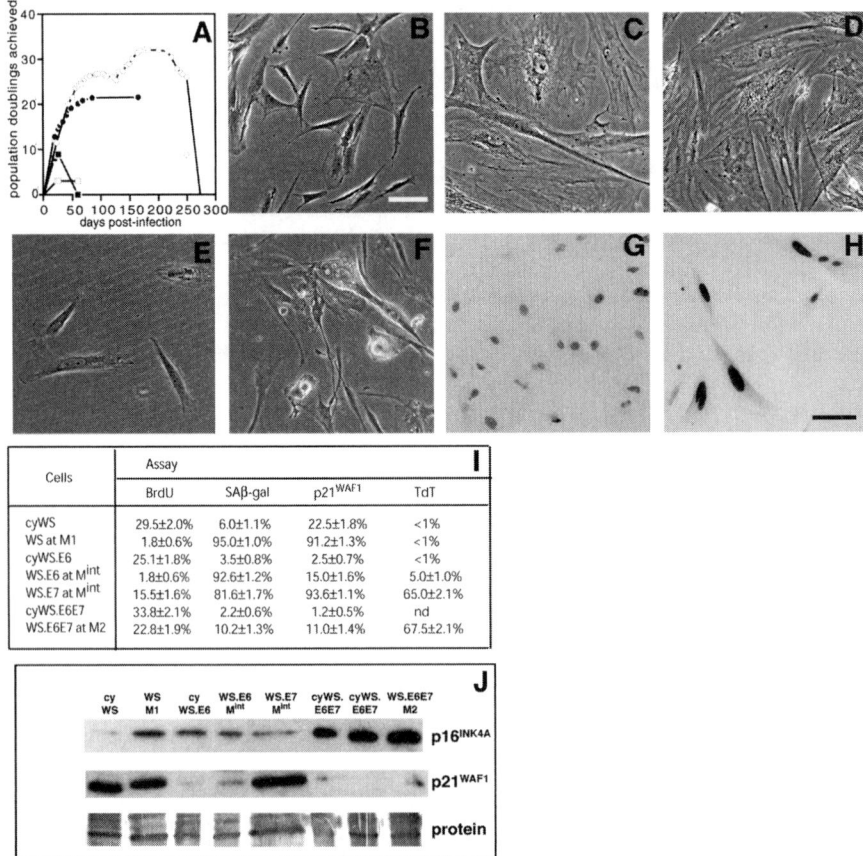

FIGURE 1. Growth of AG05229 fibroblasts. (A) Growth curve of PDs versus time: (*closed circles*) WS.E6; (*closed squares*) WS.E7; (*open circles*) WS.E6E7; (*open squares*) WS.neo control. Phase contrast of (B) young cells, (C) M1 cells, (D) WS.E6 at M^{int}, (E) WS.E7 at M^{int}, (F) WS.E6E7 at M2. $p21^{WAF1}$ staining in (G) M1 cells, (H) WS.E7 at M^{int}. Bars = 100 μm. (I) Table showing cell cycle parameters. Percentages of cells synthesizing DNA (BrdU) staining with senescence-associated β-galactosidase (SAβ-gal), $p21^{WAF1}$, and apoptosis (TdT). Figures are given as percentages ± SE in a count of 500 cells. cy = cycling cells; nd = not determined. (J) Immunoblot analysis of WS fibroblasts: the two cyWS.E6E7 samples are at PDs 24 and 27, respectively.

but at M^{int} was at a level equal to or less than that at M1. In E7-infected cells at M^{int}, the level of p16^{INK4A} was similar to that in E6-infected cells at M^{int}. In the presence of both E6 and E7 oncoproteins, the level of p16^{INK4A} increases with PDs.

CONCLUSIONS

WS fibroblasts had a short proliferative life span, with most of the senescent cells having a G_1-S content of DNA, and high levels of the CdkIs p16^{INK4a} and p21^{WAF1}. Presenescent WS fibroblasts expressing the E6 and/or E7 oncoproteins bypassed M1 and reached a second proliferative life span barrier, which strongly resembled the second life span barriers found in normal cells for growth dynamics, cellular morphology, and expression of the CdkIs p16^{INK4A} and p21^{WAF1}.[7-9] However, the nature of the senescence-inducing signal in WS cells is not known and may involve faster telomere erosion,[10] or may be caused by increased stress during S-phase transition possibly caused by replication fork stalling.[2] The strong similarity between the signaling pathways in cell cycle arrest in WS and normal fibroblasts provides support for the defect in WS causing the acceleration of a normal aging mechanism and validates the use of WS as a model for some aspects of human aging.

ACKNOWLEDGMENTS

This work was supported by the BBSRC's Science of Ageing and Exploratory Research into Ageing initiatives.

REFERENCES

1. MARTIN, G.M., J. OSHIMA, M.D. GRAY & M. POOT. 1999. What geriatricians should know about the Werner Syndrome. J. Am. Geriatr. Soc. **47:** 1136–1144.
2. RODRÍGUEZ-LÓPEZ, A.M., D.A. JACKSON, F. IBORRA & L.S. COX. 2002. Asymmetry of DNA replication fork progression in Werner's syndrome. Aging Cell **1:** 30–39.
3. WRIGHT, W.E. & J.W. SHAY. 2002. Historical claims and current interpretations of replicative aging. Nat. Biotechnol. **20:** 682–688.
4. MARTIN, G.M., C.C. SPRAGUE & C.J. EPSTEIN. 1970. Replicative life span of cultivated human cells. Lab. Invest. **23:** 86–92.
5. FARAGHER, R.G.A., I.R. KILL, J.A. HUNTER, et al. 1993. The gene responsible for Werner syndrome may be a cell division "counting" gene. Proc. Natl. Acad. Sci. USA **90:** 12030–12034.
6. WYLLIE, F.S., C.J. JONES, J.W. SKINNER, et al. 2000. Telomerase prevents the accelerated ageing of Werner syndrome fibroblasts. Nat. Genet. **24:** 16–17.
7. BOND, J.A., M.F. HAUGHTON, J.M. ROWSON, et al. 1999. Control of replicative life span in human cells: barriers to clonal expansion intermediate between M1 senescence and M2 crisis. Mol. Cell. Biol. **19:** 3103–3114.
8. DAVIS, T., S.K. SINGHRAO, F.S. WYLLIE, et al. 2003. Telomere-based proliferative life span barriers in Werner syndrome fibroblasts involve both p53-dependent and p53-independent mechanisms. J. Cell Sci. **116:** 1349–1357.
9. DULIC, V.G., E. BENEY, G. FREBOURG, et al. 2000. Uncoupling between phenotypic senescence and cell cycle arrest in ageing p21-deficient fibroblasts. Mol. Cell. Biol. **20:** 6741–6754.
10. SCHULZ, V.P., V.A. ZAKIAN, C.E. OGBURN, et al. 1996. Accelerated loss of telomere repeats may not explain accelerated replicative decline in Werner syndrome cells. Hum. Genet. **97:** 750–754.

Mechanism of Telomere Shortening by Oxidative Stress

SHOSUKE KAWANISHI AND SHINJI OIKAWA

Department of Environmental and Molecular Medicine, Mie University School of Medicine, Mie 514-8507, Japan

ABSTRACT: We investigated whether oxidative stress, which contributes to aging, accelerates the telomere shortening in human cultured cells. The terminal restriction fragment (TRF) from WI-38 fibroblasts irradiated with UVA (365-nm light) decreased with increasing of the irradiation dose. Furthermore, UVA irradiation dose-dependently increased the formation of 8-oxo-7,8-dihydro-2'-deoxyguanosine (8-oxodG) in both WI-38 fibroblasts and HL-60 cells. In order to clarify the mechanism of the acceleration of telomere shortening, we investigated site-specific DNA damage induced by UVA irradiation in the presence of endogenous photosensitizers using ^{32}P 5' end-labeled DNA fragments containing telomeric oligonucleotide (TTAGGG)$_4$. UVA irradiation with riboflavin induced 8-oxodG formation in the DNA fragments containing telomeric sequence, and Fpg protein treatment led to chain cleavages at the central guanine of 5'-GGG-3' in telomere sequence. Human 8-oxodG-DNA glycosylase introduces a chain break in a double-stranded oligonucleotide specifically at an 8-oxodG residue. The amount of 8-oxodG formation in DNA fragment containing telomere sequence [5'-CGC(TTAGGG)$_7$CGC-3'] was approximately five times more than that in the DNA fragment containing nontelomere sequence [5'-CGC(TGTGAG)$_7$CGC-3']. Furthermore, H_2O_2 plus Cu(II) caused DNA damage, including 8-oxodG formation, specifically at the GGG sequence in the telomere sequence (5'-TTAGGG-3'). It is concluded that the formation of 8-oxodG at the GGG triplet in telomere sequence induced by oxidative stress could participate in acceleration of telomere shortening.

KEYWORDS: telomere shortening; oxidative stress; aging; terminal restriction fragment (TRF); UVA irradiation; 8-oxodG

INTRODUCTION

Eukaryotic telomeres have important roles in cellular processes, including chromatin organization and control of cell proliferation. Telomere shortening has been implicated in cellular aging.[1] A study on aging in animals has revealed that telomeres shorten in the rat kidney, liver, pancreas, and lung in an age-dependent manner. In human beings, telomere shortening contributes to mortality in many age-related diseases.[2] Notably, it is reported that some alleles show almost complete loss

---

Address for correspondence: Shosuke Kawanishi, Department of Environmental and Molecular Medicine, Mie University School of Medicine, Mie 514-8507, Japan. Fax: +81-59-231-5011. kawanisi@doc.medic.mie-u.ac.jp

of TTAGGG repeats at senescence.[3] Thus, telomere shortening has been suggested to be a "molecular clock" of the aging process. Recently, von Zglinicki reported an increase of the rate of telomere shortening by oxidative stress in human fibroblasts.[4] In addition, suppression of oxidative stress by antioxidative agents, such as vitamin C, extends the replicative life span by reducing the rate of telomere shortening. However, the mechanism for increasing the telomere shortening rate by oxidative stress remains to be clarified.

Repeated exposure of human skin to solar UV irradiation leads to skin carcinogenesis and photoaging that involved cell senescence. Increasing evidence demonstrates that UVA, as well as UVB, contributes to photoaging.[5] In this study, we investigated the shortening rate of telomeres in human WI-38 fibroblasts exposed to UVA irradiation. We also examined the formation of 8-oxo-7,8-dihydro-2′-deoxyguanosine (8-oxodG) in human cultured cells by using an electrochemical detector coupled to an HPLC (HPLC-ECD). Furthermore, we investigated the mechanism for increasing the telomere shortening induced by UVA irradiation using ^{32}P 5′ end-labeled DNA fragment, including the telomeric sequence.

Aging is associated with increased rates of mitochondrial oxygen free radical production. Oxygen free radical, O_2^-, and H_2O_2 play important roles in DNA damage. In addition, nitric oxide (NO) may be one of the contributors to age-related oxidative stress. In this study, we investigated the mechanism for telomere shortening induced by oxidative stress (H_2O_2, NO plus O_2^-) using the ^{32}P 5′ end-labeled DNA fragment, including the telomeric sequence.

MATERIALS AND METHODS

Analysis of Terminal Restriction Fragment Length

WI-38 fibroblasts were cultured in minimum essential medium (GIBCO) containing 10% fetal calf serum (FCS) at 37°C under 5% CO_2 in a humidified atmosphere. The cells were irradiated with five 8-W UV lamps (365 nm, UVP, model TDM-20, San Gabriel, CA) placed at a distance of 3–5 cm. The genomic DNA, which was extracted from irradiated WI-38 fibroblasts, was digested with *Hinf* I and *Rsa* I to generate the terminal restriction fragment (TRF). The DNA samples were electrophoresed on a 0.8% agarose gel in TAE buffer. The DNA was transferred to a nylon membrane in 20× SSC overnight. After a 30-min prehybridization, the membrane was hybridized for 3 h at 42°C with telomere probe [(TTAGGG)$_3$].

Analysis of Damage to ^{32}P 5′ End-Labeled DNA by Oxidative Stress

The 48-base fragment, 5′-(TAGTAG)$_4$(TTAGGG)$_4$-3′, was phosphorylated with [γ-^{32}P]ATP and T4 polynucleotide kinase. The preferred cleavage sites were determined by direct comparison of the positions of the oligonucleotides with those produced by the procedure of Maxam and Gilbert using a DNA-sequencing system (LKB 2010 Macrophor). A laser densitometer (LKB 2222 UltroScan XL) was used for the measurement of the relative amounts of oligonucleotides from treated DNA fragments.

TABLE 1. TRF length and 8-oxodG formation in WI-38 fibroblasts irradiated with UVA

UVA (J/cm^2)	TRF (kb)	8-oxodG/10^5 dG ± SE
0	9.48	0.44 ± 0.07
2	8.53	0.72 ± 0.03*
5	7.98	0.98 ± 0.16**

NOTE: WI-38 fibroblasts (2.0×10^6 cells) were irradiated with the indicated dose of UVA light (365 nm). After irradiation, the cells were lysed, and DNA was extracted, subjected to enzyme digestion, and analyzed by Southern blot and HPLC-ECD. Results expressed as means ± SE, obtained from 3–5 independent experiments. *$P < .01$, **$P < .05$ compared with nonirradiation; t test.

RESULTS

Decrease in Telomere Length and Formation of 8-oxodG in WI-38 Fibroblasts by UVA Irradiation

To investigate the effect of UVA irradiation on telomere length, the size of the TRF from WI-38 fibroblasts irradiated with UVA was examined. The TRF was calculated as TRF = S(ODi)/S(ODi/Li), where ODi is densitometer output and Li is the length of the TRF fragment at position i according to the method described.[1] TRF dose-dependently declined with UVA irradiation. This result suggests that telomere shortening is accelerated with increasing of the irradiation dose (TABLE 1). The formation of 8-oxodG in WI-38 fibroblast cells significantly increased after UVA irradiation (TABLE 1).

Site Preference of DNA Cleavage by UVA Irradiation with Riboflavin

The patterns of DNA cleavage caused by UVA irradiation with riboflavin and subsequently treated with piperidine or Fpg protein were determined with DNA sequences by the Maxam-Gilbert procedure. The relative intensity of DNA cleavage obtained by scanning autoradiogram with a laser densitometer is shown in FIGURE 1. UVA irradiation of double-stranded DNA in the presence of riboflavin induced cleavages specifically at the central guanine of 5′-GGG-3′ in the telomere sequence region in DNA fragment [5′-(TAGTAG)$_4$(TTAGGG)$_4$-3′]. No or little cleavage was observed at the nontelomere sequence region (FIG. 1).

Site-Specific Damage of Telomeric DNA Fragments by Oxidative Stress

H_2O_2 plus Cu(II) ion efficiently caused DNA damage at the 5′ site of 5′-GGG-3′ in telomere sequence (FIG. 2A). The increased amount of oligonucleotides detected following piperidine treatment (data not shown) suggests that base alteration was induced by H_2O_2 in the presence of Cu(II).

SIN-1 was used as a model for the continuous release of NO and O_2^-. SIN-1 efficiently caused DNA cleavage at the 5′ site of 5′-GGG-3′ sequence in telomere sequence (FIG. 2B). A similar DNA cleavage pattern was observed with a combination of NO-generating agent (NOC-7) and O_2^--generating system (BQ + NADH) (data not shown). It has been reported that O_2^- is continuously generated through NADH-mediated BQ reduction.

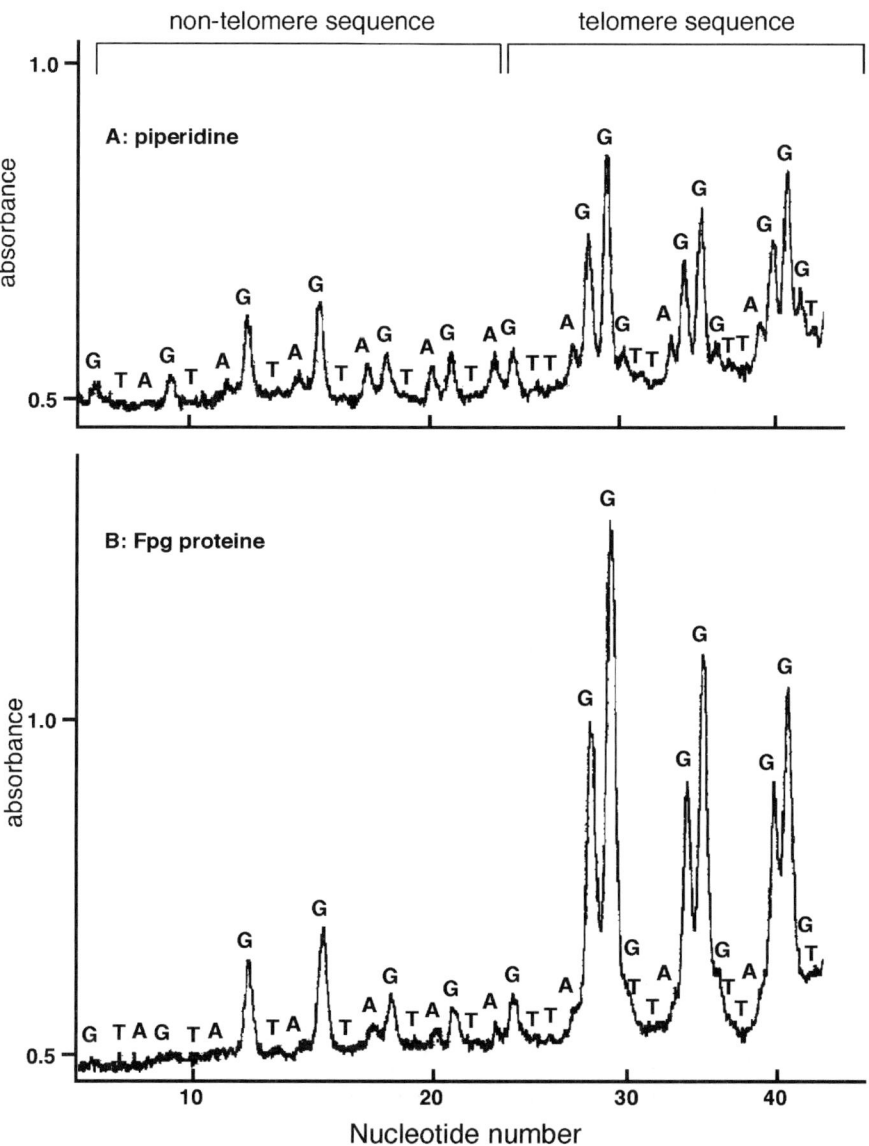

FIGURE 1. Site preference of DNA cleavage by UVA irradiation in the presence of riboflavin. The ^{32}P 5' end-labeled 48-base-pair fragment [5'-(TAGTAG)$_4$(TTAGGG)$_4$-3'] was exposed to 2 J/cm^2 UVA light (365 nm) with 20 μM riboflavin in 100 μL of 10 mM sodium phosphate buffer (pH 7.8) containing 5 μM DTPA. After piperidine **(A)** or Fpg protein **(B)** treatment, DNA fragments were electrophoresed on a 12% polyacrylamide/8 M urea gel using a DNA-sequencing system, and the autoradiogram was obtained by exposing X-ray film to the gel. The horizontal axis shows the nucleotide number.

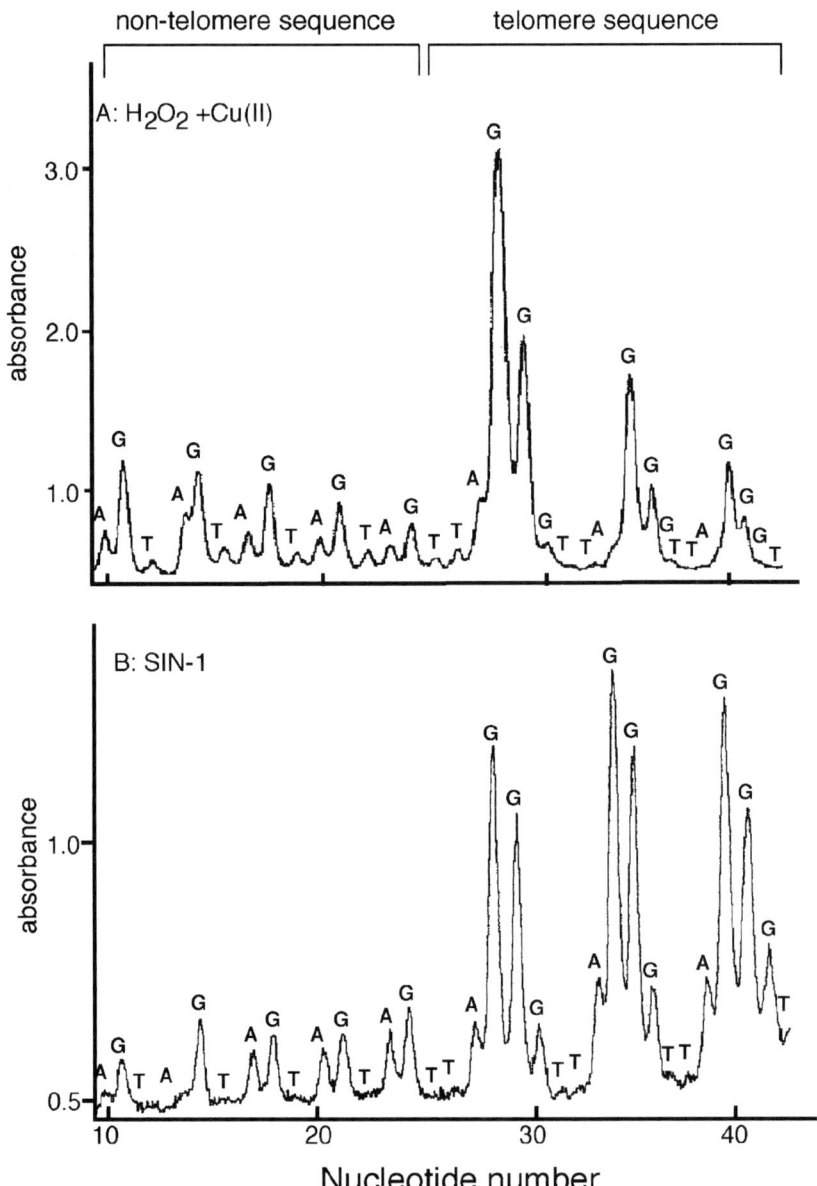

FIGURE 2. Site specificity of DNA cleavage by oxidative stress. The [32]P 5' end-labeled 48-base-pair fragment [5'-(TAGTAG)$_4$(TTAGGG)$_4$-3'] in 200 μL of 10 mM sodium bicarbonate buffer (pH 7) containing 5 μM DTPA and 20 μM per base of calf thymus DNA was incubated with 250 μM H_2O_2 in the presence of 20 μM Cu(II) **(A)** or 1 mM SIN-1 **(B)** at 37°C for 30 min. After piperidine treatment, DNA fragments were electrophoresed on a 12% polyacrylamide/8 M urea gel using a DNA-sequencing system, and the autoradiogram was obtained by exposing X-ray film to the gel.

DISCUSSION

This study demonstrated that UVA irradiation caused decreasing of telomere length, which is measured as length of TRF in WI-38 fibroblasts. Furthermore, the formation of 8-oxodG significantly increased in both WI-38 fibroblasts and HL-60 cells irradiated with UVA light dose-dependently. A progressive increase in 8-oxodG formation by UVA irradiation correlated with a decrease in TRF (TABLE 1). Human 8-oxodG-DNA glycosylase introduces a chain break in a double-stranded oligonucleotide specifically at an 8-oxodG residue base-paired with cytosine. Therefore, it is concluded that formation of 8-oxodG and piperidine-labile residues induced by UVA irradiation may participate in the increase of telomere shortening rate. In order to clarify the mechanism of the acceleration of telomere shortening, we investigated site-specific DNA damage induced by UVA irradiation in the presence of endogenous photosensitizers using DNA fragments containing the telomere sequence. UVA irradiation with riboflavin induced 8-oxodG formation specifically at the central guanine of 5'-GGG-3' in telomere sequence. The site-specific photodamage at telomeric DNA was induced through the type I mechanism. Type I mechanism involves electron transfer from DNA bases, particularly guanine, to an excited photosensitizer, resulting in formation of the guanine cation radical. Guanine has the lowest oxidation potential among the four DNA bases.

Furthermore, the present study showed that oxidative stress efficiently induced DNA damage at the 5' site of 5'-GGG-3' in telomere sequence. H_2O_2 plus Cu(II) caused predominant DNA cleavage at the 5' site of 5'-GGG-3' in the telomere sequence region in DNA fragment [5'-(TAGTAG)$_4$(TTAGGG)$_4$-3']. SIN-1, which leads to simultaneous generation of both NO and O_2^-, and NO-generating agent plus O_2^--generating system efficiently caused base alteration at the 5' site of 5'-GGG-3' sequence in telomere sequence.

Oxidative stress may function as a common trigger for activation of the senescence program. The GGG-specific DNA damage in telomere sequence induced by oxidative stress may play an important role in increasing of the rate of telomere shortening.[6,7] Telomere shortening might impact on the regenerative capacity of human tissues during aging and chronic diseases.[8] In addition, by keeping homocysteine levels low, folic acid can protect cerebral vessels and prevent accumulation of DNA damage in neurons caused by oxidative stress and facilitated by homocysteine.[9] Thus, elevated homocysteine levels may render the brain vulnerable to age-related neurodegenerative disorders. We have demonstrated that homocysteine causes sequence-specific DNA damage via reactive oxygen species generation in the presence of Cu(II).[10] These results require further study to clarify whether telomere dysfunction contributes to aging and chronic diseases.

REFERENCES

1. HARLEY, C.B., A.B. FUTCHER & C.W. GREIDER. 1990. Telomeres shorten during ageing of human fibroblasts. Nature **345**: 458–460.
2. CAWTHON, R.M., K.R. SMITH, E. O'BRIEN *et al.* 2003. Association between telomere length in blood and mortality in people aged 60 years or older. Lancet **361**: 393–395.
3. BAIRD, D.M., J. ROWSON, D. WYNFORD-THOMAS & D. KIPLING. 2003. Extensive allelic variation and ultrashort telomeres in senescent human cells. Nat. Genet. **33**: 203–207.

4. VON ZGLINICKI, T. 2002. Oxidative stress shortens telomeres. Trends Biochem. Sci. **27:** 339–344.
5. KAWANISHI, S., Y. HIRAKU & S. OIKAWA. 2001. Mechanism of guanine-specific DNA damage by oxidative stress and its role in carcinogenesis and aging. Mutat. Res. **488:** 65–76.
6. OIKAWA, S., S. TADA-OIKAWA & S. KAWANISHI. 2001. Site-specific DNA damage at the GGG sequence by UVA involves acceleration of telomere shortening. Biochemistry **40:** 4763–4768.
7. OIKAWA, S. & S. KAWANISHI. 1999. Site-specific DNA damage at GGG sequence by oxidative stress may accelerate telomere shortening. FEBS Lett. **453:** 365–368.
8. SATYANARAYANA, A., S.U. WIEMANN, J. BUER *et al.* 2003. Telomere shortening impairs organ regeneration by inhibiting cell cycle re-entry of a subpopulation of cells. EMBO J. **22:** 4003–4013.
9. MATTSON, M.P. 2003. Gene-diet interactions in brain aging and neurodegenerative disorders. Ann. Intern. Med. **139:** 441–444.
10. OIKAWA, S., K. MURAKAMI & S. KAWANISHI. 2003. Oxidative damage to cellular and isolated DNA by homocysteine: implications for carcinogenesis. Oncogene **22:** 3530–3538.

Lysosomal Redox-Active Iron Is Important for Oxidative Stress–Induced DNA Damage

TINO KURZ,[a,b] ALAN LEAKE,[a] THOMAS VON ZGLINICKI,[a] AND ULF T. BRUNK[b]

[a]*School of Clinical Medical Sciences–Gerontology, University of Newcastle upon Tyne, Newcastle General Hospital, Henry Wellcome Laboratory for Biogerontology Research, Newcastle upon Tyne NE4 6BE, United Kingdom*

[b]*Division of Pathology II, Medical Faculty, University of Linköping, SE-581 85 Linköping, Sweden*

ABSTRACT: Data show that specifically chelating lysosomal redox-active iron can prevent most H_2O_2-induced DNA damage. Lysosomes seem to contain the major pool of redox-active labile iron within the cell. Under oxidative stress conditions, this iron may then relocate to the nucleus and play an important role for DNA damage by taking part in Fenton reactions.

KEYWORDS: lysosomes; oxidative stress; desferrioxamine; telomeres

INTRODUCTION

Oxidative damage to DNA is known to involve Fenton chemistry. Transition metals, such as iron, interact with hydrogen peroxide (H_2O_2) and produce the highly reactive hydroxyl radical.[1–3] Due to its short half-life (~10^{-9} s), the hydroxyl radical can travel only 4 nm and, thus, induces site-specific damage. Therefore, in order to induce DNA damage, the redox-active iron must be in close proximity to DNA. So far, the presence of redox-active iron inside the nucleus has never been convincingly shown. Recently, lysosomes have been suggested as a major pool of redox-active iron.[4,5] Lysosomes are the sites of intracellular degradation of organelles and long-lived proteins (e.g., ferritin and many metalloproteins) and, therefore, contain a pool of loose or labile iron. Such iron can catalyze Fenton reactions in the presence of H_2O_2, resulting in rupture of lysosomal membranes and subsequent efflux of redox-active iron into the cytoplasm. From there, it may relocate to the nucleus and induce DNA damage under persistent oxidative stress. In order to prove this hypothesis, we used the iron chelator, desferrioxamine (DFO), coupled to starch, forming a high-molecular-weight complex (HMW-DFO) that can only be taken up by fluid-phase endocytosis and, consequently, localizes into lysosomes where it remains and makes the iron non-redox-active.[6,7]

Address for correspondence: Tino Kurz, School of Clinical Medical Sciences–Gerontology, University of Newcastle upon Tyne, Newcastle General Hospital, Henry Wellcome Laboratory for Biogerontology Research, Newcastle upon Tyne NE4 6BE, United Kingdom. Voice: +44-(0)-191-256-3466; fax: +44-(0)-191-256-3445.

tino.kurz@ncl.ac.uk

MATERIALS AND METHODS

Acute lymphoblastic T cells 1301 were grown in suspension in RPMI 1640 medium. Lysosomal membrane stability in the 1301 cell line was assayed using the metachromatic fluorophore, acridine orange (AO), that fluoresces red at high concentrations and green at low concentrations. AO is also a lysosomotropic base ($pK_a \approx 10$) and is retained in its charged form by proton trapping mainly inside the acidic vacuolar compartment, preferentially in secondary lysosomes (pH 4–5). AO-loaded cells show intense granular (lysosomal) red fluorescence in a moderate green cytosol with green nuclei. Flow cytofluorometry was used to monitor early lysosomal rupture and AO relocation,[8] resulting in increased green cytoplasmic and nuclear fluorescence, during oxidative stress. In other experiments, cells were stained with AO at 5 h after the end of oxidative stress and following return of the cells to standard culture conditions. In these AO uptake experiments,[8] cells with a reduced number of intact AO-accumulating lysosomes were detected by their diminished red fluorescence.

General DNA damage was measured using a semiautomated, fluorescence-detected alkaline DNA unwinding (FADU) assay.[9] DNA unwinding in alkali starts at DNA ends and strand breaks. After time-controlled partial DNA unwinding, the amount of DNA fluorescence dye (SYBR Green) incorporated into the DNA is inversely proportional to the amount of DNA strand breaks.

To assess DNA damage in telomeres, the frequency of their single-strand breaks was measured using the S1 nuclease assay.[10] Cells were subjected to a bolus dose of H_2O_2 for 30 min, embedded in agarose plugs, and digested with proteinase K. DNA was restricted with *Hinf*I and single-strand breaks converted into double-strand breaks by nuclease S1. After size separation of DNA fragments in a pulsed field gel electrophoresis, the DNA was hybridized to a ^{32}P-γ-ATP-labeled telomeric probe. Telomeric signals were visualized in a phosphoimager and average telomere length calculated by densitometry.

RESULTS AND DISCUSSION

The 1301 cells were exposed to fluorescence-labeled dextran in order to show that a high-molecular-weight complex with a similar molecular weight as HMW-DFO can only be taken up by endocytosis and remains inside lysosomes. After 3-h incubation, a distinct cytoplasmic granular staining pattern could be observed, indicating stable lysosomal localization.

The protection of lysosomes by ordinary DFO and HMW-DFO against oxidative stress using the AO relocation and uptake methods was then examined. After exposure of 1301 cells to 50 μM H_2O_2 for 30 min, a 2.5-fold increase in green fluorescence compared to control cells was observed, indicating rupture of lysosomes and release of AO into the cytoplasm. Lysosomal membranes were stabilized when cells were exposed to 1–3 mM unconjugated DFO for 1–3 h prior to oxidative stress. To achieve the same degree of lysosomal protection with conjugated DFO (HMW-DFO), a somewhat higher concentration and a longer uptake time were required (2–3 mM and 3 h). Using the AO uptake method to examine later lysosomal rupture, no difference was observed between the control and protected cells following 3-h exposure

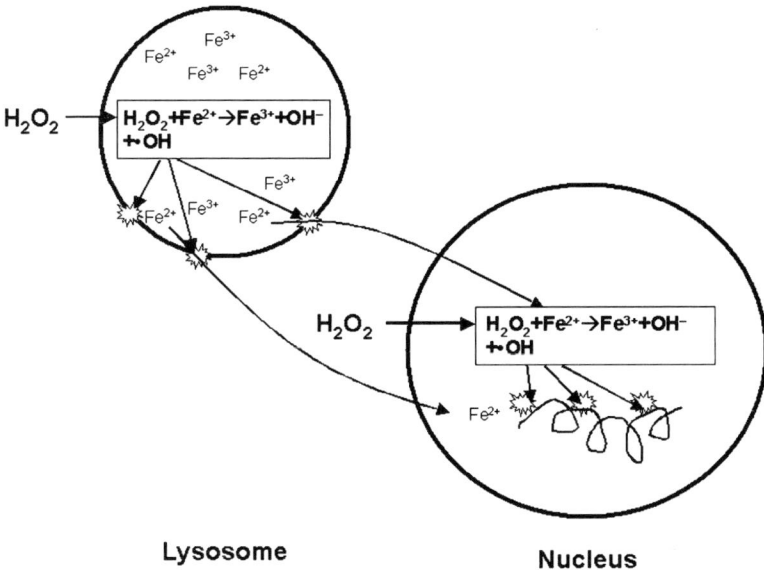

FIGURE 1. Under H_2O_2-induced oxidative stress, lysosomal redox-active iron reacts in Fenton chemistry to produce the highly reactive hydroxyl radicals, which cause lysosomal membrane rupture. Released redox-active iron may relocate to the nucleus and induce DNA damage under persistent oxidative stress.

to 3 mM DFO or HMW-DFO. Red lysosomal fluorescence was measured 5 h after exposure to different H_2O_2 concentrations.

Pretreatment of cells with DFO showed a concentration-dependent protective effect against DNA damage. A preexposure of cells to 3 mM DFO for 3 h was sufficient to almost completely protect the cells against DNA damage induced by 50 μM H_2O_2. The efficiency of HMW-DFO in protecting against DNA damage was somewhat less effective. However, prolonged preincubation (6 h) partly compensated for this.

Since telomeres are specifically vulnerable to oxidative stress and are important triggers for stress responses and senescent cell cycle arrest, we wanted to know if DFO and HMW-DFO also protect telomeres against oxidative challenge. The data show a significant protection of telomeric DNA against H_2O_2-induced single-strand breaks by both DFO and HMW-DFO after cells were preincubated with 1–3 mM DFO or HMW-DFO for 3 h. The protection by the lower concentrations of HMW-DFO is significantly less than that by DFO.

In summary, the data show that specifically chelating lysosomal redox-active iron can prevent most H_2O_2-induced DNA damage. Furthermore, lysosomes seem to contain the major pool of redox-active labile iron within the cell. Under oxidative stress conditions, this iron may then relocate to the nucleus and play an important role for DNA damage by taking part in Fenton reactions (FIG. 1).

ACKNOWLEDGMENTS

This work was supported by the Swedish Cancer Society (Grant No. 4296 to U. T. Brunk) and by UK Medical Research Council and Research into Ageing grants to T. von Zglinicki.

REFERENCES

1. HALLIWELL, B. & O.I. ARUOMA. 1991. DNA damage by oxygen-derived species: its mechanism and measurement in mammalian systems. FEBS Lett. **281:** 9–19.
2. MENEGHINI, R. 1997. Iron homeostasis, oxidative stress, and DNA damage. Free Radical Biol. Med. **23:** 783–792.
3. CHATGILIALOGLU, C. & P. O'NEILL. 2001. Free radicals associated with DNA damage. Exp. Gerontol. **36:** 1459–1471.
4. PERSSON, H.L. et al. 2003. Prevention of oxidant-induced cell death by lysosomotropic iron chelators. Free Radical Biol. Med. **34:** 1295–1305.
5. YU, Z. et al. 2003. Intralysosomal iron: a major determinant of oxidant-induced cell death. Free Radical Biol. Med. **34:** 1243–1252.
6. GRAF, E. et al. 1984. Iron-catalyzed hydroxyl radical formation: stringent requirement for free iron coordination site. J. Biol. Chem. **259:** 3620–3624.
7. LLOYD, J.B., H. CABLE & C. RICE-EVANS. 1991. Evidence that desferrioxamine cannot enter cells by passive diffusion. Biochem. Pharmacol. **41:** 1361–1363.
8. ZDOLSEK, J. et al. 1993. H_2O_2-mediated damage to lysosomal membranes of J-774 cells. Free Radical Res. Commun. **18:** 71–85.
9. BRABECK, C. et al. 2003. L-Selegiline potentiates the cellular poly(ADP-ribosyl)ation response to ionizing radiation. J. Pharmacol. Exp. Ther. **306:** 973–979.
10. VON ZGLINICKI, T., R. PILGER & N. SITTE. 2000. Accumulation of single-strand breaks is the major cause of telomere shortening in human fibroblasts. Free Radical Biol. Med. **28:** 64–74.

Low Levels of mtDNA Deletion Mutations in ETS Normal Fibers from Aged Rats

JEONG W. PAK AND JUDD M. AIKEN

*Department of Animal Health and Biomedical Sciences,
University of Wisconsin–Madison, Madison, Wisconsin 53706, USA*

ABSTRACT: The objectives were (1) to determine whether deletion mutations occur in phenotypically normal type I and type II fibers, (2) to quantify the levels of both deletion mutant and wild-type (wt) mtDNA (nondeletion) within single normal fibers containing mutant mtDNA, and (3) to quantify the amount of wt mtDNA in genotypically and phenotypically normal type I and type II fibers. Deletion mutations in normal fibers are not restricted to specific fiber types, although clonal accumulation of mtDNA deletion mutations and subsequent ETS abnormalities occur exclusively in type II fibers.

KEYWORDS: mitochondrial DNA; deletion mutations; ETS abnormality; fiber type; quantitative PCR

BACKGROUND AND OBJECTIVES

Mitochondrial DNA (mtDNA) deletion mutations can accumulate to levels that result in electron transport system (ETS) abnormal regions (cytochrome *c* oxidase negative, succinate dehydrogenase hyperreactive) in aged skeletal muscle.[1,2] The ETS abnormal phenotype is primarily observed in type II fibers. Fibers containing these enzymatic abnormalities are prone to fiber atrophy and fiber breakage, suggesting a molecular basis for age-associated muscle fiber loss.[2] MtDNA sequence analysis of microdissected portions of single fibers containing the ETS abnormal regions identified large deletion mutations. These deletion mutations were contained within the major arc of the mitochondrial genome, between the cyt *b* and COX subunit genes.[3]

We have shown that certain muscles (soleus, adductor longus) rarely have ETS abnormalities and exhibit little fiber loss with age.[4] These muscles predominantly comprise type I fibers. This lack of ETS abnormal phenotype in type I fibers could be due to an inability of these fibers to either generate or accumulate mtDNA deletion mutations. We found, however, that PCR analysis of tissue homogenates of soleus muscle identified mtDNA deletion mutations. In addition, in muscles that accumulate ETS abnormalities with age (vastus lateralis, rectus femoris), tissue homogenate analysis revealed numerous mtDNA deletion mutations including

---

Address for correspondence: Judd M. Aiken, Department of Animal Health and Biomedical Sciences, University of Wisconsin–Madison, 1656 Linden Drive, Madison, WI 53706. Voice: 608-262-7362; fax: 608-262-7420.
aiken@svm.vetmed.wisc.edu

minor arc deletions and deletion mutations that removed the light strand origin. These observations suggest that only a subset of mtDNA deletion mutations clonally accumulate to levels resulting in the ETS abnormal phenotype. Given that mtDNA deletion mutations need to be abundant (60–90%) to exhibit an ETS abnormal phenotype,[5–7] we initiated a study to examine the mtDNA deletion load in individual ETS normal fibers. Our objectives were (1) to determine whether deletion mutations occur in phenotypically normal type I and type II fibers, (2) to quantify the levels of both deletion mutant and wild-type (wt) mtDNA (nondeletion) within single normal fibers containing mutant mtDNA, and (3) to quantify the amount of wt mtDNA in genotypically and phenotypically normal type I and type II fibers.

PRINCIPAL FINDINGS

(1) About 10–25% of ETS normal fibers analyzed from aged rat skeletal muscle contained deletion mutations.
(2) Deletion mutations were clonal within a fiber.
(3) Deletion mutational loads in individual ETS normal fibers (10-μm fiber segments) were low, ranging between 0.01% and 2.17%, in both type I and type II fibers (FIG. 1a).
(4) No difference was observed in wt mtDNA levels between type I and type II fibers (FIG. 1b).
(5) The incidence of mtDNA deletion mutations is not specific for fiber type, but the accumulation and subsequent phenotypic effect of the genetic defect are dependent upon fiber type.

Using laser-capture microdissection, 96 individual ETS normal fibers were isolated from vastus lateralis and soleus muscle of 36-month-old Fischer 344 × Brown Norway F1 hybrid rats ($n = 3$). PCR and direct sequencing analyses of these phenotypically normal fibers revealed 3 deletion mutations from 28 soleus type I fibers (10.7%), 5 deletions in 28 vastus lateralis type I fibers (17.8%), 5 deletions in 20 type IIa fibers (25%), and 4 deletions in 20 type IIb fibers (20%). Generally, the deletion mutations were clonal within a fiber (i.e., in those fibers containing mtDNA deletion mutations, only a single size amplification product was found). The size of the deletion mutations varied among individual fibers. The average size of the deletions was 8.6 ± 1.4 kb. Most deletion mutations were localized to the major arc region of the mitochondrial genome, except that 3 deletions each from type I, type IIa, and type IIb fibers (vastus lateralis) removed the light strand origin, generating an ~11-kb deletion.

Real-time quantitative PCR was performed for both wt mtDNA and deletion mutant mtDNA within single normal fibers to measure mutational loads. The mean mutation loads (percentage of mutant mtDNA out of total mtDNA) were very low (0.01–2%) from these normal fibers regardless of the fiber type (FIG. 1a). Interestingly, there was no significant difference in the level of wt mtDNA between type I and type II fibers (FIG. 1b). The average copy of wt mtDNA per cell (10-μm-thick fiber segment) was ~1.0×10^5 from all skeletal muscle fiber types analyzed. It was also noted that the presence of deletion mutations did not affect the levels of wt mtDNA.

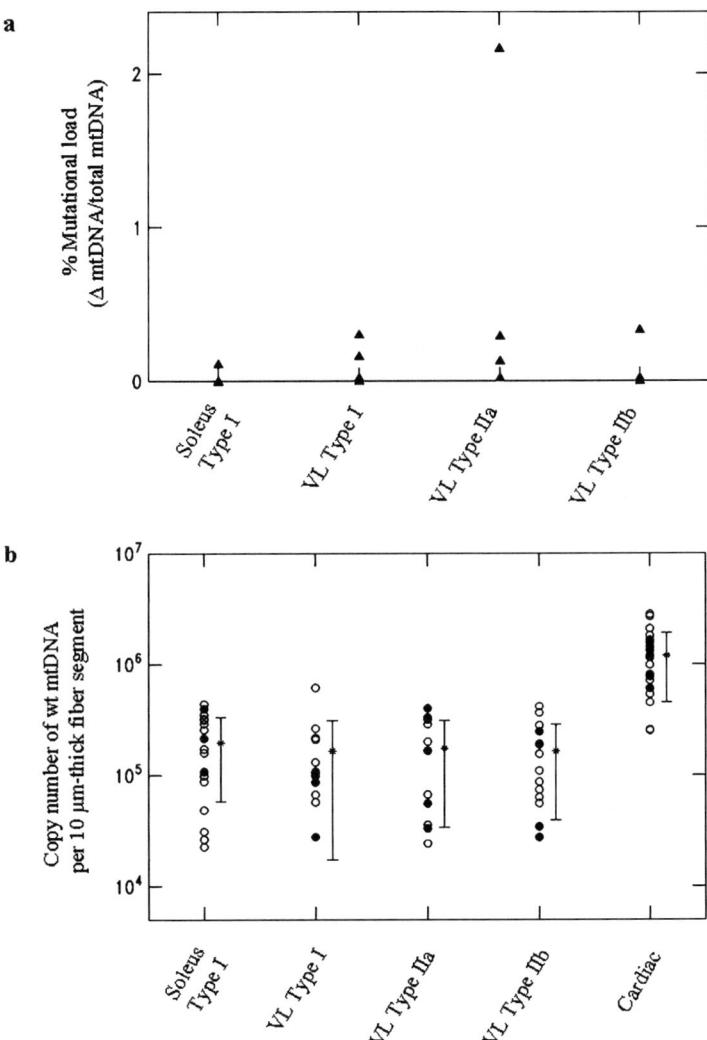

FIGURE 1. Percentage of deletion (Δ) mutant mtDNA genome **(a)** and quantitation of absolute amount of wt mtDNA **(b)** in individual ETS normal type I and type II fibers from 36-month-old rats. *Closed triangles* indicate the percent of mutant mtDNA out of total mtDNA in each normal fiber. *Open circles* represent genotypically and phenotypically normal fibers, while *closed circles* denote phenotypically normal fibers containing deletion mutations. Cardiac cells, used as a comparison to skeletal muscle fibers, contained approximately 10-fold more wt mtDNA copies than skeletal muscle fibers. Each data point is a mean value of at least triplicate measures.

CONCLUSIONS AND SIGNIFICANCE

MtDNA deletion mutations were identified in ETS normal fibers from aged rats, albeit at low abundance. To our knowledge, this is the first report on the presence of mtDNA deletion mutations in single ETS normal fibers from naturally aged rats. Previous studies showed that the mutant mtDNA genomes were absent or rare in normal fiber segments from patients with mitochondrial myopathy as well as aged rat muscle.[3,8,9] One prominent feature of the deletion mutations from the normal fibers in this work is the loss of the light strand origin of replication. These large deletions were identified in both fiber types of the normal fibers, but were not found in ETS abnormal fibers, where the deletion mutations were exclusively localized to the major arc region of the mitochondrial genome. Although deletion mutations were present in normal fibers, their abundance within a fiber was very low.

The presence and number of different deletion mutations in normal fibers are not specific for fiber type. The mutational loads in normal fibers are equally low between the fiber types. Only certain mutations in type II fibers, presumably those with a replicative advantage, selectively accumulate to reach a phenotypic threshold and result in ETS dysfunction. The rareness of ETS abnormalities in type I fibers in aged rat skeletal muscle is not due to an inability of the fibers to generate deletion mutations. Deletion mutations can be generated in type I fibers, yet these mutations do not accumulate to sufficient levels to produce the ETS abnormalities. Despite similar wt mtDNA amounts, histochemical staining for COX and SDH enzyme activities displayed higher enzymatic activities in type I/IIa fibers than in type IIb fibers. Therefore, not only the levels of mutated DNA, but also the expression levels of ETS enzymes, which vary depending on fiber types or different tissues, could be important factors affecting the cellular phenotype of deletion mutations.

REFERENCES

1. MUELLER-HOECKER, J., P. SEIBEL, K. SCHNEIDERBANGER & B. KADENBACH. 1993. Different *in situ* hybridization patterns of mitochondrial DNA in cytochrome *c* oxidase–deficient extraocular muscle fibers in the elderly. Virchows Arch. A Pathol. Anat. Histopathol. **422:** 7–15.
2. WANAGAT, J., Z. CAO, P. PATHARE & J.M. AIKEN. 2001. Mitochondrial DNA deletion mutations colocalize with segmental electron transport system abnormalities, muscle fiber atrophy, fiber splitting, and oxidative damage in sarcopenia. FASEB J. **15:** 322–332.
3. CAO, Z., J. WANAGAT, S. MCKIERNAN & J.M. AIKEN. 2001. Mitochondrial DNA deletion mutations are concomitant with ragged red regions of individual, aged muscle fibers: analysis by laser-capture microdissection. Nucleic Acids Res. **29:** 4502–4508.
4. BUA, E.A., S. MCKIERNAN, J. WANAGAT *et al.* 2002. Mitochondrial abnormalities are more frequent in muscles undergoing sarcopenia. J. Appl. Physiol. **92:** 2617–2624.
5. HAYASHI, J.I., S. OHTA, A. KIKUCHI *et al.* 1991. Introduction of disease-related mitochondrial DNA deletions into HeLa cells lacking mitochondrial DNA results in mitochondrial dysfunction. Proc. Natl. Acad. Sci. USA **88:** 10614–10618.
6. MORAES, C.T. & E.A. SCHON. 1996. Detection and analysis of mitochondrial DNA and RNA in muscle by *in situ* hybridization and single-fiber PCR. Methods Enzymol. **264:** 522–540.
7. ROSSIGNOL, R., B. FAUSTIN, C. ROCHER *et al.* 2003. Mitochondrial threshold effects. Biochem. J. **370:** 751–762.

8. SHOUBRIDGE, E.A., G. KARPATI & K.E.M. HASTINGS. 1990. Deletion mutants are functionally dominant over wild-type mitochondrial genomes in skeletal muscle fiber segments in mitochondrial disease. Cell **62:** 43–49.
9. SCIACCO, M., E. BONILLA, E.A. SCHON *et al.* 1994. Distribution of wild-type and common deletion forms of mtDNA in normal and respiration-deficient muscle fibers from patients with mitochondrial myopathy. Hum. Mol. Genet. **3:** 13–19.

Age-Related Muscle Loss and Progressive Dysfunction in Mechanosensitive Growth Factor Signaling

GEOFFREY GOLDSPINK

Division of Surgery, Royal Free and University College Medical School, Royal Free Campus, Rowland Hill Street, London NW3 2PF, United Kingdom

ABSTRACT: Loss of muscle mass and function (sarcopenia) is one of the most marked problems associated with aging because it has major healthcare as well as socioeconomic implications. The growth hormone/IGF-I axis is regarded as an important regulator of muscle mass. However, it is now appreciated that other tissues in addition to the liver express IGF-I. Also, there are local as well as systemic forms of IGF-I that have different functions. We cloned two different IGF-Is that are expressed by skeletal muscle, and both are derived from the IGF-I gene by alternative splicing. One of these is expressed in response to physical activity, which has now been called "mechanogrowth factor" (MGF). The other is similar to the systemic or liver type (IGF-IEa) and is important as the provider of mature IGF-I required for upregulating protein synthesis. MGF differs from systemic IGF-IEa in that it has a different peptide sequence that is responsible for activating muscle satellite (stem) cells. Therefore, it appears these two forms of IGF-I have different actions and that they are important regulators of muscle growth. Growth hormone treatment apparently upregulates the level of IGF-I gene expression, and when it is combined with resistance exercise more is spliced toward MGF. This results in an increase in muscle cross-sectional area in the elderly subjects who otherwise would produce less MGF. The possibility of ameliorating sarcopenia using MGF delivered as a peptide or by gene therapy will be discussed.

KEYWORDS: age-related muscle loss; IGF-I; MGF; sarcopenia; growth hormone; resistance training; young, elderly human volunteers

Loss of muscle mass and function (sarcopenia) is one of the most marked problems associated with aging because it has major healthcare as well as socioeconomic implications. One of the more obvious problems is that the elderly tend to fall over and break bones made brittle by osteoporosis. This is probably because of their poorer sense of balance but also because they cannot generate sufficient muscle power to prevent falling. Muscles generate the mechanical strain that maintains bone, and a vicious circle is established when the muscles start to produce less and less force resulting in more and more loss of bone. Because muscle generates most of the heat

Address for correspondence: Geoffrey Goldspink, Division of Surgery, Royal Free and University College Medical School, Royal Free Campus, Rowland Hill Street, London NW3 2PF, United Kingdom. Voice: +44-0-20-7830-2410; fax: +44-0-20-7830-2917.
goldspink@rfc.ucl.ac.uk

Ann. N.Y. Acad. Sci. 1019: 294–298 (2004). © 2004 New York Academy of Sciences.
doi: 10.1196/annals.1297.050

necessary for maintaining the body temperature, keeping warm is often a problem for older people with decreased muscle mass and lack of exercise. Another aspect that is less well appreciated is that muscle acts as a dynamic metabolic store, and in a traumatic situation it is muscle that produces proteins to prevent tissue cachexia and metabolites required for acid–base balance. Hence, a frail old lady may not survive major surgery or a traffic accident because of lack of muscle tissue. Animal experiments have shown that older muscles are injured more easily[1] and regenerate less successfully,[2] and this normally results in an impaired functional recovery.[3] Contraction-induced injury combined with the inability to undergo local repair is probably the reason for age-related atrophy. Denervation of muscle fibers is also a contributory problem to muscle loss during aging. Electrophysiology experiments in human subjects and animal experiments[4,5] indicate that aged muscle fiber are less likely to be reinnervated by axonal sprouting, thus resulting in a loss of muscle fibers during the aging process.

CLONING OF MUSCLE GROWTH FACTORS

The growth hormone/IGF-I axis is regarded as an important regulator of muscle mass. However, it is apparent that there must be local as well as systemic control of

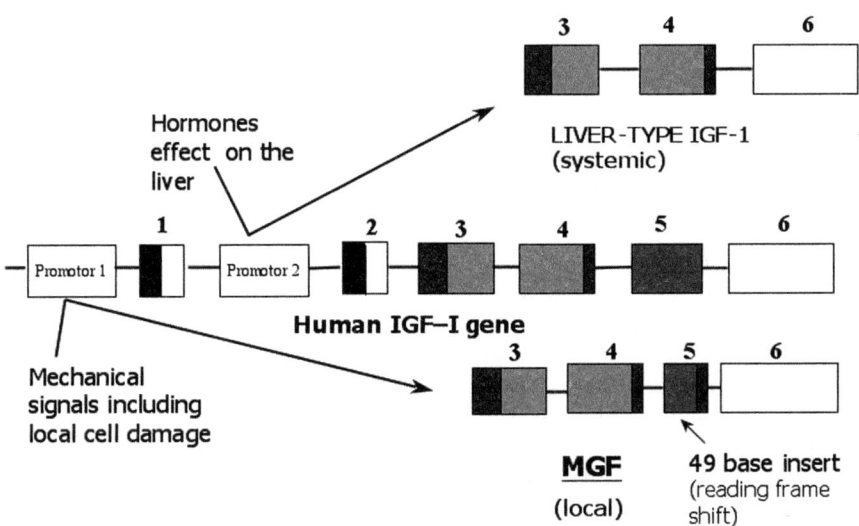

FIGURE 1. The way in which the IGF-I is spliced in muscle as a result of exercise and/or muscle damage (Promoter 1) and hormones (Promoter 2). The IGF-I receptor domain is included in all these splice variants and is encoded by exons 3 and 4. In human muscle, a 49-base insert (52-base insert in the rat) changes the reading frameshift in MGF, resulting in a different carboxy peptide. Hormones upregulate the expression of the IGF-I gene particularly the IGF-IEa, and, as recent work has shown, by combining growth hormone therapy plus resistance training, MGF can be markedly upregulated in elderly muscle.

muscle growth, because if a muscle is exercised it is that muscle that undergoes hypertrophy, not all the muscles of the body. We cloned two different growth factors that are expressed by skeletal muscle, and both are derived from the IGF-I gene by alternative splicing (FIG. 1). One of these is expressed in response to physical activity which has now been called "mechanogrowth factor" (MGF). The other is similar to the systemic or liver type (IGF-IEa) and is important as the provider of mature IGF-I required for upregulating protein synthesis. Its expression is also upregulated by exercise; this presumably explains why during intensive exercise most of the circulating IGF-I is derived from muscle rather than the liver.[6] MGF differs from systemic IGF-IEa; it has a 49-base insert in the human (52 in the rat) which results in a reading frameshift and hence a different carboxy peptide sequence. The E domain of MGF has been shown to act as a separate growth factor and is responsible for activating muscle satellite (stem) cells. Therefore, it appears these two forms of IGF-I have different roles, but they are both important regulators of muscle growth.

To determine if MGF would be effective for muscle maintenance, we inserted its cDNA into a plasmid vector and introduced this by intramuscular injection into normal mice. This resulted in a 25% increase in the mean muscle fiber size in injected muscle within 2 weeks.[7] Similar experiments by other groups have also been conducted using a viral construct containing the liver type of IGF-I. This also resulted in a 25% increase in muscle mass, but this took over 4 months to develop.[8] The probable reason why MGF is so effective in producing muscle hypertrophy in comparison with IGF-IEa is that it is responsible for the initial activation of the muscle satellite (stem) cells, and this acts as a "kick start" for the hypertrophy/repair process.

EXPRESSION OF MGF IN ELDERLY MUSCLE IN RESPONSE TO EXERCISE

In a recent study in our laboratory,[9] we used tendon ablation to overload the soleus and plantaris muscles of young, mature, and old rats. This study showed that as a result of overload MGF mRNA was three times higher in the young muscle as compared with mature muscle and five times higher than in the older muscles. IGF-IEa mRNA levels also were upregulated by the challenge but showed no clear age-related effect. The study therefore suggested an age-related reduction in the ability to upregulate the MGF isoform. Furthermore, it was suggested that the two IGF-I isoforms were differentially regulated. A similar study was performed on young (25–36 years) and elderly (76–82 years) volunteers using 10 repetitions of knee extensor exercises.[10] Muscle biopsy samples were obtained from the quadricep muscle of both the control and exercised legs 2.5 hours after completion of the exercise bout. Expression levels of the IGF-I mRNA transcripts were determined using real-time quantitative RT-PCR with specific primers. No difference was observed between the resting levels of the two isoforms between the two subject groups. High-resistance exercise resulted in a significant increase in MGF mRNA in the young, but not in the elderly subjects. No changes in IGF-IEa mRNA levels were observed as a result of exercise in either group.

GROWTH HORMONES AND EXERCISE

One of the most marked effects of aging is that at 70+ years upward our circulating growth hormone levels are only approximately one third of what it is during our late teen years.[11] GH produced by the pituitary is known to induce liver IGF-I expression, but the roles of circulating GH and circulating IGF-I are unclear. The results of gene deletion experiments using the Cre-loxP method have questioned the role of liver IGF-I and circulating IGF-I in controlling postnatal muscle growth.[12,13] The measurements of body weight made from 3 to 6 weeks, body length and individual organ weights at 6 weeks were no different between the knockout animals and their wild-type littermates, thus emphasizing the role of the local IGF-I system in this process. However, Michael Kajaer's group in Copenhagen showed that growth hormone (GH) treatment upregulates the level of IGF-I gene expression and when combined with resistance exercise more is spliced toward MGF.[14] This resulted in an increase in muscle cross-sectional area in the elderly subjects, but the response was still not as high as in young subjects. When using GH treatment combined with resistance exercise therefore, there seems to be possibility of ameliorating sarcopenia.

MECHANOTRANSDUCTION

Mechanical signals influence gene expression in several types of tissue. The mechanism via which these are detected by the cells are not known, although in certain diseases such as the muscular dystrophies the cytoskeleton system is defective and they are unable to upregulate MGF expression.[15] Recent evidence from work involving the transfer of the dystrophin gene using stem cells into dystrophic muscle indicates that dystrophin is involved in mechanotransduction as the ability to produce MGF is restored by transferring the correct gene.[16] Whether this is true for aged human muscle cells which also cannot express MGF at the same levels as in younger people is not known but needs to be further investigated. It has been shown that there is a marked decrease loss of compliance due to connective tissue changes in muscle during aging.[17] It is expected that this will affect the mechanotransduction system involved in switching on certain genes, including MGF as response to physical activity. This aspect, however, has yet to be investigated in relation to the inability to express certain genes.

REFERENCES

1. ZERBA, E., T.E. KOMOROWSKI & J.A. FAULKNER. 1990. Free radical injury to skeletal muscles of young, adult and old mice. Am. J. Physiol. **258**: C429–C435.
2. CARLSON, B.M. & J.A. FAULKNER. 1989. Muscle transplantation between young and old rats: age of host determines recovery. Am. J. Physiol. **256**: C1262–C1266.
3. BROOKS, S.V. & J.A. FAULKNER. 1990. Contraction-induced injury: recovery of skeletal muscles in young and old mice. Am. J. Physiol. **258**: C436–C442.
4. MCCOMAS, A.J. & R.E. SICA. 1978. Automatic quantitative analysis of the electromyogram in partially denervated distal muscles: comparison with motor unit counting. Can. J. Neurol. Sci. **5**: 377–383.
5. LEXELL, J., C.C. TAYLOR & M. SJOSTROM. 1988. What is the cause of the ageing atrophy? Total number, size and proportion of different fiber types studied in whole vastus lateralis muscle from 15- to 83-year-old-men. J. Neurol. Sci. **84**: 275–294.

6. BRAHM, H., K. PIEHL-AULIN, B. SALTIN & S. LJUNGHALL. 1997. Net fluxes over working thigh of hormones, growth factors and biomarkers of bone metabolism during short lasting dynamic exercise. Calcif. Tissue Int. **60:** 175–180.
7. GOLDSPINK, G. & S.Y. YANG, inventors. University College London, London (GB), assignee. 2001. USA patent 6,221,842 B1. 2001 April 24.
8. MUSARO, A., K. MCCULLAGH, A. PAUL, *et al.* 2001. Localized Igf-1 transgene expression sustains hypertrophy and regeneration in senescent skeletal muscle. Nat. Genet. **27:** 195–200.
9. OWINO, V., S.Y. YANG, & G. GOLDSPINK. 2001. Age-related loss of skeletal muscle function and the inability to express the autocrine form of insulin-like growth factor-1 (MGF) in response to mechanical overload. FEBS Lett. **505:** 259–263.
10. HAMEED, M., R.W. ORRELL, M. COBBOLD, *et al.* 2003. Expression of IGF-I splice variants in young and old human skeletal muscle after high resistance exercise. J. Physiol. **547:** 247–254.
11. RUDMAN, D., M.H. KUTNER, C.M. ROGERS, *et al.* 1981. Impaired growth hormone secretion in the adult population: relation to age and adiposity. J. Clin. Invest. **67:** 1361–1369.
12. SJORGREN, K., J.L. LIU, K. BLAD, *et al.* 1999. Liver-derived insulin-like growth factor I (IGF-I) is the principal source of IGF-I in blood but is not required for postnatal body growth in mice. Proc. Natl. Acad. Sci. USA **96:** 7088–7092.
13. YAKAR, S., J.L. LIU, B. STANNARD, et al. 1999. Normal growth and development in the absence of hepatic insulin-like growth factor I. Proc. Natl. Acad. Sci. USA **96:** 7324–7329.
14. HAMEED, M., K.H.W. LANGE, J.L. ANDERSEN, *et al.* 2004. The effect of recombinant human growth hormone and resistance training on IGF-I mRNA expression in the muscles of elderly men. J. Physiol. **555:** 231–240.
15. GOLDSPINK, G., S.Y. YANG, M. SKARLI & G. VRBOVA. 1996. Local growth regulation is associated with an isoform of IGF-I that is expressed in normal muscles but not in dystrophic muscles. J. Physiol. **495:** 162.
16. DE BARI, C., F. DELL'ACCIO, F. VANDENABEELE, *et al.* 2003. Skeletal muscle repair by adult human mesenchymal stem cells from synovial membrane. J. Cell Biol. **160:** 909–918.
17. ALNAQEEB, M.A., N.S. AL ZAID & G. GOLDSPINK. 1984. Connective tissue changes and physical properties of developing and ageing skeletal muscle. J. Anat. **139:** 677–689.

What Do Hormones Have to Do with Aging? What Does Aging Have to Do with Hormones?

S. MITCHELL HARMAN

Kronos Longevity Research Institute, Phoenix, Arizona 85016, USA

ABSTRACT: It is clear that aging results in alterations of endocrine physiology, which in turn appear to contribute to development of the senescent phenotype. How the underlying basic aging process or processes cause the endocrine cell dysfunctions leading to hormone imbalance is far from clear, but oxidative alteration of cell membranes is an attractive candidate mechanism that might be susceptible to some degree of global remediation.

KEYWORDS: hormones; aging; diet; cell; damage; oxidative stress

Aging humans lose skeletal muscle mass and strength[1] as well as aerobic capacity.[2] These changes are accompanied by diminished function, which may lead to frailty and dependency.[3] At the same time, total fat mass and percent body fat increase,[4] often accompanied by insulin resistance and greater risk of type 2 diabetes.[5,6] Negative calcium balance leads to decreased bone density, osteoporosis, and the potential for fractures.[7] There are also decreases in rate of protein synthesis, slower healing, and impaired immune system function.[8] Aging men report lower libido and reduced numbers and quality of erections.[9–11] Behavioral and psychological manifestations of aging include slower problem solving, lapses of memory, and increasing incidence of dementing illness.

At the same time these changes are occurring, serum testosterone (T) concentrations are also decreasing progressively in men,[12] as are various measures of free or bioavailable T,[13] where the latter decline is steeper due to increases in circulating sex hormone binding globulin (SHBG) with age. The decreases in T have been observed to begin in the third decade and proceed at a more-or-less constant rate into extreme old age whether measured cross-sectionally[14] or longitudinally.[15,16] Integrated 24-h growth hormone (GH) secretion and blood levels of insulin-like growth factor I are also diminished with age in both male and female rodents[17] and humans.[18–23] Responsiveness of pituitary GH secretion to various stimuli may also be reduced.[24,25] Altered metabolic responsiveness of liver, muscle, and adipose tissue to glucagon, insulin, and β-adrenergic stimuli have all been found in older humans[6,26–28] and laboratory rats.[29–31] Finally, there are age-related decreases in the number of T lymphocytes responding, as well as in the magnitude of their responses, to stimulation by antigens and cytokines in both humans and animals.[32–34]

Address for correspondence: S. Mitchell Harman, M.D., Ph.D., Kronos Longevity Research Institute, Phoenix, AZ 85016. Voice: 602-778-7499; fax: 602-778-7490.
 mitch.harman@kronosinstitute.org

The extents to which alterations in hormone balance contribute to the changes in body composition and function are not well defined. However, each of the hormonal alterations mentioned above, when present in young adults, presents a clinical picture having certain features in common with the typical age-related changes. For example, male hypogonadism is associated with loss of muscle mass and strength, increased total and especially truncal and visceral body fat (accompanied by mild insulin resistance), and reduced libido and erectile capacity. Recently, it has become clear that the decline in free/bioavailable T levels is sufficient to make a substantial fraction of men over the age of 65 hypogonadal, at least by standard serum hormone level criteria.[15]

While it is likely that hormonal alterations contribute to the aging phenotype, the underlying mechanism (or mechanisms) by which the aging process impairs hormonal regulation in a wide variety of endocrine and neuroendocrine cells is unknown. One widely held theory of aging is that accumulation of oxidative damage to, and cross-linking of, proteins, lipids, and DNA progressively compromises the function of vital cell components. Endogenous oxidative stress is a "side effect" of normal metabolic processes[35–37] due to production of ROS (superoxide, hydrogen peroxide, and hydroxyl radicals) during the cell's energy generation process. ROS can damage proteins, lipid membranes, and nucleic acids (DNA and RNA), the critical components of living cells. Evidence continues to accumulate that oxidative damage plays a role in the aging process.[38–44] If one tentatively accepts oxidative stress as an important basic aging process, one critical question arises: namely, how might this process lead to the observed age-related compromise of endocrine function?

The mechanisms of cellular responses to peptide and protein hormones and cytokines have in common their binding as specific ligands to cell membrane proteins (receptors) whose peptide chains cross the membrane so that they have both extracellular and intracellular domains. The binding of a ligand to the extracellular receptor domain alters its configuration and/or promotes association with other membrane-bound proteins to change the enzymatic activity of the intracellular domain. These changes result in a chain of intracellular events, which may include generation of messenger molecules (such as cyclic AMP), phosphorylation and dephosphorylation of various enzymes and transactivation factors, and activation of specific genes with synthesis of new protein. The process of transmembrane signal transduction has been the focus of extensive investigations in a wide variety of cell types over the past 20 years.

Investigations of alterations in transmembrane signaling responses of aged cells have generally failed to reveal changes in numbers or chemical integrity of receptors sufficient to account for the magnitude of the effects of aging on function.[45–48] Suggesting that the aging defect may be in the membrane itself are the findings that postreceptor cascades appear to be intact when stimulated by alternative pathways not requiring transmembrane signaling[49] and that T lymphocytes from aged donors demonstrate a defect in assembly of membrane-resident receptor subunits.[50] Consistent with the above hypothesis, it has been shown that aging is associated with reductions in polyunsaturated fatty acid (PUFA) content of phospholipids[51] and accumulation of peroxidized and cross-linked fatty acids, trans-fatty acids, and cholesterol esters in biological membranes.[52,53] These alterations lead to a loss of membrane fluidity,[52,54,55] which could in turn impair signaling by receptors resident in the altered membranes.

Given the above, possible strategies for clinical reversal of age-related hormone imbalance include the following:

(1) Replace deficient hormones by (*a*) administering exogenous hormones or (*b*) stimulating endogenous hormone production.
(2) Repair or remediate damage to existing secretory cell membranes to restore transmembrane signaling.
(3) Replace damaged, senescent endocrine cells with newly differentiated cells having freshly synthesized membranes.

Hormone replacement trials with T in aged men, estrogen in postmenopausal women, and GH and sex-appropriate steroid hormones in elders of both sexes have been conducted with mixed results. In one study, treatment with exogenous T for three years improved bone density in those men with the lowest T levels,[56] but failed to produce significant improvements in muscle strength, despite increases in lean body mass.[57] In other trials, androgen replacement was found to improve muscle strength[58] and was associated with significant increases in libido[59] and erectile function.[60] The combination of T and GH has been found to decrease body fat and increase lean body mass, muscle strength, and aerobic capacity in men,[61] but significant effects of GH or T alone were limited to changes in body composition. GH, but not estrogen, improved body composition in women in this study, with no effects on strength or aerobic capacity, and there were no additive effects of GH with estrogen.[61] Estrogen replacement in women has recently been reported to have an adverse risk/benefit ratio in older postmenopausal women,[62] although results in younger newly menopausal women may be more favorable.[63] Nonetheless, hormone replacement strategies have the potential for a host of adverse effects in both sexes, potentially including increased frequencies of prostate[64–66] and breast[62,67,68] cancer. Whether restoration of youthful patterns of endogenous hormone production is feasible or would have fewer adverse effects remains unknown.

The role of stem cells in aging and the concept of restoring function by replacing dysfunctional, senescent cells from the body's own store of undifferentiated precursor/stem cells or with exogenous stem cells have recently been subjects of considerable discussion,[69–72] but have received little experimental support to date. In one study,[73] a specific toxin, ethane dimethanesulfonate (EDS), was employed to destroy the Leydig cell population in testes of old, T-deficient rats. After this cell population in the old rat testes was reconstituted by new Leydig cells, presumably differentiated from the precursor cell reserve present in the interstitial compartment, their testosterone responses to gonadotrophic stimulation resembled those of young rats. Whether the principle of eliminating senescent cells to allow their replacement with fresh functional cells is applicable to other organs and systems or whether it will ever be clinically practicable is speculative. Nonetheless, this idea is intriguing.

Cell membrane fluidity can be improved by increasing dietary PUFA,[74,75] and changes in the fatty acid content of cell membranes can be achieved fairly rapidly (4–8 weeks) by altering dietary fat intake.[76–78] Moreover, it has long been known that metabolic function is affected by fatty acid composition of cell membranes. For example, as early as 1981, Awad[79] observed that glucose utilization by adipose tissue from animals fed a safflower oil diet was greater than in adipose from animals fed a stock or coconut oil diet. In 1985, Panek *et al.*[80] specifically stated the hypothesis that "… dietary manipulations alter the lipid environment of receptor proteins which may result in the perturbation of specific membrane-associated processes." These workers found that a diet high in saturated fatty acids leads to impairment of the processes of norepinephrine storage and release in sympathetic neurons. In other rat experiments, fish oil feeding improved LDL receptor activity in liver,[81] and the phentolamine-stimulated norepinephrine release in adult rat hearts was found to be greatest in coconut oil–fed animals and lowest in sunflower oil–fed animals.[82] Fish oil feeding of diabetic rats was associated with lower blood sugar levels and higher muscle cell membrane content of Glut-4 glucose transporters,[83] as well as with increased insulin-induced glucose transport into muscle.[84] In rats, the effect of thyroid hormone to increase mitochondrial membrane proton leak can be reduced by a diet that increases ω-3 PUFA content in membrane.[85] Antibody responses to rabbit gamma globulin were downregulated by gamma globulin pretreatment in mice fed diets low in PUFA, but upregulated in animals fed high PUFA diets.[86] In old rats, substitution of corn oil, which is high in ω-6 (PUFA), for 12 weeks resulted in near-normalization of the glycogenolytic response of liver cells to glucagon and of the lipolytic response of fat cells to β-adrenergic stimulation.[87] Membrane transduction of adrenergic signaling in parotid gland cells from old rats improved when membrane fluidity was increased using S-adenosylmethionine.[88] Minehira et al.[89] have found that dietary manipulation to reduce the amount of oxidized cholesterol in cell membranes of old animals improves T cell responses.

The results cited above, taken together, suggest that manipulation of membrane chemistry can partially reverse age-related changes in transmembrane signaling. Diets high in PUFA have also been shown to delay some age-associated changes in mouse[90,91] and dog[92] immune system function and reverse the age-related impairments in long-term potentiation and depolarization-induced glutamate transmitter release in rat hippocampus.[93] Various studies in humans have shown dietary ω-3 PUFA to have positive effects on some cardiovascular risk factors, including lipids[94–96] and arterial compliance,[97] but not on inflammatory proteins such as fibrinogen and PAI-1.[98,99] Diets rich in ω-3 PUFA improve cardiovascular death rate,[100] but not incidence of nonfatal stroke or myocardial infarction (MI)[101] or recurrent MI in patients with existing heart disease.[102] The latter apparent paradox is probably due to prevention of cardiac sudden death[101,103] due to stabilization of excitable membranes.[104] The improvement in excitable membrane function with ω-3 PUFA may extend to the central nervous system. Recently, beneficial effects of ω-3 fatty acids on bipolar and depressive illness have been reported.[105] It has also been suggested that high linoleic acid intake is positively associated, whereas high fish consumption is inversely associated, with cognitive impairment in older men.[106] There is also excellent evidence that ω-3 PUFAs are required for normal cognitive development in infants.[107]

A diet high in ω-3 PUFA may improve glucose tolerance in nondiabetics,[108] especially in elderly persons,[109] but has not resulted in improved insulin sensitivity or better glucose control in patients with diabetes.[94,96]

The effects of a diet high in ω-3 PUFA on endocrine regulation and immune cell function in aging humans have not been previously studied. We have recently completed the sample collection phase of a pilot study, investigating whether, in men and women older than 60 years of age, an ω-3 PUFA–enriched diet will result in reversion of transmembrane signaling–mediated responses of hormone-secreting and endocrine target organs and immune cells toward a pattern more characteristic of younger individuals. We have employed a variety of provocative tests of endocrine function to assess responsivity of transmembrane signaling before and after a diet containing nonfatty fish and with a supplement of 15 mL/day of 50:50 corn oil and olive oil, and a diet with 3 servings per week of fatty fish and with a supplement of 15 mL/day of cold-pressed fish oil containing 3–4 g of ω-3 (eicosapentoic plus docosahexanoic) fatty acids. Testing included pituitary responses to gonadotropin releasing hormone and growth hormone releasing hormone, adrenal response to ACTH, testosterone response to human chorionic gonadotropin in men, hepatic mobilization of glucose in response to glucagon, release of fatty acids and glycerol from adipose in response to catecholaminergic stimulation (graded isuprel test), and measurement of insulin sensitivity using a dynamic somatostatin-insulin suppression test. Results of this study await analysis of samples for hormone levels and will be reported in the near future.

In summary, it is clear that aging results in alterations of endocrine physiology, which in turn appear to contribute to development of the senescent phenotype. How the underlying basic aging process or processes cause the endocrine cell dysfunctions leading to hormone imbalance is far from clear, but oxidative alteration of cell membranes is an attractive candidate mechanism that might be susceptible to some degree of global remediation. Whether this is the case should be the subject of further study in both experimental animals and humans.

REFERENCES

1. KALLMAN, D.A., C. PLATO & J. TOBIN. 1990. The role of muscle loss in age-related decline in grip strength: a cross-sectional and longitudinal analysis. J. Gerontol. **45:** M82–M88.
2. FLEG, J.L. & E.G. LAKATTA. 1988. Role of muscle loss in the age-associated reduction in VO_2 max. J. Appl. Physiol. **65**(3): 1147–1151.
3. FRIED, L.P., R.A. KRONMAL, A.B. NEWMAN, et al. 1998. Risk factors for 5-year mortality in older adults: the Cardiovascular Health Study. JAMA **279**(8): 585–592.
4. SHIMOKATA, H., J.D. TOBIN, D.C. MULLER, et al. 1989. Studies in the distribution of body fat: I. Effects of age, sex, and obesity. J. Gerontol. **44:** M67–M73.
5. KOHRT, W.M., J.P. KIRWAN, M.A. STATEN, et al. 1993. Insulin resistance in aging is related to abdominal obesity. Diabetes **42:** 273–281.
6. FINK, R.I., O.G. KOLTERMAN, J. GRIFFIN & J.M. OLEFSKY. 1983. Mechanisms of insulin resistance in aging. J. Clin. Invest. **71:** 1523–1535.
7. WARK, J.D. 1996. Osteoporotic fractures: background and prevention strategies. Maturitas **23**(2): 193–207.
8. SCORDAMAGLIA, A., G. CIPRANDI, F. INDIVERI & G.W. CANONICA. 1991. The effect of aging on host defences: implications for therapy. Drugs Aging **1**(4): 303–316.
9. HELGASON, A.R., J. ADOLFSSON, P. DICKMAN, et al. 1996. Sexual desire, erection, orgasm, and ejaculatory functions and their importance to elderly Swedish men: a population-based study. Age Ageing **25**(4): 285–291.
10. MORLEY, J.E., E. CHARLTON, P. PATRICK, et al. 2000. Validation of a screening questionnaire for androgen deficiency in aging males. Metabolism **49**(9): 1239–1242.
11. KAISER, F.E., S.P. VIOSCA, J.E. MORLEY, et al. 1988. Impotence and aging: clinical and hormonal factors. J. Am. Geriatr. Soc. **36**(6): 511–519.
12. BREMNER, W.J. & P.N. PRINZ. 1983. A loss of circadian rhythmicity in blood testosterone levels with aging in normal men. J. Clin. Endocrinol. Metab. **56:** 1278–1281.
13. VERMEULEN, A. & J.M. KAUFMAN. 1995. Ageing of the hypothalamo-pituitary-testicular axis in men. Horm. Res. **43**(1–3): 25–28.

14. TENOVER, J.S., A.M. MATSUMOTO, S.R. PLYMATE & W.J. BREMNER. 1987. The effects of aging in normal men on bioavailable testosterone and luteinizing hormone secretion: response to clomiphene citrate. J. Clin. Endocrinol. Metab. **65**: 1118–1126.
15. HARMAN, S.M., E.J. METTER, J.D. TOBIN, et al. 2001. Longitudinal effects of aging on serum total and free testosterone levels in healthy men: Baltimore Longitudinal Study of Aging. J. Clin. Endocrinol. Metab. **86**(2): 724–731.
16. MORLEY, J.E., F.E. KAISER, H.M. PERRY, et al. 1997. Longitudinal changes in testosterone, luteinizing hormone, and follicle-stimulating hormone in healthy older men. Metabolism **46**(4): 410–413.
17. SONNTAG, W.E. & J. MEITES. 1988. Decline in GH secretion in aging animals and man. In Regulation of Neuroendocrine Aging, pp. 111–124. Karger. Basel.
18. VITTONE, J., M.R. BLACKMAN, M.J. BUSBY-WHITEHEAD, et al. 1997. Effects of single nightly injections of growth hormone releasing hormone (GHRH 1–29) in healthy elderly men. Metabolism **46**: 89–96.
19. CORPAS, E., S.M. HARMAN & M.R. BLACKMAN. 1993. Human growth hormone and human aging. Endocr. Rev. **14**: 20–39.
20. O'CONNOR, K.O., T.E. STEVENS & M.R. BLACKMAN. 1996. GH and aging. In Growth Hormone in Adults, pp. 323–366. Cambridge University Press. London/Cambridge/New York.
21. KELIJMAN, M. 1991. Age-related alterations of the growth hormone/insulin-like-growth-factor I axis. J. Am. Geriatr. Soc. **39**(3): 295–307.
22. HO, K.Y., W.S. EVANS, R.M. BLIZZARD, et al. 1987. Effects of sex and age on the 24-hour profile of growth hormone secretion in man: importance of endogenous estradiol concentrations. J. Clin. Endocrinol. Metab. **64**(1): 51–58.
23. O'CONNOR, K.G., J.D. TOBIN, S.M. HARMAN, et al. 1998. Serum levels of insulin-like growth factor-I are related to age and not to body composition in healthy women and men. J. Gerontol. A Biol. Sci. Med. Sci. **53**(3): M176–M182.
24. PAVLOV, E.P., S.M. HARMAN, G.R. MERRIAM, et al. 1986. Responses of growth hormone (GH) and somatomedin-C to GH-releasing hormone in healthy aging men. J. Clin. Endocrinol. Metab. **62**(3): 595–600.
25. SHIBASAKI, T., K. SHIZUME, M. NAKAHARA, et al. 1984. Age-related changes in plasma growth hormone response to growth hormone–releasing factor in man. J. Clin. Endocrinol. Metab. **58**: 212–214.
26. DUDL, R. & J. ENSICK. 1977. Insulin and glucagon relationships during aging in man. Metabolism **26**: 33–41.
27. COPELAND, K.C., R.B. COLLETTI, J.D. DEVLIN & T.L. MCAULIFFE. 1990. The relationship between insulin-like growth factor-1, adiposity, and aging. Metab. Clin. Exp. **39**: 584–587.
28. DEFRONZO, R.A. 1979. Glucose intolerance and aging: evidence for tissue insensitivity to insulin. Diabetes **28**: 1095–1101.
29. FRAEYMAN, N., E. VAN DE VELDE, A. VAN ERMEN, et al. 2000. Effect of maturation and aging on beta-adrenergic signal transduction in rat kidney and liver. Biochem. Pharmacol. **60**(12): 1787–1795.
30. KATZ, M.S., E.M. DAX & R.I. GREGERMAN. 1993. Beta adrenergic regulation of rat liver glycogenolysis during aging. Exp. Gerontol. **28**(4–5): 329–340.
31. CARVALHO, E., C. RONDINONE & U. SMITH. 2000. Insulin resistance in fat cells from obese Zucker rats—evidence for an impaired activation and translocation of protein kinase B and glucose transporter 4. Mol. Cell. Biochem. **206**(1–2): 7–16.
32. LIM, B.O., C.A. JOLLY, K. ZAMAN & G. FERNANDES. 2000. Dietary (n-6) and (n-3) fatty acids and energy restriction modulate mesenteric lymph node lymphocyte function in autoimmune-prone (NZB × NZW)F1 mice. J. Nutr. **130**(7): 1657–1664.
33. SONG, L., Y.H. KIM, R.K. CHOPRA, et al. 1993. Age-related effects in T cell activation and proliferation. Exp. Gerontol. **28**(4–5): 313–321.
34. SONG, L.J., J.E. NAGEL, F.J. CHREST, et al. 1992. Comparison of CD3 and CD2 activation pathways in T cells from young and elderly adults. Aging (Milano) **4**(4): 307–315.
35. ARKING, R. 1998. Biology of Aging: Observations and Principles. Second edition. Sinauer Associates. Sunderland, MA.

36. CUTLER, R.G. 1976. Nature of aging and life maintenance processes. *In* Interdisciplinary Topics in Gerontology, pp. 83–133. Karger. Basel.
37. CUTLER, R.G. 1982. Longevity is determined by specific genes: testing the hypothesis. *In* Testing the Theories of Aging, pp. 25–114. CRC Press. Boca Raton, FL.
38. SASTRE, J., F.V. PALLARDO, J. GARCIA DE LA ASUNCION & J. VINA. 2000. Mitochondria, oxidative stress, and aging. Free Radical Res. **32**(3): 189–198.
39. HOMMA, Y., M. TSUNODA & H. KASAI. 1994. Evidence for the accumulation of oxidative stress during cellular ageing of human diploid fibroblasts. Biochem. Biophys. Res. Commun. **203**(2): 1063–1068.
40. HAMILTON, M.L., H. VAN REMMEN, J.A. DRAKE, *et al.* 2001. Does oxidative damage to DNA increase with age? Proc. Natl. Acad. Sci. USA **98**(18): 10469–10474.
41. VAN REMMEN, H. & A. RICHARDSON. 2001. Oxidative damage to mitochondria and aging. Exp. Gerontol. **36**(7): 957–968.
42. CUTLER, R.G. 1993. Oxidative stress state in aging and longevity mechanisms. *In* Free Radicals: From Basic Science to Medicine. Birkhauser. Basel/New York.
43. STADTMAN, E.R. & B.S. BERLETT. 1998. Reactive oxygen-mediated protein oxidation in aging and disease. Drug Metab. Rev. **30**(2): 225–243.
44. FUKAGAWA, N.K. 1999. Aging: is oxidative stress a marker or is it causal? Proc. Soc. Exp. Biol. Med. **222**(3): 293–298.
45. DAX, E.M., J.S. PARTILLA, M.A. PINEYRO & R.I. GREGERMAN. 1987. Beta-adrenergic receptors, glucagon receptors, and their relationship to adenylate cyclase in rat liver during aging. Endocrinology **120**(4): 1534–1541.
46. ROTH, G.S. 1997. Age changes in signal transduction and gene expression. Mech. Ageing Dev. **98**(3): 231–238.
47. ISHIKAWA, Y., M.V. GEE, B.J. BAUM & G.S. ROTH. 1989. Decreased signal transduction in rat parotid cell aggregates during aging is not due to loss of alpha1-adrenergic receptors. Exp. Gerontol. **24**(1): 25–36.
48. ROY, D., B. KALYANARAMAN & J.G. LIEHR. 1991. Xanthine oxidase–catalyzed reduction of estrogen quinones to semiquinones and hydroquinones. Biochem. Pharmacol. **42**(8): 1627–1631.
49. GREGERMAN, R.I. 1986. Mechanisms of age-related alterations of hormone secretion and action: an overview of 30 years of progress. Exp. Gerontol. **21**(4–5): 345–365.
50. TAMIR, A., M.D. EISENBRAUN, G.G. GARCIA & R.A. MILLER. 2000. Age-dependent alterations in the assembly of signal transduction complexes at the site of T cell/APC interaction. J. Immunol. **165**(3): 1243–1251.
51. AWAD, A.B. & S.W. CLAY. 1982. Age-dependent alterations in lipids and function of rat heart sarcolemma. Mech. Ageing Dev. **19**(4): 333–342.
52. YANAGAWA, K., H. TAKEDA, T. EGASHIRA, *et al.* 1999. Age-related changes in alpha-tocopherol dynamics with relation to lipid hydroperoxide content and fluidity of rat erythrocyte membrane. J. Gerontol. A Biol. Sci. Med. Sci. **54**(9): B379–B383.
53. ANDO, K., M. BEPPU & K. KIKUGAWA. 1995. Evidence for accumulation of lipid hydroperoxides during the aging of human red blood cells in the circulation. Biol. Pharm. Bull. **18**(5): 659–663.
54. HASHIMOTO, M., S. HOSSAIN & S. MASUMURA. 1999. Effect of aging on plasma membrane fluidity of rat aortic endothelial cells. Exp. Gerontol. **34**(5): 687–698.
55. HOSSAIN, M.S., M. HASHIMOTO, S. GAMOH & S. MASUMURA. 1999. Association of age-related decrease in platelet membrane fluidity with platelet lipid peroxide. Life Sci. **64**(2): 135–143.
56. SNYDER, P.J., H. PEACHEY, P. HANNOUSH, *et al.* 1999. Effect of testosterone treatment on bone mineral density in men over 65 years of age. J. Clin. Endocrinol. Metab. **84**(6): 1966–1972.
57. SNYDER, P.J., H. PEACHEY, P. HANNOUSH, *et al.* 1999. Effect of testosterone treatment on body composition and muscle strength in men over 65 years of age. J. Clin. Endocrinol. Metab. **84**(8): 2647–2653.
58. SIH, R., J.E. MORLEY, F.E. KAISER, *et al.* 1997. Testosterone replacement in older hypogonadal men: a 12-month randomized controlled trial. J. Clin. Endocrinol. Metab. **82**(6): 1661–1667.

59. HAJJAR, R.R., F.E. KAISER & J.E. MORLEY. 1997. Outcomes of long-term testosterone replacement in older hypogonadal males: a retrospective analysis. J. Clin. Endocrinol. Metab. **82**(11): 3793–3796.
60. KUNELIUS, P., O. LUKKARINEN, M.L. HANNUKSELA, et al. 2002. The effects of transdermal dihydrotestosterone in the aging male: a prospective, randomized, double blind study. J. Clin. Endocrinol. Metab. **87**(4): 1467–1472.
61. BLACKMAN, M.R., J.D. SORKIN, T. MUNZER, et al. 2002. Growth hormone and sex steroid administration in healthy aged women and men: a randomized controlled trial. JAMA **288**(18): 2282–2292.
62. WOMEN'S HEALTH INITIATIVE. 2002. Risks and benefits of estrogen plus progestin in healthy postmenopausal women: principal results from the Women's Health Initiative randomized controlled trial. JAMA **288**(3): 321–333.
63. GRODSTEIN, F., T.B. CLARKSON & J.E. MANSON. 2003. Understanding the divergent data on postmenopausal hormone therapy. N. Engl. J. Med. **348**(7): 645–650.
64. HARMAN, S.M., E.J. METTER, M.R. BLACKMAN, et al. 2000. Serum levels of insulin-like growth factor I (IGF-I), IGF-II, IGF-binding protein-3, and prostate-specific antigen as predictors of clinical prostate cancer. J. Clin. Endocrinol. Metab. **85**(11): 4258–4265.
65. CHAN, J.M., M.J. STAMPFER, E. GIOVANNUCCI, et al. 1998. Plasma insulin-like growth factor-I and prostate cancer risk: a prospective study [see comments]. Science **279**(5350): 563–566.
66. ROLF, C. & E. NIESCHLAG. 1998. Potential adverse effects of long-term testosterone therapy. Bailliere's Clin. Endocrinol. Metab. **12**(3): 521–534.
67. BERGKVIST, L., H-O. ADAMI, I. PERSSON, et al. 1989. The risk of breast cancer after estrogen and estrogen-progestin replacement. N. Engl. J. Med. **321**(5): 293–297.
68. SCHAIRER, C., J. LUBIN, R. TROISI, et al. 2000. Menopausal estrogen and estrogen-progestin replacement therapy and breast cancer risk. J. Am. Med. Assoc. **283**(4): 485–491.
69. DE GREY, A.D. 2002. Stem cells: a cellular fountain of youth. In Advances in Cell Aging and Gerontology. Elsevier. Amsterdam/New York.
70. VAN ZANT, G. 2003. Genetic control of stem cells: implications for aging. Int. J. Hematol. **77**(1): 29–36.
71. TROSKO, J.E. 2003. Human stem cells as targets for the aging and diseases of aging processes. Med. Hypotheses **60**(3): 439–447.
72. ROCCANOVA, L. & P. RAMPHAL. 2003. The role of stem cells in the evolution of longevity and its application to tissue therapy. Tissue Cell **35**(1): 79–81.
73. CHEN, H., I. HUHTANIEMI & B.R. ZIRKIN. 1996. Depletion and repopulation of Leydig cells in the testes of aging brown Norway rats. Endocrinology **137**(8): 3447–3452.
74. MILLS, D.E., W.R. GALEY & H. DIXON. 1993. Effects of dietary fatty-acid supplementation on fatty-acid composition and deformability of young and old erythrocytes. Biochim. Biophys. Acta **1149**(2): 313–318.
75. HASHIMOTO, M., S. HOSSAIN, H. YAMASAKI, et al. 1999. Effects of eicosapentaenoic acid and docosahexaenoic acid on plasma membrane fluidity of aortic endothelial cells. Lipids **34**(12): 1297–1304.
76. MCMURCHIE, E.J., B.M. MARGETTS, L.J. BEILIN, et al. 1984. Dietary-induced changes in the fatty acid composition of human cheek cell phospholipids: correlation with changes in the dietary polyunsaturated/saturated fat ratio. Am. J. Clin. Nutr. **39**(6): 975–980.
77. STANGL, G.I., M. KIRCHGESSNER, K. EDER & A.M. REICHLMAYR-LAIS. 1994. Effect of dietary hyperlipidemic components and fish oil on concentration of lipids in liver and liver fatty acid profile of rats. Z. Ernaehrwiss. **33**(3): 195–206.
78. AWAD, T.B. & J.P. CHATTOPADHYAY. 1983. Effect of dietary fats on the lipid composition and enzyme activities of rat cardiac sarcolemma. J. Nutr. **13**(9): 1878–1883.
79. AWAD, A.B. 1981. Effect of dietary lipids on composition and glucose utilization by rat adipose tissue. J. Nutr. **111**(1): 34–39.
80. PANEK, R.L., W.R. DIXON & C.O. RUTLEDGE. 1985. Modification of sympathetic neuronal function in the rat tail artery by dietary lipid treatment. J. Pharmacol. Exp. Ther. **233**(3): 578–583.
81. TRIPODI, A., P. LORIA, M.A. DILENGITE & N. CARULLI. 1991. Effect of fish oil and coconut oil diet on the LDL receptor activity of rat liver plasma membranes. Biochim. Biophys. Acta **1083**(3): 298–304.

82. SEMAFUKO, W.E., C.O. RUTLEDGE & W.R. DIXON. 1987. Effect of dietary lipids on myocardial norepinephrine content and field stimulation-mediated release of norepinephrine from perfused neonatal and adult rat hearts. J. Cardiovasc. Pharmacol. **10**(1): 16–23.
83. GIRON, M.D., R. SALTO, P. HORTELANO, et al. 1999. Increased diaphragm expression of GLUT4 in control and streptozotocin-diabetic rats by fish oil–supplemented diets. Lipids **34**(8): 801–807.
84. SOHAL, P.S., V.E. BARACOS & M.T. CLANDININ. 1992. Dietary omega 3 fatty acid alters prostaglandin synthesis, glucose transport, and protein turnover in skeletal muscle of healthy and diabetic rats. Biochem. J. **286**(part 2): 405–411.
85. PEHOWICH, D.J. 1999. Thyroid hormone status and membrane n-3 fatty acid content influence mitochondrial proton leak. Biochim. Biophys. Acta **1411**(1): 192–200.
86. PONNAPPAN, U., B. CINADER & M.T. CLANDININ. 1988. Effect of dietary fat on antibody response and on down-regulation. Immunol. Lett. **18**(3): 205–211.
87. DAX, E.M., J.S. PARTILLA, M.A. PINEYRO & R.I. GREGERMAN. 1990. Altered glucagon- and catecholamine hormone–sensitive adenylyl cyclase responsiveness in rat liver membranes induced by manipulation of dietary fatty acid intake. Endocrinology **127**(5): 2236–2240.
88. KOWATCH, M.A., J.F. KELLY, N.A. DENISOVA & G.S. ROTH. 1995. Partial restoration of impaired alpha1-adrenergic responsiveness in parotid cells of aged rats by S-adenosylmethionine treatment. Mol. Cell. Biochem. **148**(1): 73–77.
89. MINEHIRA, K., S. INOUE, M. NONAKA, et al. 2000. Effects of dietary protein type on oxidized cholesterol-induced alteration in age-related modulation of lipid metabolism and indices of immune function in rats. Biochim. Biophys. Acta **1483**(1): 141–153.
90. CINADER, B., M.T. CLANDININ, S.W. KOH, et al. 1986. Dietary fat alters progression of some age-related changes of the immune system. Immunol. Lett. **12**(2–3): 175–179.
91. CINADER, B., M.T. CLANDININ, T. HOSOKAWA & N.M. ROBBLEE. 1983. Dietary fat alters the fatty acid composition of lymphocyte membranes and the rate at which suppressor capacity is lost. Immunol. Lett. **6**(6): 331–337.
92. KEARNS, R.J., M.G. HAYEK, J.J. TUREK, et al. 1999. Effect of age, breed, and dietary omega-6 (n-6):omega-3 (n-3) fatty acid ratio on immune function, eicosanoid production, and lipid peroxidation in young and aged dogs. Vet. Immunol. Immunopathol. **69**(2–4): 165–183.
93. MCGAHON, B.M., D.S. MARTIN, D.F. HORROBIN & M.A. LYNCH. 1999. Age-related changes in synaptic function: analysis of the effect of dietary supplementation with omega-3 fatty acids. Neuroscience **94**(1): 305–314.
94. LUO, J., S.W. RIZKALLA, H. VIDAL, et al. 1998. Moderate intake of n-3 fatty acids for 2 months has no detrimental effect on glucose metabolism and could ameliorate the lipid profile in type 2 diabetic men: results of a controlled study. Diabetes Care **21**(5): 717–724.
95. MORI, T.A., R. VANDONGEN, J.R. MASAREI, et al. 1991. Comparison of diets supplemented with fish oil or olive oil on plasma lipoproteins in insulin-dependent diabetics. Metabolism **40**(3): 241–246.
96. RIVELLESE, A.A., A. MAFFETTONE, C. IOVINE, et al. 1996. Long-term effects of fish oil on insulin resistance and plasma lipoproteins in NIDDM patients with hypertriglyceridemia. Diabetes Care **19**(11): 1207–1213.
97. MCVEIGH, G.E., G.M. BRENNAN, J.N. COHN, et al. 1994. Fish oil improves arterial compliance in non-insulin-dependent diabetes mellitus. Arterioscler. Thromb. **14**(9): 1425–1429.
98. TOFT, I., K.H. BONAA, O.C. INGEBRETSEN, et al. 1997. Fibrinolytic function after dietary supplementation with omega-3 polyunsaturated fatty acids. Arterioscler. Thromb. Vasc. Biol. **17**(5): 814–819.
99. PERSICHETTI, S., S. MAGGI, R. PONZIO, et al. 1996. Effects of omega-3 PUFA on plasma fibrinogen levels in hypertriglyceridemic hemodialysis patients. Minerva Urol. Nefrol. **48**(3): 137–138.
100. STONE, N.J. 2000. The Gruppo Italiano per lo Studio della Sopravvivenza nell'Infarto Miocardio (GISSI)–Prevenzione Trial on fish oil and vitamin E supplementation in myocardial infarction survivors. Curr. Cardiol. Rep. **2**(5): 445–451.

101. ALBERT, C.M., C.H. HENNEKENS, C.J. O'DONNELL, *et al.* 1998. Fish consumption and risk of sudden cardiac death [see comments]. JAMA **279**(1): 23–28.
102. MORRIS, J.Z., H.A. TISSENBAUM & G. RUVKUN. 1996. A phosphatidylinositol-3-OH kinase family member regulating longevity and diapause in *Caenorhabditis elegans*. Nature **382**(6591): 536–539.
103. SHEARD, N.F. 1998. Fish consumption and risk of sudden cardiac death. Nutr. Rev. **56**(6): 177–179.
104. CHRISTENSEN, J.H., J. AAROE, N. KNUDSEN, *et al.* 1998. Heart rate variability and n-3 fatty acids in patients with chronic renal failure—a pilot study. Clin. Nephrol. **49**(2): 102–106.
105. MAES, M., A. CHRISTOPHE, J. DELANGHE, *et al.* 1999. Lowered omega-3 polyunsaturated fatty acids in serum phospholipids and cholesteryl esters of depressed patients. Psychiatry Res. **85**(3): 275–291.
106. KALMIJN, S., E.J. FESKENS, L.J. LAUNER & D. KROMHOUT. 1997. Polyunsaturated fatty acids, antioxidants, and cognitive function in very old men. Am. J. Epidemiol. **145**(1): 33–41.
107. GIBSON, R.A., M.A. NEUMANN & M. MAKRIDES. 1996. Effect of dietary docosahexanoic acid on brain composition and neural function in term infants. Lipids **31**(suppl.): 177–181.
108. STORLIEN, L.H., A.D. KRIKETOS, A.B. JENKINS, *et al.* 1997. Does dietary fat influence insulin action? Ann. N.Y. Acad. Sci. **827**: 287–301.
109. FESKENS, E.J., C.H. BOWLES & D. KROMHOUT. 1991. Inverse association between fish intake and risk of glucose intolerance in normoglycemic elderly men and women. Diabetes Care **14**(11): 935–941.

Functional Efficiency of the Senescent Cells: Replace or Restore?

SANG CHUL PARK, KYUNG A. CHO, IK SOON JANG, KYUNG TAE KIM, AND SUNG JIN RYU

Department of Biochemistry and Molecular Biology, Aging and Apoptosis Research Center, Seoul National University College of Medicine, Seoul, South Korea

ABSTRACT: It is generally accepted that aging is a phenomenon of irreversibility, inevitability, and universality with parenchymal loss and functional decline. Consequently, the major goals of aging research are focused on the development of a replace strategy of the aged organs or cells, based on immortalizing tools, stem cells, or artificial substitutes. Recently, however, a new concept of functional recovery has been introduced on the basis of the functional restoration of the responsiveness of the senescent cells toward a variety of agonists, including growth factors. The aging phenotypes of hyporesponsiveness and morphological alteration are shown to be readily adjusted by modulation of the several membrane-associated molecules, named gatekeeper molecules, among which caveolin is one of the major determinants. Caveolin is the essential component of the caveolae, responsible for regulation of signal transduction, endocytosis and trancytosis, and cytoskeletal arrangement via its scaffolding domain. The caveolin status is associated strictly with cellular transformation, if depleted, and with senescent phenotype, if overexpressed. Therefore, simple reduction of caveolin status in senescent cells leads to restoration of the functional responsiveness to mitogenic stimuli and even of the cellular shape. These data strongly suggest that the gatekeeper molecules, represented by caveolin, may play the prime role in determination of the senescent phenotypes. From these results, it can be summarized that the replace principle would not necessarily be the essential one, but the restore principle can be somehow substituted for the betterment of the aged cells and organisms.

KEYWORDS: caveolin; aging; gatekeeper; restore; replace

INTRODUCTION

Aging is a universal phenomenon, characterized by structural changes and functional deterioration with time of life. The functional deterioration of an organism, especially the human organism, is primarily responsible for the decrease in quality of life, leading to a burden not only on the individual, but also on society. Such a deterioration at the level of the organism can be traced to alterations at the cellular

Address for correspondence: Sang Chul Park, Department of Biochemistry and Molecular Biology, Aging and Apoptosis Research Center, Seoul National University College of Medicine, 28 Yungon Dong, Chong No Ku, Seoul 110-799, South Korea. Voice: +82-2-740-8244; fax: +82-2-744-4534.
scpark@snu.ac.kr

level. The biological characteristics of the senescent human diploid fibroblasts (HDF) in functional aspects can be represented by replicative senescence, hyporesponsiveness, and apoptosis resistance. Growth arrest of the senescent cells is strongly associated with their attenuated responses to growth factors. The hyporesponsiveness of the senescent cells to growth factors or to other external stimuli might be the major fundamental mechanism for their physiological and phenotypic alterations.

Previously, we reported that the membrane event, working as the gate for the external stimuli, plays the most important role in determining the physiologic status of the senescent cells.[1] Therefore, we have reached a tentative hypothesis that the biological characteristics of the senescent cells, such as irreversibility and irresponsiveness, should be reevaluated for the possibility of reversibility and responsiveness.

DETERMINISTIC APPROACH TO AGING CONTROL: REPLACE PRINCIPLE

The deterministic view on the aging process has led to the development of a spectrum of therapeutic approaches based on the replace principle at the levels of genes, cells, tissues, organs, and cosmetic substitutes. However, most of the trials have met the fundamental problems. To illustrate, some genetic approaches are not validated because of the virtuality of the gerontogenes and of the wary problems of immortalizing genes; cellular approaches have trouble identifying the stem cells and their niches, and in inducing them for intact three-dimensional development; tissue approaches are also still defective for the interactive functional linkage; organ approaches, such as transplantation and artificially engineered organs, experience some immunocompatibility and effective nano-sized problems; cosmetic substitutes, such as plastic surgery and supplementary medicines, are limited and transient in their effects. Therefore, many efforts to control the aging process have not been satisfactory, and the deterministic view of the aging process, with its conceptual irreversibility that, in consequence, inevitability leads to death, predominates.

Interestingly, we have, however, observed that the old cells and organs are more resistant to physical and chemical apoptosis-inducing agents,[2,3] suggesting that aging is not necessarily prone to death, but rather to survival. From these data, we have conjectured that the senescent phenotypes would be derived not from the deterministic genetic origin, but mainly from the adaptive responsive system of the organism. If the concept of aging as the adaptive and responsive phenomena were of significance, a novel principle of aging control based on the restore policy rather than the replace approach would emerge.

NOVEL CONCEPT OF GATE SYSTEM FOR THE AGING PROCESS

Endocytosis is the major mechanism for intercellular communication, maintenance of protective functions, removal of dead and dying cells, modulation of plasma membrane composition, or entry route to pathogens. Among a variety of endocytic functions, however, the ligand-specific receptor-mediated endocytosis attracts special attention for its specific and controlled mode of action and for its significance in biological phenomena. Receptor-mediated endocytosis can be classified as the clathrin-dependent and the clathrin-independent systems, both of which are downregulated in the senescent state.[4,5] However, caveolae-mediated endocytosis, the typical clathrin-independent pathway, is more responsible for the cellular senescent phenotype, not only in the functional decay, but also in structural alterations.

Caveolae have emerged as the site of important dynamic and regulatory events at the plasma membrane, which is abundant in terminally differentiated cell types, that is, adipocytes, endothelial cells, and muscle cells.[6–9] Caveolae have been implicated in a wide range of cell activities, such as endocytosis and transcytosis of biomolecules and regulation of signal transduction efficiency. Signaling molecules are enriched in caveolae structure, where their activities are regulated.[10] Therefore, caveolae may function as subcellular compartments for the storage of signaling molecules, regulation of activities, and quantitation of cross talk between distinct signaling cascades.

The principal component of caveolae is a caveolin, a 21- to 24-kDa integral membrane protein. The mammalian caveolin gene family consists of caveolin-1, -2, and -3. Caveolin-1 and -2 are coexpressed and form a hetero-oligomeric complex in many cell types, with particularly high levels in adipocytes, whereas expression of caveolin-3 is muscle specific.[11–13] Caveolin may function as a scaffolding protein within the caveolae membrane.[10]

Growth factors, such as epidermal growth factor (EGF) and platelet-derived growth factor (PDGF), stimulate their specific cell surface receptors and the subsequent activation of the intrinsic tyrosine kinases. However, senescent cells do not respond efficiently to external growth factors, such as EGF and PDGF.[14] Age-related reductions in the numbers of PDGF binding sites or PDGF receptors (PDGFR) have also been demonstrated in several cell systems, including human smooth muscle cells and human diploid fibroblasts.[14,15] In contrast, the changes in the numbers and their binding affinity of EGF receptors to EGF in the senescent cells are controversial in rat hepatocytes or human dipliod fibroblas.[4,16–18]

Domain-mapping studies revealed that the interaction of caveolin-1 with signaling molecules is mediated via a membrane-proximal region of caveolin, termed the "caveolin-scaffolding domain."[19] Through this domain, caveolin-1 interacts with G-protein alpha-subunits, H-Ras, Src-family tyrosine kinases, PKC isoforms, EGF-R, Neu, and eNOS, resulting in suppression of their activities.[12,20–23]. It is shown that the targeted downregulation of caveolin-1 is sufficient to drive transformation of cells and hyperactivate the Erk kinase cascade.[24] In addition, caveolin levels in most cancer tissues are significantly lower than those in normal tissues, suggesting the circumvention of signal suppression by caveolin. Moreover, the coexpression of EGFR, Raf, MEK-1, or Erk-2 with caveolin-1 resulted in inhibition of signaling from the cytoplasm to the nucleus *in vivo*.[24]

In contrast, senescent HDF show an increased level of caveolin and its colocalization with EGFR. Overexpression of caveolin-1 in young HDF suppressed the activation of Erk-1/2 on EGF stimulation, indicating that caveolin has a direct role of EGF signaling.[4] Moreover, overexpression of caveolin-1 induces premature cellular senescence in primary cultures of murine fibroblasts transgenically overexpressing caveolin-1.[25] These results clearly show the central role of caveolin-1 in the suppression of mitogenic signaling and promoting cellular senescence. Therefore, it can be assumed that the receptor-mediated endocytosis system, especially the caveolin-dependent type, might be operating in the cell to control the senescent phenotype, as if it were the gate for the aging process.

FUNCTIONAL AND MORPHOLOGICAL RESTORATION OF THE SENESCENT PHENOTYPE

To clarify the role of caveolin-1 in aging, we investigated the modulation of the role of caveolin in senescent cells to determine the effect of caveolin on mitogenic signaling efficiency and cell cycling. Reduction of caveolin-1 expression could be induced by two different kinds of methods, such as antisense-oligonucleotides (AS-ON) and small intefering RNA (siRNA). Interestingly, we found that the downregulation of caveolin-1 by AS-ON or siRNA treatment led to restoration of the basal p-Erk level and Erk activation upon EGF stimulation. Moreover, the downstream activation of Elk phosphorylation upon EGF treatment also caused the resoration of the senescent HDFs. A simple reduction in the caveolin level in senescent HDF cells can induce the restoration of the Erk signaling system upon EGF stimulation, not only in terms of its phosphorylation, but also its translocation into and activation of transcriptional factors in the nuclei.[26]

CDK inhibitors, p21^{Wafl}, and p16^{INK4a}, as well as p53, are consistently present in senescent cells at highly elevated levels. These might be the molecules responsible for CDK inhibition, reduced E2F activity, and the consequent growth arrest of the senescent cells.[27] It was reported recently that caveolin-1–mediated cell cycle arrest occurs through a p53/p21^{Wafl}-dependent pathway.[28] Downregulation of caveolin-1 in senescent HDF also reduced the level of the cell-cycle inhibitors, p53 and p21. Therefore, the cell-cycle reentry of the senescent cells was examined and proven by monitoring BrdU incorporation in response to EGF stimuli after the status of caveolin was reduced.[26] These results indicate that a simple adjustment of the caveolin level in senescent cells can profoundly influence the aging phenotype. Moreover, evidence for the role of caveolin in cancer cells has been well documented,[29] wherein caveolin was suggested to be a tumor suppressor. It is apparent, therefore, that caveolin plays an important role in the regulation of both aging and cancer.

Senescent cells show morphological changes such as flat and large cell shape in addition to functional decay and growth arrest. Structural alteration of senescent cells is strongly related to the increase of focal adhesion and Rb family proteins.[30] Interestingly, caveolin-1 is associated with the focal adhesion complex through intergin in the membrane,[31,32] and the activation of focal adhesion kinase (FAK) is significantly decreased by downregulation of caveolin-1.[33] These results indicate that caveolin can play an important role in focal adhesion, and thereby participate in adhesion signal cascade. We have observed that the formation of focal adhesion and actin stress fiber is increased, anchored in membrane via interaction with caveolin-1 in senescent cells (manuscript in preparation). Therefore, reduction of caveolin-1 in senescent cells can cause the restoration of small and spindle shaped young cells through the adjustment of focal adhesion complexes. Moreover, senescent cells and the H-ras mutant expressers showed the accumulation of p-Erk1/2 in the cytoplasm with increased MEK activity and failure of its translocation into nuclei on EGF stimulation.[34] These results strongly suggest the possibility of deregulation of the Erk activation system in senescent cells. FAK is a major component of the Erk activation signal cascade. Interestingly, we have observed that the basal phosphorylated Erk level is dramatically reduced by downregulation of caveolin-1 by blocking the FAK activity in senescent cells (manuscript in preparation).

RESTORE PRINCIPLE BASED ON THE ADAPTIVE AND RESPONSIVE APPROACH TO AGING CONTROL

We have reported that the functional deterioration of the senescent cells is strongly related to the dysregulation or imbalance of the signal transduction network in an agonist-specific or in a pathway-specific manner.[1] In consequence, the senescence-associated functional decay might lead to hyporesposiveness, growth arrest, and disease-proneness of the aged organism. We reported previously that the RTK system was severely damaged, while the GPCR system was affected to a limited extent in senescent cells.[1] Major age-related defects in the RTK system of receptor-mediated endocytosis were associated with the age-related increase of caveolin and age-related decrease of amphiphysin-1.[4,5] Thereafter, we have shown that functional recovery of the receptor-mediated endocytosis can be readily induced in senescent cells simply by restoring the level of caveolin or amphiphysin-1.[1,5,35]

This possibility of the functional restoration of receptor-mediated endocytosis, either caveolae dependent or clathrin dependent, has opened a new area in aging research with respect to the conversion of senescent phenotype into a functionally active status. We found that the restoration of the receptor-mediated endocytosis in the senescent cells could not only improve the functional sensitivity to the external stimuli, but also restore the morphological appearance.

The possibility of converting the senescent phenotype into the functionally active and structurally normalized state simply by restoring the membrane signaling apparatus confirms the significance of the membrane signaling system in the aging phenomenon. Therefore, we assumed that the aging process could be initiated and regulated at the membrane by the membrane-associated signal switch system. From these results, we have proposed the gate theory of aging, in which the fundamental role of the membrane on/off switch system for a variety of signals has been emphasized.[1] We have conjectured that several different molecules could be the tentative gatekeepers of aging at the membrane. So far, however, we have observed that the simple adjustment of the status of caveolin in the senescent cells, either by transfection or by its reduction with antisense oligonucleotides or the siRNA method, can efficiently restore the physiological and morphological property to the active status. Therefore, we suggest that caveolin might be the prime gatekeeper of the cellular aging process, regulating the bilateral modes of structural and functional alterations. In addition, the new principle of the restore policy for aging control can be initiated and may substitute or complement the old principle of the replace strategy.

CONCLUSION

The molecular mechanism for age-related defective endocytosis is the imbalance or dysregulation of the signal transduction apparatus, which modulate the entry and relay of signals at the membrane level. Therefore, we have proposed the gate theory of aging, with special emphasis on the role of gatekeeper molecules at the membrane for determination of the senescent phenotype.

In addition, as a candidate molecule for the gatekeeper at the membrane for the aging phenomenon, we proposed that the caveolin would be the prime one. We have proven that the expression of caveolins increased in most of the cells and organs of the aged animals *in vitro* and *in vivo*, and through simple adjustment of caveolin status, not only can we induce premature senescence to the young cells, but we can also restore the functional and physiological response of the senescent cells. In addition, we can restore the young cell-like morphological shape from the old cells by the same procedure. Taken together, it can be shown that a senescent phenotype of either the physiological response or of the morphological property could be modulated by a simple adjustment of the gatekeeper molecule at the membrane, represented by caveolin, at least to a considerable extent, suggesting the possibility of the emerging restore principle for aging control in contrast to the conventional replace principle.

ACKNOWLEDGMENTS

This work was supported by grants from the Korea Science and Engineering Foundation (AARC RII 2002-001-01-001), the Ministry of Health and Welfare (HMP-00-PJ1-PG1-Ch16-002), VRIA of Nippon Boehringer Ingelheim, graduate program of the BK21 project from the Ministry of Education, and the Korea Research Foundation for Health Science.

REFERENCES

1. YEO, E.J. & S.C. PARK. 2002. Age-dependent agonist-specific dysregulation of membrane-mediated signal transduction: emergence of the gate theory of aging. Mech. Ageing Dev. **123**: 1563–1578.
2. YEO, E.J., Y.C. HWANG, C.M. KANG, et al. 2000. Reduction of UV-induced cell death in the human senescent fibroblasts. Mol. Cells **10**: 415–422.
3. SUH, Y., K.A. LEE, W.H. KIM, et al. 2002. Aging alters the apoptotic response to genotoxic stress. Nat. Med. **8**: 3–4.
4. PARK, W.Y., J.S. PARK, K.A. CHO, et al. 2000. Up-regulation of caveolin attenuates epidermal growth factor signaling in senescent cells. J. Biol. Chem. **275**: 20847–20852.
5. PARK, J.S., W.Y. PARK, K.A. CHO, et al. 2001. Downregulation of amphiphysin-1 is responsible for reduced receptor-mediated endocytosis in senescent cells. FASEB J. **15**: 1625–1627.
6. BRETSCHER, M.S. & S. WHYTOCK. 1977. Membrane-associated vesicles in fibroblasts. J. Ultrastruct. Res. **61**: 215–217.
7. ANDERSON, R.G. 1998. The caveolae membrane system. Annu. Rev. Biochem **67**: 1996–2003.
8. ENGELMAN, J.A., C. CHU, A. LIN, et al. 1998. Caveolin-mediated regulation of signaling along the p42/44 MAP kinase cascade in vivo. A role for the caveolin-scaffolding domain. FEBS Lett. **428**: 205–211.
9. DKAMOTO, T., A. SCHLEGEL, P.E. SCHLEGEL & M.P. SCHLEGEL. 1998. Caveolins, a family of scaffolding proteins for organizing "preassembled signaling complexes" at the plasma membrane. J. Biol. Chem. **273**: 5419–5422.

10. SARGIACOMO, M., P.E. SCHERER, Z. TANG, et al. 1995. Oligomeric structure of caveolin: implications for caveolae membrane organization. Proc. Natl. Acad. Sci. USA **92:** 9407–9411.
11. PARTON, R.G., M. WAY, N. ZORZI & E. STANG. 1997. Caveolin-3 associates with developing T-tubules during muscle differentiation. J. Cell Biol. **136:** 137–154.
12. SONG, K.S., P.E. SCHERER, Z. TANG, et al. 1996. Expression of caveolin-3 in skeletal, cardiac, and smooth muscle cells. Caveolin-3 is a component of the sarcolemma and co-fractionates with dystrophin and dystrophin-associated glycoproteins. J. Biol. Chem. **271:** 15160–15165.
13. TANG, Z., P.E. SCHERER, T. OKAMOTO, et al. 1996. Molecular cloning of caveolin-3, a novel member of the caveolin gene family expressed predominantly in muscle. J. Biol. Chem. **271:** 2255–2261.
14. YEO, E.J., I.S. JANG, H.K. LIM, et al. 2002. Agonist-specific differential changes of cellular signal transduction pathways in senescent human diploid fibroblasts. Exp. Gerontol. **37:** 871–883.
15. AOYAGI, M., N. FUKAI, K. OGAMI, et al. 1995. Kinetics of 125I-PDGF binding and down-regulation of PDGF receptor in human arterial smooth muscle cell strains during cellular senescence in vitro. J. Cell. Physiol. **164:** 376–384.
16. ISHIGAMI, A., T.D. REED & G.S. ROTH. 1993. Effect of aging on EGF stimulated DNA synthesis and EGF receptor levels in primary cultured rat hepatocytes. Biochem. Biophys. Res. Commun. **196:** 181–186.
17. PALMER, H.J., C.T. TUZON & K.E. PAULSON. 1999. Age-dependent decline in mitogenic stimulation of hepatocytes. Reduced association between Shc and the epidermal growth factor receptor is coupled to decreased activation of Raf and extracellular singal-regulated kinases. J. Biol. Chem. **274:** 11424–11430.
18. HUTTER, D., Y. YO, W. CHEN, et al. 2000. Age-related decline in Ras/ERK mitogen-activated protein kinase cascade is linked to a reduced association between Shc and EGF receptor. J. Gerontol. A Biol. Sci. Med. Sci. **55:** B125–B134.
19. COUET, J., S. LI, T. OKAMOTO, et al. 1997. Identification of peptide and protein ligands for the caveolin-scaffolding domain. Implications for the interaction of caveolin with caveolae-associated proteins. J. Biol. Chem. **272:** 6525–6533.
20. COUET, J., M. SARGIACOMO & M.P. LISANTI. 1997. Interaction of a receptor tyrosine kinase, EGF-R, with caveolins: caveolin-binding negatively regulates tyrosine and serine/threonine kinase activities. J. Biol. Chem. **272:** 30429–30438.
21. LI, S., J. COUET & M.P. LISANTI. 1996. Src tyrosine kinases, G alpha subunits and H-Ras share a common membrane-anchored scaffolding protein, caveolin. Caveolin binding negatively regulates the auto-activation of Src tyrosine kinases. J. Biol. Chem. **271:** 29182–29190.
22. LI, S., T. OKAMOTO, M. CHUN, et al. 1995. Evidence for a regulated interaction between hetero-trimeric G proteins and caveolin. J. Biol. Chem. **270:** 15693–15701.
23. CARMAN, C.V., M.P. LISANTI & J.L. BENOVIC. 1999. Regulation of G protein-coupled receptor kinases by caveolin. J. Biol. Chem. **274:** 8858–8864.
24. ENGELMAN, J.A., X. ZHANG, F. GALBIATI, et al. 1998. Molecular genetics of the caveolin gene family: implications for human cancers, diabetes, Alzheimer disease, and muscular dystrophy. Am. J. Hum. Genet. **63:** 1578–1587.
25. VOLONTE, D., K. ZHANG, M.P. LISANTI & F. GALBIATI. 2002. Expression of caveolin-1 induces premature cellular senescence in primary cultures of murine fibroblasts. Mol. Biol. Cell. **13:** 2502–2517.
26. CHO, K.A., S.J. RYU, I.S. JUNG, et al. 2003. Senescent phenotype can be reversed by reduction of caveolin status. J. Biol. Chem. **278:** 27789–27795.
27. DIMRI, G.P., M. NAKANISHIM, M.J. DESPREZ, et al. 1996. Inhibition of E2F activity by the cyclin-dependent protein kinase inhibitor p21 in cells expressing or lacking a functional retinoblastoma protein. Mol. Cell. Biol. **16:** 2987–2997.
28. GALBIATI, F., D. VOLONTÉ, O. GIL, et al. 1998. Expression of caveolin-1 and -2 in differentiating PC12 cells and dorsal root ganglion neurons: caveolin-2 is upregulated in response to cell injury. Proc. Natl. Acad. Sci. USA **95:** 10257–10262.
29. RAZANI, B., A. SCHLEGEL, J. LIU & M.P. LISANTI. 2001. Caveolin-1, a putative tumour suppressor gene. Biochem. Soc. Trans. (Review) **29:** 494–499.

30. CHEN, Q.M., V.C. TU, J. CATANIA, *et al.* 2000. Involvement of Rb family proteins, focal adhesion proteins and protein synthesis in senescent morphogenesis induced by hydrogen peroxide. J. Cell Sci. **113**(Pt. 22): 4087–4097.
31. WEI, Y., X. YANG, Q. LIU, *et al.* 1999. A role for caveolin and the urokinase receptor in integrin-mediated adhesion and signaling. J. Cell Biol. **144**: 1285–1294.
32. CHAPMAN, H.A., Y. WEI, D.I. SIMON & DA. WALTZ. 1999. Role of urokinase receptor and caveolin in regulation of integrin signaling. Thromb. Haemostasis **82**: 291–297.
33. TEIXEIRA, A., N. CHAVEROT, C. SCHRODER, *et al.* 1999. Requirement of caveolae microdomains in extracellular signal-regulated kinase and focal adhesion kinase activation induced by endothelin-1 in primary astrocytes. J. Neurochem. **72**: 120–128.
34. LIM, I.K., K. WON HONG, I.H. KWAK, *et al.* 2000. Cytoplasmic retention of p-Erk1/2 and nuclear accumulation of actin proteins during cellular senescence in human diploid fibroblasts. Mech. Ageing Dev. **119**: 113–130.
35. PARK, S.C. Functional recovery of senescent cells through restoration of receptor-mediated endocytosis. Mech. Aging Dev. **123**: 917–926.

Growth Hormone Alters Components of the Glutathione Metabolic Pathway in Ames Dwarf Mice[a]

HOLLY M. BROWN-BORG,[b] SHARLENE G. RAKOCZY,[b] AND ERIC O. UTHUS[c]

[b]*Department of Pharmacology, Physiology, and Therapeutics, University of North Dakota School of Medicine and Health Sciences, Grand Forks, North Dakota 58203, USA*

[c]*U.S. Department of Agriculture, ARS, Grand Forks Human Nutrition Research Center, Grand Forks, North Dakota 58203, USA*

ABSTRACT: Reduced signaling of the growth hormone (GH)/insulin-like growth factor-1(IGF-1)/insulin pathway is associated with extended life span in several species. Ames dwarf mice are GH and IGF-1 deficient and live 50–64% longer than wild-type littermates (males and females, respectively). Previously, we have shown that Ames mice exhibit elevated levels of antioxidative enzymes and lower oxidative damage. To further explore the relationship between GH and antioxidant expression, we administered GH or saline to dwarf mice and evaluated components of the glutathione (GSH) synthesis and degradation system. Growth hormone treatment significantly elevated kidney gamma-glutamyl-cysteine synthetase protein levels in 3- and 12-month-old dwarf mice. In contrast, the activity of the GSH degradation enzyme, gamma-glutamyl transpeptidase, was suppressed by GH administration in brain ($P < .05$), kidney ($P < .01$), heart ($P < .005$), and liver ($P < .06$). Activity levels of the detoxification enzyme, glutathione-S-transferase, were also suppressed in kidney tissues at 3 and 12 months of age and in 12-month-old dwarf liver tissues ($P < .05$). Taken together, the current results along with data from previous studies support a role for growth hormone in the regulation of antioxidative defense and, ultimately, life span in organisms with altered GH or IGF-1 signaling.

KEYWORDS: insulin-like growth factor; Ames dwarf mice; signaling

---

[a]The U.S. Department of Agriculture, Agricultural Research Service, Northern Plains Area is an equal opportunity/affirmative action employer and all agency services are available without discrimination.

Mention of a trademark or proprietary product does not constitute a guarantee of warranty of the product by the United States Department of Agriculture and does not imply its approval to the exclusion of other products that may also be suitable.

Address for correspondence: Holly M. Brown-Borg, Department of Pharmacology, Physiology, and Therapeutics, University of North Dakota School of Medicine and Health Sciences, 501 N. Columbia Road, Grand Forks, ND 58203. Voice: 701-777-3949; fax: 701-777-4490.
  brownbrg@medicine.nodak.edu

INTRODUCTION

Factors that affect aging and their regulation are not well understood. Specific components of the endocrine system exhibit predictable age-related changes. In particular, it is well known that plasma growth hormone (GH) and insulin-like growth factor-1 (IGF-1) levels decline in humans beginning around age 30 years. This decrease in youthful levels of growth-promoting proteins has been strongly implicated in physical (decreased muscle mass, increased fat mass) and biochemical changes that occur with aging.

Reduced signaling of the GH/IGF-1/insulin pathway is associated with extended life span in several species including mammals, flies, worms, and yeast. Increased resistance to oxidative stress is a characteristic common to many of these longevity mutants. Ames dwarf mice are GH and IGF-1 deficient and live 50–64% longer than wild-type littermates (males and females, respectively).[1] Previously, we have shown that Ames mice exhibit elevated levels of antioxidative enzymes, lower oxidative damage, and enhanced methionine metabolism.[2–4] To further explore the relationship between GH and antioxidant expression, we administered GH or saline to dwarf mice and evaluated components of the glutathione (GSH) synthesis and degradation system and some components of the methionine metabolic pathway.

MATERIALS AND METHODS

Ames dwarf mice were housed in a temperature-controlled environment ($22 \pm 1°C$) with *ad libitum* access to food (PMI, St. Louis, MO) and water (standard laboratory conditions). All procedures involving mice were reviewed and approved by the University of North Dakota Institutional Animal Care and Use Committee.

Three- and twelve-month-old dwarf mice received either porcine GH (50 µg total; NHPP-NIDDK) in alkaline saline mixed with 50% PVP (polyvinylpyrrolidone) or saline:PVP in two daily injections for seven days. Body and liver weights were recorded and reported as part of a larger study.[5] Tissues collected and analyzed included liver, kidney, heart, and brain. Glutathione, glutathione disulfide (GSSG), glutathione peroxidase (GPX), and glutathione reductase (GR) levels were previously measured and reported.[5]

Gamma-glutamylcysteine synthetase (GCS), the rate-limiting step in GSH biosynthesis, was measured using standard immunoblotting procedures. Gamma-glutamyltranspeptidase (GGT; E.C. 2.3.2.2) and glutathione S-transferase (GST; EC 2.5.1.18) activities were measured in tissues.[6,7]

Liver was the only tissue used for evaluation of methionine metabolism because of the very limited amounts of tissue from dwarf mice. Liver was prepared for SAM and SAH analysis and measured with a Dionex 4000i HPLC (Dionex, Sunnyvale, CA) according to previously reported procedures.[4] Methionine adenosyltransferase (MAT) activity and glycine N-methyltransferase (GNMT) activity were determined as previously described.[4]

For activity assays, analysis of variance (ANOVA) was used to determine significant differences among means. When needed, a Newman-Keuls post hoc test was used to test for specific differences. For comparison of protein levels (densitometric analysis), Student's *t* tests were used.

RESULTS

Short-term GH administration to dwarf mice induced significant body and liver weight gains compared to saline-injected dwarf mice in both 3- and 12-month-old mice (body weight changes: 3 month, 4-fold increase; 12 month, 15-fold increase).[5]

In liver tissues, GH treatment decreased MAT activity 40% and 38% in 3- and 12-month-old dwarf mice, respectively, compared with saline-treated mice ($P < .0001$ and $P = .0008$). The activity of GNMT, an enzyme that removes methyl groups from SAM, was also significantly suppressed by GH administration in both 3- (44%) and 12-month-old (43%) mice ($P = .0001$ and $P = .006$). Although levels of SAM were not altered, SAH concentrations were significantly decreased 24% and 30% by GH treatment in 3- and 12-month-old mice, respectively. The ratio of SAM:SAH was elevated in 12-month-old GH-treated mice ($P = .05$).

We previously reported that GSH and GSH:GSSG ratios were elevated in liver, brain, and muscle tissue after short-term GH treatment.[5] In addition, GPX levels were significantly reduced by GH. In the current study, we did not observe differences in protein levels of GCS after GH administration at either age examined. Regarding degradation, liver GGT activity was decreased 23% in 3-month-old GH-treated dwarf mice compared with mice receiving daily saline treatments ($P = .059$). Detoxification of compounds is accomplished by conjugation to GSH via the glutathione S-transferases. The activity of GST was suppressed 24% in 12-month-old GH-treated mice ($P = .05$) compared with age-matched saline-treated mice.

The kidney is a tissue that also plays a significant role in metabolism and detoxification. Our previous report showed that GSH levels were not affected by GH treatment, whereas GPX was markedly decreased.[5] In contrast, GR activity was elevated in this tissue. The protein involved in *de novo* synthesis of GSH, GCS, was elevated 64% and 46% in kidney tissues from GH-injected dwarf mice at 3 and 12 months of age, respectively ($P = .0003$ and $P = .02$). The activity of GGT was not affected by treatment; however, GST activity was reduced 33% and 16% in 3- and 12-month-old mice compared with saline-injected control ($P = .0008$ and $P = .04$).

Protein levels of GCS in hearts of GH-treated mice were nearly half (52%) that of mice receiving saline ($P = .0008$) at 12 months of age. Similar to kidney, GH administration to GH-deficient dwarf mice reduced GGT activity in heart tissue by 31% in 3-month-old mice ($P = .005$).

Effects of GH treatment on whole-brain tissue were less pronounced compared with peripheral tissues. Brain GSH and GSH:GSSG levels were elevated by GH treatment, whereas GPX was depressed.[5] Brain levels of GCS protein were unaffected by GH treatment. In agreement with other tissues, though, GGT activity was suppressed 15% by 7 days of GH injections in 3-month-old mice ($P = .05$). The level of GST activity was similarly decreased (17%) by GH treatment at this age relative to the levels in saline-injected mice ($P = .03$).

DISCUSSION

The area of hormonal regulation of the aging process is under intense investigation. Reduced signaling of the GH/IGF-1/insulin pathway is a well-conserved mechanism that exerts a major influence over antioxidative defense, in particular, and extends life span in multiple species. In this study, GH-deficient dwarf mice were used to evaluate specific effects of GH replacement on GSH and methionine metabolism. Our results indicate first that the responses of various components of GSH metabolism to GH treatment were tissue dependent. Levels of GCS protein, a protein that catalyzes the rate-limiting step in GSH biosynthesis, were altered in kidney and heart tissues only, although not in the same direction. In contrast, both the activities of GGT and GST were always reduced by GH treatment when a change was observed. These data suggest that the elevated levels of GSH in tissues of GH-treated mice may be partially caused by downregulation of the initial step in GSH degradation. At the same time, GH appears to suppress GSH conjugation activity (via GST) possibly reducing the ability to combat challenges by toxins. Second, we showed that GH downregulates MAT and GNMT activities in liver tissue of GH-deficient mice. Previously, we reported that the activities of these enzymes were significantly elevated in Ames mice compared with wild-type mice.[5] These new data suggest that GH may be involved in regulation of methionine metabolism, thus affecting nucleic acid methylation and subsequent gene expression. Taken together, the current results along with data from previous studies support a role for growth hormone in the regulation of antioxidative defense and, ultimately, life span in organisms with altered GH or IGF-1 signaling.

REFERENCES

1. BROWN-BORG, H.M., K.E. BORG, C.J. MELISKA & A. BARTKE. 1996. Dwarf mice and the aging process. Nature **384**: 33.
2. BROWN-BORG, H.M. & S.G. RAKOCZY. 2000. Catalase expression in delayed and premature aging mouse models. Exp. Gerontol. **35**: 199–212.
3. BROWN-BORG, H.M., W.T. JOHNSON, S.G. RAKOCZY & M.A. ROMANICK. 2001. Mitochondrial oxidant production and oxidative damage in Ames dwarf mice. J. Am. Aging Assoc. **24**: 85–96.
4. UTHUS, E.O. & H.M. BROWN-BORG. 2003. Altered methionine metabolism in long-living Ames dwarf mice. Exp. Geron. **38**: 491–498.
5. BROWN-BORG, H.M. & S.G. RAKOCZY. 2003. Growth hormone administration to long-living dwarf mice alters multiple components of the antioxidative defense system. Mech. Age. Dev. **124**: 1013–1024.
6. TATE, S.S. & A. MEISTER. 1974. Interaction of gamma-glutamyl transpeptidase with amino acids, dipeptides, and derivatives and analogs of glutathione. J. Biol. Chem. **249**: 7593–7602.
7. HABIG, W.H., M.J. PABST & W.B. JAKOBY. 1974. Glutathione S-transferases. J. Biol. Chem. **249**: 7130–7139.

Age-Related Endocrine Dysfunction in Nonhuman Primates

N. D. GONCHAROVA AND B. A. LAPIN

Laboratory of Endocrinology, Research Institute of Medical Primatology, Russian Academy of Medical Sciences, Sochi-Adler, Russia, 354376

ABSTRACT: Peculiarities of functioning of some parts of the endocrine system (the pineal gland, pancreatic gland, hypothalamic-pituitary-adrenal axis, and hypothalamic-pituitary-testicular axis) in an aging nonhuman primate model (*Papio hamadryas* and *Macaca mulatta*) are described in this article. It has been established that basal activity of some endocrine functions (glucocorticoid, corticotropic, pancreatic, male estradiol producing) varies little with age. Other functions significantly decrease (DHEA/DHEAS-producing, pineal, testicular) or increase (male gonadotropic) with age. In contrast with basal activity, pronounced age-related changes in response to specific stimuli were detected in all endocrine functions. Old baboons and rhesus monkeys exhibited a delay of the normalization of the pituitary-testicular axis, adrenal cortex, and pancreatic gland function after their activation in response to specific stimuli, such as LHRH, CRH, ACTH, and glucose. Old monkeys also demonstrate decreased HPA axis sensitivity to glucocorticoid regulation by negative feedback and the HPT axis to inhibitory effect of prolonged administration of LHRH agonist. Age-related changes in reactions of endocrine functions in response to specific stimulating and inhibiting stimuli indicate impaired resiliency of these functions. Age-related endocrine changes perhaps play a pathophysiological role in age function disorders of hormonocompetent tissues and organs and age pathology.

KEYWORDS: endocrine system; primate; glucose; aging

The endocrine system plays a role in the organization of complex forms of behavior; nonspecific adaptation to environmental stress factors; and regulation of reproduction, homeostasis, thermoregulation, immune status, and higher nervous system activity, that is, the processes most often disturbed during aging. It can be expected that age-related changes in the functioning of the endocrine system underlie age-related disturbances of various functions. Considerable rejuvenation of some age-related diseases in modern society characterized by a wide spectrum of stress factors indicates the important role of endocrine disorders in the pathogenesis of accelerated aging. Species-specific differences in the functioning of some endocrine glands make the choice of experimental model for endocrinology aging study a particularly important problem. The purpose of this investigation was studying the changes in the

Address for correspondence: Dr. Goncharova, Laboratory of Endocrinology, Research Institute of Medical Primatology, Russian Academy of Medical Sciences, Sochi-Adler, Russia, 354376. Voice: +7-8622-422862; fax: +7-8622-422239.
iprim@sochi.net

Ann. N.Y. Acad. Sci. 1019: 321–325 (2004). © 2004 New York Academy of Sciences.
doi: 10.1196/annals.1297.054

pineal gland, pancreatic gland, and hypothalamic-pituitary-adrenal (HPA) axis and hypothalamic-pituitary-testicular (HPT) axis functioning during aging in a nonhuman primate model.

MATERIALS AND METHODS

Forty male baboons (*Papio hamadryas*) and 70 female rhesus monkeys (*Macaca mulatta*) were observed for the HPA and HPT systems, and pancreatic and pineal gland functioning in different age periods (6–8 years old, young adults; 10–15 years old, mature age; and 20–27 years old, old age) at basal conditions and during their specific stimulation by administration of corticotrophin-releasing hormone (CRH), short-acting corticotrophin (ACTH), luteinizing hormone-releasing hormone (LHRH), and glucose. Plasma hormone levels were determined by specific radioimmunoassay and immunoenzyme methods.

RESULTS

Basal activity of some endocrine functions (glucocorticoid, corticotropic, pancreatic, male estradiol producing) varies little with age, that of other functions (dehydroepiandrosterone/dehydroepiandrosterone sulfate [DHEA/DHEAS]–producing, pineal, testicular) significantly decreases with aging, and the activity of other functions (male gonadotropic) increases. Marked hormonal imbalance was formed in peripheral blood plasma of aged monkeys because of unequal changes of different endocrine functions.[1–5] Note that there was a considerable increase in cortisol/DHEA and cortisol/DHEAS molar ratios in particular. This fact may have an important physiological meaning because these corticosteroid fractions are antagonists in their influence on some physiological systems, for example, immune and nervous. Furthermore, the estradiol/testosterone plus 5-alpha-dihydrotestosterone molar ratio increased in old male baboons, and an index of free plasma testosterone fraction increased in aged female monkeys because of the decrease of estrogen secretion and decrease of maximum binding capacity of sex hormone binding globulin in comparison with that in young monkeys. The latter disturbances have important pathophysiological consequences for age-related reproductive diseases. Note also that the circadian profile of pineal and glucocorticoid function activity was clearly flattened in old monkeys due to the impairment of the nocturnal secretion of melatonin and elevation of cortisol (F) plasma level in the evening and nighttime.[3,5]

In contrast with basal activity, pronounced age-related changes were detected in the reaction of all endocrine functions to specific stimuli. FIGURE 1 demonstrates age-related changes in the dynamics of serum F and insulin level in response to, respectively, CRH or glucose administration in the rhesus monkeys of two age groups. The young animals exhibited a sharp decrease in the F level within 90 min after the peak concentrations had been reached (i.e., 60 and 120 min after CRH administration). In contrast, the aged animals did not exhibit any F decrease in this period; their F concentration even continued to increase. Similar age-related changes were observed in the dynamic of serum insulin level in response to glucose administration in monkeys of different age groups (see FIG. 1), but in another time period. In young

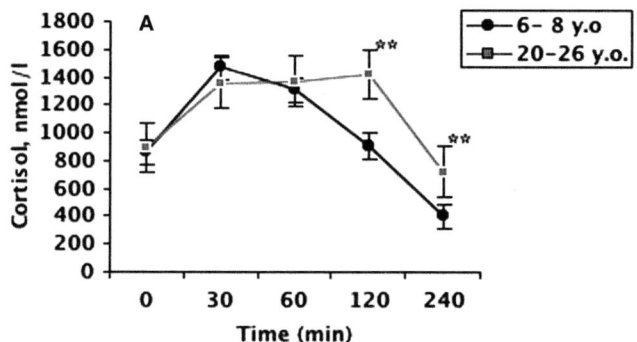

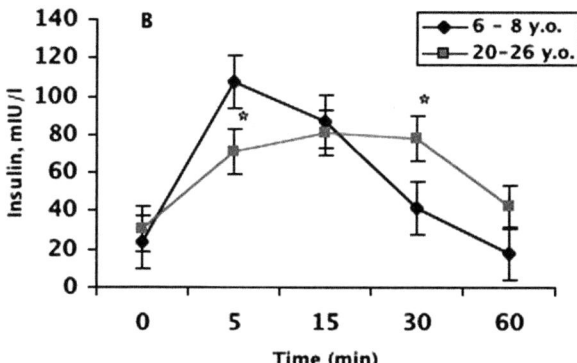

FIGURE 1. The dynamics of plasma cortisol in response to CRH administration (at 03:00 p.m., bovine, synthetic, Sigma, 0.8 μg/kg b.w., i.v., **A**) and the dynamics of plasma insulin in response to glucose administration (at 09:00 a.m., 300 mg/kg b.w., i.v., **B**) in female rhesus monkeys of different age (mean ± SEM). *$P < .05$, **$P < .01$ (vs. relative values in young animals).

monkeys, insulin concentration attained the peak values 5 min after glucose administration and then sharply decreased, returning to initial levels within 30 min. In old monkeys, the serum insulin concentration remained maximal 10 and 25 min after it had reached the peak (15 and 30 min after glucose administration). A similar picture of age-related changes in plasma F, testosterone, and luteinizing hormone levels was observed in monkeys of different ages in response to, respectively, a single injection of short-acting ACTH and LHRH.[2,4,5] The old baboons and rhesus monkeys exhibited a delay of the normalization of the pituitary-testicular axis and adrenal cortex function after their activation in response to specific stimuli. The old monkeys also demonstrated decreased HPA axis sensitivity to glucocorticoid regulation by a negative feedback mechanism and the HPT axis to inhibitory effect of a prolonged course of LHRH agonist (buserelin, Hoechst A.G.).[1,2,4,5] Age-related changes in reaction to the endocrine functions in response to specific stimulating and inhibiting stimuli indicate impaired resiliency of these functions.

CONCLUSIONS

This study demonstrates significant age-related endocrine dysfunction in nonhuman primates both in basal conditions and in conditions of the endocrine gland activations or inhibitions. Main endocrine dysfunctions revealed in nonhuman primates are similar to those in humans.[1,5,6,7] Some disturbances in the endocrine gland functioning (e.g., the delay of processes of restoration of initial endocrine gland activity after their stimulation by specific stimuli and age-related changes of circadian rhythms of melatonin and F) can be explained by age disorders in the tonus of central nervous pathways, for example, adrenergic, serotoninergic, and cholinergic. These pathways, as it is known, take part in regulation of the HPA axis, HPT system activity, and also of insulin and melatonin secretion.[7–9] Age-related changes in the tonus of central nervous pathways can depend on age-related changes in neurotransmitter level and in the distribution and density of their receptors in the central nervous system.[10,11]

Presumably, the deviations revealed can be of pathophysiological significance for age-associated dysfunction of hormone-competent cells, tissues, and organs and for the development of age-associated diseases. Thus, hormonal imbalance forming in the peripheral blood in basal conditions perhaps (in particular, a progressive decrease of DHEA, DHEAS) plays an important role in the development of neurodegenerative diseases, atherosclerosis, increased insulin tolerance, reproductive dysfunction, and higher incidence of tumors. The slowing down of processes of restoration of the initial level of activity of the HPA system, the HPT system, and the pancreatic gland leads to prolonged elevation of F, testosterone, and insulin concentrations. The latter may be important for the pathogenesis of disorders in adaptation to changing environmental conditions and may increase the risk of cardiovascular and neurodegenerative diseases, diabetes mellitus, and some age-related diseases of the reproductive system. The decreased secretion of melatonin during aging seems to be an important factor for the pathogenesis of many mental and somatic diseases. Early correction of endocrine disorders may become an important component for the therapy of age-associated diseases and for prevention of premature and/or accelerated aging.

REFERENCES

1. GONCHAROVA, N.D. 1997. Zh. Evolyuts. Biokhim. Fiziol. **33:** 44–51.
2. GONCHAROVA, N.D. & B.A. LAPIN. 2000. J. Med. Primatol. **29:** 26–35.
3. GONCHAROVA, N.D., V.KH. KHAVINSON & B.A. LAPIN. 2001. Byull. Eksp. Biol. Med. **131:** 466–468.
4. GONCHAROVA, N.D. & B.A. LAPIN. 2002. Mech. Ageing Dev. **123:** 1191–1201.
5. GONCHAROVA, N.D., B.A. LAPIN & V.KH. KHAVINSON. 2002. Byull. Eksp. Biol. Med. **134:** 417–421.
6. FERRARI, E., L. CRAVELLO, B. MUZZONI, et al. 2001. Eur. J. Endocrinol. **144:** 319–329.
7. REITER, R.J. 1998. Progr. Neurobiol. **56:** 359–384.

8. KAUFMAN, J.M. & A. VERMEULEN. 1989. J. Clin. Endocrinol. Metab. **68:** 219–222.
9. AL-DAMLUJU, S., P. BOULOUX, A. WHITE & M. BESSER. 1990. Neuroendocrinology **51:** 76–81.
10. BIGHAM, M.H. & M.S. LIDOW. 1995. Neurobiol. Aging **16:** 91–104.
11. PETERS, A. 2002. Neurosci. Biobehav. Rev. **26:** 733–741.

Secretion of Melatonin in Healthy Elderly Subjects: A Longitudinal Study

N. M. K. NG YING KIN, N. P. V. NAIR, G. SCHWARTZ, J. X. THAVUNDAYIL, AND L. ANNABLE

Department of Psychiatry, McGill University and Douglas Hospital Research Centre, Verdun, Quebec, Canada, H4H 1R3

ABSTRACT: We report on a 10-year longitudinal study on 24-h serum melatonin secretion (AUC) in healthy human subjects. Fifty women and 53 men (aged 42–83 yr) participated in the study initially. Of these, 18 women and 15 men were followed for 6 consecutive years. Results: (a) *Cross-sectional analysis (n = 103)*: A significant ($R = -.49$, $P = .0001$) decline in AUC melatonin with age was found in women, but not in men. (b) *Longitudinal analysis (n = 33)*: Repeated-measure ANOVAs for women ($n = 18$): Time: linear $F_{1,17} = 5.14$, $P = .037$. The AUC increased by about 40% over the six-year period. In men, there were no significant changes. Conclusion: In agreement with most cross-sectional studies, an inverse relationship was found between melatonin secretion and age. However, the longitudinal study showed an increase in melatonin secretion, indicating the presence of putative compensatory mechanisms during healthy aging. Changes in melatonin secretion were gender specific, occurring in women only.

KEYWORDS: melatonin; aging; gender; longitudinal study

Melatonin, a hormone secreted by the pineal gland, is thought to be involved in the aging process.[1] Most reports, including our own, described an age-related decline in the hormone secretion in human subjects.[2–5] Animal studies[6] also supported these findings. However, Zeitzer *et al.*[7] saw no significant difference between two groups of young and elderly subjects, respectively. All these reports were based on cross-sectional studies. Hitherto, a longitudinal study has not been reported in humans. We believe such a study could provide a more physiological assessment of the relationship between aging and changes in melatonin secretion. Here, we report on the results of our study that was carried out over a period of 10 years. Since our study population was almost equally divided between men and women subjects, it also allowed us to investigate the putative role of gender in melatonin secretion.

Address for correspondence: N.P.V. Nair, Department of Psychiatry, McGill University and Douglas Hospital Research Centre, 6875 LaSalle Blvd., Verdun, Quebec, Canada, H4H 1R3. Voice: 514-762-3035, ext. 3428; fax: 514-762-3020.
vasavan.nair@douglas.mcgill.ca

METHODS

Initially, 102 physically healthy subjects (50 women, age 42–73 yr; 53 men, age 51–83 yr) participated in the study, and were assessed yearly. Of these, 33 subjects (18 women; age 55–73 yr; 15 men, age 57–74 yr) were studied for six consecutive years. Psychiatric abnormality was ruled out by a formal clinical interview and a battery of neuropsychological tests designed to detect cognitive deficit. All participating subjects were also given a complete physical examination by a general practitioner, and had the following laboratory tests: electrocardiography, electroencephalography, computerized axial tomography scans, and blood tests for kidney, liver, and thyroid functions, vitamin B12, and folate levels. Informed consents were obtained from all participants.

All subjects entered the Clinical Investigation Unit of the Research Centre before 8 a.m. and stayed indoors for the next 24 hours. Upon arrival, an indwelling intravenous catheter with a 0.3% heparin solution was installed in the subject's forearm. Blood samples were collected at hourly intervals over the next 24 hours. Throughout the course of sampling, illumination was maintained at 300 lux during the "daytime" (0700–2300 h) and at 50 lux during the "nighttime" (2300–0700 h). The blood sample (7 mL each), drawn into a Vacutainer tube, was allowed to clot for 30 min at room temperature. Blood sera were isolated using a refrigerated centrifuge, and stored at $-20°$ until analyzed for melatonin, using a validated radio-immunoassay method (Stockgrand, Guildford, Surrey, U.K.). The 24-h secretion of melatonin was calculated from the area under the time-concentration curve (AUC).

Statistical Procedures

Repeated-measure ANOVAs, with Greenhouse-Geisser corrections, if required, were carried out on AUC values over time. Pearson correlations between AUC and age were calculated. All significant tests were two-tailed and subjected to Bonferroni correction, where required, to maintain an overall Type 1 error of 0.05.

RESULTS

Cross-Sectional Analysis on the 102 Subjects

In Women (N = 49)

A significant (Pearson $R = -.51$, $P < .0001$) inverse correlation was found between AUC melatonin and age in female subjects. This was also the case when peak melatonin levels were measured (Pearson $R = -.43$, $P < .002$). When the subjects were divided into two groups, aged 65 yr or under, the older subjects, $N = 16$, had significantly ($P < .01$) lower AUC melatonin secretion when compared to the younger ones ($N = 33$), mean ± SD: 312 ± 101 v/s 456 ± 198 pg-h/mL.

In Men (N = 53)

There was no significant relationship between age and AUC melatonin or between age and peak melatonin levels (in both cases, the Pearson $R = 0$).

Longitudinal Analysis on the 33 Subjects

In Women (N=18)

Repeated-measures ANOVA showed a linear increase in AUC melatonin over time ($F_{1,17} = 5.14$, $P = .037$). The AUC increased from 356 ± 142 to 494 ± 267 pg-h/mL (40%) over the 6-yr period. The increase over the first 5 years was 73% (from 356 ± 142 to 616 ± 412 pg-h/mL) followed by a decline of 20 percent.

In Men (N=15)

There was a nonsignificant directional trend for an increase in melatonin secretion over the 6-yr period, from 373 ± 172 to 597 ± 692 pg-h/mL (60%) (repeated-measure ANOVAs: linear $F_{1,14} = 2.18$, $P = .16$).

DISCUSSION AND CONCLUSION

In agreement with most of the studies reported so far, an inverse relationship was found between melatonin secretion and age.[2-5] However, Zeitzer et al.[7] recently reported that that there was no relationship between melatonin secretion and aging. The results of the present study showing that a gender-specific decline in melatonin secretion in women may explain this discrepancy. The study of Zeitzer et al. consisted mostly of young men: 98 men aged 18–30 yr, 14 men aged 64–75 yr, and 20 women aged 65–81 yr.

While the cross-sectional studies clearly show a decline in melatonin secretion in older women, results of this six-year longitudinal study showed an increase in melatonin secretion. This probably indicates the presence of a putative compensatory mechanism during healthy aging. We believe that in age-related disorders such as Alzheimer disease (AD), this mechanism is flawed, resulting in a continuing decline in melatonin secretion during aging. Previous studies have described the abnormal secretions of melatonin in AD.[5,8,9] The present findings highlight the importance of defining gender when studying the relationship between melatonin and age-related disorders such as AD, a condition more prevalent in women than in men.

REFERENCES

1. PIERPAOLI, W. et al. 1991. The pineal control of aging. The effects of pineal grafting on the survival of older mice. Ann. N.Y. Acad. Sci. **621:** 291–313.
2. NAIR, N.P.V. et al. 1986. Plasma melatonin—An index of brain aging? Biol. Psychiatry **21:** 141–150.
3. WETTERBERG, L. et al. 1999. Normative melatonin excretion: a multinational study. Psychoneuroendocrinology **24:** 209–226.
4. TARQUINI, B. et al. 1997. Chronome assessment of circulating melatonin in humans. In Vivo **6:** 473–484.
5. LIU, R.Y. et al. 1999. Decreased melatonin levels in postmortem cerebrospinal fluid in relation to aging, Alzheimer's disease, and apolipoprotein E epsilon4/4 genotype. J. Clin. Endocrinol. & Metab. **84:** 323–327.
6. SELMAOUI, B. & Y. TOUITOU. 1999. Age-related differences in serum melatonin and pineal NAT activity and in the response of rat pineal to a 50-Hz magnetic field. Life Sci. **64:** 2291–2297.

7. ZIETZER, J.M. *et al.* 1999. Do plasma melatonin concentrations decline with age? Am. J. Med. **107:** 432–436.
8. MISHIMA, K. *et al.* 1999. Melatonin secretion rhythm disorders in patients with senile dementia of Alzheimer's type with disturbed sleep-waking. Biol. Psychiatry **45:** 417–421.
9. NAIR, N.P.V. *et al.* 1998. Circadian rhythms of cortisol and melatonin secretion in Alzheimer's disease and normal elderly subjects. *In* Biological Clocks. Mechanisms and Applications. Y. Touitou, Ed.: 357–360. Elsevier. Amsterdam.

The Proinflammatory Phenotype of Senescent Cells

The p53-Mediated ICAM-1 Expression

DIMITRIS KLETSAS,[a] HARRIS PRATSINIS,[a] GIORGOS MARIATOS,[b] PANAYOTIS ZACHARATOS,[b] AND VASSILIS G. GORGOULIS[b]

[a]*Laboratory of Cell Proliferation and Ageing, Institute of Biology, NCSR "Demokritos," 15310 Athens, Greece*

[b]*Department of Histology and Embryology, Molecular Carcinogenesis Group, Medical School, University of Athens, 11527 Athens, Greece*

ABSTRACT: Senescent cells are characterized by the activation of the tumor suppressor protein p53 and consequently their inability to proliferate. However, their phenotype is not restricted to the exhaustion of their replicative potential, as they also exhibit a proinflammatory phenotype, which could possibly contribute to the aging process. Intercellular adhesion molecule-1 (ICAM-1) is one of the molecules involved in inflammatory response that is overexpressed in senescent cells and aged tissues. Although the role of the nuclear factor-kappaB (NF–κB) signaling cascade is crucial in ICAM-1 activation, we have shown that p53 directly activates the expression of ICAM-1 in an NF–kB-independent manner. This may link p53 to ICAM-1 function and consequently to the aging process and to various age-related pathologies.

KEYWORDS: p53; cellular senescence; proinflammatory phenotype; ICAM-1

In contrast to tumor cell lines, which can proliferate *ad infinitum,* most normal cells when cultured *in vitro* do not divide indefinitely, but exhibit a finite number of cell divisions before they enter a nondividing state referred to as cellular (or replicative) senescence.[1,2] Accordingly, the most widely accepted interpretation for the biological function of replicative senescence is that it represents an obstacle against tumorigenesis. Nevertheless, several lines of evidence indicate a connection between cellular and organismal aging, probably most important being the much shorter life span of the cells derived from patients with premature aging syndromes.[1] In this regard, it must be mentioned that the senescent phenotype is not restricted to the exhaustion of the replicative potential, as senescent cells also exhibit a less fibrogenic and a pronounced inflammatory phenotype that could possibly contribute to the aging process. However, the mechanism underlying the connection between the senescent state and inflammation needs to be elucidated.

Address for correspondence: Dr. D. Kletsas, Laboratory of Cell Proliferation and Ageing, Institute of Biology, National Centre of Scientific Research "Demokritos," Athens, Greece. Voice: +30-210-6503565; fax: +30-210-6511767.
 dkletsas@bio.demokritos.gr

The p53 protein is a multifunctional transcriptional regulator that is activated in response to several stresses, and regulates a plethora of biological processes, such as apoptosis, DNA repair, and cell cycle progression.[3] Its importance as a tumor suppressor can be deduced from the estimation that nearly 80% of human cancers have defects in p53 signaling.[2] On the other hand, in senescent cells p53 exhibits an increased DNA binding and transcriptional activity and, in addition, p53 overexpression can induce a senescent-like phenotype in a number of different cellular contexts.[2] Recently, a mutant mouse line has been generated that expresses a modestly overactive p53 form. These mice, as expected, exhibit enhanced resistance to spontaneous tumorigenesis, but they also display premature onset of aging-associated phenotypes, thus also implicating p53 in organismal aging.[4] Hence, our goal was to understand the role of p53 in the development of some features of senescent cells, and in particular of those linked with their proinflammatory phenotype.

Among the several molecules found to be overexpressed in senescent cells is the intercellular adhesion molecule-1 (ICAM-1 or CD54),[5] a member of the immunoglobulin gene superfamily, which binds to several surface molecules and is involved in the initiation of the immune reaction.[6] ICAM-1 is induced by cytokines and various stress stimuli, such as hypoxia, ultraviolet, and ionizing radiation. Although the role of the nuclear factor–kappaB (NF–κB) signaling cascade is pivotal in ICAM-1 activation, NF–κB-independent pathways may also participate, predominantly in stress-inducing stimuli. Given that similar stimuli are potent inducers of p53,[7] we investigated whether p53 could represent an alternative activator of ICAM-1.

Initially, we examined whether the activation of the p53 pathway could induce ICAM-1. For this purpose we used the tetracycline-inducible p53 Saos-2 cell line (Saos-2-Tet-hp53)[8] and found that upon treatment with tetracycline the ICAM-1 mRNA and protein levels were highly elevated, indicating that endogenous ICAM-1 is induced by p53 at the transcriptional level.[6] A comparable increase was observed in mRNA of the classic p53-target genes p21^{WAF-1} and MDM-2. In order to rule out the possibility that the observed effect could represent an NF–κB-mediated result after p53 activation, we treated the cells with the well-characterized MEK1 inhibitor PD98059, which efficiently blocks NF–κB activation via the Raf/MAPK/pp90^{rsk} pathway.[8] The observed increase of ICAM-1 mRNA and protein levels remained unaffected in these cells after administration of PD98059, favoring an NF–κB-independent p53 effect. Subsequently, we examined the ability of endogenous p53 to activate ICAM-1 within a physiological cellular context. To address this issue, we developed primary human diploid dermal fibroblasts (HDFs) and explored the status of ICAM-1 after activation of p53 in response to a potent genotoxic stress stimulus, that is, γ-irradiation. Exposure of HDFs to ionizing radiation resulted in an intense increase of ICAM-1 expression. To exclude the possibilty that ICAM-1 was induced by other p53-independent pathways, we incubated the cells with the specific p53 inhibitor pifithrin-α (PFT-α) prior to irradiation. Treatment with PFT-α reduced ICAM-1 and p21^{WAF-1} mRNA expression to baseline levels, clearly demonstrating that the p53 pathway is directly involved in ICAM-1 induction.[6]

In silico examination of the ICAM-1 genomic sequence revealed three potential p53 responsive elements (p53REs) in the first and second introns. Electrophoretic mobility-shift assay analysis revealed that the predicted DNA elements are indeed specific p53-binding sites. In addition, all the elements conferred inducibility specifically by p53 in *cis* to a heterologous promoter when introduced into the human p53-null osteosarcoma cell line Saos-2, confirming that these REs may function as active p53-binding sites. Finally, we have analyzed the interaction of p53 with the putative p53REs by chromatin immunoprecipitation (ChIP) experiments and found that p53 interacts specifically with two of them. Thus, our findings collectively indicate that p53 activates directly the expression of ICAM-1, in an NF–κB-independent manner, that may link p53 to the ICAM-1 function in various pathophysiologies.[6]

Subsequently, we have investigated ICAM-1 expression in senescent cells. To this end, we have used two cell assay systems: (a) human skin fibroblasts that have undergone senescence after serial subculturing in vitro, and (b) human vascular smooth muscle cells (designated SM1) stably transfected with a nonreplicative retroviral vector containing a temperature-sensitive (tsA58) mutant of SV40 large T-antigen. SM1 cells, while at the permissive temperature of 36°C can proliferate indefinitely, at the nonpermissive temperature of 39°C (where large T-antigen expression is downregulated) acquire a senescent phenotype.[9] Senescent fibroblast and SM1 cells strongly overexpress ICAM-1, at both the mRNA and protein levels. In the presence of the specific p53 inhibitor PFT-α, the ICAM-1 upregulation in senescent cells is severely attenuated. These data indicate that ICAM-1 overexpression in senescent cells is (at least in part) p53-mediated.

The preceding findings fit well within the hypothesis of "antagonistic pleiotropy," predicting that during the course of evolution several genes have been selected for the maintenance of homeostasis in young individuals, but can have deleterious effects in the elderly.[10] Thus, although p53 has probably evolved to suppress tumorigenesis, it can also induce the appearance of certain proinflammatory features, such as ICAM-1 overexpression, which can accelerate the aging process.

ACKNOWLEDGMENT

This work was partially supported by the IPE-Cyprus ("Atheroma" Project) and the European Union (Contract No. QLK6-CT-2002-02582).

REFERENCES

1. CAMPISI, J. 1997. Aging and cancer: the double-edged sword of replicative senescence. J. Am. Geriatr. Soc. **45:** 482–488.
2. DONEHOWER, L.A. 2002. Does p53 affect organismal aging? J. Cell. Physiol. **192:** 23–33.
3. ITAHANA, K., G. DIMRI & J. CAMPISI. 2001. Regulation of cellular senescence by p53. Eur. J. Biochem. **268:** 2784–2791.
4. TYNER, S.D. et al. 2002. p53 mutant mice that display early ageing-associated phenotypes. Nature **415:** 45–53.
5. SHELTON, D.N. et al. 1999. Microarray analysis of replicative senescence. Curr. Biol. **9:** 939–945.
6. GORGOULIS, V.G. et al. 2003. p53 activates ICAM-1 (CD54) expression in an NF-kappaB-independent manner. EMBO J. **22:** 1567–1578.
7. PRIVES, C. & P.A. HALL. 1999. The p53 pathway. J. Pathol. **187:** 112–126.
8. RYAN, K.M. et al. 2000. Role of NF-kappaB in p53-mediated programmed cell death. Nature **404:** 892–897.
9. HSIEH, J.K. et al. 2000. p53, p21(WAF1/CIP1), and MDM2 involvement in the proliferation and apoptosis in an in vitro model of conditionally immortalized human vascular smooth muscle cells. Arterioscler. Thromb. Vasc. Biol. **20:** 973–981.
10. KIRKWOOD, T.B. & S.N. AUSTAD. 2000. Why do we age? Nature **408:** 233–238.

Short-Term Caloric Restriction and Sites of Oxygen Radical Generation in Kidney and Skeletal Muscle Mitochondria

RICARDO GREDILLA,[a] SHARON PHANEUF,[b] COLIN SELMAN,[b] SUMA KENDAIAH,[b] CHRISTIAAN LEEUWENBURGH,[b] AND GUSTAVO BARJA[a]

[a]*Department of Animal Biology–II (Animal Physiology), Faculty of Biology, Complutense University, 28040 Madrid, Spain*

[b]*Biochemistry of Aging Laboratory, College of Health and Human Performance, University of Florida, Gainesville, Florida 32611, USA*

ABSTRACT: Mitochondrial free radical generation is believed to be one of the principal factors determining aging rate, and complexes I and III have been described as the main sources of reactive oxygen species (ROS) within mitochondria in heart, brain, and liver. Moreover, complex I ROS generation of heart and liver mitochondria seems especially linked to aging rate both in comparative studies between animals with different longevities and in caloric restriction models. Caloric restriction (CR) is a well-documented manipulation that extends mean and maximum longevity. One of the factors that appears to be involved in such life span extension is the reduction in mitochondrial free radical generation at complex I. We have performed two parallel investigations, one studying the effect of short-term CR on oxygen radical generation in kidney and skeletal muscle (gastrocnemius) mitochondria and a second one regarding location of mitochondrial ROS-generating sites in these same tissues. In the former study, no effect of short-term caloric restriction was observed in mitochondrial free radical generation in either kidney or skeletal muscle. The latter study ruled out complex II as a principal source of free radicals in kidney and in skeletal muscle mitochondria, and, similar to previous investigations in heart and liver organelles, the main free radical generators were located at complexes I and III within the electron transport system.

KEYWORDS: reactive oxygen species; mitochondria; caloric restriction

INTRODUCTION

Mitochondria are the most important sources of reactive oxygen species (ROS) in healthy tissues because the main generator, the electron transport chain, is located at the inner mitochondrial membrane. They are also important targets of oxidative damage and are considered one of the main determinants of aging.[1–5] Mitochondrial

Address for correspondence: Dr. Gustavo Barja, Departmento de Biología Animal–II, Facultad de Biología, Universidad Complutense, Madrid 28040, Spain. Voice: +34-91-394-49-19; fax: +34-91-394-490-35.
gbarja@bio.ucm.es

free radical generation and the ensuing accumulation of oxidative damage can be responsible for the age-related decline in maximum functional capacities of tissues.

Caloric restriction (CR) is the only known nongenetic manipulation that extends maximum longevity in a wide variety of animals. In the last years, new insights about the underlying mechanism involved in the CR life-extension effect have been reported. Thus, CR decreases oxidative damage and its deleterious effects during aging, at least in part by decreasing mitochondrial oxygen radical production.[6–9] The magnitude of such reduction seems to depend on implementation time and the specific tissue, probably due to sensitivity differences to CR regimen.[10–13]

Although there is general agreement pointing to mitochondrial free radical generation as one of the principal causes of aging, controversy still exists concerning the sources of those reactive species within mitochondria.

Pioneer studies on the location of mitochondrial ROS-generating sites specially emphasized complex III as the major contributor to mitochondrial ROS production,[14] although contribution of complex I was suggested by others based on studies in submitochondrial particles.[15] During many decades, the view that complex III was the main or even the only source of ROS within mitochondria prevailed. However, recent investigations unequivocally show that complex I generates ROS in intact functional mitochondria;[16–21] see Barja[4] for review). Furthermore, complex I seems to play a decisive role in aging as deduced from caloric restriction investigations and comparative studies between birds and mammals. We have reported recently that the decrease in mitochondrial free radical production observed in animals subjected to CR takes place exclusively at complex I both in heart and liver mitochondria.[7–9] Regarding comparative studies, the lower mitochondrial ROS generation observed in long-lived birds versus short-lived rodents also was reported to occur mainly at complex I.[16–18] The importance of complex I ROS generation is also supported by its implication in the development of age-related pathologies such as Parkinson disease[22,23] However, most of the investigations described above were performed in tissues like heart (mainly) and liver, and almost no information exists in skeletal muscle (a postmitotic tissue) and kidney (the other mainly responsible for age related death in rodents).

In the current investigation, we studied the effect of short-term caloric restriction on mitochondrial free radical generation in kidney and skeletal muscle as well as the location of free radical generators sites.

MATERIALS AND METHODS

Animals and Experimental Design

Caloric Restriction Study

Both *ad libitum* and caloric restricted male Fischer 344 rats were obtained from the National Institute of Aging colony (Indianapolis, IN, USA) at 4 months of age. Caloric restriction was started at 3.5 months of age (10% restriction), increased to 25% restriction at 3.75 months of age, and maintained from 4 months at 40% restriction until the termination of the experiment at 6 months of age. From 4 months onward, all animals were housed individually under a 12-hour-light/12-hour-dark photoperiod and an ambient temperature of 18–20°C. After 8 weeks of acclimation, two animals per day (one *ad libitum* and one caloric restricted) were killed after anesthesia with haloperidol.

Location Study

Male Fischer 344 rats were obtained from Iffa Credo (Lyon, France) several weeks before being killed. Rats were fed *ad libitum* and caged individually under a 12-hour-light/12-hour-dark photoperiod and an ambient temperature of 18–20°C. Animals were killed by decapitation at 6 months of age.

Mitochondrial Isolation

Mitochondria were subsequently isolated from kidney and gastrocnemius muscle by differential centrifugation. Gastrocnemious muscles were immediately dissected and minced after decapitation. Homogenization was performed in isolation buffer A (225 mM mannitol, 75 mM sucrose, 1 mM EDTA, 0.2% BSA, pH 7.4) in a 1:10 dilution (wt/vol). The homogenate was centrifuged at 700g for 10 minutes, and the resulting supernatant was centrifuged twice at 8,000 g for 10 minutes. The mitochondrial pellet was resuspended in isolation buffer A without BSA. Kidneys were rapidly removed and homogenized in isolation buffer B (210 mM Mannitol, 70 mM sucrose, 5 mM Hepes, 1 mM EDTA, pH 7.35). The procedure performed to obtain the mitochondrial pellet was the same used in skeletal muscle. The mitochondrial pellet was resuspended in isolation buffer B without EDTA. All the isolation procedures were performed at 4°C. Mitochondrial protein was measured by the Biuret method.

Mitochondrial H_2O_2 Generation and Oxygen Consumption

The rate of mitochondrial H_2O_2 production was assayed measuring the increase in fluorescence (excitation at 312 nm, emission at 420 nm) due to oxidation of homovanillic acid by H_2O_2 in the presence of horseradish peroxidase.[32] The assays were performed in incubation buffer (145 mM KCl, 30 mM HEPES, 5 mM KH_2PO_4, 3 mM $MgCl_2$, 0.1 mM EGTA, 0.1% BSA, pH 7.4), and the reaction conditions were 0.25 mg/mL of mitochondrial protein, 6 U/mL of horseradish peroxidase, and 0.1 mM homovanillic acid (total volume 1.5 mL). The reactions were started by the addition of 2.5 mM pyruvate/2.5 mM malate or 5 mM succinate as substrates. Some of the assays with succinate were performed in the presence of 2 μM rotenone to avoid the backward flow of electrons to complex I. In some assays, 2 μM antimycin A and 11 μM thenoyltrifluoroacetone (TTFA) were added to succinate + rotenone-supplemented mitochondria, and 2 μM rotenone was added to pyruvate/malate-supplemented mitochondria to determinate the maximum rates of H_2O_2 production of complexes III, II, and I, respectively. After 15 min of incubation at 37°C, the reaction was stopped transferring the samples to a cold bath and adding 0.5 mL of 0.1 M glycine containing 25 mM EDTA-NaOH (pH 12.0). Known amounts of H_2O_2 produced by glucose oxidase with glucose as substrate were used as standards. In the CR study, fluorescence was determined using a fluorescent microplate reader (GeminiXS; Molecular Devices, Sunnyvale, CA), whereas in the location study the fluorescence of the total reaction volume (2 mL) was measured using a LS50B Perkin Elmer fluorometer (Buckinghamshire, UK).

Mitochondrial oxygen consumption was measured in a Clark-type O_2 electrode (Oxygraph, Hansatech, Norfolk, UK) in the absence (State 4) and in the presence (State 3) of ADP (500 µM) in the same conditions used for H_2O_2 measurements. All the assays were performed within 2 hours after the isolation of mitochondria.

Statistical Analyses

Comparisons were statistically analyzed with Student's t tests. The minimum level of statistical significance was set at $P < .05$ for all the analyses.

RESULTS

Caloric Restriction: Mitochondrial ROS Generation and Oxygen Consumption

Well-coupled mitochondria were isolated from kidney and skeletal muscle as indicated by the respiratory control ratio (RCR). In pyruvate/malate-supplemented skeletal muscle mitochondria, RCR values were 10.94 ± 1.65 and 11.46 ± 1.35 for *ad libitum* and CR group, respectively; in kidney, RCR values were 14.74 ± 1.07 in *ad libitum* and 14.03 ± 1.59 in the restricted group. Caloric restriction did not change oxygen consumption in either state 4 or state 3 in kidney or skeletal muscle mitochondria (data not shown). Mitochondrial ROS generation was measured in skeletal muscle mitochondria respiring with complex I–linked substrates (pyruvate/malate). However, because we did not detect ROS production in kidney mitochondria using pyruvate/malate as substrates, we supplemented those particular mitochondrial suspensions with a complex II–linked substrate (succinate). No changes in H_2O_2 production were found between the two dietary groups either in skeletal muscle or in kidney mitochondria (data not shown).

Location of ROS-Generating Sites within Mitochondria

Detectable amounts of H_2O_2 were released by kidney and skeletal muscle mitochondria in basal conditions when pyruvate/malate or succinate were added as substrates (FIGS. 1 and 2). Measurement of mitochondrial oxygen consumption allowed us to test that the mitochondrial suspensions were well coupled (TABLE 1).

When rotenone was added to pyruvate/malate supplemented mitochondria, ROS generation was significantly increased in both tissues ($P < .001$; FIG. 1A, B). Further

TABLE 1. Location study: oxygen consumption of pyruvate/malate-supplemented mitochondria in kidney and skeletal muscle (gastrocnemius)

	State 4	State 3	RCR
Skeletal muscle	15.63 ± 1.60	131.68 ± 3.86	8.68 ± 0.85
Kidney	18.19 ± 3.34	119.36 ± 22.73	6.53 ± 0.35

[a]Results are means ± SEM from four different animals and were expressed in nmoles O_2/min·mg protein.

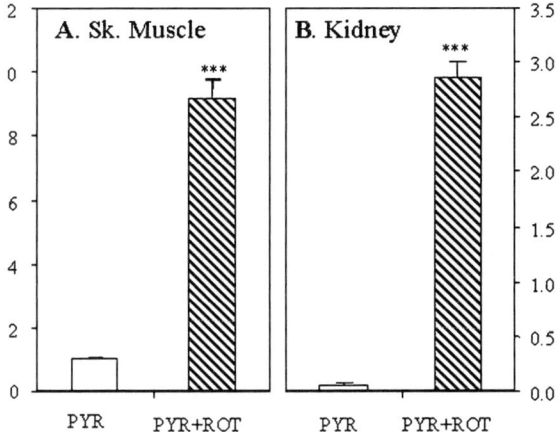

FIGURE 1. Location study. Effect of rotenone (ROT) on the basal rates of H_2O_2 production (nmoles H_2O_2/min · mg prot) with pyruvate/malate (PYR) as substrate in skeletal muscle (**A**) and kidney (**B**) mitochondria. Results are means ± SEM from four different animals. Asterisks represent statistical significance comparing H_2O_2 production with and without rotenone (ROT) in the same tissue and substrate. $*P < .05$; $**P < .01$; $***P < .001$.

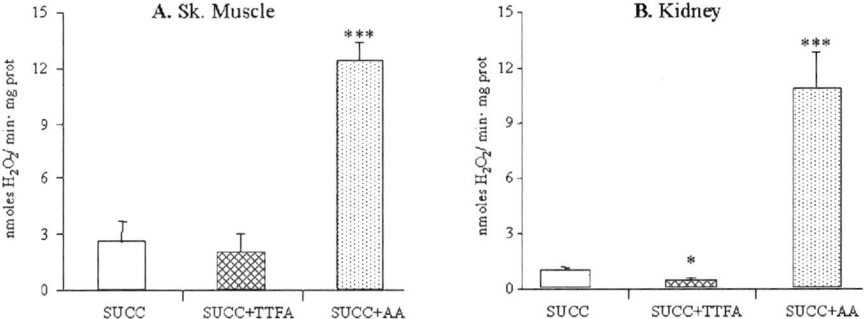

FIGURE 2. Location study. Effect of thenoyltrifluoroacetone (TTFA) and antimycin A (AA) on the basal rates of H_2O_2 production with succinate (SUCC) as substrate in skeletal muscle (**A**) and kidney (**B**) mitochondria. Rotenone was added with succinate in all the assays. Results are means ± SEM from four different animals. Asterisks represent statistical significance comparing H_2O_2 production with and without AA or TTFA in the same tissue and substrate. $*P < .05$; $**P < .01$; $***P < .001$.

indications about the role of complex I in ROS generation were obtained after supplementing mitochondria with succinate. Similar to what has been observed previously,[4] H_2O_2 production was strongly decreased when rotenone was added to succinate-supplemented kidney or skeletal muscle mitochondria (data not shown). ROS generation was not increased after the addition of TTFA to succinate plus srotenone-supplemented mitochondria in either kidney or skeletal muscle (FIG. 2A, B); it was not changed in skeletal muscle, and it was even decreased in kidney after TTFA addition. Finally, Antimycin A strongly increased H_2O_2 generation when added to succinate plus rotenone-supplemented mitochondria (FIG. 2A, B) in both tissues.

DISCUSSION

Long-term caloric restriction has been shown to extend maximum life span, at least in part, by decreasing mitochondrial free radical generation.[6,8,9,24] It is noteworthy that whenever CR was implemented in long-term experiments by different investigators, a decrease in the rate of ROS generation has been always observed (see Barja[5] for review). However, when short-term CR has been studied, different results have been reported in free radical generation rate depending on the tissue. Thus, significant decreases in mitochondrial ROS production has been described to occur in liver,[7] whereas the trends to decrease were observed in heart after 6 weeks[8] and 4 months[12] of CR did not reach statistical significance. In this investigation, short-term caloric restriction (2 months) was not enough to decrease ROS generation either in kidney or skeletal muscle mitochondria.

Because we did not detect any H_2O_2 production in kidney mitochondria in the CR study, when pyruvate/malate was used as substrate, we supplemented mitochondria with succinate. Mitochondrial ROS generation with succinate in the absence of rotenone has been reported to be higher than with pyruvate/malate as substrate.[9,21,25] The lack of detectable amounts of mitochondrial H_2O_2 production in kidney could be caused by a sensitivity problem because the assays of the CR study were performed in a fluorescent microplate reader and only a fraction of the total reaction volume (300 µL out of 2,000) could be used in the measurements. This decreases sensitivity by sevenfold. Indeed, free radical generation in pyruvate/malate-supplemented kidney mitochondria was detected when we investigated the location of ROS-generating sites within mitochondria. In this location study, we read the fluorescence of the whole reaction volume (2 mL) in a fluorometer cuvette. This suggests that the whole volume of reaction should be used to avoid sensitivity losses, especially when rates of free radical generation are low. When using succinate in the absence of rotenone, electrons flow from complex II to complex III but also to complex I through reverse electron flow. In such conditions, possible sensitivity problems were avoided, and we could study the effects of the CR regimen on ROS generation at complexes I and III.

The only previous study investigating dietary restriction and ROS generation in kidney mitochondria used succinate as substrate without rotenone addition in mice.[6] Although in that study decreases in mitochondrial ROS generation were observed in CR animals, the implementation times were longer than those used in the current investigation. It has been reported that the implementation time has a strong effect in dietary restriction studies.[10,11] The lack of effect on H_2O_2 generation observed here after only 8 weeks can be because of such time dependence.

Concerning skeletal muscle, a previous investigation reported a decrease in superoxide production after long-term CR in mice submitochondrial particles.[24] However, a recent study in functional isolated mitochondria showed that caloric restriction only tended (nonsignificantly) to lower H_2O_2 generation in skeletal muscle of the restricted rats.[26] The current study reports no significant changes in mitochondrial ROS generation in skeletal muscle after 2 months of restriction. However, the mitochondrial rate of H_2O_2 generation observed in restricted animals was 11% lower than in *ad libitum* fed rats. The magnitude of such reduction interestingly is very similar to that found in rat heart mitochondria after 6 weeks or 4 months (15% and 13%, respectively) of CR.[12] It is possible that tissues differ in their sensitivity to CR implementation times; decreases on mitochondrial free radical generation after short-term CR would be easily observed in organs such as the liver (more affected by digestive and metabolic changes), whereas in heart and skeletal muscle such decrease would not reach statistical significance. Thus, longer CR time periods would be needed to observed statistical significant decreases in those muscular tissues.

Regarding the sites where mitochondrial ROS generation took place, results were similar to previous studies in other tissues. Various respiratory chain inhibitors were used to localize the free radical generator sites. The rate of free radical production in the respiratory chain increases as a function of the degree of reduction of the autoxidizable electron carriers.[27] When the respiratory chain is blocked with an inhibitor, the degree of reduction of the electron carriers situated on the substrate side strongly increases, whereas those on the oxygen side become oxidized. Thus, an increase in ROS production after the addition of an inhibitor indicates that the free radical generator site is located on the substrate side in relation to the inhibitor. On the other hand, a decrease in ROS production after the addition of an inhibitor means that the free radical generator is situated on the oxygen side.

In this investigation, we report that complexes I and III are the main sites of free radical generation. Complex I generates radicals because the addition of rotenone largely increased ROS generation in pyruvate/malate-supplemented mitochondria and strongly decreased it in succinate plus rotenone-supplemented mitochondria. Moreover, when antimycin A was added to mitochondria oxidizing succinate (plus rotenone) the mitochondrial rate of H_2O_2 generation also was increased, thus indicating complex III ROS generation. TTFA did not increase the rate of free radical generation in succinate plus rotenone-supplemented mitochondria, ruling out complex II as a principal source of ROS in rat kidney and skeletal muscle mitochondria.

One of the characteristics of aging is its universality.[28,29] The mechanisms causing aging are probably similar, especially in closely related species of the same phylogenetic group. Several lines of evidence support the mitochondrial free radical theory of aging. This theory postulates that aging rate is determined, at least in part, by the rate of mitochondrial free radical production.[4,5] Therefore, it makes sense that the main mitochondrial ROS generator sites are the same in different tissues within a species and in different species of the same phylogenetic group. It has been described that the main source of ROS related to aging in heart and brain is located at complex I in a wide group of mammalian species.[8,30] Recent studies indicate that complex I is a main site of free radical generation in liver, heart, and brain mitochondria.[8,9,16,17,19–21] However, previous controversial results had been reported when kidney was studied,[25] questioning the role of complex I on ROS production of kidney mitochondria. In such investigation, the addition of rotenone to NADH-linked supplemented kidney mitochondria did not increase H_2O_2 generation; this led to ruling out complex I as a main source of free radicals. However, when we added rotenone to succinate-supplemented kidney mitochondria a strong decrease in the H_2O_2 generation was observed, supporting the role of complex I in ROS generation in those conditions. This conclusion agrees with other investigations reporting that the rate of H_2O_2 production of succinate-supplemented mitochondria seems to come mainly from complex I (not from complex III) because of reverse electron flow from complex II to complex I.[9,21,31] This explains why succinate-supported H_2O_2 production is largely blocked after addition of rotenone. Our results support the role of complex I in free radical generation in kidney mitochondria, not only when the organelles oxidize complex II–linked substrates, but also when supplementing them with complex I–linked substrates. Because similar results were obtained in skeletal muscle mitochondria, the present investigation supports the idea that complex I is a main ROS generator in many different tissues, suggesting that complex I plays an important role in ROS generation and, possibly, in the determination of the rate of aging.

Together with previous information,[4,5,33] these results are consistent with an important role of complex I ROS generation in the determination of aging rate in at least heart, brain, kidney, and skeletal muscle.

ACKNOWLEDGMENTS

We are grateful to Young Mok Jang and Alberto Sanz for their help during these experiments. This research was supported by two grants from the National Institutes of Health and the National Institute on Aging, USA (AG 17994 and AG 21042) to Christiaan Leeuwenburgh and a grant from the Spanish Ministry of Science and Technology (SAF 2002-01635) to Gustavo Barja. Ricardo Gredilla was supported by a predoctoral fellowship from the Education Council of the Madrid Community (CAM), Spain.

REFERENCES

1. HARMAN, D. 1972. The biologic clock: the mitochondria? J. Am. Geriatr. Soc. **20**: 145–147.
2. MIQUEL, J. 1988. An integrated theory of aging as a result of mitochondrial-DNA mutation in differentiated cells. Arch. Gerontol. Geriatr. **12**: 99–117.
3. SOHAL, R.S. & R. WEINDRUCH. 1996. Oxidative stress, caloric restriction and aging. Science **273**: 59–63.
4. BARJA, G. 1999. Mitochondrial free radical generation: sites of production in states 4 and 3, organ specificity and relationship with aging rate. J. Bioenerg. Biomembr. **31**: 347–366.
5. BARJA, G. 2003. Aging in vertebrates, and the effect of caloric restriction: a mitochondrial free radical production-DNA damage mechanism? Biol. Rev. **78**: 1–17.
6. SOHAL, R.S., H.H. KU, S. AGARWAL, et al. 1994. Oxidative damage, mitochondrial oxidant generation and antioxidant defenses during aging and in response to food restriction in the mouse. Mech. Ageing Dev. **74**: 121–133.

7. GREDILLA, R., G. BARJA & M. LÓPEZ-TORRES. 2001. Effect of short-term caloric restriction on H_2O_2 production and oxidative DNA damage in rat liver mitochondria, and location of the free radical source. J. Bioenerg. Biomembr. **33:** 279–287.
8. GREDILLA, R., A. SANZ, M. LÓPEZ-TORRES & G. BARJA. 2001. Caloric restriction decreases mitochondrial free radical generation at complex I and lowers oxidative damage to mitochondrial DNA in the rat heart. FASEB J. **15:** 1589–1591.
9. LÓPEZ-TORRES, M., R. GREDILLA, A. SANZ & G. BARJA. 2002. Influence of aging and long-term caloric restriction on oxygen radical generation and oxidative DNA damage in rat liver mitochondria. Free Radic. Biol. Med. **32:** 882–889.
10. YU, B.P. 1996. Aging and oxidative stress: modulation by dietary restriction. Free Radic. Biol. Med. **21:** 651–668.
11. WEINDRUCH, R. & R.L. WALFORD. 1988. The retardation of aging and disease by dietary restriction. Thomas. Springfield, IL.
12. GREDILLA, R., M. LÓPEZ-TORRES & G. BARJA. 2002. Effect of time of restriction on the decrease in mitochondrial H2O2 production and oxidative DNA damage in the heart of food-restricted rats. Microsc. Res. Tech. **59:** 273–277.
13. GREDILLA, R. & G. BARJA. 2003. Mitochondrial oxidative stress and caloric restriction. Adv. Cell Aging Gerontol. **14:** 105–122.
14. BOVERIS, A., E. CADENAS & A.O.M. STOPPANI. 1976. Role of ubiquinone in the mitochondrial generation of hydrogen peroxide. Biochem. J. **156:** 435–444.
15. TAKESHIGE, K. & S. MINAKAMI. 1979. NADH- and NADPH-dependent formation of superoxide anions by bovine heart submitochondrial particles and NADH-ubiquinone reductase preparation. Biochem. J. **180:** 129–135.
16. BARJA, G. & A. HERRERO. 1998. Localization at complex I and mechanism of the higher free radical production of brain nonsynaptic mitochondria in the short-lived rat than in the longevous pigeon. J. Bioenerg. Biomembr. **30:** 235–243.
17. HERRERO, A. & G. BARJA. 1997. Sites and mechanisms responsible for the low rate of free radical production of heart mitochondria in the long-lived pigeon. Mech. Ageing Dev. **98:** 95–111.
18. HERRERO, A. & G. BARJA. 1998. H2O2 production of heart mitochondria and aging rate are slower in canaries and parakeets than in mice: sites of free radical generation and mechanisms involved. Mech. Ageing Dev. **103:** 133–146.
19. GENOVA, M.L., B. VENTURA, G. GIULIANO, *et al.* 2001. the site of production of superoxide radical in mitochondrial complex I is not a bound ubisemiquinone but presumably iron-sulfur cluster N2. FEBS Lett. **505:** 364–368.
20. KUSHNAREVA, Y., A.N. MURPHY & A. ANDREYEV. 2002. Complex I-mediated reactive oxygen species generation: modulation by cytochrome c and NAD(P)+ oxidation-reduction state. Biochem. J. **368:** 545–553.
21. LIU, Y., G. FISKUM & D. SCHUBERT. 2002. Generation of reactive oxygen species by the mitochondrial electron transport chain. J. Neurochem. **80:** 780–787.
22. GREENAMYRE, J.T., T.B. SHERER, R. BETARBET & A.V. PANOV. 2001. Complex I and Parkinson's disease. IUBMB Life **52:** s135–s141.
23. BETARBET, R., T.B. SHERER, G. MACKENZIE, *et al.* 2000. Chronic systemic pesticide exposure reproduces features of Parkinson's disease. Nat. Neurosci. **3:** 1301–1306.
24. LASS, A., B.H. SOHAL, R. WEINDRUCH, *et al.* 1998. Caloric restriction prevents age-associated accrual of oxidative damage to mouse skeletal muscle mitochondria. Free Radic. Biol. Med. **25:** 1089–1097.
25. KWONG, L.K. & R.S. SOHAL. 1998. Substrate and site specificity of hydrogen peroxide generation in mouse mitochondria. Arch. Biochem. Biophys. **350:** 118–126.
26. DREW, B., S. PHANEUF, A. DIRKS, *et al.* 2003. Effects of aging and caloric restriction on mitochondrial energy production in gastrocnemius muscle and heart. Am. J. Physiol. Regul. Integr. Comp. Physiol. **284:** R474–R480.
27. BOVERIS, A. & B. CHANCE. 1973. The mitochondrial generation of hydrogen peroxide. General properties and effect of hyperbaric oxygen. Biochem. J. **134:** 707–716.
28. STREHLER, B.L. 1962. Time, cells and aging. Academic Press. New York.
29. BARJA, G. 2000. The flux of free radical attack through mitochondrial DNA is related to aging rate. Aging Clin. Exp. Res. **12:** 342–355.

30. HERRERO, A. & G. BARJA. 2000. Localization of the site of oxygen radical generation inside the complex I of heart and nonsynaptic brain mammalian mitochondria. J. Bioenerg. Biomembr. **32:** 609–615.
31. VOTYAKOVA, T.V. & I.J. REYNOLDS. 2001. DeltaPsi(m)-dependent and -independent production of reactive oxygen species by rat brain mitochondria. J. Neurochem. **79:** 266–277.
32. BARJA, G. 2002. The quantitative measurement of H2O2 generation in isolated mitochondria. J. Bioenerg. Biomembr. **34:** 227–233.
33. BARJA, G. 1998. Mitochondrial free radical production and aging in mammals and birds. Ann. N.Y. Acad. Sci. **854:** 224–238.

Mechanism of Superoxide-Mediated Damage
Relevance to Mitochondrial Aging

I. B. AFANAS'EV

Vitamin Research Institute, Moscow, Russia

ABSTRACT: The damaging effects of superoxide in mitochondria leading to pathological disorders and aging are well documented and usually ascribed to superoxide's role as a precursor of reactive free radical species. However, the latest findings point out the importance of the nucleophilic properties of superoxide and its ability to regulate heterolytic enzymatic processes. Hypothetical mechanisms of superoxide mediation of phosphorylation and dephosphorylation reactions with participation of protein kinases and the apoptotic protein BAD are considered.

KEYWORDS: superoxide; mitochondria; hypertensive rats

Mitochondrial overproduction of superoxide is considered to be one of the major factors of aging and many pathological disorders. The damaging effect of superoxide has been shown in many studies, although its mechanism is not always clear. Notwithstanding its distinguished name, superoxide by itself is not a "superoxidant," and its destructive activity is thought to be caused by conversion into the other, much more active oxygen species: hydroxyl or hydroxyl-like free radicals formed by the famous Fenton reaction or peroxynitrite formed by the interaction with NO. However, the last developments demonstrate both the inhibitory and stimulatory effects of superoxide, which are difficult to explain because of their role as precursors of reactive species. For example, it has been shown[1] that superoxide enhanced the hydrolysis of phosphatidylinositol (PIP) to inositol 1,4,5-tris-phosphate (IP_3) and inhibited cGMP formation in rat aortic smooth muscle cells, especially in spontaneously hypertensive rats:

$$PIP \Rightarrow (O_2^{\cdot-}) \Rightarrow IP_3. \qquad (1)$$

Kang *et al.*[2] also has reported that high glucose induced apoptosis in mesangial cells by an oxidant (superoxide)–dependent mechanism via the inhibition of phosphorylation of serine-threonine kinase Akt, which in turn activated proapoptotic protein BAD. Noshita *et al.*[3] has found that the expression of phosphorylated Akt kinase enhanced after cerebral ischemia in SOD1 transgenic (Tg) mice, that is, a decrease in superoxide production in Tg mice, decreased BAD activation.

Address for correspondence: I. B. Afanas'ev, Vitamin Research Institute, Moscow, Russia. iafan@aha.ru

These findings may be relevant to an important role of superoxide in mitochondrial aging. However, the effects of superoxide on the phosphorylation of Akt are not always inhibitory. Recently, Dong-Yun et al.[4] demonstrated that the low concentrations of superoxide stimulated Akt activity in human hepatoma cells apparently by increasing the phosphatidylinositol 3-kinase (PI3K)–catalyzed phosphorylation of Akt because PI3K inhibitor wortmannin inhibited superoxide-dependent Akt phosphorylation.

These contradictory signaling effects of superoxide are difficult to understand on the basis of traditional free radical mechanisms. It is well known that a major characteristic of free hydroxyl radicals is indiscriminate interaction with neighboring molecules. The same is true for peroxynitrite, which slowly decomposes to hydroxyl radicals during reactions with organic molecules. However, the above examples point out highly specific and probably reversible reactions of superoxide. We believe that it might be explained by one now well-forgotten property of superoxide.

Not being a "superoxidant," superoxide, nonetheless, has another "super" quality, being a supernucleophil, whose reactivity excels the reactivity of the hydroxyl ion in the heterolytic processes.[5] Thus, superoxide easily hydrolyzes esters by mechanisms:

$$O_2^{\bullet-} + RCOOR' \Rightarrow RC(O)OO^{\bullet} + R'O^- \qquad (2)$$

$$RC(O)OO^{\bullet} + O_2^{\bullet-} \Rightarrow RC(O)OO^- + O_2. \qquad (3)$$

Another important heterolytic reaction of superoxide is the interaction with proton donors:

$$O_2^{\bullet-} + ROH \Rightarrow RO^- + HOO^{\bullet} \qquad (4)$$

$$HOO^{\bullet} + O_2^{\bullet-} \Rightarrow HOO^- + O_2. \qquad (5)$$

We suppose that both heterolytic reactions, hydrolysis of esters, and deprotonation can be the highly selective steps of superoxide signaling. For example, it has been suggested that superoxide stimulated apoptosis by the inhibition of phosphorylation of proapoptotic protein BAD by protein kinase B.

Antiapoptotic process:

$$PI3K \xrightarrow{phosphorylation} phosphoAkt \xrightarrow{phosphorylation} phosphoBAD.$$

Apoptotic process: The suppression of BAD phosphorylation by superoxide.

(PI3K is phosphatidylinositol 3-kinase; PKB or Akt is protein kinase B; BAD is proapoptotic protein.) Because phosphate esters must be hydrolyzed by superoxide even more easily than organic esters, the following mechanisms of BAD dephosphorylation might be suggested:

$$BAD[OP(O)(OR)_2] + O_2^{\bullet-} \Rightarrow BAD[O^-] + {}^{\bullet}OOP(O)(OR)_2 \qquad (6)$$

$$^\bullet\text{OOP(O)(OR)}_2 + \text{O}_2^{\bullet-} \Rightarrow {}^-\text{OOP(O)(OR)}_2 + \text{O}_2. \tag{7}$$

On the other hand, a deprotonation reaction may be the origin of accelerating phosphorylation in the presence of low superoxide concentration:[4]

$$\text{Akt[OH]} + \text{O}_2^{\bullet-} \Rightarrow \text{Akt[O}^-] + \text{HOO}^\bullet \tag{8}$$

$$\text{Akt[O}^-] + \text{P(O)(OR)}_3 \Rightarrow \text{Akt[OP(O)(OR)}_2] + \text{RO}^-. \tag{9}$$

CONCLUSIONS

Two types of reactions, namely, free radical and heterolytic reactions of superoxide can be responsible for superoxide signaling in cells. Free radical mechanisms of signaling occur through the formation of highly reactive oxygen and nitrogen species (hydroxyl radicals, hydroxyl-like radicals, and peroxynitrite) and lead to irreversible damage in cells. Heterolytic mechanisms depend on hydrolysis and deprotonation reactions due to the "super"-nucleophilic activity of superoxide and may stimulate both proapoptotic and antiapoptotic effects.

REFERENCES

1. WU, L. & J. DE CHAMPLAIN. 1999. Hypertension **34:** 1247–1253.
2. KANG, P.S., S. FRENCHER, V. REFFY, et al. 2003. Am. J. Physiol. Renal Physiol. **284:** F455–F466.
3. NOSHITA, N., T. SUGAWARA, A. LEWEN, et al. 2003. Stroke **34:** 1513–1518.
4. DONG-YUN, S., D. YU-RU, L. SHAN-LIN, et al. 2003. FEBS Lett. **542:** 60–64.
5. AFANAS'EV, I.B. 1989. Superoxide Ion: Chemistry and Biological Implications. Vol. 1. CRC Press. Boca Raton, FL.

Glutathione Metabolism during Aging and in Alzheimer Disease

HONGLEI LIU,[a] HONG WANG,[a] SWAPNA SHENVI,[b] TORY M. HAGEN,[b] AND RUI-MING LIU[c]

[a]*Department of Immunology School of Medicine, University of Alabama at Birmingham, Birmingham, Alabama 35294-0022, USA*

[b]*Linus Pauling Institute, Oregon State University, Corvallis, Oregon, USA*

[c]*Department of Environmental Health Sciences School of Public Health, University of Alabama at Birmingham, Birmingham, Alabama 35294-0022, USA*

> ABSTRACT: The concentration of glutathione (GSH), the most abundant intracellular nonprotein thiol and important antioxidant, declines with age and in some age-related diseases. The underlying mechanism, however, is not clear. The previous studies from our laboratory showed that the age-dependent decline in GSH content in Fisher 344 rats was associated with a downregulation of glutamate cysteine ligase (GCL), the rate-limiting enzyme in *de novo* GSH synthesis. Our recent studies further indicated that the activity and mRNA content of glutathione synthase (GS), which catalyzes the second reaction in *de novo* GSH synthesis, were also decreased with age in some tissues. No age-associated change was observed in glutathione reductase or γ-glutamyl transpeptidase activities. Also, although GSH content declined with age in both male and female mice, male mice experienced more dramatic age-associated decline in many tissues/organs than female mice. Furthermore, we found that GSH content was significantly decreased in the red blood cells from male Alzheimer disease patients, which was associated with decreases in GCL and GS activities. Finally, we showed that estrogen increased GSH content, GS and GR activities, and GCL gene expression in the liver of both male and female mice. Taken together, our results suggest that (1) GCL plays a critical role in maintaining GSH homeostasis under both physiological and pathological conditions; (2) decreased GSH content may be involved in AD pathology in humans; and (3) estrogen increases GSH content in mice by multiple mechanisms.
>
> KEYWORDS: glutathione; aging; gender; glutamate cysteine ligase; γ-glutamylcysteine synthetase; Alzheimer disease; estrogen

The mechanism underlying aging, an inevitable biological process that affects most living organisms, is still an area of significant controversy and so is the mechanism for neurodegenerative diseases. Reactive oxygen species (ROS), generated endogenously or exogenously, cause damages to DNA, RNA, lipids, and proteins. Accumu-

---

Address for correspondence: Rui-Ming Liu, Ph.D., Department of Environmental Health Sciences, UAB School of Public Health, 1665 University Boulevard, Birmingham, AL 35294-0022. Voice: 205-934-7028; fax: 205-975-6341.
   rliu@uab.edu

lated evidence indicates that oxidative damage of these macromolecules increases with age, which may contribute importantly to the aging process and the pathogeneses of age-associated diseases.[1–5] Although intensive studies have been done, the mechanism underlying such increased oxidative damage of the macromolecules in aged animals and in age-related neurodegenerative diseases has not been completely elucidated.

Glutathione (GSH), the most abundant intracellular nonprotein thiol, participates in many important biological processes. The most important function of this tripeptide, perhaps, is to detoxify oxidants and electrophiles. Although many studies, including those from this laboratory, have shown that GSH content decreases with age in many tissues from different animal species, the underlying mechanism is not clear. It is also not clear whether there is any difference between genders in terms of GSH metabolism during the aging process.

In the past few years, we have systematically explored the mechanism underlying the age-associated decline in GSH content in rats and mice. Our results showed that GSH content was decreased in many tissues of old rats and mice, including liver, kidney, lung, red blood cells, cerebral cortex, and cerebellum in rats as well as liver, spleen lymphocytes, lung (male), cortex, and brainstem in mice.[6–9] The activities of γ-glutamyl transpeptidase (GGT), the enzyme initiating the degradation of extracellular GSH to prove cells with substrates for the *de novo* GSH synthesis, and glutathione reductase (GR), the enzyme catalyzing the redox cycling of oxidized glutathione, were not significantly different between aged and young rats in any tissues/organs examined. There was no significant age-associated decline in cysteine, another rate-limiting factor in *de novo* GSH synthesis, or age-associated increase in GSSG content in any of the rat or mouse organs/tissues examined. These data suggest that the age-associated decline in GSH content in rats and mice is not caused by increased oxidative stress or decreased availability of cysteine. On the other hand, it was found that the activity of glutamate cysteine ligase (GCL), the enzyme catalyzing the first and the rate-limiting step in *de novo* GSH synthesis, was decreased with age in all the tissues in rats, in which an age-associated decline in GSH content has been observed. GSH synthase activity also was decreased with age in the lung and kidney of rats. Such a decrease in GCL and GS activities was associated with a downregulation of GCL and GS gene expression. These data suggest that the age-associated decline in GSH content in mouse and rat is mainly caused by the downregulation of the gene expression of two enzymes involved in *de novo* GSH synthesis.

Further, although there was no significant difference in the GSH content between young male and female mice in most tissues examined, and GSH content decreased with age in both male and female mice, male mice seemed to be more vulnerable to such age-associated decline than female mice in most tissues/organs except the liver. The age-dependent decline in GSH content in both male and female mice was also associated with a downregulation of GCL gene expression. These results may reveal an important basis underlying the gender-associated differences in the longevity and the susceptibility to certain age-related diseases.

Plasma concentration of estrogen, a sex hormone, decreases with age in both women and men. Such age-associated decline in estrogen level has been suggested to play a role in several age-related diseases such as osteoporosis, cardiovascular diseases, and Alzheimer disease. Importantly, estrogen replacement therapy has been shown to be able to prevent cardiovascular disease and retard the development and severity of AD in postmenopausal women.[10–12] Although several hypotheses have been proposed to explain protective effects of estrogen against the age-related diseases, the exact underlying mechanism remains unclear. In this study, we showed that GSH concentration was decreased in the uterus of ovariectomized mice as compared with sham mice. However, no change was observed in the GSH content in the liver, heart, brainstem, cortex, or hippocampus after ovariectomy. Furthermore, we showed that estrogen treatment increased GSH content in the liver and uterus of female mice as well as in the liver of male mice. However, it had no effect on the GSH content in any of other tissues/organs examined including heart and brain. The increase in GSH content in the liver was associated with increased activities of GR and GS, indicating that increased synthesis and redox cycling may contribute to the estrogen-induced increase in GSH content.

An alteration in GSH metabolism has been shown in Parkinson disease, an age-related neurodegenerative disease. Whether GSH metabolism is altered in Alzheimer disease (AD), another age-related neurodegenerative disease, is not clear. We compared GSH content in the blood from AD patients and age-matched controls. The results showed that GSH content was not significantly different in the plasma, white blood cells, or red blood cells between female patients and female controls. There was also no difference in GSH content in the plasma and white blood cells between male patients and male controls. However, GSH concentration was significantly decreased in the red blood cells from male patients as compared with that from age-matched male controls. Further studies showed that both GCL and GS activities were significantly lower in the red blood cells from male AD patients as compared with those from male controls. These data suggest that GSH depletion may contribute to the pathogenesis of AD in males.

In summary, GSH concentration declines with age in both rat and mouse tissues, and a more dramatic age-associated decline was observed in most tissues of male mice as compared with female mice. Decreased synthetic capacity due to the down-regulation of GCL and GS, the two enzymes involved in *de novo* GSH synthesis, may underlie the age-associated decline in GSH content in Fisher 344 rats and C57BL mice. Estrogen increases GSH in mouse liver and uterus; however, ovariectomy causes a decrease in GSH content only in the uterus. Therefore, the age-associated decline in GSH content in female mice may not result from estrogen deficiency. Furthermore, we found that GSH content was decreased in the red blood cells from male but not female AD patients as compared with age- and gender-matched controls. The biological significance of such decrease in GSH content in red blood cells of male AD patients needs to be explored further.

REFERENCES

1. TIAN, L., Q. CAI & H. WEI. 1998. Alterations of antioxidant enzymes and oxidative damage to macromolecules in different organs of rats during aging. Free Radic. Biol. Med. **24:** 1477–1484.
2. MIRO, O., J. CASADEMONT, E. CASALS, *et al.* 2000. Aging is associated with increased lipid peroxidation in human hearts, but not with mitochondrial respiratory chain enzyme defects. Cardiovasc. Res. **47:** 624–631.

3. HAMILTON, M.L., H. VAN REMMEN, J.A. DRAKE, et al. 2001. Does oxidative damage to DNA increase with age? Proc. Natl. Acad. Sci. USA **98:** 10469–10474.
4. PERRY, G., A. NUNOMURA, K. HIRAI, et al. 2002. Is oxidative damage the fundamental pathogenic mechanism of Alzheimer's and other neurodegenerative diseases? Free Radic. Biol. Med. **33:** 1475–1479.
5. ZEEVALK, G.D., L.P. BERNARD & W.J. NICKLAS. 1998. Role of oxidative stress and the glutathione system in loss of dopamine neurons due to impairment of energy metabolism. J. Neurochem. **70:** 1421–1430.
6. LIU, R.-M. & J. CHOI. 2000. Age-associated decline of gamma-glutamylcysteine synthetase gene expression in rats. Free Radic. Biol. Med. **28:** 566–574.
7. LIU, R.M. 2002. Down-regulation of gamma-glutamylcysteine synthetase regulatory subunit gene expression in rat brain tissue during aging. J. Neurosci. Res. **68:** 344–351.
8. LIU, R.M. & D.A. DICKINSON. 2003. Decreased synthetic capacity underlies the age-associated decline in glutathione content in Fisher 344 rats. Antioxid. Redox Signal **5:** 529–536.
9. WANG, H., H. LIU & R.M. LIU. 2003. Gender difference in glutathione metabolism during aging in mice. Exp. Gerontol. **38:** 507–517.
10. VAN DEN BELD, A.W., F.H. DE JONG, D.E. GROBBEE, et al. 2000. Measures of bioavailable serum testosterone and estradiol and their relationships with muscle strength, bone density, and body composition in elderly men. J. Clin. Endocrinol. Metab. **85:** 3276–3282.
11. CARLSON, L.E. & B.B. SHERWIN. 2000. Higher levels of plasma estradiol and testosterone in healthy elderly men compared with age-matched women may protect aspects of explicit memory. Menopause **7:** 168–177.
12. DENTI, L., G. PASOLINI, L. SANFELICI, et al. 2000. Aging-related decline of gonadal function in healthy men: correlation with body composition and lipoproteins. J. Am. Geriatr. Soc. **48:** 51–58.

Alpha–Lipoic Acid Increases $Na^+K^+ATPase$ Activity and Reduces Lipofuscin Accumulation in Discrete Brain Regions of Aged Rats

P. ARIVAZHAGAN[a,b] AND C. PANNEERSELVAM[a]

[a]*Department of Biochemistry, Dr. ALM Post Graduate Institute of Basic Medical Sciences, University of Madras, Chennai, 600 113, India*

[b]*Department of Biochemistry, Kihara Institute for Biological Research, Yokohama City University, Maioka-cho 641-12, Totsuka-ku, Yokohama 244-0813, Japan*

ABSTRACT: A convincing link between oxidative stress and neurodegenerative diseases has been found with the knowledge that it actually damages neuronal cells in culture. We analyzed the effect of DL-α-lipoic acid on lipofuscin and Na^+K^+ ATPase in discrete brain regions of young and aged rats. In aged rats, the level of lipofuscin was increased, and the activity of $Na^+K^+ATPase$ was decreased. Intraperitoneal administration of lipoic acid to aged rats led to a duration-dependent reduction and elevation in lipofuscin and enzyme activity, respectively, in the cortex, cerebellum, striatum, hippocampus, and hypothalamus of the brain. These results suggest that lipoic acid, a natural metabolic antioxidant, should be useful as a therapeutic tool in preventing neuronal dysfunction in aged individuals.

KEYWORDS: aging; brain regions; lipoic acid

INTRODUCTION

Several lines of experimental evidence support the idea that many aspects of aging, including degeneration of the central nervous system may be, at least in part, related to cellular damage inflicted by oxygen free radicals and their intermediates. Generation of free radicals itself may increase during the normal process of aging due to a decrease in the ability to erase oxidative stress by antioxidant enzymes. Resulting net increase in free radicals in the intracellular environments may accelerate cell damage and lead to the pathophysiological changes associated with aging.[1] One cytological index of the oxidative cellular damage is accumulation of lipofuscin pigment in the nerve cells. Peroxidation of membrane lipids may lead to an increase in mitochondrial ionic permeability, which causes a decline ATP synthesis.[2] Age-related decrease in $Na^+K^+ATPase$ activity is, in turn, shown to be highly correlated with increase in the content of lipofuscin in several brain regions.[3]

Address for correspondence: C. Panneerselvam, Department of Biochemistry, Dr. ALM Post Graduate Institute of Basic Medical Sciences, University of Madras, Chennai, 600 113, India. Fax: +91-44-24926709.
panneerselvam@eth.net

Many efforts have been made to identify an agent that may have a possible therapeutic effect in combating diseases caused by oxidative stress. One such agent, lipoic acid, recently has received considerable attention as an antioxidant[4] because it seems to have powerful antioxidant effects on neural tissues.[5] Therefore, we have been testing its potential use as an antioxidative drug with various promising results, including our own. Here, we report several novel findings as regards the effect of α-lipoic acid on the level of lipofuscin and the activity of Na^+K^+ATPase in discrete brain regions of aged rats.

MATERIALS AND METHODS

Experiments were performed on male albino rats of Wistar strain weighing approximately 130–160 g (young) and 380–410 g (aged). The animals were divided into two groups. Group I consisted of normal young rats (3–4 months old) and Group II normal aged rats (>22 months old). Each group was further subdivided into three groups: one control group (Groups Ia and IIa) and two experimental groups administered with lipoic acid for 7 days (Groups Ib and IIb) and 14 days (Groups Ic and IIc). Lipoic acid (100 mg/kg body weight/day) was dissolved in alkaline saline and injected intraperitoneally to the animals. Control young and aged rats received vehicle alone in the similar manner. Upon completion of lipoic acid administration, animals were killed by cervical decapitation. The brain was immediately excised and immersed in ice-cold physiological saline, and specific brain regions were separated. Lipofuscin and Na^+K^+ATPase activity were measured according to the methods described elsewhere.[6,7]

STATISTICAL ANALYSIS

Values are represented as mean ± SD for results obtained with six rats in each group, and the significance of differences between values was determined by one-way analysis of variance coupled with the Student-Newman-Kuel multiple comparison test. P values of less than .05 were considered to be significant. Statistical significance of the differences between the young control (Group Ia) and aged control (Group IIa) were determined by Student's t test. The levels of significance were evaluated with P values.

RESULTS

We examined the effect of lipoic acid on the content of lipofuscin and the activity of Na^+K^+ATPase in the cortex, cerebellum, striatum, hippocampus, and hypothalamus of young and aged rats (TABLE 1). Lipofuscin were increased 50–65% ($P < .001$) in the regions of aged rat brains (Group IIa) compared with the young counterparts (Group Ia). Intraperitoneal administration of lipoic acid to the aged rats duration-dependently decreased their levels to almost control levels of the young rat brains. The same treatment also reduced the lipofuscin levels in the young rats

TABLE 1. Effect of DL-α-lipoic acid on lipofuscin and Na$^+$K$^+$ATPase activity in various brain regions of young and aged rats

Parameters	Young Rats				Aged Rats		
	Group Ia (Control)	Group Ib (7 days)	Group Ic (14 days)	Group IIa (Control)	Group IIb (7 days)	Group IIc (14 days)
Lipofuscin (fluorescent units/g tissue)							
Cortex	3.54 ± 0.31	3.32 ± 0.29	3.08 ± 0.28^a	5.71^b ± 0.48***	4.52 ± 0.42^c	3.63 ± 0.32^{c,d}
Cerebellum	2.43 ± 0.28	2.25 ± 0.25	1.95 ± 0.22^a	3.61^b ± 0.33***	3.10 ± 0.29^c	2.67 ± 0.26^{c,d}
Striatum	2.93 ± 0.31	2.67 ± 0.28	2.42 ± 0.27^a	4.57^b ± 0.39***	3.82 ± 0.30^c	3.07 ± 0.27^{c,d}
Hippocampus	3.02 ± 0.29	2.82 ± 0.28	2.60 ± 0.26^a	4.68^b ± 0.42***	3.92 ± 0.36^c	3.23 ± 0.25^{c,d}
Hypothalamus	2.16 ± 0.21	1.93 ± 0.19	1.82 ± 0.20^a	3.52^b ± 0.33***	2.93 ± 0.27^c	2.30 ± 0.20^{c,d}
Na$^+$K$^+$ATPase (mmoles of Pi liberated/min/mg protein)							
Cortex	0.247 ± 0.018	0.263 ± 0.022	0.280 ± 0.020^a	0.197^b ± 0.015***	0.220 ± 0.018^c	0.241 ± 0.021^c
Cerebellum	0.423 ± 0.032	0.441 ± 0.033	0.462 ± 0.031	0.350^b ± 0.030**	0.373 ± 0.027	0.414 ± 0.031^{c,d}
Striatum	0.398 ± 0.031	0.429 ± 0.033	0.447 ± 0.035^a	0.348^b ± 0.020**	0.371 ± 0.029	0.390 ± 0.033^c
Hippocampus	0.239 ± 0.020	0.247 ± 0.021	0.263 ± 0.025	0.196^b ± 0.016**	0.212 ± 0.018	0.223 ± 0.023^c
Hypothalamus	0.268 ± 0.021	0.270 ± 0.025	0.289 ± 0.023	0.221^b ± 0.019**	0.245 ± 0.017^c	0.263 ± 0.023^c

NOTE: Values are expressed as mean ± SD for six rats in each group. When comparing Group Ia with Group IIa, *$P<.05$, **$P<.01$, ***$P<.001$.
^{a}Group Ia compared with Ib and Ic; ^{b}Group Ia compared with IIa; ^{c}Group IIa compared with IIb and IIc; ^{d}Group IIb compared with IIc.

duration-dependently (Groups Ib–c). However, its effects were marginal because the changes were very small in the young rats.

The activity of Na^+K^+ATPase was found to be decreased by approximately 20% ($P < .001$) in the brain regions of the aged rats examined (Group IIa) compared with the young counterparts (Group Ia). Administration of lipoic acid to the aged rats duration-dependently returned their levels to control levels in the young rats. In the young rats (Groups IIb–c), it increased the enzyme activity duration-dependently. These results demonstrate that exogenously supplied lipoic acid prevents the proceedings of two aging parameters examined.

DISCUSSION

Lipofuscin is a structurally complex compound, consisting mainly of lipids and proteins, and sugars. It disrupts lysosomal membrane, which, in turn, releases hydrolytic enzymes into the cytoplasm and impairs the functions of mitochondria, thereby releasing free radicals. This age-dependent pigmentation also may be responsible for loss of neurons. In the current study, lipoic acid was shown to prevent accumulation of lipofuscin in various regions of the brain in aged rats. Because lipid peroxide greatly contributes to the formation of lipofuscin, the reduced level of lipofuscin found in aged rats given lipoic acid can be explained by reduction of lipid peroxides by α-lipoic acid. Earlier studies have demonstrated that lipoic acid reduces the level of lipid peroxidation and increases those of antioxidants and neurotransmitters in discrete regions of brain in aged rats.[8,9]

In the current study, the activity of Na^+K^+ATPase was found to be decreased in various regions of the brain in aged rats. This is in line with earlier studies showing decreases in the enzyme activity during aging.[3] This phenomenon may be explained by the progressive increase in the lipofuscin contents in the brain because it damages the mitochondrial lipid bilayer containing Na^+K^+ATPase. This enzyme is known to be highly susceptible to changes in the composition of membrane lipids. Thus, lipoic acid is thought to have restored the environments surrounding the enzyme by lowering peroxidation of membrane lipids. Further, α-lipoic acid might have prevented other age-dependent mitochondrial dysfunction and subsequently increased the availability of ATP.[10]

Normal functions of mitochondria appear to be essential for neuronal cells. It is believed that reduced levels of ATP caused by mitochondrial dysfunction cannot drive the ion pumps to maintain depolarization of neurons. Upon depolarization of the neuronal membrane, magnesium that normally blocks NMDA receptor channel is extruded, and an ambient extracellular level of glutamate may become lethal to neurons via NMDA receptor mechanism.[2] Along these lines of evidence, it seems likely that lipoic acid could enhance mitochondrial functions by scavenging free radicals or increase the reduced forms of antioxidants such as glutathione and ascorbate that might play roles as potent neuroprotective agents.

In conclusion, our observations suggest that lipoic acid treatment significantly attenuates the age-related parameters, the accumulation of lipofuscin, and the decrease in Na^+K^+ATPase activity. The mechanism by which lipoic acid affects these parameters may involve maintaining membrane integrity or preventing the accumulation of oxidative compounds generated as metabolic by-products in the discrete brain regions. More detailed consideration of the mechanism merits further investigation. Lipoic acid treatment appears beneficial in preventing aging of the brain, an important target of antiaging. This raises a promising and potential use of lipoic acid as an antiaging drug.

REFERENCES

1. OKATANI, Y. *et al.* 2002. Melatonin reduces oxidative damage of neural lipids and proteins in senescence-accelerated mouse. Neurobiol. Aging **23:** 639–644.
2. LIU, J. *et al.* 2002. Memory loss in old rats is associated with brain mitochondrial decay and RNA/DNA oxidation: partial reversal by feeding acetyl-L-carnitine and/or R-α-lipoic acid. Proc. Natl. Acad. Sci. USA **99:** 2356–2361.
3. KAUR, J. *et al.* 2001. Aceyl-L-carnitine enhances Na^+,K^+-ATPase, glutathione-S-transferase and multiple unit activity and reduces lipid peroxidation and lipofuscin concentration in aged rat brain regions. Neurosci. Lett. **301:** 1–4.
4. PACKER, L. *et al.* 1997. Neuroprotection by the metabolic antioxidant α-lipoic acid. Free Rad. Biol. Med. **22:** 359–378.
5. LYNCH, M.A. 2001. Lipoic acid confers protection against oxidative injury in non-neuronal and neuronal tissue. Nutr. Neurosci. **4:** 419–438.
6. FLETCHER, B.L. *et al.* 1973. Measurement of fluorescent lipid peroxidation products in biological systems and tissues. Anal. Biochem. **52:** 1–9.
7. BONTING, S.L. 1970. Sodium-potassium activated adenosine triphosphatase and cation transport. *In* Membrane Iron Transport. E.E. Bitter, Ed.: 257–263. Interscience. Chichester, UK.
8. ARIVAZHAGAN, P. *et al.* 2002. Effect of DL-α-lipoic acid on the status of lipid peroxidation and antioxidant enzymes in various brain regions of aged rats. Exp. Gerontol. **37:** 803–811.
9. ARIVAZHAGAN, P. & C. PANNEERSELVAM. 2002. Neurochemical changes related to ageing in the rat brain and the effect of DL-α-lipoic acid. Exp. Gerontol. **37:** 1489–1494.
10. ZIMMER, G. *et al.* 1991. Dihydrolipoic acid activates oligomycin-sensitive thiol groups and increases ATP synthesis in mitochondria. Arch. Biochem. Biophys. **288:** 609–613.

The Bud Scar–Based Screening System for Hunting Human Genes Extending Life Span

CUIYING CHEN AND ROLAND CONTRERAS

Fundamental and Applied Molecular Biology, Ghent University and Flanders Interuniversity Institute for Biotechnology, B-9052 Zwijnaarde, Belgium

ABSTRACT: We developed a high-throughput screening system that allows identification of genes prolonging life span in the budding yeast *Saccharomyces cerevisiae*. The method is based on isolating yeast mother cells with an extended number of cell divisions as indicated by the increased number of bud scars on their surface. Fluorescently labeled wheat germ agglutinin (WGA) was used for specific staining of bud scars. Screening of a human HepG2 cDNA expression library in yeast resulted in the isolation of several yeast transformants with a potentially prolonged life span. The budding yeast *S. cerevisiae*, one of the favorite models used to study aging, has been studied extensively for the better understanding of the mechanisms of human aging. Because human disease genes often have yeast counterparts, they can be studied efficiently in this organism. One interesting example is the *WRN* gene, the human DNA helicase, which participates in the DNA repair pathway. The mutation of the *WRN* gene causes Werner syndrome showing premature-aging phenotype. Budding yeast contains WRN homologue, SGS1, and its mutation results in shortening yeast life span. The knowledge gained from the studies of budding yeast will benefit studies in humans for better understanding of aging and aging-related disease.

KEYWORDS: aging; budding yeast; WGA; bud scar; life span

We have developed a unique screening system that allows identification of genes that modulate the life span of *Saccharomyces cerevisiae* cells. The bud scar sorting (BSS) screening system involves biotin labeling the cell wall of a Mother-cell (M-cell) population, which allows for successive rounds of purification and regrowth of the M-cells. After the desired generations of growth, the M-cells are collected and cells with extended life spans are sorted and separated by flow cytometry based on increased numbers of bud scars.

THE BUD SCAR SORTING SCREENING SYSTEM

To study yeast aging, the first step is to isolate the mother cell from its progenies or daughters. It has been observed that daughter cells (D-cells) do not have detect-

Address for correspondence: Cuiying Chen, Fundamental and Applied Molecular Biology, Ghent University and Flanders Interuniversity Institute for Biotechnology, Technologiepark 927, B-9052 Zwijnaarde, Belgium. Voice: +32-9331-3625; fax: +32-9331-3502.
chitty.chen@dmbr.UGent.be

able wall remnants of M-cells, so that a labeled M-cell wall is not transferred to later generations. Therefore, covalent binding of biotin to the primary amines on the cell wall hallmarked the M-cells throughout the entire period of growth and facilitated separation from the D-cell population. Smeal et al.[1] demonstrated successful isolation of M-cells based on the biotinylation of initial mothers but noticed a poor viability and low recovery. To overcome this problem, we modified the method in a critical step by using microbeads (50 nm diameter). Because of their small size, microbeads did not affect cell physiology and therefore bead detachment was not necessary. To start each experiment, we used approximately 3×10^7 biotinylated yeast cells at early log phase as M-cells. During subsequent growth, the percentage of initial labeled M-cells in the population declines exponentially in every generation. For example in their 20 generations, total cell number will increase 2^{20} fold. To allow M-cells to reach a high number of cell cycles under optimal, nonstationary phase conditions huge culture volumes would be required, which is practically impossible. Therefore, after an intermediary growth cycle number (usually 7), the M-cells are collected by a magnet based on biotin binding microbeads and regrowth in a fresh medium.

The yeast replicative life span is defined as the number of cell divisions or daughter cells that mother cells produce in their life. During yeast growth, each cell division leaves a circular bud scar on the surface of the M-cell, specifically at the site of division. Thus, the age (counted in generations) of an M-cell can simply be determined by counting the number of bud scars on its surface. Yeast cells often are stained with high concentration of Calcofluor white M2R for visualization of bud scars. However, this reagent is not bud scar specific because it is known to bind to other cell wall components, such as other polysaccharides. To find a suitable bud scar–specific dye, we tested whether wheat germ agglutinin (WGA) (binding with high specificity to chitin polymers) can be used as a marker for specific labeling of bud scars because the bud scar rings are rich in chitin. To do so, we collected yeast cells at different generations and stained them with WGA conjugated with fluorescent dye. We found that the fluorescent dye (FITC) clearly confined to the bud scar rings and was hardly detectable on other cell wall parts. The intensity of the fluorescence signal detected by flow cytometry indeed correlated with the number of bud scars on each individual cell, allowing the sorter to separate and collect cells with a desired number of bud scars. Biotin-specific staining with streptavidin conjugated with R-phycoerythrin (PE) was applied simultaneously to distinguish M-cells from contaminating D-cells. M-cells were double-stained and recognized according to multicolor fluorescence (FITC green and PE orange) by the flow cytometer, whereas D-cells were only stained with WGA-FITC.

APPLICATION OF BUD SCAR SORTING FOR SCREENING OF A HUMAN cDNA LIBRARY

It has been reported that (over)expression of certain human genes in yeast might have an influence on the growth characteristics of the population. This (over)expression of a single mammalian gene modulating the longevity in a single-cell system could provide valuable information for understanding basic cellular processed in human aging. Our BSS screening system could allow us to screen human genes that

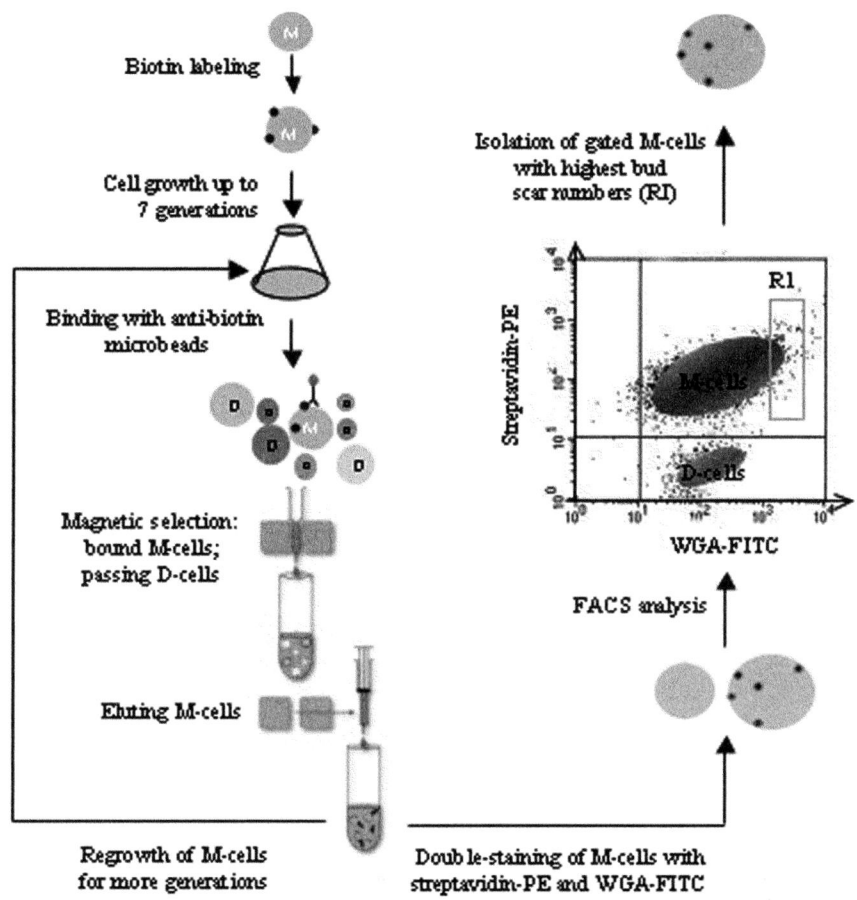

FIGURE 1. Scheme of the bud scar sorting (BSS) system for old yeast M-cells. The BSS system contains two major steps. The first step is at the left side of the figure: magnetic sorting of biotinylated M-cells and regrowth of sorted M-cells to higher generation numbers when needed. The second step is at the right side of the figure: WGA staining of bud scars and sorting of longer living M-cells according to bud scar staining using the FACS. This figure is adapted from Chen et al.[12]

might be involved in aging processes. We therefore constructed a cDNA library from stressed hepatoma (HepG2) cells and applied BSS screening on the library. The expression of the human gene is driven by either yeast GAL10 promoter or cytochrome c promoter. Screening of a human HepG2 cDNA expression library in yeast resulted in the isolation of several yeast transformants with a potentially prolonged life span. Among selected genes, some of them have been documented to play a role in aging and/or antioxidant. For example, two human clones HSP70 (NM_006597; BC018740) and antioxidants protein 2 (BC025421) have been documented as important modification factors in cellular responses to a variety of physiologically relevant conditions such as hyperthermia, oxidative stress, metabolic change, and aging.[2–5] HSP70 extended longevity phenotype has been documented in *Drosophila melanogaster*,[6] *Caenorhabditis elegans*,[7] and rat.[8] It has been reported that the human apoA-I (NM_000039) plays a role as antioxidant in mice and HepG2 cells.[9,10] The function of ferritin light chain (BC004245) as an antioxidant has been documented in various mammalians (see review by Gosslau & Rensing[11]).

CONCLUSION

A frequently used strategy to search for genes responsible for aging is to select survivors after exposure of cells to stress. The question remains whether such genes are picked up in response to a stress treatment or because of their direct effect on aging. The screening method described here provides an alternative that allows direct hunting of human genes that confers longevity. Our BSS screening system also can be used for screening genes with potential antiaging functions from various libraries or library combinations of eukaryotes in more natural growth conditions. The process is high-throughput, efficient, sensitive, rapid, user friendly, and reliable. The isolated genes should permit the rational design of drugs and the development of therapies in the field of age-related diseases.

ACKNOWLEDGMENTS

The authors acknowledge support from the Concerted Research Action of the Ghent University, the Fund for Scientific Research-Flanders, and the European Commission.

REFERENCES

1. SMEAL, T., J. CLAUS, B. KENNEDY, *et al.* 1996. Loss of transcriptional silencing causes sterility in old mother cells of *S. cerevisiae*. Cell **84:** 633–642.
2. KREGEL, K.C. 2002. Heat shock proteins: modifying factors in physiological stress responses and acquired thermotolerance. J. Appl. Physiol. **92:** 2177–2186.
3. FATMA, N., D.P. SINGH, T. SHINOHARA & L.T. CHYLACK, Jr. 2001. Transcriptional regulation of the antioxidant protein 2 gene, a thiol-specific antioxidant, by lens epithelium-derived growth factor to protect cells from oxidative stress. J. Biol. Chem. **276:** 48899–48907.
4. STUHLMEIER, K.M. *et al.* 2003. Antioxidant protein 2 prevents methemoglobin formation in erythrocyte hemolysates. Eur. J. Biochem. **270:** 334–341.
5. PHELAN, M.W. *et al.* 2001. Botulinum toxin urethral sphincter injection to restore bladder emptying in men and women with voiding dysfunction. J. Urol. **165:** 1107–1110.
6. AIGAKI, T., K. SEONG & T. MATSUO. 2002. Longevity determination genes in *Drosophila melanogaster*. Mech. Ageing Dev. **123:** 1531–1541.
7. YOKOYAMA, K. *et al.* 2002. Extended longevity of *Caenorhabditis elegans* by knocking in extra copies of hsp70F, a homolog of mot-2 mortalin /mthsp70/Grp75. FEBS Lett. **516:** 53–57.
8. HELFERT, R.H., F.R. GLATZ, III, T.S. WILSON, *et al.* 2002. Hsp70 in the inferior colliculus of Fischer-344 rats: effects of age and acoustic stress. Hear Res. **170:** 155–165.
9. HAYEK, T., J. OIKNINE, G. DANKNER, *et al.* 1995. HDL apolipoprotein A-I attenuates oxidative modification of low density lipoprotein: studies in transgenic mice. Eur. J. Clin. Chem. Clin. Biochem. **33:** 721–725.

10. TAM, S.P., X. ZHANG, C. CUTHBERT, *et al.* 1997. Effects of dimethyl sulfoxide on apolipoprotein A-I in the human hepatoma cell line, HepG2. J. Lipid. Res. **38:** 2090–2102.
11. GOSSLAU, A. & L. RENSING. 2002. [Oxidative stress, age-dependent (correction of age-related) cell damage and antioxidative mechanisms]. Z. Gerontol. Geriatr. **35:** 139–150.
12. CHEN, C., S. DEWAELE, B. BRAECKMAN, *et al.* 2003. A high-throughput screening system for genes extending life-span. Exp. Gerontol. **38:** 1051–1063.

Senescence Marker Protein–30 as a Novel Antiaging Molecule

DONGYUN FENG,[a,b] YOSHITAKA KONDO,[a,c] AKIHITO ISHIGAMI,[a] MASASHI KURAMOTO,[a] TAKEO MACHIDA,[b] AND NAOKI MARUYAMA[a]

[a]*Department of Molecular Pathology, Tokyo Metropolitan Institute of Gerontology, Tokyo, Japan*

[b]*Department of Regulation Biology, Faculty of Science, Saitama University, Saitama, Japan*

[c]*School of Medicine, Tokyo Medical and Dental University, Tokyo, Japan*

ABSTRACT: Senescence marker protein–30 (SMP30), composed of 299 amino acids, has an approximate molecular mass of 32–34 kDa and has a pI 4.9 in charge. The amino acid alignment from various animal species revealed a highly conserved structure. SMP30 has an enzyme activity hydrolyzing sarin, soman, and tabun, known as lethal toxic nerve chemicals. We analyzed the organophosphatase activity of SMP30 using DFP as a substrate. This DFPase activity is revealed in a dose-dependent manner in the presence of magnesium ions. We investigated the intracellular localization of SMP30. It is localized in both the cytoplasm and nucleus. To confirm the presence of SMP30 in the nucleus, we prepared nuclear and cytoplasmic extracts from isolated cultured hepatocytes. Western blotting showed that SMP30 was detected in both extracts. Because the expression is reduced by carbon tetrachloride, one can speculate that the expression is modulated by oxidative stress increased with aging.

KEYWORDS: SMP30; DFPase; aging

INTRODUCTION

After the postgenome era, proteomic analysis became one of the powerful tools for aging study. This methodology provided us with new insight into gerontology. During a survey of age-associated changes in soluble proteins of rat liver, we discovered a novel molecule that is designated as senescence marker protein–30 (SMP30).[1] Subsequently, we established an SMP30-knockout (SMP30-KO) mouse to seek for its biological functions. The experiments using the strain provided us information on significance of SMP30 for geriatric diseases. To understand the biological function of SMP30 further, we have been studying the molecular characteristics of SMP30.

Address for correspondence: Naoki Maruyama, M.D., Department of Molecular Pathology, Tokyo Metropolitan Institute of Gerontology, 35-2 Sakaecho, Itabashi-ku, Tokyo 173-0015, Japan. Voice: +813-3964-3241; fax: +813-3579-4776.

maruyama@center.tmig.or.jp

Ann. N.Y. Acad. Sci. 1019: 360–364 (2004). © 2004 New York Academy of Sciences.
doi: 10.1196/annals.1297.062

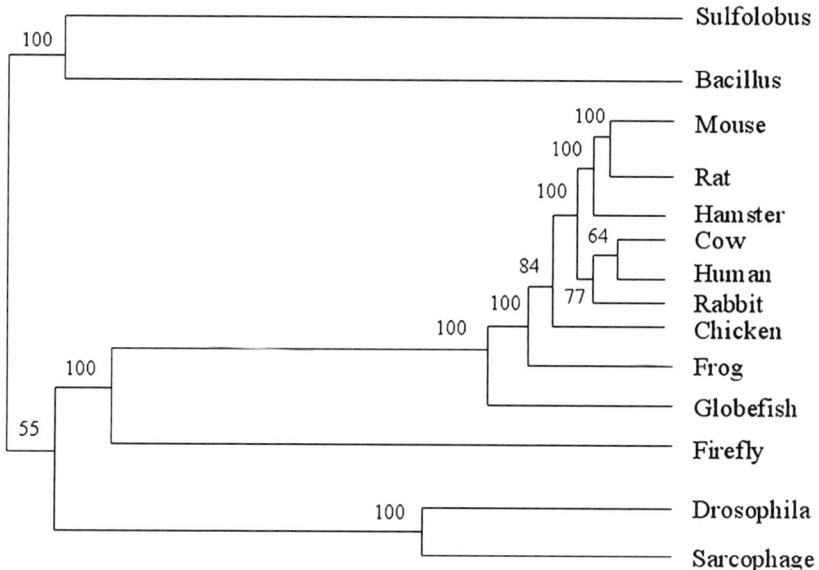

FIGURE 1. Molecular evolution of SMP30. Phylogenic tree of the SMP30 family is reconstructed with the neighbor-joining method. The numbers above lines are the bootstrap values of 100.

HIGHLY CONSERVED STRUCTURE OF SMP30

The expression of SMP30 is decreased with aging in a sex-independent manner. The transcripts have been detected in multiple tissues, including the liver, kidney, brain, lung, adrenal gland, stomach, ovary, uterus, testis, and epidermis. This molecule has a molecular mass of approximately 32–34 kDa and has a pI 4.9 in charge. SMP30 is composed of 299 amino acids. The amino acid alignment of SMP30 from various animal species revealed a highly conserved structure.[2] This suggests that SMP30 may have important biological roles. Recently, several SMP30 homologues were discovered in various species including nonvertebrates. One of the interesting homologues is luciferin-regenerating enzyme (LRE) discovered in firefly light organ.[3] However, no homologue has been detected in *C. elegans*. The phylogenic tree of SMP30 may stress the importance of this molecule (FIG. 1). There is a wide choice of animal species for aging studies. At the discovery of SMP30, there was information available on known functional domain in the database. Later, we found a sequence with similarity of the mouse SMP30 (51 amino acids, residues 150–200) to a yeast (*Sacchcromyces cerevisiae*) RNA polymerase subunit RPO26 and a bacterial (*Bacillus subtilis*) RNA polymerase.[4] Little similarity was found between SMP30 and mammalian RNA polymerase. The function of this domain is not elucidated.

ENZYME ACTIVITY

As in the firefly, the SMP30 homologue in insects has enzyme activity. It is important to define the new enzyme activity in mammalian SMP30. Billecke *et al.* isolated a molecule having organophosphatase activity from rat liver.[5] This molecule has an enzyme activity hydrolyzing sarin, soman, and tabun, known as lethal toxic nerve chemicals. The amino acid analysis showed that the molecule is identical with SMP30. We analyzed the organophosphatase activity of SMP30 using DFP as a substrate. This DFPase activity shows dose-dependent manner in the presence of magnesium ions. We compared requirements of several ions to show the DFPase activity of SMP30. In addition to magnesium, manganese and cobalt are required to show DFPase activity of SMP30. Although these three divalent cationic ions are required for organophosphatase activity of SMP30, calcium ion was not required.

Because firefly LRE is an SMP30 homologue, we have compared the LRE and rat SMP30. Although LRE has DFPase activity, rat SMP30 does not have LRE activity. The precise comparison of domain structures is reserved for further studies.

CHARACTERISTICS OF SMP30 MOLECULE

After our discovery, another research group reported an identical molecule as a calcium-binding protein, named regucalcin.[6] However, the experiments by Nakajima and Natori using AFP as SMP30 homologue of flesh fly showed no binding to calcium.[7] Our aforementioned result that there is no requirement of calcium ion for DFPase activity of SMP30 also raised the argument on the binding trait of calcium ion. To confirm the calcium binding activity of mammalian SMP30, we performed calcium binding assay. Calmodulin bound radioactive calcium well. In contrast, no binding activity of rat SMP30 to calcium was detected. These results confirmed that SMP30 is not a calcium binding protein. However, this molecule has the very important function of keeping intracellular calcium homeostasis.[8]

We investigated the intracellular localization of SMP30. SMP30 is localized in both the cytoplasm and nucleus. To confirm the presence of SMP30 in nucleus, we prepared nuclear and cytoplasmic extracts from isolated cultured hepatocytes. Western blotting showed that SMP30 was detected in both extracts.[4] However, there is no signal sequence for nuclear translocation of SMP30 in its structure. One of the possibilities for the explanation of nuclear translocation is the phosphorylation. Thus, we developed Western blot analysis of SMP30 using antiphosphorylated tyrosine antibody. The results suggested the phosphorylation of SMP30 in both extracts.

In the amino acid sequence of SMP30, there are many candidate sites for phosphorylation. To determine the phosphorylation sites, we developed a proteomic analysis using highly purified rat SMP30. After application of rat SMP30 to proteomics analysis, we found several shifts in electric charge of the molecules. To confirm that the serial spots are derived from the same molecule, we performed immunostaining of the spots. By using anti–SMP30 antiserum, we identified six spots with identical molecular weights and different *pI* values. Four of them are phosphorylated. Subsequently, we purified each spot and applied MALDI-TOF mass spectrometry. Three phosphorylated candidate residues were identified. Those are highly conserved among various animal species.

EXPRESSION OF SMP30

The expression of SMP30 is decreased with aging. One can speculate that the expression is modulated by oxidative stress increased with aging. In our previous study, the treatment of carbon tetrachloride as acute oxidative stress markedly suppresses the expression of SMP30 in liver.[9] On the contrary, the dietary restriction enhances the SMP30 expression. Because dietary restriction reduces the oxidative stress, the elongation of life span resulted. Those results suggested that SMP30 expression is modulated by oxidative stress.

CONCLUSION

Our studies revealed the phosphorylation of SMP30 and phosphorylated sites. This phenomenon could be associated with nuclear localization of SMP30. From the nuclear localization of SMP30 and its similarity to the RNA polymerase subunit, we speculate that besides Ca^{2+}-pumping and anticell proliferative roles, SMP30 may act in the regulation of gene expression such as in transcription.

The molecular traits of SMP30 have been elucidated after its discovery. Those studies suggest that SMP30 is a multifunctional molecule. Combining with the results of the SMP30-KO mouse study, this molecule seems to be pivotal to keep cellular and physical homeostasis during life span.[10] Our recent studies suggested that SMP30 suppresses the generation of reactive oxygen species in hepatocytes. These results strongly suggested that SMP30 has antioxidant properties protecting cells from oxidative stress. Therefore, the generation of SMP30 can be regarded as an antiaging molecule.

ACKNOWLEDGMENTS

This work is supported by a grant from the Health Science Research Grants for Comprehensive Research on Aging and Health supported by the Ministry of Health Labor and Welfare, Japan, and a grant from the Ministry of Education, Science, and Culture, Japan.

REFERENCES

1. FUJITA, T., T. SHIRASAWA, K. UCHIDA, et al. 1992. Isolation of cDNA clone encoding rat senescence marker protein-30 (SMP30) and its tissue distribution. Biochim. Biophys. Acta **1132**: 297–305.
2. FUJITA, T., J.T. MANDEL, T. SHIRASAWA, et al. 1995. Isolation cDNA clone encoding human senescence marker protein-30 (SMP30) and its location on the X chromosome. Biochim. Biophys. Acta **1263**: 249–252.
3. GOMI, K., K. HIROKAWA & N. KAJIYAMA. 2002. Molecular cloning and expression of the cDNA encoding luciferin-regenerating enzyme from *Luciola cruciata* and *Luciola lateralis*. Gene **294**: 157–166.
4. ISHIGAMI, A., S. HANDA, N. MARUYAMA, et al. 2003. Nuclear localization of senescence marker protein-30, SMP30, in cultured mouse hepatocytes and its similarity to RNA polymerase. Biosci. Biotechnol. Biochem. **67**: 158–160.

5. BILLECKE, S.S., S.L. PRIMO-PARMO, C.S. DUNLOP, *et al.* 1999. Characterization of a soluble mouse liver enzyme capable of hydrolyzing diisopropyl phosphorofluoridate. Chem. Biol. Interact. **119-120:** 251–256.
6. SHIMOKAWA, N. & M. YAMAGUCHI. 1993. Molecular cloning and sequencing of the cDNA coding for a calcium-binding protein regucalcin from rat liver. FEBS Lett. **327:** 251–255.
7. NAKAJIMA, Y. & S. NATORI. 2000. Identification and characterization of an anterior fat body protein in an insect. J. Biochem. **127:** 901–908.
8. FUJITA, T., H. INOUE, T. KITAMURA, *et al.* 1998. Senescence marker protein-30 (SMP30) rescues cell death by enhancing plasma membrane Ca^{2+}-pumping activity in Hep G2 cells. Biochem. Biophys. Res. Commun. **250:** 374–380.
9. ISHIGAMI, T., T. FUJITA, G. SIMBULA, *et al.* 2001. Regulatory effects of senescence marker protein 30 on the proliferation of hepatocytes. Pathol. Int. **51:** 491–497.
10. ISHIGAMI, A., T. FUJITA, S. HANDA, *et al.* 2002. Senescence marker protein-30 knockout mouse liver is highly susceptible to TNF-α- and Fas-mediated apoptosis. Am. J. Pathol. **161:** 1273–1281.

Iron Accumulation during Cellular Senescence

DAVID W. KILLILEA,[a,b] STEPHANIE L. WONG,[b] HENDRY S. CAHAYA,[b] HANI ATAMNA,[a] AND BRUCE N. AMES[a,b]

[a]*Children's Hospital Oakland Research Institute, Oakland, California 94609, USA*

[b]*Molecular and Cellular Biology, University of California at Berkeley, Berkeley, California 94720, USA*

ABSTRACT: Iron accumulates as a function of age and is associated with the pathology of numerous age-related diseases. These changes may be caused by altered iron homeostasis at the cellular level, yet this is poorly understood. Therefore, changes in iron content in primary human fibroblasts were studied in culture models of cellular senescence. Total iron content increased exponentially during cellular senescence, reaching ~10-fold higher levels than young cells. Increasing intracellular iron levels through iron-citrate supplementation or decreasing intracellular iron levels using iron-selective chelators had little effect on cellular life span and markers of cellular senescence when used at subtoxic doses. However, accelerating cellular senescence with low-dose H_2O_2 also accelerated senescence-associated iron accumulation. Delaying cellular senescence with *N-tert*-butyl-hydroxylamine (NtBHA) attenuated senescence-associated iron accumulation. Furthermore, H_2O_2 or NtBHA had no effect on iron intracellular levels in immortalized fibroblasts. Thus, iron accumulation is not a cause, but a consequence of normal cellular senescence *in vitro*. Senescence-associated iron accumulation may contribute to the increased oxidative stress and cellular dysfunction seen in senescent cells.

KEYWORDS: cellular senescence; iron; oxidative stress; fibroblasts; hydroxylamine

Iron accumulates as a function of age in many tissues, a condition exaggerated in numerous age-related pathologies.[1] This is of interest because iron can catalyze formation of oxidants that damage biological macromolecules,[2] and oxidative stress is widely reported to increase with age.[3] Thus, altered iron homeostasis may play a role in age-related decay of tissue function. The molecular basis of age-related iron accumulation is not known, but it may be caused by a loss of iron homeostasis at the cellular level. Therefore, we examined the relationship between intracellular iron content and cellular senescence *in vitro*.[4]

Primary human fibroblast (IMR-90) and endothelial cells (HUVECs) were analyzed for metal content as a function of time in culture using inductively coupled plasma spectrometry. Intracellular iron content increased exponentially in both cell

---

Address for correspondence: Dr. Bruce N. Ames, Nutritional Genomics Center, Children's Hospital Oakland Research Institute, 5700 Martin Luther King, Jr. Way, Oakland, CA 94609. Voice: 510-450-7627; fax: 510-450-7910.

bames@chori.org

types such that iron levels were 10-fold higher in IMR-90s and 50-fold higher in HUVECs at the end of replicative life span. The intracellular content of potassium, magnesium, manganese, and zinc also increased in both primary cell types; however, these increases were modest and may be related to the concomitant increases in total protein content and cellular volume with senescence. Iron accumulation occurred earlier and to a greater extent than other measured metals, exceeding changes in cellular protein and volume levels.

We then attempted to determine causality to the relationship between iron and cellular senescence. Previous work in *Drosophila* has shown that increased iron intake decreased life span, whereas reducing iron intake prolonged life span.[5,6] This suggested life span can be influenced by changing iron status, although the contribution of oxidative stress related to excess iron was not fully assessed in that work. Also, the cells in *Drosophila* are postmitotic; little work has been reported in proliferating cells. Therefore, intracellular iron levels of IMR-90s were increased by weekly administration of ferrous iron citrate or reduced by desferrioxamine or salicyladehyde isonicotinoyl hydrazone, metals chelators with high selectivity for iron. Doses of iron or chelators were chosen that did not induce toxicity as determined by vital dye exclusion or tetrazolium dye assays. Exogenous iron supplementation dose-dependently stimulated growth rates and increased intracellular iron content up to 10-fold (like that of senescent IMR-90s) after only 2–3 weeks; replicative capacity, however, of the iron-treated cultures was not significantly shorter than control cultures. Iron chelators reduced intracellular iron content by up to 50% in 2–3 weeks, although replicative capacity of the chelator-treated cultures was not significantly longer than control cultures; repeated treatment of higher doses reduced replicative capacity. Changing intracellular iron levels did not appear to affect time to replicative senescence in these cells.

We then tested how altering cellular senescence would affect iron homeostasis. First, SV-40 transformed, immortalized IMR-90s were tested for changes in iron content under the same conditions as primary cells. SV-40 transformation leads to inactivation of p53 and Rb, the major integration points for the molecular mechanisms that drive senescence. SV-IMR-90s demonstrated no change in the intracellular content of iron or other measured metals over six months in culture; all metal levels remained similar to that of young primary IMR-90s.

Additionally, we have reported pharmacological approaches to altering senescence in human cell cultures. IMR-90s treated weekly with low-dose H_2O_2 demonstrated accelerated senescence, whereas treatment with the mitochondrial antioxidant *N-tert*-butyl-hydroxylamine (NtBHA) delayed senescence.[7] We determined the affect of these models on intracellular iron levels. Low-dose H_2O_2 dose-dependently accelerated intracellular iron accumulation concomitantly with accelerated senescence. Likewise, NtBHA dose-dependently attenuated intracellular iron accumulation concomitantly with delayed senescence. NtBHA also lowered H_2O_2-induced iron accumulation even when NtBHA was added to cultures 24 hours after oxidant stress, indicating that NtBHA could reverse oxidant stress–mediated changes in cellular phenotype. This activity may play a role in the antisenescence properties of NtBHA. Furthermore, there was no change in intracellular iron content in SV-IMR-90s when treated with either H_2O_2 and/or NtBHA, illustrating the requirement for intact mechanisms of replicative senescence to lead to altered iron homeostasis.

These data suggest that changes in iron homeostasis result from, not cause, the processes that drive cellular senescence in cultured human cells. The specific mechanisms that drive senescence-related iron accumulation are under investigation. One possibility is that oxidative stress uncouples iron homeostatic regulation by activating iron response proteins, which serve as master regulators of iron balance.[8] Another possibility is that heme deficiency, induced by aging-related oxidative stress and mitochondrial decay, may lead to disturbances in cellular iron homeostasis.[9] In addition, iron accumulation may result from age-related changes in lysosome function and turnover as recently described.[10] The functional consequences of senescence-related iron accumulation are also unknown. This accumulation of iron may contribute to the increased oxidative stress and cellular dysfunction seen in senescent cells. However, it is unclear how relevant iron accumulation *in vitro* is to iron accumulation in human tissues *in vivo* during normal aging and in age-related pathologies.

REFERENCES

1. WALTER, P.B, K.B. BECKMAN & B.N. AMES. 1999. The role of iron and mitochondria in aging. *In* Understanding the Process of Aging. E. Cadenas & L. Packer, Eds.: 203–227. Marcel Dekker. New York.
2. HALLIWELL, B. & J.M.C. GUTTERIDGE. 1999. Free radicals in biology and medicine. Oxford University Press. Oxford.
3. BECKMAN, K.B. & B.N. AMES. 1998. The free radical theory of aging matures. Physiol. Rev. **78:** 547–581.
4. KILLILEA, D.W., H. ATAMNA, C. LIAO & B.N. AMES. 2003. Iron accumulation during cellular senescence in human fibroblasts *in vitro*. Antioxid. Redox Signal. **5:** 507–516.
5. MASSIE, H.R., V.R. AIELLO & T.R. WILLIAMS. 1985. Iron accumulation during development and ageing of Drosophila. Mech. Ageing Dev. **29:** 215–220.
6. MASSIE, H.R., V.R. AIELLO & T.R. WILLIAMS. 1993. Inhibition of iron absorption prolongs the life span of Drosophila. Mech. Ageing Dev. **67:** 227–237.
7. ATAMNA, H., A. PALER-MARTINEZ & B.N. AMES. 2000. N-t-Butyl hydroxylamine, a hydrolysis product of alpha-phenyl-N-t-butyl nitrone, is more potent in delaying senescence in human lung fibroblasts. J. Biol. Chem. **275:** 6741–6748.
8. PANTOPOULOS, K. & M.W. HENTZE. 1995. Rapid responses to oxidative stress mediated by iron regulatory protein. EMBO J. **14:** 2917–2924.
9. ATAMNA, H., D.W. KILLILEA, A.N. KILLILEA & B.N. AMES. 2002. Heme deficiency may be a factor in the mitochondrial and neuronal decay of aging. Proc. Natl. Acad. Sci. USA **99:** 14807–14812.
10. BRUNK, U.T. & A. TERMAN. 2002. Lipofuscin: mechanisms of age-related accumulation and influence on cell function. Free Radic. Biol. Med. **33:** 611–619.

Investigations on the Nature of the Cost of Reproduction

Susceptibility to Heat Stress in Fruitflies

JALAL KOOCHMESHGI, SHADI LADONNI, AND
SEYED MEHDI HOSSEINI-MAZINANI

National Research Center for Genetic Engineering and Biotechnology, Tehran, Iran

> ABSTRACT: Studies in various species have shown that changes in reproductive activity result in inverse changes in life span. It is interesting to know how this "cost of reproduction" is incurred. It is possible that reproductive activity renders the organism more vulnerable to stress and that accumulated damage has a role in the observed decrease in life span. Previously, other investigators had shown that mated female fruitflies have significantly shorter life spans than virgin females. We compare mated and virgin young fruitflies for susceptibility to lethal heat stress. Preliminary results suggest that mated fruitflies are significantly more susceptible to heat stress than virgin ones.
>
> KEYWORDS: cost of reproduction; fruitfly; heat stress

Studies in various species have shown an inverse relationship between reproductive capacity and life span. Factors like age at maturity, mating, and reproductive yield are shown to inversely affect life span. This inverse relationship has been demonstrated in a plethora of species, from fruitflies to humans, and coined "cost of reproduction."[1–3]

What is the nature of this cost of reproduction? Why and how are reproductive factors and life span related? The answers to these questions are likely to have far-reaching theoretical and practical implications in biomedical sciences. The phenomenon traditionally has been studied by ecologists and in an evolutionary context, and it has been formalized in life-history theory. The prevailing view holds that at the heart of the phenomenon is the issue of allocation of limited available resources to competing demands of reproduction and survival. This concept has been developed in detailed mathematical models.[4–6]

Yet, it is equally interesting, and important, to know how this "cost of reproduction" is incurred. A possibility is that reproductive activity renders an organism more vulnerable to various types of stress and that the accumulated damage has a role in the observed decrease in life span. From this point of view, death is regarded as the end result of accumulated damage sustained by organism. The rate of this damage accumulation is modulated by organism's level of susceptibility to various kinds of

---

Address for correspondence: Jalal Koochmeshgi, National Research Center for Genetic Engineering and Biotechnology, P.O. Box 14155-6343, Tehran, Iran.
jkoochmeshgi@yahoo.co.uk

stress. Types of stress commonly occurring in organism's life are primary candidates for study.

The fruitfly is a suitable model organism to investigate this possibility. Earlier, investigators had shown that mated female fruitflies have significantly shorter life span than virgin females.[7] Recently, it has been demonstrated that mated young fruitflies are significantly more susceptible to oxidative stress and starvation than virgin ones.[8] We compared mated and virgin young fruitflies for susceptibility to another type of stress, heat stress.

Fruitflies, which were kept under standard laboratory conditions, were sexed within 2 hours after eclosion. Half of fruitflies were kept together and were allowed to mate freely. The other half were segregated according to sex and kept in separate bottles for virgin males and virgin females. After five days, fruitflies were incubated at 40°C and each individual was closely observed until death. Preliminary results and analysis of survival data suggest that mated fruitflies are significantly more susceptible to heat stress than virgin ones.

Stress susceptibility assays, including assays for susceptibility to heat stress, can be useful in studying the nature of the cost of reproduction. Although, to gain more comprehensive results, lethal, acute exposure to stressors should be complemented with sublethal and chronic exposure.

ACKNOWLEDGMENTS

J.K. thanks the Wellcome Trust for a travel award to attend IABG10.

REFERENCES

1. WILLIAMS, G.C. 1966. Natural selection, the cost of reproduction, and a refinement of Lack's principle. Am. Nat. **100**: 687–690.
2. WILLIAMS, G.C. 1975. Sex and Evolution. Princeton University Press. Princeton, NJ.
3. RICKLEFS, R.E. & G.L. MILLER. 2000. Ecology. Fourth edition. W. H. Freeman and Company. New York.
4. HAMILTON, W.D. 1966. The moulding of senescence by natural selection. J. Theor. Biol. **12**: 12–45.
5. ROFF, D.A. 1992. The evolution of life histories. Chapman & Hall. New York.
6. STEARNS, S.C. 1992. The evolution of life histories. Oxford University Press. Oxford.
7. FOWLER, K. & L. PARTRIDGE. 1989. A cost of mating in female fruitflies. Nature **338**: 760–761.
8. SALMON, A.B., D.B. MARX & L.G. HARSHMAN. 2001. A cost of reproduction in *Drosophila melanogaster*: stress susceptibility. Evolution **55**: 1660–1608.

Alternative Pathways Might Mediate Toxicity of High Concentrations of Superoxide Dismutase

AXEL KOWALD AND EDDA KLIPP

Kinetic Modelling Group, Max Planck Institute for Molecular Genetics, Berlin, Germany

ABSTRACT: One of the most important antioxidant enzymes is superoxide dismutase (SOD), which catalyzes the dismutation of superoxide radicals to peroxide. The gene for CuZnSOD lies in humans on chromosome 21, and its activity is increased in patients with Down syndrome. However, instead of being beneficial, increased lipid peroxidation is associated with this increased expression, and also studies on bacteria and transgenic animals show that high levels of SOD actually lead to increased lipid peroxidation and hypersensitivity to oxidative stress. Using mathematical models, we investigated the question of how overexpression of SOD can lead to increased oxidative stress, although it is an antioxidant enzyme. We considered several possibilities that have been proposed in the literature, such as CuZnSOD-catalyzed hydroxyl radical formation, superoxide-mediated inhibition of membrane peroxidation, and short-circuiting of the Cu(I)ZnSOD/Cu(II)ZnSOD redox cycle. We found that one of the proposed mechanisms under certain circumstances is able to explain the increased oxidative stress caused by SOD. Furthermore, we identified an additional mechanism that agrees well with experimental observations. We call it the "alternative pathway" mechanism, because it depends on superoxide radicals having alternative pathways besides their reaction with SOD. The alternative pathway mechanism is a very general explanation for SOD-associated oxidative stress, because it does not depend on the specific type of SOD, nor on the redox status of the cell. We therefore think that it might be the common mechanism for the detrimental effects seen in cells and organisms with increased levels of the different forms of superoxide dismutase.

KEYWORDS: antioxidants; aging; free radicals; transgenics

INTRODUCTION

One of the most important antioxidant enzymes is superoxide dismutase (SOD), which catalyzes the dismutation of superoxide radicals to hydrogen peroxide:

$$O_2^{\bullet -} \xrightarrow{SOD} H_2O_2 \xrightarrow{cat/GPX} H_2O.$$

Address for correspondence: Axel Kowald, Kinetic Modelling Group, Max Planck Institute for Molecular Genetics, Ihnestrasse 73, 14195 Berlin, Germany. Voice: +49-30-8413-1670; fax: +49-30-8413-1176.
kowald@molgen.mpg.de

The gene for CuZnSOD lies in humans on chromosome 21 and its activity is increased in patients with Down syndrome.[1] However, instead of being beneficial, increased lipid peroxidation is associated with this increased expression,[2] and also studies on bacteria and transgenic animals show that high levels of SOD actually lead to increased lipid peroxidation and hypersensitivity to oxidative stress.[3–6] The most popular explanation, that increased amounts of SOD simply produce more product (H_2O_2), cannot be correct because under steady state conditions the rate of superoxide consumption is exactly identical to its generation rate, independent of the concentration of SOD. More SOD lowers the level of superoxide, but cannot yield more H_2O_2.

Here, we investigate the question of how overexpression of SOD can lead to increased oxidative stress although it is an antioxidant enzyme by modeling three proposals from the literature:

- Normally, SOD cycles between a reduced and oxidized state [Cu(1)ZnSOD/Cu(2)ZnSOD]. At low superoxide levels, the intermediates might interact with other cellular redox partners and increase the superoxide reductase (SOR) activity of SOD. The standard reaction of SOD, $2\,O_2^{\bullet-} + 2H^+ \rightarrow H_2O_2 + O_2$, generates one molecule of hydrogen peroxide for two molecules of superoxide. By short-circuiting the SOD cycle, this ratio could increase to 1:1 and thus lead to an increased hydrogen peroxide production. For CuZnSOD (but not for MnSOD), it has been shown experimentally that such a short-circuiting is possible.[7]

- $O_2^{\bullet-}$ radicals might reduce membrane damage by reacting with lipid peroxyl radicals and thus acting as chain breakers: $LOO^\bullet + O_2^{\bullet-} + H^+ \rightarrow LOOH + O_2$.[8]

- It has been proposed that CuZnSOD can react with H_2O_2 leading to hydroxyl radicals ($OH^\bullet$).[9]

To investigate the above ideas, we constructed a reaction network that encompasses the necessary reactions. This network then was translated into a system of seven coupled differential equations that has been solved numerically using Mathematica. In this network $O_2^{\bullet-}$ is produced by the cellular metabolism at a fixed rate and can then undergo several different reactions. It can react with Cu(II)ZnSOD and react to O_2 (the SOO part of the dismutation cycle); it can react with Cu(I)ZnSOD and react to H_2O_2 (the SOR part of the dismutation cycle); together with H_2O_2 it can cause $OH^\bullet$ radicals via the iron-catalyzed Haber-Weiss reaction; it can react with lipid peroxyl radicals interrupting the lipid peroxidation cycle; and it stands in fast equilibrium with its conjugated base, the perhydroxyl radical, $HO_2^\bullet$.

The possibility of shortcutting the SOD cycle (proposal one) is realized by introducing reactions that directly connect the oxidized and the reduced form of SOD. By manipulating the rate constants of these reactions, either superoxide oxidase or superoxide reductase activity is favored.

To test proposal 2, reactions describing the lipid peroxidation cycle have to be implemented. In the model $OH^\bullet$ and $HO_2^\bullet$ can start the chain reaction by forming lipid carbon radicals ($L^\bullet$). Under aerobic conditions, these react with oxygen to produce lipid peroxyl radical ($LOO^\bullet$). Peroxyl radicals are capable of abstracting protons from other lipid molecules, leading to a lipid hydroperoxide and another $L^\bullet$.

This represents the propagation stage of lipid peroxidation. This chain reaction can be interrupted in two ways. Either two LOO• molecules can react with each other in a process of self-termination or, as proposed, lipid peroxyl radicals can interact with superoxide, which now acts as chain breaker.

Further, as proposed, the SOD peroxidase activity is implemented as possible production of hydroxyl radicals from H_2O_2. Finally, hydrogen peroxide is removed from the system by the enzymatic action of catalase or glutathione peroxidase. For simplicity, this is represented as the action of a single enzyme.

RESULTS AND DISCUSSION

Short-circuiting the Superoxide Dismutase Cycle

To study the effects of shortcutting the SOD cycle, we increased the superoxide reductase activity of SOD and then calculated the steady state concentrations of the various oxygen species for SOD concentrations ranging from 10^{-7} M to 10^{-5} M. As predicted, increasing levels of SOD now lead to an increasing H_2O_2 concentration. However, the opposite effect is also possible. If the intracellular conditions are such that superoxide oxidase activity is favored, then increasing SOD levels actually lead to decreasing hydrogen peroxide equilibrium concentrations.

Termination of Lipid Peroxidation

According to the second idea, superoxide radicals can be beneficial if they react with lipid peroxyl radicals and thus interrupt the propagation stage of lipid peroxidation. If there is overscavenging of superoxide (caused by large amounts of SOD), the chain length of the lipid autoxidation process might increase and thus lead to increasing oxidative stress. However, our model simulations have shown that this idea is flawed. It turns out that the lipid peroxyl concentration is completely independent of superoxide. The critical point is that both termination *and* initiation of lipid peroxidation are influenced by differences in the $O_2^{\bullet-}$ concentration and both effects cancel out.

Superoxide Dismutase as Radical Generator

Also, the last proposal cannot explain the increased oxidative stress associated with SOD overexpression. It turns out that the hydroxyl radical level does vary substantially (approximately ninefold), but the equilibrium concentrations of all other variables change by less than 0.01%. The reason is that the hydroxyl radical steady state concentration is many orders of magnitude below the concentrations of the other molecular species. Also, although it is extremely reactive, it seems that the main damage to lipids is not caused by the hydroxyl radical, but by the perhydroxyl radical that exists in much higher concentrations.

"Alternative Pathway" Mechanism

However, studying the described reaction model shown, we discovered a new mechanism that might account for the elevated oxidative stress. We call it the

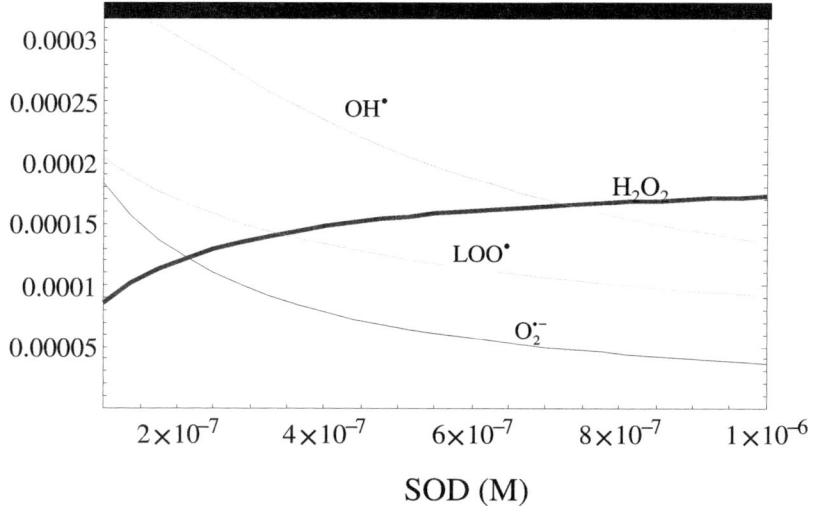

FIGURE 1. Alternative pathway mechanism leading to increased H_2O_2 steady state concentrations. For this simulation the concentration of superoxide dismutase was varied from 10^{-7} M to 10^{-6} M, and the resulting steady state concentrations of the other variables are shown (in arbitrary units). Because of the existence of alternative reaction pathways for $O_2^{\bullet-}$ radicals, increasing SOD levels are accompanied by increasing hydrogen peroxide concentrations.

"alternative pathway" mechanism because it depends on superoxide radicals having alternative pathways besides their reaction with SOD.

In the model under investigation the alternative pathway of $O_2^{\bullet-}$ is the reaction with lipid molecules (initiation and termination of damage). FIGURE 1 shows how the steady state concentrations depend on the amount of SOD. Increasing SOD leads to a decline of superoxide and hydroxyl radicals, but to an increase of hydrogen peroxide. To understand this behavior, we used a heavily simplified version of the full model. The complete lipid peroxidation part has been omitted and also the rest has been simplified as much as possible. In contrast with the standard reactions of SOD and catalase, the model contains an additional alternative pathway for superoxide radicals (via k_{10}):

$$\frac{dO_2^{\bullet-}}{dt} = k_1 - O_2^{\bullet-} - k_2 \cdot SOD \cdot O_2^{\bullet-} \qquad O_2^{\bullet-} = \frac{k_1}{k_{10} + k_2 \cdot SOD}$$

$$\frac{dH_2O_2}{dt} = k_2 \cdot SOD \cdot O_2^{\bullet-} - k_3 \cdot cat \cdot H_2O_2 \qquad H_2O_2 = \frac{k_1 \cdot k_2 \cdot SOD}{(k_{10} + k_2 \cdot SOD) \cdot k_3 \cdot cat}$$

Without alternative pathway ($k_{10} = 0$), SOD cancels out of the expression for the H_2O_2 equilibrium concentration. With alternative pathway, however, the dependency remains and increasing levels of superoxide dismutase lead to increased steady state concentrations of hydrogen peroxide.

The alternative pathway mechanism is a very general explanation for SOD-associated oxidative stress because it does not depend on a special cell state (SOR activity favored over SOO activity) nor on specific properties of superoxide dismutase enzymes (peroxidase activity of CuZnSOD, but not MnSOD). We therefore think that it might be the common mechanism for the detrimental effects seen in cells and organisms with increased levels of the different forms of superoxide dismutase.

REFERENCES

1. SINET, P.M. 1982. Metabolism of oxygen derivatives in Down's syndrome. Ann. N.Y. Acad. Sci. **396:** 83–94.
2. BROOKSBANK, B.W.L. & R. BALAZS. 1984. Superoxide dismutase, glutathione peroxidase and lipoperoxidation in Down's syndrome fetal brain. Dev. Brain Res. **16:** 37.
3. ORR, W.C. & R.S. SOHAL. 1993. Effects of Cu-Zn superoxide dismutase overexpression on life span and resistance to oxidative stress in transgenic *Drosophila melanogaster*. Arch. Biochem. Biophys. **301:** 34–40.
4. REVEILLAUD, I. et al. 1991. Expression of bovine superoxide dismutase in *Drosophila melanogaster* augments resistance to oxidative stress. Mol. Cell. Biol. **11:** 632–640.
5. SCOTT, M.D., S.R. MESHNICK & J.W. EATON. 1987. Superoxide dismutase rich bacteria. Paradoxidal increase in oxidant toxicity. J. Biol. Chem. **262:** 3640–3645.
6. SIWECKI, G. & O.R. BROWN. 1990. Overproduction of superoxide dismutase does not protect *Escherichia coli* from stringency-induced growth inhibition by 1 mM paraquat. Biochem. Int. **20:** 191–200.
7. LIOCHEV, S.I. & I. FRIDOVICH. 2000. Copper- and zinc-containing superoxide dismutase can act as a superoxide reductase and a superoxide oxidase. J. Biol. Chem. **275:** 38482–38485.
8. NELSON, S.K., S.K. BOSE & J.M. MCCORD. 1994. The toxicity of high-dose superoxide dismutase suggests that superoxide can both initiate and terminate lipid peroxidation in the reperfused heart. Free Radic. Biol. Med. **16:** 195–200.
9. YIM, M.B., P.B. CHOCK & E.R. STADTMAN. 1993. Enzyme function of copper, zinc superoxide dismutase as a free radical generator. J. Biol. Chem. **268:** 4099–4105.

No Increase in Senescence-Associated β-Galactosidase Activity in Werner Syndrome Fibroblasts after Exposure to H_2O_2

JOÃO PEDRO DE MAGALHÃES,[a] VALÉRIE MIGEOT,[a]
VÉRONIQUE MAINFROID,[a] FRANÇOISE DE LONGUEVILLE,[b]
JOSÉ REMACLE,[b] AND OLIVIER TOUSSAINT[a]

[a]*Research Unit on Cellular Biology, University of Namur, B-5000 Namur, Belgium*

[b]*Eppendorf Array Technologies, B-5000 Namur, Belgium*

ABSTRACT: Normal human diploid fibroblasts (HDFs) exposed to a single H_2O_2 subcytotoxic stress display features of premature senescence, termed stress-induced premature senescence (SIPS). In this work, our aim was to study SIPS in Werner syndrome (WS) fibroblasts, derived from a patient with WS, a disease resembling accelerated aging. The subcytotoxic dose for WS fibroblasts was found to be inferior to that of normal HDFs, indicating WS fibroblasts are more sensitive to hydrogen peroxide than normal HDFs. SA β-gal activity has been shown to occur both *in vitro* and *in vivo*, and we studied the proportion of WS cells positive for SA β-gal. Intriguingly, the percentage of positive cells did not increase with the dose of H_2O_2 used. Contrary to other HDFs, the DNA-binding activity of p53 in WS fibroblasts did not increase in SIPS. We found, based on our results, that WS fibroblasts feature an altered stress response and do not reach SIPS from H_2O_2. We suggest that the proportion of cells that in normal HDFs would enter SIPS instead die in WS fibroblasts. Last, we propose that aging derives from a loss of integrity of the chromatin structure, which occurs faster in WS patients.

KEYWORDS: aging; cellular senescence; stress; Werner syndrome

Werner syndrome (WS) is an autosomal recessive disease resembling accelerated aging. The pathology of WS involves multiple organs, including skin changes, gray hair, alopecia, cataracts, and cancer susceptibility. The mutated gene, *WRN*, encodes a member of the RecQ helicase family unique in also featuring exonuclease activity. WRN interacts with several proteins involved in DNA metabolism. Alternate DNA structures serve as substrate to WRN, which is able to resolve aberrant DNA structures. Cells derived from patients with WS have a shorter proliferative capacity, an extended S phase, increased telomere loss, and feature genomic instabilities. WS fibroblasts are also hypersensitive to topoisomerase inhibitors and 4-nitroquinoline 1-oxide, but not to other DNA-damaging agents such as ultraviolet light. The accel-

Address for correspondence: Olivier Toussaint, University of Namur (FUNDP), Research Unit on Cellular Biology (URBC), Rue de Bruxelles, 61, B-5000 Namur, Belgium. Voice: +32-81-724132; fax: +32-81-724135.
olivier.toussaint@fundp.ac.be

erated aging seen in tissues of patients with WS suggests that the premature *in vitro* senescence of cells derived from WS patients may be related events.[1]

Normal human diploid fibroblasts (HDFs) exposed to a single H_2O_2 subcytotoxic stress display features of premature senescence. After at least 48 hours of recovery, cells exhibit senescence-associated β-galactosidase (SA β-gal) activity, a senescent morphology, and the overexpression of a number of genes. This long-term response is termed stress-induced premature senescence (SIPS) and has been demonstrated in a wide variety of human cell lines. Understanding the mechanisms of SIPS may have implications for aging and cancer research.[2] In this work, our aim was to study SIPS in WS fibroblasts.

We obtained AG00780 WS dermal fibroblasts from ATCC, and cells were cultured in Eagle basal medium + 10% fetal calf serum at 37°C with 5% CO_2. Confluent cultures at population doubling (PD) 16 were exposed for 2 hours to H_2O_2 doses ranging from 10 to 500 μM diluted in medium plus serum. We determined the cytotoxic mortality using the Cytotoxicity Detection Kit from Roche (Basel, Switzerland). The subcytotoxic dose for AG00780 fibroblasts was calculated to be 75 μM, which is inferior to the subcytotoxic dose used in normal HDFs such as AG04431, BJ, IMR-90, and WI-38: respectively, 300, 1,200, 150, and 300 μM. These results indicate that WS fibroblasts are more sensitive to hydrogen peroxide than normal HDFs.

SA β-gal activity has been shown to occur both *in vitro* and *in vivo*, and we studied the proportion of WS cells positive for SA β-gal as described.[3] Previous reports indicated that SA β-gal activity increases drastically in AG00780 fibroblasts from PD 10.9 to PD 32.5.[4] The percentage of SA β-gal–positive cells also increases in HDFs at early PD under SIPS.[2] Our results show that although the percentage of WS fibroblasts positive for SA β-gal in the controls was relatively low (10.4 ± 3.8%), when compared with, for instance, senescent HDFs, the percentage of cells positive for SA β-gal staining did not increase with the dose of H_2O_2 used. For example, in foreskin BJ HDFs the SA β-gal activity in controls and at the subcytotoxic dose was respectively 9.7 ± 2.6% and 24.4 ± 0.3%. In addition, the WS fibroblasts grew slowly and showed the morphology of old cells both before and after a single H_2O_2 stress, which suggests an uncoupling between SA β-gal and the senescent morphogenesis.

One important pathway in SIPS and cellular senescence involves the activation of p53 in response to DNA damage. Indeed, recent results indicate that, as happens in normal HDFs, p53 plays a key role in the telomere-mediated signaling of senescence in WS fibroblasts.[5] Therefore, we used the TransAM kit from ActiveMotif (San Diego, CA, USA) to determine the influence of a single H_2O_2 stress on the DNA-binding activity of p53. Nuclear extracts were added to a 96-well plate, and the DNA-binding activity of p53 was determined according to the manufacturer's specifications. Our results suggest that the DNA-binding activity of p53 does not increase significantly in WS fibroblasts after a single H_2O_2 stress at either 24 or 72 hours after the stress: respectively, 39 ± 46% and 26 ± 41%. This is in contrast with other cell lines; for example, in BJ and hTERT-BJ1 cells p53's DNA-binding activity increases approximately twofold at 24 and 72 hours after a single subcytotoxic H_2O_2 stress (J.P. de Magalhaes *et al.*, in preparation).

We also used DNA microarrays to compare gene expression patterns between WS fibroblasts and BJ HDFs at early (young) and late (old) PD. We used the DualChip Human General from Eppendorf (Hamburg, Germany) containing 202 genes involved in basic cellular processes. Although AG00780 and BJ cell lines were derived from the skin, alterations in gene expression may be caused by differences between the cell lines. Even so, we found a higher percentage of genes differentially expressed between WS fibroblast and young BJ HDFs than between senescent BJ HDFs and WS fibroblasts: 20% versus 12%. Genes affected by WRN included SHC1, SM22, CAV1, PKM2, PAI2, and PCNA, which were overexpressed in WS fibroblasts, and IL11RA, MSRA, NCOR1, and GSTP1, which were underexpressed. These results suggest that the WS fibroblasts' gene expression patterns are more closely related to senescent BJ cells than to BJ cells at early PD. The results are being further analyzed.

Based on our results, WS fibroblasts feature an altered stress response. Interestingly, p53-dependent apoptosis is attenuated in WS fibroblasts.[6] Our data confirm previous reports that WS fibroblasts are more sensitive to oxidative stress than normal cells. We propose that the proportion of cells that in normal HDFs would enter SIPS instead die in WS fibroblasts, perhaps through a p53-independent event such as necrosis.

The response to DNA damage is altered in WS fibroblasts, which helps explain the increased genomic instability. WRN functions as a key factor in resolving aberrant DNA structures and can induce p53 in response to DNA damage.[1,7] Recent results suggest that WRN plays a structural role in DNA repair independent of its enzymatic activities.[8] Herein, we propose that aging derives from a loss of integrity of the chromatin structure, which occurs faster in WS patients.

WRN may detect damage or changes in unusual DNA structures, facilitate the access of the DNA repair machinery to unusual DNA structures, or help maintain the integrity of the chromatin structure after repair. Indeed, WS fibroblasts are hypersensitive to topoisomerase inhibitors.[1] Changes in chromatin structure affect the expression of certain genes; DNA damage and repair are altered in regions where the chromatin structure changes, in turn disrupting the cell's response to stress/insults. Results from yeast already have implicated chromatin changes in aging and similar mechanism may operate in WS.[9] For example, it has been shown that changes in chromatin remodeling genes make yeast more susceptible to stress.[10] We propose that changes in chromatin structure, for example, condensation, accumulate with age, making our cell's ability to cope with insults decrease with age and thus resulting in an increase in age-related vulnerability. In patients with WS, the accumulation is presumably faster.

ACKNOWLEDGMENTS

J. P. de Magalhães' work is funded by the FCT, Portugal. O. Toussaint is a Research Associate of the FNRS, Belgium. We also thank the European Union, 5th Framework Programme, for the "Cellage" (CRAFT' 1999-71628) project and the Région Wallonne for the "Modelage," "Arrayage," and ToxiSIPS Projects.

REFERENCES

1. FRY, M. 2002 (April 3). The Werner syndrome helicase-nuclease—one protein, many mysteries. Science's SAGE KE, http://sageke.sciencemag.org/cgi/content/full/sageke;2002/13/re2/.

2. TOUSSAINT, O. et al. 2002. Stress-induced premature senescence or stress-induced senescence-like phenotype: one in vivo reality, two possible definitions? Sci. World J. **2:** 230–247.
3. DIMRI, G.P. et al. 1995. A biomarker that identifies senescent human cells in culture and in aging skin in vivo. Proc. Natl. Acad. Sci. USA **92:** 9363–9367.
4. CHOI, D. et al. 2001. Telomerase expression prevents replicative senescence but does not fully reset mRNA expression patterns in Werner syndrome cell strains. FASEB J. **15:** 1014–1020.
5. DAVIS, T. et al. 2003. Telomere-based proliferative lifespan barriers in Werner-syndrome fibroblasts involve both p53-dependent and p53-independent mechanisms. J. Cell Sci. **116:** 1349–1357.
6. SPILLARE, E.A. et al. 1999. p53-mediated apoptosis is attenuated in Werner syndrome cells. Genes Dev. **13:** 1355–1360.
7. BLANDER, G. et al. 2000. The Werner syndrome protein contributes to induction of p53 by DNA damage. FASEB J. **14:** 2138–2140.
8. CHEN, L. et al. 2003. WRN, the protein deficient in Werner syndrome, plays a critical structural role in optimizing DNA repair. Aging Cell **2:** 191–199.
9. GUARENTE, L. 1997. Chromatin and ageing in yeast and in mammals. Ciba Found. Symp. **211:** 104–107; discussion, 107–111.
10. TSUKIYAMA, T. et al. 1999. Characterization of the imitation switch subfamily of ATP-dependent chromatin-remodeling factors in *Saccharomyces cerevisiae*. Genes Dev. **13:** 686–697.

Aging and Vitamin E Deficiency Are Responsible for Altered RNA Pathways

MANUELA MALATESTA,[a] CARLO BERTONI-FREDDARI,[b]
PATRIZIA FATTORETTI,[b] BEATRICE BALDELLI,[a] STANISLAV FAKAN,[c]
AND GIANCARLO GAZZANELLI[a]

[a]*Istituto di Istologia e Analisi di Laboratorio,
University of Urbino "Carlo Bo," Urbino, Italy*

[b]*Neurobiology of Aging Laboratory, INRCA Research Department, Ancona, Italy*

[c]*Centre of Electron Microscopy, University of Lausanne, Switzerland*

ABSTRACT: Fibrillar centers (FCs), dense fibrillar (DFC) and granular (GC) components in nucleoli, and perichromatin granules (PGs) in nucleoplasm were measured by morphometry. FC size and their nucleolar surface fraction significantly decreased in aging and vitamin E deficiency. The GC and DFC nucleolar fraction was unchanged in adult and old rats, but in vitamin E–deficient animals GC increased and DFC decreased significantly. PG density significantly increased in aging and decreased in vitamin E deficiency. The quantitative evaluation of immunolabeled transcription and splicing factors revealed that polymerase II and SC-35 significantly decreased in old and vitamin E–deficient versus adult animals. Fibrillarin and snRNPs did not change between adult and old rats, but were significantly lower in vitamin E–deficient rats. These data document altered RNA pathways in aging and vitamin E deficiency. Considering the antioxidant role of vitamin E, they lend further support to the importance of free radical production and control in the aging process.

KEYWORDS: aging; vitamin E deficiency; hepatocyte; nucleus; nucleolus; RNA

A defective control of oxygen reactions, at the level of oxidative phosphorylation, is reported to result in the production of free radicals, which are responsible for significant cellular damage occurring not only close to the site of free radical generation, but also on molecules located at distant cellular compartments, that is, the nucleus. Specific cellular processes and antioxidant compounds counteract the deleterious effects of free radical attacks; thus, the balance between damage and cellular defense strategies appears to play a critical role in the occurrence of cellular alterations with advancing age. Vitamin E (α-tocopherol) is a biological antioxidant able to quench the free radical–mediated lipid peroxidation chain.[1] Conceivably, the absence of this molecule from the diet of young laboratory animals results in the lack of protection from free radical injury and may lead to aging-like alterations.[2] In the interphase nucleus, some components have been structurally identified and functionally char-

---

Address for correspondence: Dr. Carlo Bertoni-Freddari, Neurobiology of Aging Laboratory, INRCA Research Department, Via Birarelli 8, 60121 Ancona, Italy. Voice: +39-071-800-4153; fax: +39-071-206791.
 c.bertoni@inrca.it

acterized. These include perichromatin fibrils (PFs), perichromatin granules (PGs), dense fibrillar component (DFC), granular component (GC), and fibrillar centers (FCs). From a functional standpoint, the above-mentioned structural components, while individually reporting on specific aspects of RNA transcription, splicing and storage, when taken together, provide reliable information on RNA processing. To verify the role of an increased oxidative stress and aging on the above RNA structural constituents, we conducted morphometric and immunocytochemical studies on hepatocyte nuclei of adult, old, and vitamin E–deficient rats.

Female Wistar rats were used. Animals of 9 (adult) and 28 (old) months of age received a standard diet *ad libitum*. A third group of animals was fed a vitamin E–deficient diet from 1 to 12 months of age, at which time they were killed. The rats were anesthetized with an intraperitoneal injection of 2,2,2-tribromoethanol (20 mg/100 g b.w.) and then intracardiacally perfused with a 0.09% NaCl solution followed by 4% paraformaldehyde in 0.1 M Sörensen buffer, pH 7.4. Liver samples were kept in the same fixation solution for 2 h at 4°C, dehydrated, and embedded in LR White resin. To reveal nuclear ribonucleoprotein (RNP) constituents, we stained ultrathin sections by the EDTA method.[3] Morphometric analysis was conducted on 90 electron micrographs (×20,000) of hepatocyte nuclei (10 micrographs/animal). The areas of nuclei and nucleoli and of each nucleolar component (FCs, DFC, and GC) were measured by a computer-assisted image analyzer. The nucleoplasmic area and the percentage of FC, DFC, or GC area/nucleolar area were calculated. PGs were counted and their density was expressed as number of PGs/μm^2 of nucleoplasm. The fine distribution of some transcription and splicing factors was investigated by using monoclonal antibodies against polymerase II (Research Diagnostics Inc.), snRNPs (small nuclear RNPs; LabVision), non-snRNP splicing factor SC-35 (Sigma-Aldrich), and the nucleolar protein fibrillarin (Cytoskeleton Inc.), revealed by secondary 12-nm gold-conjugated antibodies (Jackson ImmunoResearch Laboratories Inc.). The labeling density (number of gold grains/μm^2) over cytoplasm, nucleoplasm, and nucleolus was evaluated. Kruskal-Wallis one-way ANOVA test was applied for statistical comparisons.

The results of our study are summarized in TABLE 1. FC size and the percentage of nucleolar surface occupied by FCs significantly decreased during aging and vitamin E deficiency. The percentage of nucleolar surface occupied by GC and DFC remained unchanged in adult and old rats, but in vitamin E–deficient animals GC increased and DFC decreased significantly. PG density was significantly increased in aging and significantly decreased in vitamin E–deficient rats versus the adult controls, respectively. The intranuclear localization of transcription factors was quite similar in adult, old, and vitamin E–deficient rats. However, the quantitative evaluation of immunolabeling revealed that polymerase II and SC-35 significantly decreased in old and vitamin E–deficient rats in comparison with adult animals, whereas snRNPs and fibrillarin did not change between adult and old rats but was significantly lower in vitamin E–deficient rats. The current findings document that nucleoplasmic and nucleolar modifications occur in aging and vitamin E deficiency. We observed that PFs, which represent the *in situ* forms of pre-mRNA transcription and splicing,[4] were very abundant in old rats; however, the low presence of nucleoplasmic transcription and splicing factors (3.07 ± 0.18 grains/μm^2 in old vs. 5.90 ± 0.37 in adult rats for polymerase II, 2.57 ± 0.21 in old vs. 3.10 ± 0.17 in adult rats for snRNPs, and 0.83 ± 0.11 in old vs. 3.43 ± 0.68 in adult rats for SC-35) suggests

TABLE 1. Morphometric and immunolabeling results on RNA structural constituents in aging and vitamin E deficiency: adult (A), old (O), vitamin E–deficient (–E) rats

Nuclear and Nucleolar Parameters

	Nuclear Area (μm^2)	Nucleolar Area (μm^2)	PG density (PG/μm^2)	GC%	DFC%	FC%	FC Area (μm^2)
A	43.45 ± 1.37	1.61 ± 0.20	5.24 ± 0.21•	52.18 ± 2.86	42.76 ± 5.38	5.75 ± 0.74	0.036 ± 0.004
O	44.40 ± 1.48	1.41 ± 0.17	9.18 ± 0.23•	52.91 ± 2.21	44.55 ± 5.40	2.95 ± 0.38*	0.016 ± 0.003*
–E	43.94 ± 1.61	1.62 ± 0.12	2.66 ± 0.11•	76.20 ± 2.80•	22.88 ± 2.29•	3.29 ± 0.68*	0.017 ± 0.001*

Immunolabeling Studies

Anti-polymerase II antibody | Anti-(Sm)snRNP antibody

	Cytoplasm	Nucleoplasm	Nucleolus		Cytoplasm	Nucleoplasm	Nucleolus
A	3.99 ± 1.08	5.90 ± 0.37	0.21 ± 0.11	A	0.70 ± 0.31	3.10 ± 0.17	0.91 ± 0.36
O	1.27 ± 0.45*	3.07 ± 0.18*	0.26 ± 0.13	O	1.16 ± 0.36	2.57 ± 0.21	0.68 ± 0.30
–E	2.63 ± 0.78*	3.44 ± 0.36*	0.29 ± 0.18	–E	0.70 ± 0.36•	1.55 ± 0.17•	0.63 ± 0.22

Anti-SC-35 antibody | Anti-fibrillarin antibody

	Cytoplasm	Nucleoplasm	Nucleolus		Cytoplasm	Nucleoplasm	Nucleolus
A	1.46 ± 0.68	3.43 ± 0.68	0.13 ± 0.08	A	0.64 ± 0.29	13.18 ± 1.59	45.54 ± 9.75
O	0.81 ± 0.36*	0.83 ± 0.11*	0.11 ± 0.06	O	0.76 ± 0.12	12.27 ± 1.89	39.99 ± 9.19
–E	0.74 ± 0.23*	0.82 ± 0.07*	0.27 ± 0.18	–E	0.74 ± 0.38	6.92 ± 1.02•	42.91 ± 9.14

* $P < .05$ vs. the adult value; • $P < .05$ vs. the other values.

that many PFs could be functionally inactive or even abortive ones. The density of PGs also was increased in old versus adult rats. PGs represent storage and/or transport sites of spliced mRNA, and it is documented that an accumulation of PFs and PGs occurs because of altered pre-mRNA processing or impaired intranuclear or nucleus-cytoplasmic transport.[5] Considering the striking abundance of PFs and PGs together with the low amounts of nucleoplasmic transcription and splicing factors, altered mRNA pathways in aging can be reliably suggested. In vitamin E–deficient rats the scant presence of PFs and PGs is matched by the low amounts of transcription and splicing factors found in these animals (3.44 ± 0.36 grains/μm^2 for polymerase II, 1.55 ± 0.17 for snRNPs, and 0.82 ± 0.07 for SC-35), indicating a low mRNA transcriptional rate. Accordingly, the deficiency of α-tocopherol in the diet of young laboratory animals is reported to lead to an impairment of RNA transcription.[6]

With reference to the nucleolus, in both aging and vitamin E deficiency, FCs containing inactive rDNA[7] significantly decrease. In vitamin E–deficient rats, DFC, the site of transcription and early splicing of pre-rRNA,[7,8] and fibrillarin, involved in the early splicing of rRNA, also decreased (6.92 ± 1.02 grains/μm^2 in vitamin E–deficient vs. 13.18 ± 1.59 in adult rats), whereas GC, containing preribosomal particles, increased in vitamin E–deficient animals. All these modifications are consistent with changes in rRNA processing[9] and an altered nucleolar activity in both aging and vitamin E deficiency. Taken together, the current morphometric and immunocytochemical data indicate the occurrence of morphofunctional changes of nuclear constituents during aging and vitamin E deficiency which may correlate with a decay of nuclear responsiveness to cellular metabolic needs and protein synthesis.[10] Considering the antioxidant action of α-tocopherol, our data lend further support to the importance of free radical production and control in the aging process.

REFERENCES

1. BURTON, G.W. & K.U. INGOLD. 1989. Vitamin E as in vitro and in vivo antioxidant. Ann. N.Y. Acad. Sci. **570:** 7–22.
2. BERTONI-FREDDARI, C., P. FATTORETTI, U. CASELLI, et al. 1995. Vitamin E deficiency as a model of precocious brain aging: assessment by X-ray analysis and morphometry. Scanning Microsc. **9:** 289–302.
3. BERNHARD, W. 1969. A new staining procedure for electron microscopic cytology. J. Ultrastruct. Res. **27:** 250–265.
4. FAKAN, S. 1994. Perichromatin fibrils are in situ forms of nascent transcriptions. Trends Cell Biol. **4:** 86–90.
5. VAZQUEZ-NIN, G.H., O.M. ECHEVERRIA & J. PEDRON. 1979. Effects of estradiol on the ribonucleoprotein constituent of the nucleus of endometrial epithelial cells. Biol. Cell. **35:** 221–228.
6. SUMMERFIELD, F.W. & A.L. TAPPEL. 1984. Effects of dietary polyunsaturated fats and vitamin E on ageing and peroxidative damage to DNA. Arch. Biochem. Biophys. **233:** 408–416.
7. BIGGIOGERA, M., M. MALATESTA, S. ABOLHASSANI-DADRAS, et al. 2001. Revealing the unseen: the organizer region of the nucleolus. J. Cell Sci. **114:** 3199–3205.
8. CMARKO, D., P.J. VERSCHURE, L.I. ROTHBLUM, et al. 2000. Ultrastructural analysis of nucleolar transcription in cells microinjected with 5-bromo-UTP. Histochem. Cell Biol. **113:** 181–187.
9. SCHWARZACHER, H.G. & F. WACHTLER. 1993. The nucleolus. Anat. Embryol. **188:** 515–536.
10. FRAGA, C.G., R. ZAMORA & A.L. TAPPEL. 1989. Damage to protein synthesis concurrent with lipid peroxidation in rat liver slices: effect of halogenated compounds, peroxides, and vitamin E. Arch. Biochem. Biophys. **270:** 84–91.

Senescence Marker Protein–30 Knockout Mouse as an Aging Model

NAOKI MARUYAMA, AKIHITO ISHIGAMI, MASASHI KURAMOTO, SETSUKO HANDA, SACHIHO KUBO, TOSHIYUKI IMASAWA, KUNIAKI SEYAMA, TATSUO SHIMOSAWA, AND YASUSHI KASAHARA

Department of Molecular Pathology, Tokyo Metropolitan Institute of Gerontology, Tokyo, Japan

ABSTRACT: A mouse strain lacking SMP30 can be regarded as a strain showing ultimate decrease of the SMP30 molecule. After three months of age, SMP30-KO mice had an increased mortality rate, compared with the SMP30-WT mice, all of which remained alive. Electron microscopic observation of the hepatocytes from 12-month-old SMP30-KO mice revealed many empty vacuoles, presumably lipid droplets, abnormally enlarged mitochondria with indistinct cristae, and exceptionally large lysosomes filled with electron-dense bodies. The total hepatic triglyceride concentration of SMP30-KO mice was approximately 3.6-fold higher than that of the age-matched wild type. Similarly, the total hepatic cholesterol of SMP30-KO mice reached an approximate 3.3-fold greater value than that of the comparative group. Total hepatic phospholipids of SMP30-KO mice achieved an approximately 3.7-fold higher level compared with that of the wild-type mice. The cells from SMP30-KO mice were sensitive to apoptotic reagents. Those results supported the idea that SMP30 has an antiapoptotic function with wide spectrum. These findings indicate that SMP30-KO mice are highly susceptible to various harmful reagents. This strain might be a useful tool for aging and biological monitoring.

KEYWORDS: SMP30; SMP30-KO; aging; life span

INTRODUCTION

During a survey of age-associated changes in soluble proteins of rat liver, we discovered a novel molecule that is designated as senescence marker protein–30 (SMP30).[1] Expression of SMP30 is decreased with aging in a sex-independent manner. The transcripts have been detected in multiple tissues, including the liver, kidney, brain, lung, adrenal gland, stomach, ovary, uterus, testis, and epidermis. The amino acid alignment of SMP30 from various animal species revealed a highly conserved structure.[2] This trait suggests that SMP30 may have important biological roles.

Address for correspondence: Naoki Maruyama, M.D., Department of Molecular Pathology, Tokyo Metropolitan Institute of Gerontology, 35-2 Sakaecho, Itabashi-ku, Tokyo 173-0015 Japan.
maruyama@center.tmig.or.jp

ESTABLISHMENT OF SMP30 KNOCKOUT MOUSE

To analyze the functions of SMP30, we established a mouse strain lacking SMP30. The SMP30 knockout (SMP30-KO) mouse can be regarded as a strain showing the ultimate decrease of the SMP30 molecule. We destroyed the third exon of SMP30 gene on the X chromosome.[3] Using Western blot analysis, we found that SMP30-KO mice showed a complete lack of SMP30. Heterozygous female mice showed mosaic expression of SMP30 in liver because of the X chromosome inactivation of the gene. This feature is critical in the clinical application. In heterozygous mice, half of the cells lack SMP30.

SHORT LIFE SPAN IN SMP30-KO MICE

We evaluated the weight and life span of SMP30-KO mice. Comparison of body weights showed that SMP30-KO mice weighed ~20% less than wild-type (SMP30-WT) mice. At 3, 6, and 12 months of age, the mean body weights of SMP30-KO mice were approximately 10, 15, and 20% lower than that of SMP30-WT mice, respectively. After 3 months of age, SMP30-KO mice had an increased mortality rate, compared with the SMP30-WT mice, all of which remained alive. Subsequently, the cumulative survival period of SMP30-KO mice gradually decreased. The 50% survival rate of these SMP30-KO mice was ~6 months. Although pathological analysis during the survival interval of SMP30-KO mice uncovered no obvious abnormalities, immediate postmortem examination revealed marked atrophy in almost all their abdominal organs.

MORPHOROLOGICAL FEATURES IN LIVER

Electron microscopic observation of the hepatocytes from 12-month-old SMP30-KO mice revealed many large and small empty vacuoles, presumably lipid droplets, abnormally enlarged mitochondria with indistinct cristae, and exceptionally large lysosomes filled with electron-dense bodies. Moreover, no well-developed, rough-surfaced endoplasmic reticulum was apparent in SMP30-KO hepatocytes. The large lipid droplets and abnormal mitochondria and lysosomes of SMP30-KO were not found in hepatocytes from 12-month-old wild-type mice.

Liver specimens from SMP30-KO and wild-type mice sampled at 3, 6, and 12 months of age were stained with Sudan black B. Black lipid-stained droplets were found around the central vein in livers from SMP30-KO mice but were not nearly as visible in livers from the wild type. Moreover, the size and number of lipid droplets were markedly increased with aging in livers from SMP30-KO mice. Of added interest, the central vein in livers from SMP30-KO mice enlarged markedly in diameter with aging when compared with those of wild-type mice.

ACCUMULATION OF LIPID CONTENTS IN LIVER

To determine intracellular neutral lipid concentrations, we extracted total lipids from the livers of SMP30-KO and wild-type mice at 12 months of age. Total triglyceride and cholesterol amounts were quantified by enzymatic methods. The total hepatic triglyceride concentration of SMP30-KO mice was approximately 3.6-fold higher than that of the age-matched wild type. Similarly, the total hepatic cholesterol of SMP30-KO mice reached an approximate 3.3-fold greater value than that of the comparative group. Total hepatic phospholipids of SMP30-KO mice achieved an approximately 3.7-fold higher level compared with that of the wild-type mice. To investigate whether the SMP30 deficiency affected the composition of these phospholipids, we analyzed lipid extracts by thin-layer chromatography. Several phospholipids in livers of SMP30-KO mice reached a noticeably higher level than that in wild-type mice. One of the noteworthy increases was in cardiolipin. This increase might be associated with mitochondria degradation previously described.

MORPHOLOGICAL FEATURES IN KIDNEY

In laboratory animal models, one of the major sites of aging is the kidney. We observed morphological features of kidney in aged SMP30-KO mice (12 months old). The most prominent characteristic was deposition of lipofuscin as an aging marker in renal tubular epithelial cells.[4] In addition electron microscopic analysis showed a marked degeneration of mitochondria like as in liver. Moderate fusion of the foot processes of glomerular epithelial cells also was observed. This feature is associated with albuminuria in aged individuals.[5]

INCREASED SUSCEPTIBILITY TO APOPTOSIS

Our previous study showed that the SMP30 molecule is associated with intracellular calcium homeostasis. We investigated the sensitivity to apoptotic triggering. Treatment of sublethal amounts of anti-Fas antibody induced a massive hemorrhage in SMP30-KO mice liver. Numbers of apoptotic cells indicated by TUNEL assay also were increased. SMP30-WT mice showed almost normal morphological features. Using TNFα and calcium ionophore, we evaluated the sensitivity to other apoptotic reagents. The cells from SMP30-KO mice were sensitive to these reagents. Those results supported the idea that SMP30 has an antiapoptotic function with wide spectrum. When we developed TNFα apoptosis in SMP30-KO mice, only the proapoptotic pathway was activated. The antiapoptotic pathway was not suppressed. Our preliminary studies suggest that antiapoptotic function is dependent on the activities of plasma membrane ATPase enhanced by SMP30 (FIG. 1).[6,7]

APPLICATION OF SMP30-KO MOUSE

SMP30 may protect the cells/organs from various injuries during the life span. This mouse strain is a useful tool for aging studies. There are several reports on the

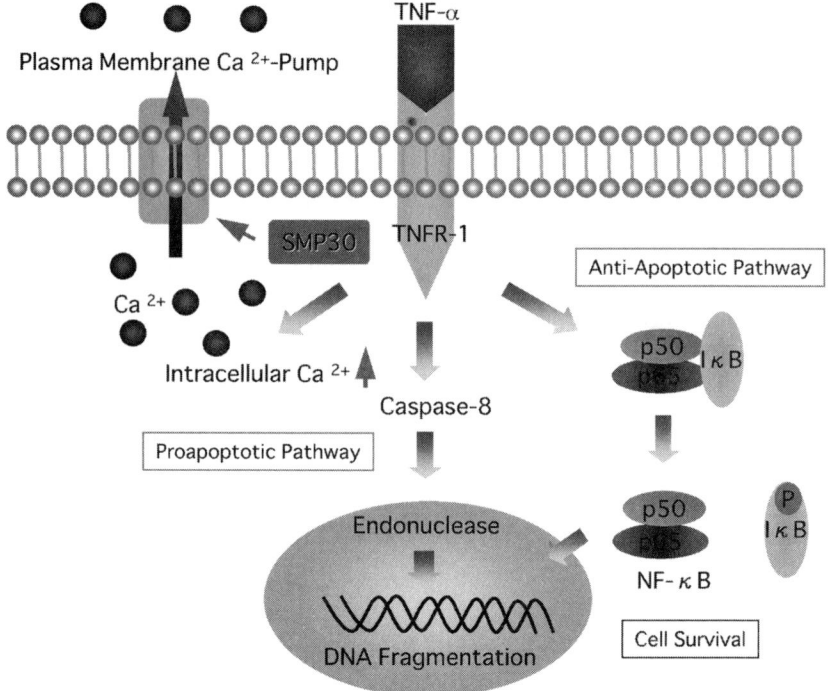

FIGURE 1. Hypothetical role of SMP30 to rescue the cells from apoptosis. TNFα activates the two pathways in the downstream triggering on the membrane. SMP30 does not affect proapoptotic and antiapoptotic pathways. Increase of intracellular calcium level by TNFα stimulation activates the plasma membrane calcium pump to excrete the calcium ion in the presence of SMP30. This mechanism may rescue the cells from apoptosis.

quantitative modulation of the SMP30 expression in animal models. Huang *et al.* reported that cisplatin as an anticancer drug reduces SMP30 expression.[8] They suggested that the decrease of SMP30 is caused by oxidative stress by cisplatin. We evaluated the renal injury induced by cisplatin in SMP30-KO mice. We observed the numerous nuclear degenerations of renal tubular epithelial cell in SMP30-KO mice. Because SMP30 is expressed in bronchial epithelial cells, we have done smoking experiments using SMP30-KO mice. Smoking induced marked apoptosis of bronchial cells in SMP30-KO mice. These findings indicate that SMP30-KO mice are highly susceptible to various harmful reagents. This strain might be a useful tool for biological monitoring.

CONCLUSIONS

SMP30 is pivotal for maintaining cellular function based on intracellular calcium homeostasis. SMP30 has an antiapoptotic function that resulted in keeping cells from various injuries during life span. Several studies suggested that the age-associated decrease of SMP30 is caused by oxidative stress. Establishment of SMP30-KO mice as the ultimate decrease of this molecule revealed the critical roles of this molecule. With aging, most organs of this strain show various phenomena such as lipid deposition, degeneration of mitochondria, prominent lysosomes, and lipofuscin granules in comparison with the wild-type strain. Thus, the SMP30-KO mouse is a useful model for aging studies.

ACKNOWLEDGMENTS

This work was supported by a grant from the Health Science Research Grants for Comprehensive Research on Aging and Health supported by Ministry of Health Labor and Welfare, Japan, and a grant from the Ministry of Education, Science, and Culture, Japan.

REFERENCES

1. FUJITA, T., T. SHIRASAWA, K. UCHIDA, et al. 1992. Isolation of cDNA clone encoding rat senescence marker protein-30 (SMP30) and its tissue distribution. Biochim. Biophys. Acta **1132:** 297–305.
2. FUJITA, T., J.T. MANDEL, T. SHIRASAWA, et al. 1995. Isolation cDNA clone encoding human senescence marker protein-30 (SMP30) and its location on the X chromosome. Biochim. Biophys. Acta **1263:** 249–252.
3. ISHIGAMI, A., T. FUJITA, S. HANDA, et al. 2002. Senescence marker protein-30 knockout mouse liver is highly susceptible to TNF-α- and Fas-mediated apoptosis. Am. J. Pathol. **161:** 1273–1281.
4. MELK, A., W. KITTIKOWIT, I. SANDHU, et al. 2003. Cell senescence in rat kidneys in vivo increases with growth and age despite lack of telomere shortening. Kidney Int. **63:** 2134–2143.
5. YUMURA, W., N. SUGINO, R. NAGASAWA, et al. 1989. Age-associated changes in renal glomeruli of mice. Exp. Gerontol. **24:** 237–249.
6. FUJITA, T., H. INOUE, T. KITAMURA, et al. 1998. Senescence marker protein-30 (SMP30) rescues cell death by enhancing plasma membrane Ca^{2+}-pumping activity in Hep G2 cells. Biochem. Biophys. Res. Commun. **250:** 374–380.
7. INOUE, H., T. FUJITA, T. KITAMURA, et al. 1999. Senescence marker protein-30 (SMP30) enhances the calcium efflux from renal tubular epithelial cells. Clin. Exp. Nephrol. **3:** 261–267.
8. HUANG, Q., R.T. DUNN, II, S. JAYADEV, et al. 2001. Assessment of cisplatin-induced nephrotoxicity by microarray technology. Toxicol. Sci. **63:** 196–207.

Lack of Correlation between Mitochondrial Reactive Oxygen Species Production and Life Span in *Drosophila*

SATOMI MIWA,[a] KUMARS RIYAHI,[b] LINDA PARTRIDGE,[b] AND MARTIN D. BRAND[a]

[a]*MRC Dunn Human Nutrition Unit, Hills Road, Cambridge CB2 2XY, United Kingdom*

[b]*Department of Biology, University College London, Gower Street, London WC1E 6BT, United Kingdom*

ABSTRACT: The free radical theory of aging proposes that mitochondrial production of reactive oxygen species (ROS) determines the rate of aging. Supporting this hypothesis, longer-lived species produce fewer ROS than shorter-lived ones, and calorically restricted rodents live longer and produce fewer ROS than controls. We studied such correlation in *Drosophila melanogaster* in caloric restriction and in mutant flies overexpressing the mitochondrial adenine nucleotide translocase (ANT). Caloric restriction extended life span, but there was no significant difference in mitochondrial ROS production compared with controls. ANT overexpressers had significantly lower ROS production (because they had lower membrane potential), but their life span was not extended compared to wild type. Our results show two examples in which mitochondrial ROS production and life span are not correlated.

KEYWORDS: mitochondria; *Drosophila*; ROS; life span

The life span of an organism can be influenced by genetic and environmental factors. With advances in scientific knowledge, life span has been successfully manipulated in model organisms, such as worms and flies, by genetic engineering. It also has been discovered that various environmental factors, such as temperature and diet, can modify life span in laboratory animals. Despite such knowledge and considerable research effort, the factors that control aging and cause death are poorly understood. The free radical theory of aging is currently the most broadly accepted postulation to explain causal factors of aging; reactive oxygen species (ROS) produced by mitochondria as by-products of normal aerobic respiration can attack and damage surrounding macromolecules, and accumulation of such damage is thought to be responsible for aging and degenerative diseases.[1,2] This idea was first presented almost 50 years ago, but it has still not been proved despite several lines of supportive experimental evidence. They include the observations that longer lived species have lower mitochondrial ROS production than shorter lived species,[3–6] and rodents

Address for correspondence: Satomi Miwa, MRC Dunn Human Nutrition Unit, Hills Road, Cambridge CB2 2XY, UK. Voice: +44-1223-252-806; fax: +44-1223-252-805.
sm@mrc-dunn.cam.ac.uk

placed under caloric restriction (CR), which extends life span in a variety of species, have lower mitochondrial ROS production and rates of accumulation of oxidatively damaged molecules than controls.[7,8] Accordingly, it is widely assumed that mitochondrial ROS production is an important determinant of life span.

However, the available data are merely correlative and do not provide information on causality, which is required to verify the theory. Nonetheless, if the theory is correct, the following should be satisfied: (1) Organisms with experimentally increased life span should have lower mitochondrial ROS production compared with controls. (2) Experimentally lowered mitochondrial ROS production should increase life span.

The fruitfly, *Drosophila melanogaster*, is an excellent model organism with which to study aging. The flies are cheap and easy to culture and have a short life span, and their tissues mostly consist of postmitotic cells, which is important if one wants to study the effects of aging on tissues. They also have a well-defined genetic background, and a variety of mutants with altered life span are available.

We recently have characterized mitochondrial ROS production by *Drosophila* mitochondria.[9] Rates of ROS production in isolated *Drosophila* flight muscle mitochondria were measured fluorometrically as hydrogen peroxide. Using glycerol 3-phosphate as a physiological substrate, complex I and glycerol 3-phosphate dehydrogenase produced ROS under native conditions (i.e., without inhibitors). Approximately one-third of total ROS was from complex I, following reversed electron flow, and was exclusively directed to the matrix side of the mitochondrial inner membrane. This component was particularly sensitive to a small decrease in membrane potential, because reversed electron flow is heavily dependent on proton motive force. The remainder was from glycerol 3-phosphate dehydrogenase, which produced ROS toward the cytosolic side of the membrane, but some appeared on the matrix side. There was no detectable native ROS production with complex I–linked substrate (pyruvate plus proline). In addition, center *o* of complex III, when fully reduced by addition of antimycin A, had a capacity to produce ROS.

To test the above two statements, we studied the relationship between life span and mitochondrial ROS production in flies using two different models, namely, the CR model and the adenine nucleotide translocase (ANT) overexpresser model.

ANIMALS WITH EXPERIMENTALLY INCREASED LIFE SPAN SHOULD HAVE LOWER MITOCHONDRIAL ROS PRODUCTION COMPARED WITH CONTROLS (CR MODEL)

CR in flies is performed by food dilution.[10] Soon after hatching, female flies were divided into two groups; one on a CR diet (0.65 times normal laboratory food concentration) and the other on a control (ad libitum, AL) diet (1.5 times normal laboratory food concentration). The CR group showed increased mean and maximum life span compared with the AL group. Mitochondrial ROS production was measured from the two groups at three time points: 10, 20, and 30 days. With glycerol 3-phosphate as substrate, there was no significant difference in native ROS production between the CR and control groups at any time points. Thus, extension of life span was not necessarily linked to decreased mitochondrial ROS production in flies.

EXPERIMENTALLY LOWERED MITOCHONDRIAL ROS PRODUCTION SHOULD INCREASE THE ANIMAL'S LIFE SPAN (ANT OVEREXPRESSER MODEL)

ANT overexpression in flies increases the proton conductance of the mitochondrial inner membrane and appears to change mitochondrial membrane potentials (unpublished observation). Because one of the factors affecting *in vitro* ROS production in mitochondria is membrane potential, it is predicted that mitochondrial ROS production in flies overexpressing ANT will be lower. We compared mitochondrial ROS production between wild-type flies and two different lines of ANT overexpressing flies. Both of the ANT overexpresser groups had significantly lower mitochondrial ROS production compared with wild-type controls. There was no difference in mitochondrial ROS production between the two ANT overexpresser groups. They had almost identical mean and maximum life spans; however, they were shorter than those of wild-type controls. It is not known whether the mutants aged faster or whether the mutations *per se* were detrimental to health and caused premature death, independent of aging. However, the results suggest that decreased mitochondrial ROS production does not necessarily cause life span extension in flies.

Overall, our results provide two examples in which mitochondrial ROS production and life span are not correlated, weakening the hypothesis that mitochondrial ROS production is an important determinant of life span. Perhaps a distinction between aging and life span may be important to interpret our result: aging might still be dependent on mitochondrial ROS production, whereas life span may not. Furthermore, this study was conducted in isolated mitochondria, which may not necessarily reflect their *in vivo* environment; therefore, investigation of cellular or *in vivo* ROS production may prove enlightening.

REFERENCES

1. SOHAL, R.S. & R. WEINDRUCH. 1996. Oxidative stress, caloric restriction, and aging. Science **273:** 59–63.
2. SHIGENAGA, M.K., T.M. HAGEN & B.N. AMES. 1994. Oxidative damage and mitochondrial decay in aging. Proc. Natl. Acad. Sci. USA **91:** 10771–10778.
3. SOHAL, R.S., I. SVENSSON & U.T. BRUNK. 1990. Hydrogen peroxide production by liver mitochondria in different species. Mech. Ageing Dev. **53:** 209–215.
4. SOHAL, R.S., L.A. ARNOLD & B.H. SOHAL. 1990. Age-related changes in antioxidant enzymes and prooxidant generation in tissues of the rat with special reference to parameters in two insect species. Free. Radic. Biol. Med. **9:** 495–500.
5. BARJA, G. 1998. Mitochondrial free radical production and aging in mammals and birds. Ann. N.Y. Acad. Sci. **854:** 224–238.
6. KU, H.H., U.T. BRUNK & R.S. SOHAL. 1993. Relationship between mitochondrial superoxide and hydrogen peroxide production and longevity of mammalian species. Free. Radic. Biol. Med. **15:** 621–627.
7. LOPEZ-TORRES, M., R. GREDILLA, A. SANZ & G. BARJA. 2002. Influence of aging and long-term caloric restriction on oxygen radical generation and oxidative DNA damage in rat liver mitochondria. Free. Radic. Biol. Med. **32:** 882–889.
8. SOHAL, R.S., H.H. KU, S. AGARWAL, *et al.* 1994. Oxidative damage, mitochondrial oxidant generation and antioxidant defenses during aging and in response to food restriction in the mouse. Mech. Ageing Dev. **74:** 121–133.

9. MIWA, S., J. ST-PIERRE, L. PARTRIDGE & M.D. BRAND. 2003. Superoxide and hydrogen peroxide production by *Drosophila* mitochondria. Free. Radic. Biol. Med. **35:** 938–948.
10. CHAPMAN, T. & L. PARTRIDGE. 1996. Female fitness in *Drosophila melanogaster*: an interaction between the effect of nutrition and of encounter rate with males. Proc. R. Soc. Lond. B Biol. Sci. **263:** 755–759.

Malondialdehyde and Measures of Antioxidant Activity in Subjects from the Belfast Elderly Longitudinal Free-Living Aging Study

I. M. REA,[a] D. McMASTER,[b] J. DONNELLY,[a] L. T. McGRATH,[a] AND I. S. YOUNG[c]

[a]Department of Geriatric Medicine, Queens University,
Belfast BT9 7BL, United Kingdom

[b]Department of Medicine, Queens University, Belfast BT9 7BL, United Kingdom

[c]Department of Clinical Chemistry, Queens University, Belfast BT9 7BL, United Kingdom

ABSTRACT: Glutathione and glutathione peroxidase activity are important components in the complex body defense against oxidative damage. In this study, we have measured malondialdehyde (MDA) as a marker of oxidative stress, the antioxidant glutathione (GSH), and activity of the antioxidant enzyme (GSHPx), in a cohort of free-living elderly subjects from the Belfast Elderly Longitudinal Free-living Aging STudy (BELFAST), hypothesizing that free-living Senieur-approximated nonagenarians might demonstrate enhanced antioxidant defense mechanisms. The main finding in the BELFAST octo/nonagenarians was that plasma antioxidant glutathione increased in nonagenarian compared with septo/octogenarian subjects ($P = .015$), whereas conversely antioxidant glutathione peroxidase activity fell in the nonagenarian group ($P < .0001$). In the same subject group, malondialdehyde, a measure of lipid peroxidation, showed no change across the age groups ($P = .73$). These results might overall represent a situation in which elderly survivors in the BELFAST study have evolved a sort of free radical/antioxidant equilibrium as a mechanism of successful aging.

KEYWORDS: aging; glutathione; glutathione peroxidase; malondialdehyde

INTRODUCTION

The body has evolved a complex defense strategy to minimize the damaging effects of various oxidants. Central to this defense is a wide array of nonenzymatic and enzymatic antioxidant defenses, including glutathione and glutathione peroxidase activity which can protect against oxidative damage to lipids, proteins, and DNA. Accumulating evidence suggests that alterations in these defensive systems may contribute to the development of chronic diseases such as atherosclerosis and neurodegenerative disorders.

Address for correspondence: Dr. I. M. Rea, Department of Geriatric Medicine, Whitla Medical Building, Queens University Belfast, Belfast BT9 7BL, United Kingdom. Voice: +44-289-027-2156; fax: +44-289-032-5839.
i.rea@qub.ac.uk

One of the most frequently used biomarkers giving an indication of overall lipid peroxidation is malondialdehyde (MDA). Because cellular membranes house the production apparatus of oxyradicals and because membranes suffer damage from these radicals, modification of membrane lipids may play a role in aging. Although the relationships between lipid peroxidation and aging have been investigated, the studies have produced conflicting results. Glutathione (GSH) is a ubiquitous cellular antioxidant with physiological functions including protecting cells against damaging reactive oxygen species, detoxifing drugs, and maintaining red cell membrane stability. Glutathione depletion can enhance oxidative stress which has been implicated in normal aging and in neurodegenerative disorders. Naturally occurring glutathione is decreased in models of aging and correction of low tissue glutathione increased longevity.[1] Glutathione peroxidase (GSHPx), one of the most prolific and effective antioxidant enzymes, is a selenium-dependent enzyme which catalyzes the removal of hydrogen peroxide using GSH, thus protecting cells, including endothelial cells against oxidative damage.

In this study, we have measured MDA as a measure of oxidative stress, the antioxidant GSH, and the antioxidant enzyme GSHPx in a cohort of free-living elderly from the Belfast Elderly Longitudinal Free-Living Aging Study (BELFAST),[2] hypothesizing that free-living "Senieur"-approximated[3] nonagenarians might demonstrate enhanced antioxidant defense mechanisms.

METHODS

Subjects

Elderly subjects were an early consecutive cohort enlisted from the BELFAST study, aged 65–100 years of age.[2] Glutathione peroxidase activity was measured in 160 subjects (40 subjects >90 years, 89 subjects 80–80 years, 31 subjects 70–79 years), malondialdehyde in 94 subjects (38 subjects >90 years, 17 subjects 80–89 years, 39 subjects 65–79 years), and glutathione in 125 subjects (39 subjects >90 years, 46 subjects 80–89 years, 40 subjects 70–79 years).

Malondialdehyde

Fasting heparinized whole blood was centrifuged, and lipoproteins were precipitated, aliquoted, and stored at −70°C. Lipid peroxidation was measured by thiobarbituric acid reactive substances (TBARS) and spectrophotometry.[4]

GSH

Blood samples, collected into metaphosphoric acid–containing tubes, were transported in liquid nitrogen and stored at −7°C until analysis by high-performance liquid chromatography.

Glutathione Peroxidase

GSHPx was measured in serum using a modification of the coupled assay of Paglia and Valentine as described by McMaster et al.[5]

TABLE 1. Serum measurements of malondialdehyde (MDA), glutathione (GSH), and glutathione peroxidase activity (GSHPx) in elderly subjects from the BELFAST study

Age group	65–79 yr	80–89 yr	>90 yr	ANOVA
MDA (94)	1.28 (0.68)	1.33 (0.49)	1.21 (0.47)	$P = .73$
GSH (125)	9.4 (1.7)	9.0 (2.1)	10.8 (2.3)	$P = .015$
GSHPx (160)	271.7 (81.3)	252.9 (67.0)	229.9 (61.5)	$P = .0001$

RESULTS

The results for serum malondialdehyde, glutathione, and glutathione peroxidase activity for the various age groups are shown in TABLE 1 with statistical analysis across the age groups by ANOVA.

DISCUSSION

The main finding in the BELFAST study was that plasma antioxidant glutathione increased in nonagenarians compared to septo/octogenarians, whereas conversely antioxidant glutathione peroxidase activity fell in the oldest group. In the same subject group, malondialdehyde, a measure of lipid peroxidation, showed no change across the age groups.

It has been speculated that glutathione status could be an indicator of health and functional age. In a study of women aged 60–101 years rigorously selected for high health status,[6] all had high blood glutathione levels similar to our nonagenarian group. In a second study, Julius et al.[7] reported that glutathione concentration correlated positively with age and good health. In this and other studies, people with chronic conditions such as diabetes had lower levels than those with no disease. These studies, however, do not accord with animal studies which showed that glutathione decreased with age.

There is conflicting evidence as to the effect of increasing age on GSHPx activity. In the French PAQUID study,[8] there was no change in GSHPx with age. In institutionalized and presumably frailer old subjects, Ducros[9] showed a decline in GSHPx with age which is similar to findings in our apparently well free-living nonagenarians in Belfast. However, an important question is the relative importance of serum GSHPx (measured in this study) versus whole-blood GSHPx, because GSHPx in red blood cells provides >95% of GSHPx-related antioxidant activity.

Increased lipid peroxidation and decreased antioxidant protection frequently occur but are not universal features of aging. In interpreting the evidence of other published MDA studies, we found that the size of the studies, the selection of subjects, and the quality of the MDA assay must be considered. Similar to our study in Belfast, studies of elderly cohorts in Paris, Turkey, and Spain showed no change in lipid peroxidation with age, whereas in the large EVA study[10] TBARS increased.

Persons older than 85 years are the fastest growing sector of Western societies, yet we know relatively little about this group. In this preliminary cross-sectional study of elderly subjects living in Belfast, serum glutathione was higher in nonagenarians, and the TBARs measure of lipid peroxidation was unchanged but serum glutathione peroxidase activity decreased. It is unclear whether these changes represent a physiological age-related change or whether they could be harmful. Conversely, they might represent a situation in which elderly survivors are in a sort of equilibrium, with lipid peroxidation stable, the antioxidant glutathione uncompromised, and glutathione peroxidase activity low, because the hosts remain in free radical/antioxidant balance and have adapted a nonthreatening equilibrium as a mechanism for successful survival.

REFERENCES

1. RITCHIE, J.P., JR., B.J. MILLS & C.A. LANG. 1987. Correction of a glutathione deficiency in ageing mosquito increases in longevity. Proc. Soc. Exp. Biol. Med. **184:** 113–117.
2. REA, I.M., D. MCMASTER, J.V. WOODSIDE, et al. 2000. Community-living nonagenarians in Northern Ireland have lower plasma homocysteine but similar methylenetetrahydrofolate reductase thermolabile genotype prevalence compared to 70–89-year-old subjects. Atherosclerosis **149:** 207–214.
3. LIGTHART, G.L., J.X. CORBERAND, C. FOURNIER, et al. 1984. Admission criteria for immunogerontological studies in man. The Senieur protocol. Mech. Ageing Dev. **28:** 47–55.
4. YOUNG, I.S & E.R. TRIMBLE. 1991. Measurement of malondialdehyde in plasma by high performance liquid chromatography with fluorimetric detection. Ann. Clin. Biochem. **28:** 504–508.
5. MCMASTER, D., D. BELL, P. ANDERSON, et al. 1980. Automated measurements of 2 indicators of human selenium status and applicability to population studies. Clin. Chem. **36:** 211–216.
6. LANG, C.A., B.J. MILLS, H.L. LANG, et al. 2002. High blood glutathione levels accompany excellent physical and mental health in women ages 60 to 103 years. J. Lab. Clin. Med. **140(6):** 413–417.
7. JULIUS, M., C.A. LANG, L. GLEIBERMAN, et al. 1994. Glutathione and morbidity in a community-based study of elderly. J. Clin. Epidemiol. **47:** 1021–1026.
8. BERR, C., A. NICOLE, J. GODIN, et al. 1993. Selenium and oxygen-metabolising enzymes in elderly community residents. A pilot epidemiological study. J. Am. Geriatr. Soc. **41:** 143–148.
9. DUCROS, V., P. FAURE, M. FERRY, et al. 1997. The sizes and the exchangeable pools of selenium in elderly women and their relation to institutionalization. Br. J. Nutr. **78:** 379–396.
10. COUDRAY, C., A.M. ROUSSEL, J. ARMAUD, et al. 1997. Selenium and antioxidant vitamin and lipoperoxidation levels in presaging French population. EVA study group Etude de viellessment arteriel. Biol. Trace Elem. Res. **57:** 183–190.

Regenerative Medicine: Antagonic-Stress® Therapy in Distress and Aging

I. Preclinical Synthesis—2003

D. RIGA,[a] S. RIGA,[a] AND F. SCHNEIDER[b]

[a]*Department of Stress Research and Prophylaxis, "Al. Obregia" Clinical Hospital of Psychiatry, RO-041914 Bucharest 8, Romania*

[b]*Center for Applied Physiology and Molecular Biology, "Vasile Goldis" Western University, RO-310396 Arad, Romania*

ABSTRACT: Repetitive and cumulative distress (acute and/or chronic, psychic and/or biologic) and aging processes (impairment phenomena, agglomerated, and accumulated with the passing of life and senescence periods), as well as distress ⇔ aging reciprocal amplification–accelerating–aggravation relationships require strong and rational (etiopathogenic) therapeutic interventions. Therefore, the drug, Antagonic-Stress® (AS)—a new integrative therapy, with specific synergistic formula, being patented worldwide—becomes an important solution in distress, senescence, and their related pathologies. In acute (contention) stress, AS treatment significantly decreased rat mortality, number and surface of stomach ulcerations, nonesterified fatty acids (NEFAs), and increased superoxide dismutase (SOD) from blood. In chronic psychic stress, live nerve cells selectively isolated from rat cerebral cortex were highly protected by the administration of AS. In addition, antistress and antiaging homeostatic actions of AS were demonstrated in accelerated senescence (aging + distress) at multiple brain levels: on functional anabolism [increase in total ribonucleic acids (RNA), total proteins (TP), and water-soluble proteins (WSP)]; on functional catabolism [decrease in water-insoluble proteins (WIP)]; on structural anabolism (increased regeneration of free ribosomes, rough endoplasmic reticulum, mitochondria, and Nissl bodies); on structural catabolism (lipofuscinolysis and ceroidolysis, neurono-glial transfer of lipopigment continuously processed and dissoluted, and finally capillary elimination). Preclinical research with AS demonstrated important regenerative processes in the key organs (liver, heart, and brain), which mostly suffer due to both distress and senescence.

KEYWORDS: regenerative medicine; preclinical studies; synthesis; antistress and antiaging therapy

Address for correspondence: D. Riga, Department of Stress Research and Prophylaxis, "Al. Obregia" Clinical Hospital of Psychiatry, 10 Berceni Road, Sector 4, RO-041914 Bucharest 8, Romania. Voice: +40-21-461-0755; fax: +40-21-230-9579.
d_s_riga@yahoo.com

INTRODUCTION

Experimental researches in both distress and aging demonstrated certain common and simultaneous mechanisms: hypoanabolism, hypercatabolism, and accumulation of insoluble products of oxidative stress catabolism. Decrease in RNA and protein biosynthesis and accumulation of lipofuscin (age)/ceroid pigments (final product of free radical attack and oxidative stress) are common in animals as well as in humans and are more evident in neurons. Therefore, distress and aging become antihomeostatic, incapacitating and impairment phenomena in the whole body, but especially in the brain, because distress accelerates the aging processes, aging decreases the ability to survive stress, distress (hyperadrenergic state) plays an important role in cerebral and cardiac atherogenesis, and distress (by sustained elevated glucocorticoids) causes neurodegeneration in the hippocampus during aging. In addition, the cumulative consequences of distress with aging and the distress ⇔ aging reciprocal amplification-accelerating relationships permanently yield negative results and reciprocal increases in their severity.

According to this etiopathologic approach, for rational therapeutic intervention in distress and aging processes, we have developed an advanced integrative therapy with specific synergistic formula, the drug, Antagonic-Stress® (AS), which is protected worldwide by 25 patents.[1]

Therefore, AS can be a complementary alternative to the next future therapies—strategies for engineered negligible senescence.[2]

MATERIALS AND METHODS

Laboratory animals (rats, mice, and guinea pigs) were divided into normal adult groups (control); groups for distress biology: acute stress, chronic psychic stress, chronic biological stress; groups for brain aging patterns: accelerated aging by chronic sociosensory deprivation; and antistress and antiaging treated groups with AS, and meclofenoxate (MF), orotic acid (OA), nicotinic acid (NA), respectively.

Followed parameters and methodologies were in accordance with distress and aging type:

- For acute stress (psychic ⊕ ulcer ⊕ oxidative), by contention stress, Selye method: animal survival; number, surface, and percentage/surface of gastric ulcerations in ulcer stress; blood nonesterified fatty acids (NEFAs) and superoxide dismutase (SOD) in oxidative stress.

- For chronic psychic stress, by chronic painful emotion, the Desiderato method: selective isolation of live nerve cells (Norton and Poduslo method); neuromorphology (phase-contrast microscopy).

- For accelerated aging (peroxidative ⊕ oxidative stresses), by chronic stress (long-term sociosensory deprivation), and by accumulative consequences of both distresses and aging—**neurobiochemistry:** regional brain nucleic acid assays: total DNA and total RNA; regional brain protein assays: total proteins (TP), water-soluble proteins (WSP), and water-insoluble proteins (WIP); their ratios; **neuromorphology:** qualitative microscopy: light, fluorescence, and

TABLE 1. AS for preclinical research[a]

Bioactive substance	Dose (mg/kg body weight)
2 mL intraperitoneally/rat	
= rapid absorption, correspondent to	
= gastrosoluble capsule in human use	
Meclofenoxate	80
Methionine	50
Magnesium aspartate	30
Fructose	3
Vitamin B_1	2.5
Vitamin B_6	3.5
Nicotinic acid	4
Zinc sulfate	0.4
2 mL subcutaneously/rat	
= slow absorption, correspondent to	
= enterosoluble capsule in human use	
Orotic acid	50
Fructose	1.5
Nicotinic acid	16
Dipotassium phosphate	12
Magnesium oxide	3.5
Lithium carbonate	0.4
Potassium iodide	0.02

[a]One of the six pharmaceutical examples from patent description; complementary composition administration and absorption: fast + slow; frequency: daily; duration: days–2 months.

- electron microscopies; quantitative microscopy: fluorescence and electron microscopies.
- For chronic biological stress (alcohol consumption ⊕ oxidative stress), by chronic intoxication with ethanol: the same parameters and methods as for accelerated aging.

Composition and administration of the AS[1,3] are presented in TABLE 1.

RESULTS AND DISCUSSION

In acute (contention) stress, AS significantly decreased (to 2.85%), whereas MF (to 12.12%) or NA (to 12.50%) significantly increased rat mortality. AS considerably diminished the ulcerations in number, surface, and percentage/stomach surface, significantly decreased NEFAs (increased by stress), and increased SOD (reduced by stress).[4]

In chronic psychic stress, live nerve cells selectively isolated from rat cerebral cortex (pyramidal neurons and protoplasmic astrocytes) showed wide neurosomal vacuolations and gliosomal tumefaction, with simplification of dendritic arborization, because of the fragility of the neurosomas and gliosomas and of cytomembranes. AS antistress treatment induced protection and stabilization of the neurosomas and gliosomas, as well as of the cytomembranes.[1]

Antistress and antiaging homeostatic actions of AS were demonstrated in accelerated aging (aging + distress) at multiple brain levels—functional anabolism: increase in total RNA, TP, and WSP and in ratios RNA/DNA and RNA/TP; functional catabolism: decrease in WIP and DNA/TP, and in (WIP/TP) × 100; structural anabolism: anabolic revitalization by increased regeneration of free ribosomes, rough endoplasmic reticulum, mitochondria, and Nissl bodies; structural catabolism: lipofuscinolysis/ceroidolysis, neuronoglial transfer, LP continuous processing and dissolution, with finally lysis in endothelial cells and capillary elimination.[1]

Antistress and antiaging treated group with AS presented totally different neuromorphological configurations in comparison with old stressed group (accelerating aging by chronic stress). Extensive perinuclear accumulations and large unipolar and bipolar clusters of neuronal and glial lipofuscin-ceroid pigments (LPs) from the old stressed group, at old stressed group treated with AS, by a marked reduction and lysis, were transformed into scattered structure and smaller blocks.[5]

The AS administration produced an intense, general, and selective decrease of LPs in old stressed animals at brain tissue level. LP lysis was conspicuous in the cerebral cortex (48.1%, 39.6%), the hippocampus (47.5%), the brainstem reticular formation (47.3–37.2%), the hypothalamus (38.8%), and the Purkinje cell layer (34.1%), regions with very strong decreases of LPs.[5]

The same aspects of LP dissolution and LP lysis were confirmed by qualitative[6,7] and quantitative[3] electron microscopy. Decreases in number, area, and complexity of LP conglomerates were observed especially in the neurons, but also in glia cells. In addition, the amplification of LP internal structure with a tendency for dispersal and ultrastructural configuration typical of LP processing were constantly found in neurons.[6] Perineuronal, but especially pericapillary glias constantly showed highly processed LPs by both strong lipofuscinolysis and ceroidolysis actions.[7]

In chronic biological stress, AS antistress, antidamage, antiaging, and regenerative actions were in the same neurobiochemical and neuromorphological directions as in accelerated aging. The differences were in parameters, regions, and intensities.[1]

AS therapeutically activates the natural homeostatic mechanisms: regenerative hyperanabolism; decrease of hypercatabolism and oxidative stress products and damages; and diminution, removal, and elimination of subcellular waste conglomerates.[3]

Moreover, by processing old lysosomes (overloaded with lipofuscin/ceroid pigments) and increase of functional/structural anbolism,[3,5-7] AS becomes an important and efficient therapeutic tool for regeneration and rejuvenation of the lysosomal system.[4]

By its original synergistic biological composition, with new cell-trophic–regenerative and antioxidative-neurometabolic–cerebrovasoactive properties,[1,4,8] AS has concomitant antistress, antiimpairment, and antiaging therapeutic actions.[8-10]

CONCLUSIONS

Independent and the present authors' preclinical studies using the new drug Antagonic-Stress® have proved the following—highly specific, pluripotent, multilevel and conjugated antistress, antidamages, and antiaging actions (AS vs. control:

ulcer/oxidative stresses and brain aging biochemistry/morphology); multiple efficacy and superiority of the AS synergistic formula (multitherapy) vs. monotherapies (MF, OA, NA).

These biogerontological experiments recommend this advanced orthomolecular drug as an innovative strategy in regenerative medicine, as well as for prevention, therapy, and recovery in stress, geriatrics, neuropsychiatry, and related disorders.

REFERENCES

1. RIGA, D. & S. RIGA. 1998–2004. Twenty-five patents worldwide of the Antagonic-Stress® drug: AU Pat. (1998), KR Pat. (1999), EUR Pat. (1999) for 16 Eur. States, RU Pat. (2000), US Pat. (2001), CN Pat. (2001), RO Pat. (2001), CA Pat. (2002), JP Pat. (2003), and BR Pat. (2004).
2. DE GREY, A.D.N.J. et al. 2002. Bioremediation meets biomedicine: therapeutic translation of microbial catabolism to the lysosome. Trends Biotechnol. **20**: 452–455.
3. RIGA, S. & D. RIGA. 1995. An antistress and antiaging neurometabolic therapy. Accelerated lipofuscinolysis and stimulated anabolic regeneration by the Antagonic-Stress synergistic formula. Ann. N.Y. Acad. Sci. **771**: 535–550.
4. RIGA, D. & S. RIGA. 1998. Anti-stress and anti-aging neurometabolic antioxidative therapy. I. Preclinical synthesis. 2nd World Congress Stress. Melbourne, Australia.
5. RIGA, S. & D. RIGA. 1994. Antagonic-Stress: a therapeutic composition for deceleration of aging. I. Brain lipofuscinolytic activity demonstrated by light and fluorescence microscopy. Arch. Gerontol. Geriatr. **19**(Suppl. 4): 217–226.
6. RIGA, D. & S. RIGA. 1994. Antagonic-Stress: a therapeutic composition for deceleration of aging. II. Brain lipofuscinolytic activity demonstrated by electron microscopy. Arch. Gerontol. Geriatr. **19**(Suppl. 4): 227–234.
7. RIGA, D. & S. RIGA. 1995. Brain lipofuscinolysis and ceroidolysis. In Lipofuscin and Ceroid Pigments. State of the Art 1995. K. Kitani, G.O. Ivy & H. Shimasaki, Eds.: 271–280. Karger. Basel, Switzerland.
8. RIGA, D. & S. RIGA. 1998. Correlations between lipofuscin accumulation and aging neuropathology. Ann. N.Y. Acad. Sci. **854**: 495.
9. RIGA, D. & S. RIGA. 2000. Stress, oxidative stress, aging and neuro-psychiatric pathology. In Textbook of Mental Health. Vol. 1. D. Prelipceanu, R. Mihailescu & R. Teodorescu, Eds.: 211–225. Encyclopaedic Press. Bucharest, Romania.
10. RIGA, S., D. RIGA & F. SCHNEIDER. 2003. Prolongevity medicine: Antagonic-Stress® drug in stress, aging, and related diseases. II. Clinical review. Biogerontology **4**(Suppl. 1): 82.

Prolongevity Medicine: Antagonic-Stress® Drug in Distress, Geriatrics, and Related Diseases

II. Clinical Review—2003

S. RIGA,[a] D. RIGA,[a] AND F. SCHNEIDER[b]

[a]*Department of Stress Research and Prophylaxis, "Al. Obregia" Clinical Hospital of Psychiatry, RO-041914 Bucharest 8, Romania*

[b]*Center for Applied Physiology and Molecular Biology, "Vasile Goldis" Western University, RO-310396 Arad, Romania*

ABSTRACT: Distress and senescence, their reciprocal aggravating–quickening connections, and their related pathologies have a large worldwide impact on healthcare systems in this new millennium. For this reason, Antagonic-Stress® (AS)—an advanced integrative therapy, with specific synergistic composition, and patented internationally—represents a significant strategy in health, aging, and longevity. Clinical research with AS proves the drug's efficacy in the management of distress (neurotic, stress-related, and affective disorders; behavioral syndromes associated with physiological disturbances and physical factors; mental and behavioral disorders due to psychoactive substance uses) and psychogeriatrics [organic, including symptomatic, mental disorders (OMD)]. Specific multiaxial psychopathological instruments and psychometric tests in multiple assessments used for gerontopsychiatry demonstrated strong improvements after AS administration in early-moderate stages of Alzheimer or vascular dementia, as well as in other OMD. In addition, comparative clinical studies evinced the superiority of AS (synergistic multitherapy) versus monotherapy [meclofenoxate (MF), piracetam (PA), pyritinol (PT), and nicergoline (NE), respectively]. These comparative clinical trials agreed closely with comparative preclinical research and confirmed AS synergistic homeostatic, adaptogenic, antioxidative, cerebrovascular, neurometabolic, and nootropic actions. Also, the AS protective actions against oxidative stress recommend this orthomolecular therapy in stress, aging, and free radical pathology.

KEYWORDS: prolongevity medicine; clinical studies; synthesis; antistress and antiaging therapy

---

Address for correspondence: S. Riga, Department of Stress Research and Prophylaxis, "Al. Obregia" Clinical Hospital of Psychiatry, 10 Berceni Road, Sector 4, RO-041914 Bucharest 8, Romania. Voice: +40-21-461-0755; fax: +40-21-230-9579.
 d_s_riga@yahoo.com

INTRODUCTION

In a global world, the great increase of distress phenomena and mental disorders (such as depression) and the general extension of total life (aging of populations) become major health problems in all countries. Therefore, the extended incidence and prevalence of stress-dependent disorders (mental and psychosomatic); of chronic, progressive, and degenerative diseases; and of accelerated and pathological aging, age-related impairments, and polypathology of the elderly require new and innovative strategies.

In addition, simultaneous rational therapeutics against distress and aging become necessary because distress is correlated with multiple pathology, accelerated aging, and the expanding vulnerability to stress of the elderly (amplification-aggravating interrelationships) and because the aging process has multicausal/multifactorial etiopathogenic mechanisms. Moreover, aging being a three-stage process, metabolism, damage, and pathology,[1] the efficient interventions in metabolic/subcellular waste levels diminish the aging pathology.

For this reason, we successively developed a new conception and advanced synergistic therapy: Antagonic-Stress® drug (AS), with worldwide international protection by 25 patents.[2]

PATIENTS AND METHODS

Antistress and Antiaging Treatments

AS represents a therapeutic strategy in the management of distress, geriatrics, and related diseases. The advanced technological process for AS manufacturing ensures the pharmaceutical stability, maximum bioavailability, and therapeutic efficiency, with the prolongation of its effects. The bioactive substances with synergistic actions were designed/distributed into complementary compositions/capsules, in two pharmaceutical units: gastrosoluble and enterosoluble[2] (TABLE 1).

TABLE 1. AS complementary composition and pharmaceutical technology: one of six examples from patent description

GASTROsoluble capsule identification color: blue		ENTEROsoluble capsule identification color: yellow	
Aminoethanol phenoxy-acetates	31.0%–33.1%	Hydrooxopyrimidine carboxylates	18.8%–20.0%
Methionine	18.0%–19.1%	Fructose	0.6%–0.7%
Aspartate	9.7%–10.6%	Nicotinic acid with prolonged release	4.1%–5.3%
Fructose	1.1%–1.3%		
Vitamin B$_1$	0.9%–1.3%	Lithium	0.025%–0.033%
Vitamin B$_6$	1.2%–1.5%	Potassium	2.5%–2.9%
Nicotinic acid with fast release	1.1%–1.3%	Magnesium	0.3%–0.4%
		Iodide	0.005%–0.007%
Magnesium	1.2%–1.5%	Monoacide phosphate	2.6%–3.5%
Zinc	0.3%–0.7%		
Sulfate	0.5%–1.0%		

The percentages of the active substances are expressed to 100 g of the minimal active dose/daily (two gastro- and one enterosoluble capsules). The dose is used to prophylactically treat stress and to bring about longevity. The therapeutic and recovery necessary daily dose, as a function of the disease (nature and seriousness), is two to four times the minimal active dose.

Comparative antistress and antiaging treatments were represented by known modern drugs (monotherapy) with multiple actions, nootropic, neurometabolic, psychotonic, scavenger, cerebral vasodilator, and geriatric—meclofenoxate (MF), piracetam (PA), pyritinol (PT), nicergoline (NE)—International Nonproprietary Names (INN) denomination.

CLINICAL DESIGN, ASSESSMENTS, AND STATISTICS

AS drug efficacy in mental and behavioral disorders connected to distress, psychogeriatrics, and related diseases was demonstrated in accordance with the international classification and clinical and diagnostic guidelines: ICD-10, Ch.V(F), WHO, Geneva, 1992; DSM-IV, APA, Washington, 1994, and DSM-IV-TR, APA, Washington, 2000.

Clinical design included double-blind, randomized, and comparative trials: AS versus placebo (PL) and AS versus monotherapy (MF, PA, PT, NE). The homogeneity of all groups was ensured by inclusion, severity, and exclusion criteria. Multiple groups of patients were investigated: adults and old, nonhospitalized (at work/in stress conditions), ambulatory, and hospitalized persons.

For gerontopsychiatry, we used specific multiaxial psychopathological instruments and psychometric tests in multiple assessments: Sandoz Clinical Assessment-Geriatric (SCAG) scale; Self-Assessment Scale-Geriatric (SASG); Hamilton Depression Scale; Hamilton Anxiety Scale; Digit symbol of WAIS; Wechsler Memory Scale (WMS)–memory quotient (MQ); Wechsler Adult Intelligence Scale (WAIS)–intelligence quotient (IQ).

Statistical analysis was made with SPSS package. Multiple comparisons were made by ANOVA (post- vs. pretreatments) and ANCOVA (for different treatments).

RESULTS AND DISCUSSION

AS homeostatic-regenerative antistress/antiaging actions have been confirmed by multiple, comparative, independent, and the present authors' research in preclinical animal studies[3] and also in multicenter clinical human trials[4,5] in stress medicine, as well as in mental, behavioral, and senescence disorders:[6,7] (1) neurotic and stress-related disorders: F43 reaction to severe stress and adjustment disorders (F43.1, F43.2) and F48 other neurotic disorders (F48.0); (2) mood (affective) disorders: F32 depressive episode (F32.0, F32.1, F32.2) and F33 recurrent depressive disorder (F33.0, F33.1, F33.3); (3) behavioral syndromes associated with physiological disturbances and physical factors: F52 sexual dysfunction, not caused by organic disorder or disease (F52.0, F52.1, F52.2, F52.3, F52.5, F52.6); (4) mental and behavioral disorders due to psychoactive substance use: F10–alcohol , F13–sedatives or hypnotics, F15–other stimulants, including caffeine, F17–tobacco/nicotine; (5)

organic, including symptomatic, mental disorders (OMD): F00 dementia in Alzheimer disease (F00.1), F01 vascular dementia (F01.1), F04 organic amnesic syndrome not induced by alcohol/other psychoactive substances, F06 other OMD due to brain damage and dysfunction and to physical disease (F06.32, F06.4, F06.6, F06.7).

A selection of therapeutic results in gerontoneuropsychiatry, Alzheimer dementia with late onset (uncomplicated F00.10/290.00 and with depression F00.13/290.21), demonstrated superiority of AS (synergistic multitherapy) versus geriatric MF and NE monotherapy[8-10] at $P < .05-.001$ significance level (ANCOVA).[9]

Important decrease of geriatric psychopathology: SCAG total score was reduced by (−)25.1 AS, (−)16.3 MF, (−)16.0 NE, from the superior limit of mild to moderate, to mild intensity; comparative remissions in five SCAG subscales scores were as follows—cognitive: (−)5.0AS, (−)4.0MF, (−)3.9NE; interpersonal: (−)6.5AS, (−)3.7MF, (−)4.6NE; affective: (−)5.6AS, (−)3.6MF, (−)3.2NE; apathy: (−)3.5AS, (−)2.4MF, (−)2.2NE; and somatic: (−) 4.4AS, (−)2.6MF, (−)2.1NE. SASG total score and five SASG subscale scores were diminished in the same manner and equivalent intensity.

Significant restoration of psychometric tests: improvements in visual–motor processing attention–concentration and in short-term memory (digit symbol of WAIS) (+)4.0AS, (+)1.6 MF, (+)1.8 NE; were associated with substantial amelioration of the memory–learning process (WMS-MQ) (+)27.3AS, (+)18.1MF, (+)17.2NE; improvements in cognitive performance–general intelligence (WAIS) were as follows—full IQ: (+)21.2AS, (+)7.8MF, (+)10.3NE; performance IQ: (+)23.2AS, (+)9.3MF, (+)9.4NE; verbal IQ: (+)16.7AS, (+)9.1MF, (+)7.5NE; superiority of AS cognitive amelioration was in performance IQ: more than 2.5 times versus MF or NE; in full IQ: more than 2.7 times versus MF, more than 2.1 times versus NE; decreases in the impairment of cognitive functions (deterioration index of WAIS) were (−)8.7AS, (−)4.0MF, (−)5.2NE; superiority in AS reversal of deterioration was more than 2.2 times versus MF, more than 1.7 times versus NE.

CONCLUSIONS

Both patents and preclinical, clinical, comparative, the present authors', and independent studies demonstrated that Antagonic-Stress® is an innovative therapy and a new strategy in stress/aging medicine, for stress-related disorders, psychosomatics, neuropsychiatry, geriatrics, and associated pathology.

Its multiple homeostatic, adaptogenic, antioxidative, cerebrovascular, neurometabolic, and nootropic actions recommend AS, an advanced pluripotent synergistic formula in modern antistress/antiaging therapies, prophylaxis, and recovery, and in regenerative and prolongevity medicine.

REFERENCES

1. DE GREY, A.D.N.J. *et al.* 2002. Time to talk SENS: critiquing the immutability of human aging. Ann. N.Y. Acad. Sci. **959:** 452–462.
2. RIGA, D. & S. RIGA. 1998–2004. Twenty-five patents worldwide of the Antagonic-Stress® drug: AU Pat. (1998), KR Pat. (1999), EUR Pat. (1999) for 16 Eur. States, RU Pat. (2000), US Pat. (2001), CN Pat. (2001), RO Pat. (2001), CA Pat. (2002), JP Pat. (2003), and BR Pat. (2004).

3. RIGA, D., S. RIGA & F. SCHNEIDER. 2003. Regenerative medicine: Antagonic-Stress® therapy in distress and aging. I. Preclinical synthesis—2003. Biogerontology **4**(Suppl. 1): 81.
4. RIGA, S. & D. RIGA. 1998. Nootropic antioxidative therapy in stress, aging and related disorders. II. Clinical review—1998. 2nd World Congress Stress. Melbourne, Australia.
5. RIGA, S. & D. RIGA. 2000. Modern therapies of anti-stress and anti-aging cerebral activation. *In* Textbook of Mental Health. Vol. 1. D. Prelipceanu, R. Mihailescu & R. Teodorescu, Eds.: 415–440. Encyclopaedic Press. Bucharest, Romania.
6. RIGA, S. & D. RIGA. 1997. Antagonic-Stress® a new therapeutic system for anti-aging, anti-impairment and anti-stress management. 16th World Congress International Association of Gerontology (Aging beyond 2000: one world one future). Book of Abstracts, Abst. 653: 215. Adelaide, Australia.
7. RIGA, S. & D. RIGA. 1998. Synergistic multitherapy as rational strategy in aging: multifactorial process. Ann. N.Y. Acad. Sci. **854**: 477.
8. PREDESCU, V. *et al*. 1994. Antagonic-Stress: a new treatment in gerontopsychiatry and for a healthy productive life. Ann. N.Y. Acad. Sci. **717**: 315–331.
9. POPA, R. *et al*. 1994. Antagonic-Stress superiority versus meclofenoxate in gerontopsychiatry (Alzheimer type dementia). Arch. Gerontol. Geriatr. **19**(Suppl. 4): 197–206.
10. SCHNEIDER, F. *et al*. 1994. Superiority of Antagonic-Stress composition versus nicergoline in gerontopsychiatry. Ann. N.Y. Acad. Sci. **717**: 332–342.

Delaying the Mitochondrial Decay of Aging

BRUCE N. AMES

University of California, Berkeley, California 94720, and Children's Hospital Oakland Research Institute, Oakland, California 94609, USA

ABSTRACT: Mitochondrial dysfunction may be a principal underlying event in aging, including the degenerative diseases of aging such as brain degeneration. Mitochondria provide energy for basic metabolic processes, and their decay with age impairs cellular metabolism and leads to cellular decline. Progress over the last decade in delaying the mitochondrial decay of aging is reviewed.

KEYWORDS: acetyl carnitine; lipoic acid; reversing genetic disease; high-dose B-vitamin; vitamin, minerals, and aging; heme deficiency; zinc deficiency; biotin deficiency; vitamin B6; pantothenic acid; copper deficiency

DELAYING THE MITOCHONDRIAL DECAY OF AGING

Oxidative mitochondrial decay is a major contributor to aging.[1–7] We are making progress in reversing some of this decay in older rats by feeding them the normal mitochondrial metabolites acetyl-L-carnitine (ALC) and alpha-lipoic acid (LA). One mechanism is that, with age, increased oxidative damage to protein causes deformation of the structure of key enzymes, with consequent lessening of affinity (K_m) for the enzyme substrate.[8] The effect of age on enzyme binding affinity can be mimicked by reacting it with malondialdehyde (a lipid peroxidation product that increases with age). Feeding the substrate ALC with LA, a mitochondrial antioxidant, restores the velocity of the reaction, K_m for ALC transferase, and mitochondrial function.[8]

In old rats (vs. young rats), mitochondrial membrane potential, cardiolipin level, respiratory control ratio, and cellular O_2 uptake are lower; oxidants/O_2, neuron RNA oxidation, and mutagenic aldehydes from lipid peroxidation are higher.[8–15] Ambulatory activity and cognition decline with age.[14,15] Feeding old rats ALC plus LA for a few weeks restores mitochondrial function, lowers oxidants, neuron RNA oxidation, and mutagenic aldehydes, and increases rat ambulatory activity and cognition (as assayed with the Skinner box and Morris water maze).[8,14,15]

THE K_M CONCEPT AND METABOLISM

As many as one-third of mutations in a gene result in the corresponding enzyme having an increased Michaelis constant, or K_m (decreased binding affinity) for a coenzyme, resulting in a lower rate of reaction.[16] Therefore, the 50 human genetic diseases caused by defective enzymes can be remedied or ameliorated in some carriers by administration of high doses of the B-vitamin component of the corresponding coenzyme, which increases levels of the coenzyme and at least partially restores enzymatic activity.[16] Several single-nucleotide polymorphisms, in which the variant amino acid reduces coenzyme binding and thus enzymatic activity, are likely to be remediable by increasing cellular concentrations of the cofactor through high-dose vitamin therapy. Examples include the (C677T; Ala222Val) methylenetetrahydrofolate reductase (NADPH) and the cofactor FAD (in relation to cardiovascular disease, migraines, and rages); the (C609T; Pro187Ser) mutation in NAD(P):quinone oxidoreductase 1 (NQO1) and FAD (in relation to cancer); the (C131G; Ala44Gly) mutation in glucose-6-phosphate 1-dehydrogenase and NADP (in relation to favism and hemolytic anemia); and the (Glu487Lys) mutation (present in ~50% of Asians) in aldehyde dehydrogenase and NAD (in relation to alcohol intolerance, Alzheimer disease, and cancer). The K_m concept is likely to be relevant not only for human nutrition, but also for ameliorating deformed proteins with altered K_m formed during mitochondrial aging. Feeding a high dose of each B vitamin to humans markedly increases the corresponding coenzyme level in mitochondria as well as cytoplasm.[16]

COMMON MICRONUTRIENT DEFICIENCIES ACCELERATE MITOCHONDRIAL DECAY

Considerable evidence suggests that diets deficient in various micronutrients can accelerate mitochondrial decay and thus contribute to neurodegeneration. We discuss iron, zinc, biotin, vitamin B6, pantothenate, and copper deficiency, in particular. Both iron deficiency and iron excess damage mitochondria and mitochondrial DNA in rats.[17] Approximately two billion people, mainly women and children, are iron deficient. We examined the effects of iron deficiency and supplementation on rats. Mitochondrial functional parameters and mitochondrial DNA (mtDNA) damage were assayed in iron-deficient (≤5 µg/day) and iron-normal (800 µg/day) rats and in both groups after daily high-iron supplementation (8000 µg/day) for 34 days. This high dose is equivalent to the daily dose commonly given to iron-deficient humans. Iron-deficient rats had lower liver mitochondrial respiratory control ratios and increased levels of oxidants in polymorphonuclear leukocytes, as assayed by DCFH ($P < .05$). Rhodamine 123 fluorescence of polymorphonuclear leukocytes also increased ($P < .05$). Lowered respiratory control ratios were found in daily high-iron–supplemented rats regardless of the previous iron status ($P < .05$). mtDNA damage was observed in both iron-deficient rats and rats receiving daily high-iron supplementation, compared with iron-normal rats ($P < .05$). Both inadequate and excessive iron ($10 \times$ nutritional need) cause significant mitochondrial malfunction. Although excess iron has been known to cause oxidative damage, the observation of oxidant-induced damage to mitochondria from iron deficiency has been unrecognized previously. Untreated iron deficiency and excessive-iron supplementation are deleterious and emphasize the importance of maintaining optimal iron intake.[17]

Heme deficiency was shown to selectively interrupt assembly of mitochondrial complex IV in human fibroblasts.[18] Heme deficiency was studied in young and old normal human fibroblasts (IMR90). Regardless of age, heme deficiency increased the steady state level of oxidants and lipid peroxidation and sensitized the cells to fluctuations in intracellular Ca^{2+}. Heme deficiency selectively decreased the activity and protein content of mitochondrial complex IV (cytochrome C oxidase) by 95%, indicating a decrease in successful assembly. Complexes I–III and catalase remained intact under conditions of heme deficiency, whereas ferrochelatase was upregulated. Complex IV is the only heme-protein in the cell that contains heme-α, which may account for its susceptibility. The rate of removal and assembly of complex IV declines with age. The major contribution to heme deficiency is likely to be the worldwide iron deficiency of women and children. Iron deficiency also could contribute to the age-related decline in complex IV in Alzheimer disease patients.[18]

The role of heme and iron-sulfur clusters in mitochondrial biogenesis, maintenance, and decay with age has been reviewed.[19] Mitochondria decay with age from oxidative damage and loss of protective mechanisms. Resistance, repair, and replacement mechanisms are essential for mitochondrial preservation and maintenance. Iron plays an essential role in the maintenance of mitochondria, through its two major functional forms: heme and iron-sulfur clusters. Both iron-based cofactors are formed and used in the mitochondria and then distributed throughout the cell. This is an important function of mitochondria that is not directly related to the production of ATP. Heme and iron-sulfur clusters are important for the normal assembly and for the optimal activity of the electron transfer complexes. Loss of mitochondrial cytochrome C oxidase, integrity of mtDNA, and function can result from abnormal homeostasis of iron.

Heme deficiency may be a factor in the mitochondrial and neuronal decay of aging.[20] Heme, a major functional form of iron in the cell, is synthesized in the mitochondria by ferrochelatase inserting ferrous iron into protoporphyrin IX. Heme deficiency was induced with N-methylprotoporphyrin IX, a selective inhibitor of ferrochelatase, in two human brain cell lines, SHSY5Y (neuroblastoma) and U373 (astrocytoma), as well as in rat primary hippocampal neurons. Heme deficiency in brain cells decreases mitochondrial complex IV, activates nitric oxide synthase, alters amyloid precursor protein, and corrupts iron and zinc homeostasis. The metabolic consequences resulting from heme deficiency seem similar to dysfunctional neurons in patients with Alzheimer disease. Heme-deficient SHSY5Y or U373 cells die when induced to differentiate or to proliferate, respectively. The role of heme in these observations could result from its interaction with heme regulatory motifs in specific proteins or secondary to the compromised mitochondria. Common causes of heme deficiency include aging, deficiency of iron and vitamin B6, and exposure to toxic metals such as aluminum. Iron and B6 deficiencies are especially important because they are widespread, but they are also preventable with supplementation. Iron deficiency in children is associated with difficulties in performing cognitive tasks and retardation in the development of the central nervous system.[21,22] Thus, heme deficiency or dysregulation may be an important and preventable component of the neurodegenerative process.[20]

Zinc deficiency induces oxidant accumulation and oxidative DNA damage, disrupts p53, NFκB, and AP1 DNA-binding, and affects DNA repair in a rat glioma cell line.[23,24] Approximately 10% of the U.S. population ingests <50% of the current recommended daily allowance for zinc. We investigated the effect of zinc deficiency on DNA damage, expression of DNA repair enzymes, and downstream signaling events in a cell culture model. Low zinc inhibited cell growth of rat glioma C6 cells and increased oxidative stress. Low intracellular zinc increased DNA single-strand breaks (comet assay). Zinc-deficient C6 cells also exhibited an increase in the expression of the zinc-containing DNA repair proteins p53 and apurinic endonuclease (APE). Repletion with zinc restored cell growth and reversed DNA damage. APE is a multifunctional protein that not only repairs DNA, but also controls DNA-binding activity of many transcription factors that may be involved in cancer progression. The ability of the transcription factors p53, nuclear factor κB, and activator protein 1 (AP1) to bind to consensus DNA sequences was decreased markedly with zinc deficiency. Thus, low intracellular zinc status causes oxidative DNA damage and induces DNA repair protein expression, but binding of p53 and important downstream signals leading to proper DNA repair are lost without zinc.[23,24] Mitochondrial decay due to heme deficiency is a plausible explanation for the oxidative stress.[23,24] δ-Aminolevulinate dehydratase (δ-ALA-D) contains eight zinc atoms and catalyzes the asymmetric condensation of two δ–aminolevulinic acids (δ-ALA) molecules to yield porphobilinogen in the cytoplasm (43), an intermediate in heme biosynthesis. Deficiency of zinc has been linked to cognitive defects in humans.[25]

Biotin deficiency, which is quite common in the population, especially during pregnancy,[26,27] also causes decline in mitochondrial function and oxidant leakage (Atamna, Erlitski, and Ames, in preparation). Biotin is a prosthetic group in four biotin-dependent carboxylases,[28] three of which are strictly mitochondrial enzymes. All three of these enzymes catalyze anaplerotic reactions (i.e., reactions that replenish an intermediate) in the Krebs cycle. The Krebs cycle is the donor for succinyl-CoA, the precursor for heme. A biotin deficiency decreases the activity of these enzymes. In addition, during biotin deficiency methylcrotonyl-CoA accumulates in the mitochondria and reacts with glycine,[28] which may result in depletion of this amino acid from the mitochondrial matrix. Thus, biotin deficiency may cause a decrease in both mitochondrial succinyl-CoA and glycine, and hence heme deficiency.

Vitamin B6 is converted to the coenzyme pyridoxal 5′-phosphate (PLP), which is directly involved in heme synthesis, as a cofactor for δ-aminolevulinic acid synthetase (δ-ALAS),[29] and results in a shortage of heme. Approximately 10% of the U.S. population consumes less than half of the recommended daily allowance of vitamin B6.[30]

Pantothenic acid is the precursor of coenzyme A (CoA) and thus is important for the production of acetyl-CoA. A deficiency of pantothenic acid depresses heme synthesis in monkeys and causes anemia.[31] Pantothenic acid deficiency in *Neurospora crassa* decreases complex IV[32] and the iron content of complex IV.[32] We assume that the level of heme and heme-α were decreased as a result of deficiency in pantothenic acid, which led to loss of complex IV. Clinical pantothenic acid deficiency in humans is very rare, although the frequency of marginal deficiency or age-related deficiency has not been investigated. Both lipoic acid and pantothenic acid are micronutrients essential for the normal supply of succinyl-CoA, the precursor for heme biosynthesis; a deficiency of either may reduce heme synthesis through a mechanism similar to that produced by a biotin deficiency.

Copper deficiency alters heme metabolism. Copper deficiency causes a selective decrease in mitochondrial complex IV, likely by decreasing its assembly[33] because copper is a prosthetic group in complex IV.[34] It has been suggested that deficiency of copper also impairs the insertion of heme-α into complex IV.[33] Copper is essential for efficient heme synthesis;[35] therefore, copper deficiency may affect complex IV also by decreasing heme content in the cell and affecting the synthesis of heme-α.[36]

A rat model for Wilson disease, a disorder of copper transport, exhibits abnormal heme metabolism,[37] supporting the connection between copper and heme synthesis.

ACKNOWLEDGMENTS

This study was supported by the Wheeler Foundation Fund of the University of California, National Institute on Aging Grant AG17140, Ellison Medical Foundation Grant sS-0422-99, National Institute of Environmental Health Sciences Center Grant P30-ES01896, and The National Center for Complementary and Alternative Medicine Research Scientist Award K05-AT001323.

REFERENCES

1. HARMAN, D. 1983. Free radical theory of aging: consequences of mitochondrial aging. Age **6**: 86–94.
2. MIQUEL, J. & J.E. FLEMING. 1984. A two-step hypothesis on the mechanisms of in vitro cell aging: cell differentiation followed by intrinsic mitochondrial mutagenesis. Exp. Gerontol. **19**: 31–36.
3. SHIGENAGA, M.K., T.M. HAGEN & B.N. AMES. 1994. Oxidative damage and mitochondrial decay in aging. Proc. Natl. Acad. Sci. USA **91**: 10771–10778.
4. HAGEN, T.M., D.L. YOWE, J.C. BARTHOLOMEW, *et al.* 1997. Mitochondrial decay in hepatocytes from old rats: membrane potential declines, heterogeneity and oxidants increase. Proc. Natl. Acad. Sci. USA **94**: 3064–3069.
5. BECKMAN, K.B. & B.N. AMES. 1998. Mitochondrial aging: open questions. Ann. N.Y. Acad. Sci. **854**: 118–127.
6. BECKMAN, K.B. & B.N. AMES. 1998. The free radical theory of aging matures. Physiol. Rev. **78**: 547–581.
7. HELBOCK, H.J., K.B. BECKMAN, M.K. SHIGENAGA, *et al.* 1998. DNA oxidation matters: the HPLC-EC assay of 8-oxo-deoxyguanosine and 8-oxo-guanine. Proc. Natl. Acad. Sci. USA **95**: 288–293.
8. LIU, J., D. KILLILEA & B.N. AMES. 2002. Age-associated mitochondrial oxidative decay: improvement of carnitine acetyltransferase substrate binding affinity and activity in brain by feeding old rats acetyl-L-carnitine and/or R-α-lipoic acid. Proc. Natl. Acad. Sci. USA **99**: 1876–1881.
9. HAGEN, T.M., R.T. INGERSOLL, C.M. WEHR, *et al.* 1998. Acetyl-L-carnitine fed to old rats partially restores mitochondrial function and ambulatory activity. Proc. Natl. Acad. Sci. USA **95**: 9562–9566.
10. HAGEN, T.M., C.M. WEHR & B.N. AMES. 1998. Mitochondrial decay in aging. Reversal through dietary supplementation of acetyl-L-carnitine and N-*tert*-butyl-α-phenylnitrone. Ann. N.Y. Acad. Sci. **854**: 214–223.
11. HAGEN, T.M., R.T. INGERSOLL, J. LIU, *et al.* 1999. (*R*)-α-Lipoic acid–supplemented old rats have improved mitochondrial function, decreased oxidative damage, and increased metabolic rate. FASEB J. **13**: 411–418.
12. LYKKESFELDT, J., T.M. HAGEN, V. VINARSKY & B.N. AMES. 1998. Age-associated decline in ascorbic acid concentration, recycling and biosynthesis in rat hepatocytes—reversal with (*R*)-α-lipoic acid supplementation. FASEB J. **12**: 1183–1189.
13. HAGEN, T.M., V. VINARSKY, C.M. WEHR & B.N. AMES. 2000. *(R)*-α-Lipoic acid reverses the age-associated increase in susceptibility of hepatocytes to *tert*-butylhydroperoxide both *in vitro* and *in vivo*. Antiox. Redox Signal. **2**: 473–483.
14. HAGEN, T.M., J. LIU, J. LYKKESFELDT, *et al.* 2002. Feeding acetyl-L-carnitine and lipoic acid to old rats significantly improves metabolic function while decreasing oxidative stress. Proc. Natl. Acad. Sci. USA **99**: 1870–1875.
15. LIU, J., E. HEAD, A.M. GHARIB, *et al.* 2002. Memory loss in old rats is associated with brain mitochondrial decay and RNA/DNA oxidation: partial reversal by feeding acetyl-L-carnitine and/or R-α-lipoic acid. Proc. Natl. Acad. Sci. USA **99**: 2356–2361.

16. AMES, B.N., I. ELSON-SCHWAB & E.A. SILVER. 2002. High-dose vitamins stimulate variant enzymes with decreased coenzyme-binding affinity (increased Km): relevance to genetic disease and polymorphisms. Am. J. Clin. Nutr. **75:** 616–658.
17. WALTER, P.W., M.D. KNUTSON, A. PALER-MARTINEZ, *et al.* 2002. Iron deficiency and iron excess damage mitochondria and mitochondrial DNA in rats. Proc. Natl. Acad. Sci. USA **99:** 2264–2269.
18. ATAMNA, H., J. LIU & B.N. AMES. 2001. Heme deficiency selectively interrupts assembly of mitochondrial complex IV in human fibroblasts: relevance to aging. J. Biol. Chem. **276:** 48410–48416.
19. ATAMNA, H., P.W. WALTER & B.N. AMES. 2002. The role of heme and iron-sulfur clusters in mitochondrial biogenesis, maintenance, and decay with age. Arch. Biochem. Biophys. **397:** 345–353.
20. ATAMNA, H., D.W. KILLILEA, A.N. KILLILEA & B.N. AMES. 2002. Heme deficiency may be a factor in the mitochondrial and neuronal decay of aging. Proc. Natl. Acad. Sci. USA **99:** 14807–14812.
21. BENTON, D. 2001. Micro-nutrient supplementation and the intelligence of children. Neurosci. Biobehav. Rev. **25:** 297–309.
22. TAMURA, T., R.L. GOLDENBERG, J. HOU, *et al.* 2002. Cord serum ferritin concentrations and mental and psychomotor development of children at five years of age. J. Pediatr. **140:** 165–170.
23. HO, E. & B.N. AMES. 2002. Low intracellular zinc induces oxidative DNA damage, disrupts p53, NFκB, and AP1 DNA-binding, and affects DNA repair in a rat glioma cell line. Proc. Natl. Acad. Sci. USA **99:** 16770–16775.
24. HO, E., C. COURTEMANCHE & B.N. AMES. 2003. Zinc deficiency induces oxidative DNA damage and increases P53 expression in human lung fibroblasts. J. Nutr. **133:** 2543–2548.
25. SANDSTEAD, H.H., C.J. FREDERICKSON & J.G. PENLAND. 2000. History of zinc as related to brain function. J. Nutr. **130:** 496S–502S.
26. MOCK, D.M., J.G. QUIRK & N.I. MOCK. 2002. Marginal biotin deficiency during normal pregnancy. Am. J. Clin. Nutr. **75:** 295–299.
27. MOCK, D.M., C.L. HENRICH, N. CARNELL & N.I. MOCK. 2002. Indicators of marginal biotin deficiency and repletion in humans: validation of 3-hydroxyisovaleric acid excretion and a leucine challenge. Am. J. Clin. Nutr. **76:** 1061–1068.
28. MOCK, D.M. 1989. Biotin. International Life Sciences Institute. Washington, D.C.
29. SCHOLNICK, P.L., L.E. HAMMAKER & H.S. MARVER. 1972. Soluble-aminolevulinic acid synthetase of rat liver. II. Studies related to the mechanism of enzyme action and hemin inhibition. J. Biol. Chem. **247:** 4132–4137.
30. WAKIMOTO, P. & G. BLOCK. 2001. Dietary intake, dietary patterns, and changes with age: an epidemiological perspective. J. Gerontol. A Biol. Sci. Med. Sci. **56:** 65–80.
31. PLESOFSKY-VIG, N. 1996. Pantothenic Acid. ILSI Press. New York.
32. BRAMBL, R. & N. PLESOFSKY-VIG. 1986. Pantothenate is required in *Neurospora crassa* for assembly of subunit peptides of cytochrome c oxidase and ATPase/ATP synthase. Proc. Natl. Acad. Sci. USA **83:** 3644–3648.
33. ROSSI, L., G. LIPPE, E. MARCHESE, *et al.* 1998. Decrease of cytochrome *c* oxidase protein in heart mitochondria of copper-deficient rats. Biometals **11:** 207–212.
34. STEFFENS, G.C., R. BIEWALD & G. BUSE. 1987. Cytochrome c oxidase is a three-copper, two-heme-A protein. Eur. J. Biochem. **164:** 295–300.
35. WILLIAMS, D.M., F.S. KENNEDY & B.G. GREEN. 1985. The effect of iron substrate on mitochondrial haem synthesis in copper deficiency. Br. J. Nutr. **53:** 131–136.
36. KEYHANI, E. & J. KEYHANI. 1980. Identification of porphyrin present in apo-cytochrome *c* oxidase of copper-deficient yeast cells. Biochim. Biophys. Acta **633:** 211–227.
37. NAKAYAMA, K., A. TAKASAWA, I. TERAI, *et al.* 2000. Spontaneous porphyria of the Long-Evans cinnamon rat: an animal model of Wilson's disease. Arch. Biochem. Biophys. **375:** 240–250.

Development of Calorie Restriction Mimetics as a Prolongevity Strategy

DONALD K. INGRAM, R. MICHAEL ANSON,[a] RAFAEL DE CABO,
JACEK MAMCZARZ, MIN ZHU, JULIE MATTISON, MARK A. LANE,[b]
AND GEORGE S. ROTH

*Laboratory of Experimental Gerontology, Gerontology Research Center,
National Institute on Aging, National Institutes of Health,
Baltimore, Maryland 21224, USA*

ABSTRACT: By applying calorie restriction (CR) at 30–50% below *ad libitum* levels, studies in numerous species have reported increased life span, reduced incidence and delayed onset of age-related diseases, improved stress resistance, and decelerated functional decline. Whether this nutritional intervention is relevant to human aging remains to be determined; however, evidence emerging from CR studies in nonhuman primates suggests that response to CR in primates parallels that observed in rodents. To evaluate CR effects in humans, clinical trials have been initiated. Even if evidence could substantiate CR as an effective antiaging strategy for humans, application of this intervention would be problematic due to the degree and length of restriction required. To meet this challenge for potential application of CR, new research to create "caloric restriction mimetics" has emerged. This strategy focuses on identifying compounds that mimic CR effects by targeting metabolic and stress response pathways affected by CR, but without actually restricting caloric intake. Microarray studies show that gene expression profiles of key enzymes in glucose (energy) handling pathways are modified by CR. Drugs that inhibit glycolysis (2-deoxyglucose) or enhance insulin action (metformin) are being assessed as CR mimetics. Promising results have emerged from initial studies regarding physiological responses indicative of CR (reduced body temperature and plasma insulin) as well as protection against neurotoxicity, enhanced dopamine action, and upregulated brain-derived neurotrophic factor. Further life span analyses in addition to expanded toxicity studies must be completed to assess the potential of any CR mimetic, but this strategy now appears to offer a very promising and expanding research field.

KEYWORDS: metabolism; body temperature; stroke; MPTP; 2-deoxyglucose; metformin; insulin

---

Address for correspondence: Donald K. Ingram, Acting Chief, Laboratory of Experimental Gerontology, Gerontology Research Center, National Institute on Aging, NIH, 5600 Nathan Shock Drive, Baltimore, MD 21224. Voice: 410-558-8180; fax: 410-558-8302.

ingramd@grc.nia.nih.gov

[a]Current address: R. Michael Anson, St. George's University School of Medicine, Grenada, West Indies.

[b]Current address: Mark A. Lane, Merck and Company, Rahway, NJ 07065.

CALORIE RESTRICTION

The most robust and reproducible prolongevity intervention in laboratory rats and mice is to reduce caloric intake by 30–50% below *ad libitum* (AL) levels over their adult life span. Evidence has emerged from hundreds of rodent studies that such calorie restriction (CR) regimens can significantly increase mean and maximum life span, reduce the incidence and age of onset of age-related diseases, increase resistance to numerous stressors and toxins, and maintain function later into life.[1–3] Although much less investigated in nonrodent species, the CR paradigm has been used to demonstrate its prolongevity effects in several other invertebrate species, including daphnia, nematodes, fruit flies, and spiders, and short-lived vertebrate species, including fish and reptiles.[2]

Recent studies of CR in rhesus monkeys have not yet generated definitive conclusions regarding effects on mortality and morbidity in a long-lived primate species, but it is clear that CR in monkeys produces physiological effects that parallel those observed in rodents.[4–6] Moreover, established risk factors for diabetes and heart disease are also reduced in monkeys on CR.[5,6] If the findings in these primate studies continue to produce evidence that aging can be retarded in a species closely related to humans, then the relevance of CR as an intervention in human aging will be strongly supported.

Abundant epidemiological data have been reported to demonstrate that caloric intake is related to the incidence of many chronic diseases, including cardiovascular disease, cancer, and diabetes, as well as neurodegenerative disorders.[7–12] However, experimental evidence that CR can retard aging processes in humans has not been established. A study of a small group of volunteers confined to Biosphere 2 confirmed that CR could be imposed for two years and would produce many of the physiological, hormonal, and morphological effects expected.[13] To further evaluate this feasibility of CR intervention in humans,[14] recent clinical studies of CR sponsored by the National Institute on Aging have been initiated at three sites—Washington University, Tufts University, and the Pennington Center at Louisiana State University. These studies will provide valuable information on physiological responses to CR over a short term (3–5 years), as well as greatly needed information on procedures to obtain and maintain compliance for such regimens.

Considering the epidemiological studies reporting an association between disease and caloric intake and assuming future results from the clinical trials under way will be positive, the foremost question will remain whether CR can alter the rate of aging in humans. If we can assume that the answer to the question is positive, then the overarching question is the following: even if CR was a well-established intervention to retard aging and age-related disease, would it be a practical antiaging prescription? Given the documented difficulty in Western culture to maintain low calorie diets for a prolonged period,[15] much less a major portion of the lifetime, the application of CR to humans could be problematic due to the severity and length of restriction required. Thus, we need to pose the following question: are there alternatives to CR that can provide its antiaging benefits without actually having to drastically reduce caloric intake?

CALORIE RESTRICTION MIMETICS

To address this question, we have developed a research program to assess interventions designed as "CR mimetics." The intent of this strategy is to produce the same prolongevity effects that CR provides, but without substantially reducing caloric intake or otherwise inhibiting food intake.[16–18] CR mimetics can be pharmaceuticals, nutraceuticals, hormones, diets, or even genetic manipulations that provide the benefits of CR without its dietary demands. In our consideration of this concept, we have steered away from other possible means of reducing caloric intake. For example, CR could be induced by restricting the digestive tract (e.g., stomach stapling) or it might be achieved by successful appetite suppression through pharmaceutical means. Instead, we have directed our efforts to interventions that target specific metabolic pathways involved in mediating the effects of CR. In effect, by activating protective mechanisms that are activated in CR, the organism could be "tricked" into a CR state when its actual caloric consumption had not been changed or changed to much less extent than conventional CR regimens would dictate.

If actual reduction in dietary calories is assumed to be the major factor driving the prolongevity effects of CR, then what would be the appropriate mechanism(s) to target for a CR mimetic? Regarding mechanisms of CR, several hypotheses have been proposed, including reducing oxidative stress,[19] controlling inflammatory responses,[20] and protecting against glycation of macromolecules.[21] Interventions that protected against these deleterious processes might have prolongevity effects. From our perspective, however, it would be more appropriate to target a broadly acting mechanism, such as enhancing stress responses to condition the organism to handle all these deleterious processes.

POSTULATED PROLONGEVITY MECHANISMS

One compelling hypothesis to explain the prolongevity effects of CR is that it induces an evolutionarily conserved stress response that conditions the organism toward enhanced stress protection.[22–26] Some investigators have invoked the concept of hormesis from toxicology, which implies that small doses of a toxin might have long-term beneficial consequences as a means of conditioning the organism toward enhanced stress responses.[25,27,28] From an evolutionary perspective, the disposable soma theory of aging proposes that, during times of low energy availability, the organism must shift away from energy investment in growth and reproductive processes to energy investment in somatic maintenance and repair.[29] The essential feature of this hypothesis is that it is adaptive for the organism under CR to use available means to protect itself and thus enhance its stress protective mechanisms. Hormonal evidence that CR induces stress is manifested in higher levels of glucocorticoids.[25] Increased stress responses of rodents on CR have been demonstrated in numerous paradigms.[25] Several studies assessing response to neurotoxins in rats and mice on various regimens of CR have shown increased protection.[30–33]

A well-studied example of the adaptive strategy of CR is the diapause observed in the nematode, *Caenorhabditis elegans*. When exposed to low energy environments, this organism converts to its dauer state in which development and reproduction are arrested. Within the dauer state, this roundworm is more stress resistant and can markedly exceed the life span of its normal adult form.[34,35] Several key genes have been identified that appear to regulate conversion to the dauer form, among them age-1, daf-2, daf-16, daf-18, akt-1, and akt-2.[36] This signal transduction pathway appears to be homologous to an insulin/insulin growth factor-1 (IGF-1) pathway in mammals.[34,35,37,38] Selected mutations of genes regulating this pathway, for example, daf-2, can reduce signaling such that the worm does not transform to the dauer form, but does have markedly extended life span associated with increased stress protection.[37,38] Mammalian models of reduced signaling through the insulin/IGF-1 pathways have also produced evidence of prolongevity effects.[39] Specifically, knockout mice for the IGF-1 receptor exhibit increased life span and increased resistance to oxidative stress. There appears to be little other phenotypic effects observed in this mouse as their energy metabolism, nutrient uptake, physical activity, fertility, and reproduction do not differ substantially from normal littermates. Similar prolongevity findings have been found in transgenic rats[40] and mutant dwarf mice[41] in which the growth hormone/IFG-1 pathway has been affected, but which differ along other phenotypic parameters from their normal controls.

2-DEOXYGLUCOSE

Studies in invertebrate and vertebrate models of prolongevity point to a logical strategy of inducing stress resistance by manipulating systems involved in energy sensing, regulation, and metabolism. Thus, as an initial target for our CR mimetic strategy, we focused on glucose metabolism. We hypothesized that inhibition of glycolytic pathways could mimic CR without altering food intake. As an initial approach,[16] rats and mice were fed a diet containing 2-deoxy-D-glucose (2DG), which inhibits the enzyme, phosphohexose isomerase, and thus reduces glycolytic processing. Previous studies revealed that 2DG injections could inhibit tumor growth[42] and produce torpor[43] and increase glucocorticoids,[44] all of which paralleled effects of CR.

In the initial study,[16] young male Fischer-344 (F344) rats were fed diets supplemented (by weight) with 0.2%, 0.4%, or 0.6% 2DG, which was approximately 100–150, 250–300, or 400–450 mg/kg, respectively. The high dose proved to be toxic as a couple of deaths were observed after a few weeks, so this group was then fed the 0.6% diet every other week, which appeared to be generally well tolerated. Acute toxicity would be expected at some 2DG dose because of insufficient cellular energy due to an intolerably high degree of glycolysis inhibition. The major end points of the study were physiological. As observed in FIGURES 1 and 2, the 2DG diet reduced plasma insulin and body temperature at the 0.4% and 0.6% concentrations, without significant reduction in plasma glucose. Although all doses initially reduced food intake and body weight, the 0.2% and 0.4% groups caught up to controls after a few weeks so that, by the end of the study at 6 months, they did not differ significantly from controls. Thus, because two major biomarkers of CR had been affected in this study, specifically reduced insulin and body temperature, we concluded that 2DG was a promising candidate as a CR mimetic.

The validity of these biomarkers of CR was further confirmed in a recent analysis of survival data in human males derived from the Baltimore Longitudinal Study of

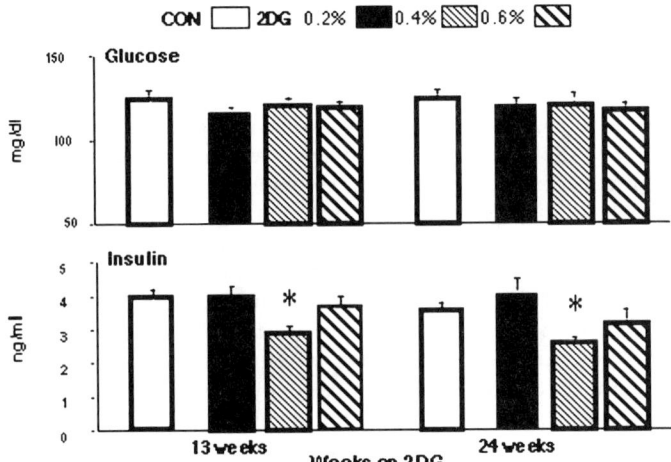

FIGURE 1. Mean (SEM) plasma concentrations of glucose and insulin in male F344 rats fed control (CON) diet or diet supplemented with 2-deoxyglucose (2DG) in three concentrations. *Significantly different from CON group.

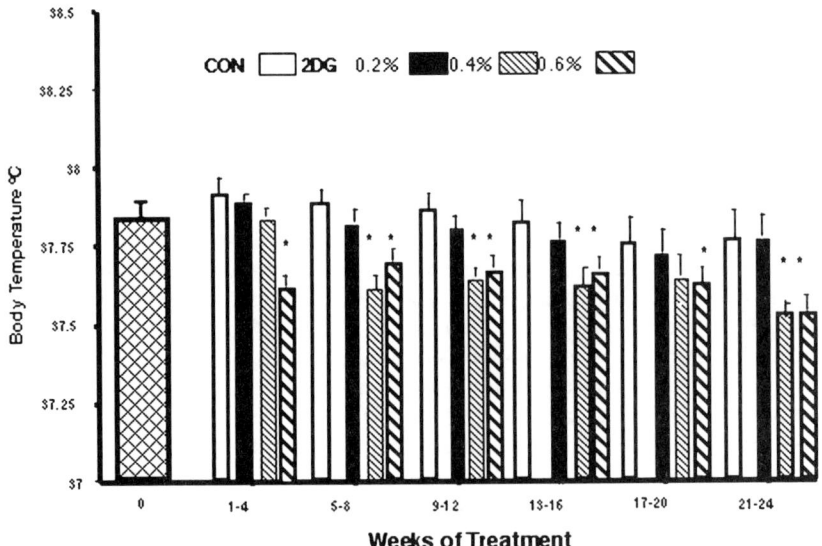

FIGURE 2. Mean (SEM) body temperature recorded in male F344 rats fed control (CON) diet or diet supplemented with 2-deoxyglucose (2DG) in three concentrations. *Significantly different from CON group.

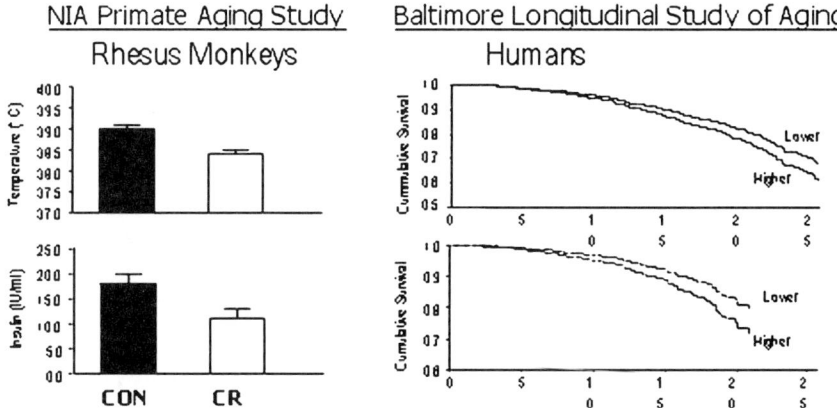

FIGURE 3. (*Left*) Mean (SEM) plasma insulin and body temperature of male rhesus monkeys on control (CON) or calorie restricted (CR) diets, and (*right*) survival probability curves of healthy males enrolled in the Baltimore Longitudinal Study of Aging based on whether in the top or bottom half of the distributions for body temperature and plasma insulin.

Aging (BLSA). Specifically, as presented in FIGURE 3, we examined the probability of survival in a healthy sample of men and found that those with the lowest temperature and plasma insulin levels had the lowest mortality risk.[45]

In vitro analysis of 2DG effects confirmed the ability of the compound to enhance protection against a number of stressors. For example, 2DG protected fetal hippocampal neurons against glutamate excitotoxicity.[46] Upregulation of heat shock protein-70 (HSP-70) and glutamate responsive protein-78 (GRP-78) was observed in the 2DG-treated cultures to confirm that stress pathways induced in CR rats could be duplicated. When rats were given 2DG injections for seven days, their cortical synaptosomes showed greater protection against iron and amyloid-β-peptide, and HSP-70 and GRP-78 were increased compared to control synaptosome preparations.[47] In an *in vivo* model of focal ischemia using middle cerebral artery occlusion-reperfusion, 2DG feeding attenuated damage similar to the effects of CR.[48] Mice injected with the neurotoxin, 1-methyl-4-phenyl-1,2,3,6-tetrahydropyridine (MPTP), exhibit marked motor impairments related to depletion of dopamine (DA) resulting from neuronal loss in the substantia nigra; however, 2DG injections provided greater protection and faster behavioral recovery.[49] Again, the stress proteins, HSP-70 and GRP-78, were increased in DA-rich brain regions in 2DG fed mice. A recent long-term study in rats comparing 2DG feeding to CR also noted many similarities.[50] Compared to AL controls, serum glucose and insulin were reduced in both CR and 2DG fed groups. Body temperature was also consistently lower in CR rats, but not so consistently lower in 2DG fed rats. However, heart rate and blood pressure were markedly decreased in both groups. In this study, all the physiological effects of CR, except body temperature, were reproduced in 2DG fed rats, for which food intake and body weight were similar to controls.

Given evidence of such robust effects of this compound, additional studies have addressed how the stress responses could be mediated. Of particular interest was how the brain might be involved. Recent studies have indicated the involvement of a neurotrophic factor, brain-derived neurotrophic factor (BDNF), which can be neuroprotective.[51] BDNF is also involved in enhancing DA neurotransmission. Past studies have demonstrated that short-term CR (e.g., 2 weeks) can increase DA-related locomotor responses.[52] Specifically, when challenged with the DA agonist, amphetamine, rats show hyperactivity, and this response is enhanced when rats are on CR. In recent studies, we have found that rats on CR for 4 months have enhanced locomotor response to amphetamine, and this response is also observed in rats fed 2DG.[53] Previously, it has been noted that CR can attenuate the age-related loss of striatal dopamine D2 receptors.[54] It would be interesting to determine if long-term 2DG feeding could produce similar results.

A variety of findings revealed a highly favorable profile for 2DG as a CR mimetic. What remained to be accomplished then was a long-term study to evaluate its effects on mortality and morbidity. To this end, we initiated a study of 2DG feeding in 6-month-old male F344 rats. We used the dose of 0.4%, which proved effective in the previous study, and a dose of 0.25%. Unfortunately, after about 2 months on the diet, deaths began to occur in the higher dose group, and these accelerated with time. A primary cause of death was congestive heart failure. In preliminary pathological analyses, we have found that rats on both 2DG doses had enlarged hearts with a marked vacuolization. We are currently completing this long-term study, but the results do not appear encouraging regarding this possible life-threatening pathology observed in 2DG fed rats. What this line of investigation demonstrates is that a useful screen for CR mimetics can be established, but the long-term studies must still be undertaken to prove the prolongevity effects of a candidate mimetic.

OTHER CALORIE RESTRICTION MIMETIC CANDIDATES

The number of possible CR mimetics would comprise a very long list. In addition to inhibiting glucose metabolism, another possible pathway to manipulate is insulin signaling. Again, many candidates could be suggested, but we have recently focused on the biguanides, specifically metformin. Metformin acts to reduce liver glucose production as well as acts as an insulin sensitizer. Known as glucophage, it is a highly prescribed medication in the treatment of type 2 diabetes.[55] Although we had not conducted much research with this compound, we were aware of previous positive life span studies using a related compound, phenformin, in mice.[56] In a recent *in vitro* study, phenformin was shown to increase resistance to glutamate toxicity in primary neuronal cultures.[57] Recently, we have undertaken a survival study in male F344 rats fed metformin (300 mg/kg). Preliminary findings indicate that this dose can reduce body temperature and plasma insulin, but without significant effects on body weight or food intake, similar to findings with 2DG.

Another inhibitor of glycolysis, iodoacetate acid (IAA), has also shown some promise. Pretreatment of fetal hippocampal neurons with IAA protected them against various stresses, including glutamate, iron, and trophic factor withdrawal, and upregulated heat shock proteins, HSP-70 and HSP-90.[58] Other possible candidates as CR mimetics could be found among the thiazolidinediones, which are agonists for peroxisome proliferator activated receptors (PPARs). Recently, in diabetic monkeys, a PPARδ agonist markedly improved the lipid and insulin profiles,[59] and these compounds are now being assessed in several clinical trials. Pharmacological inhibition of IGF-1 signaling has also been suggested as a logical candidate for CR mimetics.[8]

DIET REGIMEN

As another approach to developing CR mimetics, we have been conducting studies of other regimens that might not require a severe degree of CR. A major tenet of the CR literature is that reduction in calories is required to achieve the age-retarding benefits of this intervention.[1–3] Because few investigators have compared different regimens of CR, such as feeding every other day versus limited daily feeding, we have begun such comparative studies. The major hypothesis being evaluated is that it is an adaptation to periods of food deprivation, rather than CR per se, that provides the protective effect. Moreover, we are interested in determining the role of the central nervous system as the initiator and mediator of these responses.

Although we had conducted many previous studies showing that intermittent feeding (IF), specifically feeding every other day (EOD), was an effective intervention for extending life span and retarding aging processes in rats and mice,[60–62] no studies had directly compared IF to CR imposed every day, that is, limited daily feeding (LDF). In a recent study,[63] IF in male C57BL/6J was found to be equally effective as LDF (40%) in providing protection against neurotoxicity induced by hippocampal injections of kainic acid (KA). FIGURE 4 shows that neuronal loss was

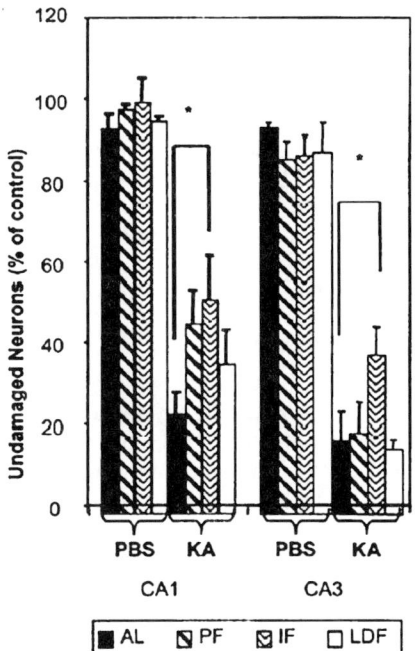

FIGURE 4. Percent reduction from controls in number of undamaged neurons in CA1 and CA3 hippocampal regions in response to injections of saline (PBS) or kainic acid (KA) in mice fed *ad libitum* (AL), intermittently fed (IF), pair-fed (PF) to the IF group, or fed 40% less daily (LDF). *Significantly different from AL group.

attenuated in both diet groups compared to KA-induced damage in AL fed controls. Indeed, in the CA3 region of the hippocampus, IF provided greater protection compared to LDF. The comparison between IF and LDF took on major significance when it was noted that the levels of restriction and body weight loss were modest in IF mice (~10%) compared to AL, yet insulin and glucose levels as well as neuroprotection were generally equivalent to the 40% LDF group. An interesting difference between IF and LDF was that serum IGF-1 levels were reduced as expected in LDF, but elevated in IF, whereas ketone bodies were increased in sera of IF and reduced in LDF mice compared to AL controls. Results of this experiment have led us to consider further that the regimen of CR, rather than the level of CR, might be the major factor for inducing the beneficial responses observed.

FUTURE DIRECTIONS

Because the number of candidate CR mimetics could be large, further development of CR mimetics would be accelerated by establishing a battery of assays to screen candidates. We have already mentioned the measurement of body temperature and plasma insulin levels as two important physiological screens. Examination of other hormonal responses, including glucocorticoids and thyroid hormones, as well as measurement of lipokines, such as leptin and adiponectin, could be added to the screen. Effects on tumor growth in experimental models could also make a highly relevant contribution to the screen. Other investigators have advocated the use of DNA microarrays to determine if a candidate CR mimetic produced, in a particular tissue, a pattern of gene expression that was highly similar to that produced by CR.[64] Many of the responses to CR, both genetic and physiological, are likely to be incidental to the prolongevity effect. The use of arrays in a comparison of the two different feeding paradigms, IF and LDF, offers a tool for eliminating many of the incidental effects and emphasizing those that are causally related to prolongevity.

The recent development in our laboratory of an *in vitro* model of CR could also be a highly useful component in a screening process for CR mimetics.[65] Specifically, a candidate compound could be provided to rats and mice, blood could be withdrawn, and subsequently extracted serum could be evaluated in a stress challenge. Serum derived from CR rats and monkeys has been shown to protect cells in culture from heat stress and oxidative stress provided by exposure to hydrogen peroxide. Thus, it stands to reason that serum derived from rats or mice treated with a candidate CR mimetic should afford cells grown *in vitro* greater protection against various stresses.

Prior to this *in vivo* screen, compounds could also be tested *in vitro* regarding their ability to protect cells against various stressors. This was the approach taken to evaluate phenformin and IAA as CR mimetics.[57,58] Even with a screen in place, any candidate CR mimetic would still need to be validated ultimately by demonstrating its beneficial effects on mortality and morbidity in a relevant animal model. Our experience in evaluating 2DG has shown the absolute necessity of such demonstration.

We believe that the concept of CR mimetics has opened up many new possibilities as a prolongevity strategy. We anticipate that many new approaches will be taken and many new candidates identified in many different laboratories as this strategy becomes increasingly popular and research directed toward this concept accelerates.

REFERENCES

1. MASORO, E.J. 2000. Caloric restriction and aging: an update. Exp. Gerontol. **35:** 299–305.
2. WEINDRUCH, R. & R.L. WALFORD. 1988. The Retardation of Aging and Disease by Dietary Restriction. Thomas. Springfield, IL.
3. WEINDRUCH, R. & R.S. SOHAL. 1997. Seminars in medicine of the Beth Israel Deaconess Medical Center: caloric intake and aging. N. Engl. J. Med. **337:** 986–994.
4. RAMSEY, J.J., R.J. COLMAN, N.C. BINKLEY, et al. 2000. Dietary restriction and aging in rhesus monkeys: The University of Wisconsin Study. Exp. Gerontol. **35:** 1131–1149.
5. MATTISON, J.A., M.A. LANE, G.S. ROTH & D.K. INGRAM. 2003. Calorie restriction in rhesus monkeys. Exp. Gerontol. **38:** 35–46.
6. ROTH, G.S., D.K. INGRAM & M.A. LANE. 2001. Caloric restriction in primates and relevance to humans. Ann. N.Y. Acad. Sci. **928:** 305–315.
7. ASTRUP, A. 2001. Healthy lifestyles in Europe: prevention of obesity and type II diabetes by diet and physical activity. Public Health Nutr. **4:** 499–515.
8. HURSTING, S.D., J.A. LAVIGNE, D. BERRIGAN, et al. 2003. Calorie restriction, aging, and cancer prevention: mechanisms of action and applicability to humans. Annu. Rev. Med. **54:** 131–152.
9. KRITCHESKY, D. 2001. Caloric restriction and cancer. J. Nutr. Sci. Vitaminol. **47:** 13–19.
10. LOGROSCINO, G., K. MARDER, L. COTE, et al. 1996. Dietary lipids and antioxidants in Parkinson's disease: a population-based, case-control study. Ann. Neurol. **39:** 89–94.
11. MAYEUX, R., R. COSTA, K. BELL, et al. 1999. Reduced risk of Alzheimer's disease among individuals with low calorie intake. Neurology **59:** S296–S297.
12. WILLET, W.C. 2000. Nutritional epidemiology issues in chronic disease at the turn of the century. Epidemiol. Rev. **22:** 82–86.
13. WALFORD, R.L., D. MOCK, R. VERDERY & T. MACCALLUM. 2002. Calorie restriction in Biosphere 2: alterations in physiologic, hematologic, hormonal, and biochemical parameters in humans restricted for a 2-year period. J. Gerontol. A Biol. Sci. Med. Sci. **57:** B211–B224.
14. HEILBRONN, L.K. & E. RAVUSSIN. 2003. Calorie restriction and aging: reviews of the literature and implications for studies in humans. Am. J. Clin. Nutr. **78:** 361–369.
15. BURKE, L.E., J.M. DUNBAR-JACOB & M.N. HILL. 1997. Compliance with cardiovascular disease prevention strategies: a review of the research. Ann. Behav. Med. **19:** 239–263.
16. LANE, M.A., D.K. INGRAM & G.S. ROTH. 1998. 2-Deoxy-D-glucose feeding in rats mimics physiological effects of calorie restriction. J. Anti-Aging Med. **1:** 327–337.
17. LANE, M.A., D.K. INGRAM & G.S. ROTH. 2002. Easy to swallow: the serious search for an anti-aging pill. Sci. Am. **287:** 24–29.
18. MATTSON, M.P., W. DUAN, J. LEE, et al. 2001. Progress in the development of caloric restriction mimetic supplements. J. Anti-Aging Med. **4:** 225–232.
19. SOHAL, R.S. & R. WEINDRUCH. 1996. Oxidative stress, caloric restriction, and aging. Science **273:** 59–63.
20. CHUNG, H.Y., H.J. KIM, J.W. KIM & B.P. YU. 2001. The inflammation hypothesis of aging: molecular modulation by calorie restriction. Ann. N.Y. Acad. Sci. **928:** 327–335.
21. SELL, D.R., M.A. LANE, W.A. JOHNSON, et al. 1996. Longevity and the genetic determination of glycooxidation kinetics in mammalian senescence. Proc. Natl. Acad. Sci. USA **93:** 485–490.
22. FRAME, L.T., R.W. HART & J.E. LEAKEY. 1998. Caloric restriction as a mechanism mediating resistance to environmental disease. Environ. Health Perspect. **106**(Suppl. 1): 313–324.
23. KIRKWOOD, T.L., P. KAPAHI & D.P. SHANLEY. 2000. Evolution, stress, and longevity. J. Anat. **197**(part 4): 587–590.
24. MATTSON, M.P. 2000. Neuroprotective signaling and the aging brain: take away my food and let me run. Brain Res. **886:** 47–53.
25. MASORO, E.J. 1996. Possible mechanisms underlying the antiaging actions of caloric restriction. Toxicol. Pathol. **24:** 738–741.
26. YU, B.P. & H.Y. CHUNG. 2001. Stress resistance by caloric restriction for longevity. Ann. N.Y. Acad. Sci. **928:** 39–47.

27. RATTAN, S.I. 2001. Applying hormesis in aging research and therapy. Hum. Exp. Toxicol. **20:** 281–285.
28. TURTURRO, A., B.S. HASS & R.W. HART. 2000. Does caloric restriction induce hormesis. Hum. Exp. Toxicol. **19:** 320–329.
29. SHANLEY, D.P. & T.B. KIRKWOOD. 2000. Calorie restriction and aging: a life-history analysis. Evol. Int. J. Org. Evol. **54:** 740–750.
30. CALINAGASAN, N.Y. & G.E. GIBSON. 2000. Dietary restriction attenuates the neuronal loss, induction of heme oxygenase-1, and blood-brain barrier breakdown induced by impaired oxidative metabolism. Brain Res. **885:** 62–69.
31. BRUCE-KELLER, A.J., G. UMBERGER, R. MCFALL & M.P. MATTSON. 1999. Food restriction reduces brain damage and improves behavioral outcome following excitotoxic and metabolic insults. Ann. Neurol. **45:** 8–15.
32. ZHU, H., Q. GUO & M.P. MATTSON. 1999. Dietary restriction protects hippocampal neurons against the death-promoting action of a presenilin-1 mutation. Brain Res. **842:** 224–229.
33. DUAN, W., J. LEE, Z. GUO & M.P. MATTSON. 2001. Dietary restriction stimulates BDNF production in the brain and thereby protects neurons against excitotoxic injury. J. Mol. Neurosci. **16:** 1–12.
34. JOHNSON, T.E., E. DE CASTRO, S. HEGI DE CASTRO, et al. 2001. Relationship between increased longevity and stress resistance as assessed through gerontogene mutations in *Caenorhabditis elegans*. Exp. Gerontol. **36:** 1609–1617.
35. LITHGOW, G.J. & G.A. WALKER. 2002. Stress resistance as a determinate of *C. elegans* lifespan. Mech. Ageing Dev. **123:** 765–771.
36. VANFLETEREN, J.R. & B.P. BRAECKMAN. 1999. Mechanisms of life span determination in *Caenorhabditis elegans*. Neurobiol. Aging **20:** 487–502.
37. TATAR, M., A. BARTKE & A. ANTEBI. 2003. The endocrine regulation of aging by insulin-like signals. Science **299:** 1346–1351.
38. GEMS, D. & L. PARTRIDGE. 2001. Insulin/IGF signaling and ageing: seeing the bigger picture. Curr. Opin. Genet. Dev. **122:** 673–693.
39. HOLZENBERGER, M., J. DUPONT, B. DUCOS, et al. 2003. IGF-1 receptor regulates lifespan and resistance to oxidative stress in mice. Nature **421:** 182–187.
40. SHIMOKAWA, I., Y. HIGAMI, M. UTSUYAMA, et al. 2002. Life span extension by reduction in growth hormone–insulin-like growth factor-1 axis in a transgenic rat model. J. Pathol. **160:** 2259–2265.
41. BARTKE, A., H. BROWN-BORG, J. MATTISON, et al. 2001. Prolonged longevity of hypopituitary dwarf mice. Exp. Gerontol. **36:** 21–28.
42. GRIDLEY, D.S., R.L. NUTTER, J.D. KETTERING, et al. 1985. Mouse neoplasia and immunity: effects of radiation, hyperthermia, 2-deoxy-D-glucose, and *Corynebacterium parvum*. Oncology **42:** 391–398.
43. DARK, J., D.R. MILLER & I. ZUCKER. 1994. Reduced glucose availability induces torpor in Siberian hamsters. Am. J. Physiol. **267:** 496–501.
44. WEIDENFELD, J., A.P. CORCOS, A. WOHLMAN & S. FELDMAN. 1994. Characterization of the 2-deoxyglucose effect on the adrenocortical axis. Endocrinology **134:** 1924–1931.
45. ROTH, G.S., M.A. LANE, D.K. INGRAM, et al. 2002. Biomarkers of caloric restriction may predict longevity in humans. Science **297:** 881.
46. LEE, J., A.J. BRUCE-KELLER, Y. KRUMAN, et al. 1999. 2-Deoxy-D-glucose protects hippocampal neurons against excitotoxic and oxidative injury: evidence for the involvement of stress proteins. J. Neurosci. Res. **57:** 48–61.
47. GUO, Z. & M.P. MATTSON. 2000. *In vivo* 2-deoxyglucose administration preserves glucose and glutamate transport and mitochondrial function in cortical synaptic terminals after exposure to amyloid β-peptide and iron: evidence for a stress response. Exp. Neurol. **166:** 173–179.
48. YU, Z.F. & M.P. MATTSON. 1999. Dietary restriction and 2-deoxyglucose administration reduce focal ischemic brain damage and improve behavioral outcome: evidence for a preconditioning mechanism. J. Neurosci. Res. **57:** 830–839.
49. DUAN, W. & M.P. MATTSON. 1999. Dietary restriction and 2-deoxyglucose administration improve behavioral outcome and reduce degeneration of dopaminergic neurons in models of Parkinson's disease. J. Neurosci. Res. **57:** 195–206.

50. WAN, R., S. CAMANDOLA & M.P. MATTSON. 2003. Intermittent fasting and dietary supplementation with 2-deoxy-D-glucose improve functional and metabolic cardiovascular risk factors in rats. FASEB J. **17:** 1133–1134.
51. HYMAN, C., M. HOFER, Y-A. BARDE, et al. 1991. BDNF is a neurotrophic factor for dopaminergic neurons of the substantia nigra. Nature **350:** 230–232.
52. FUEMAYOR, L.D. & S. DIAZ. 1984. The effect of feeding on the stereotyped behaviour induced by amphetamine and by apomorphine in the albino rat. Eur. J. Pharmacol. **99:** 153–158.
53. MAMCZARZ, J. 2003. Unpublished observations.
54. LEVIN, P., J.K. JANDA, J.A. JOSEPH, et al. 1981. Dietary restriction retards the age-associated loss of rat striatal dopaminergic receptors. Science **214:** 561–562.
55. KIRPICHNIKOV, D., S.I. MCFARLANE & J.R. SOWERS. 2002. Metformin: an update. Ann. Intern. Med. **137:** 25–33.
56. DILMAN, V.M. & V. ANISIMOV. 1980. Effect of treatment with phenformin, diphenylhydantoin, or l-dopa on life span and tumour incidence in C3H/Sn mice. Gerontology **26:** 241–246.
57. LEE, J., S.L. CHAN & M.P. MATTSON. 2002. Phenformin protects hippocampal neurons against excitotoxicity by suppressing NMDA receptor–mediated calcium influx. Exp. Neurol. **175:** 161–167.
58. GUO, Z., J. LEE, M. LANE & M. MATTSON. 2001. Iodoacetate protects hippocampal neurons against excitotoxic and oxidative injury: involvement of heat-shock proteins and Bcl-2. J. Neurochem. **79:** 361–370.
59. OLIVER, W.R., JR., J.L. SHENK, M.R. SNAITH, et al. 2001. A selective peroxisome proliferator-activated receptor delta agonist promotes reverse cholesterol transport. Proc. Natl. Acad. Sci. USA **98:** 5306–5311.
60. GOODRICK, C.L., D.K. INGRAM, M.A. REYNOLDS, et al. 1982. Effects of intermittent feeding upon growth and lifespan in rats. Gerontology **28:** 233–241.
61. GOODRICK, C.L., D.K. INGRAM, M.A. REYNOLDS, et al. 1983. Effects of intermittent feeding upon growth, activity, and lifespan in rats allowed voluntary exercise. Exp. Aging Res. **9:** 203–209.
62. GOODRICK, C.L., D.K. INGRAM, M.A. REYNOLDS, et al. 1990. Effects of intermittent feeding upon body weight and lifespan in inbred mice: interaction of genotype and age. Mech. Ageing Devel. **55:** 69–87.
63. ANSON, A., Z. GUO, R. DECABO, et al. 2003. Periodic fasting dissociates beneficial effects of dietary restriction from calorie intake. Proc. Natl. Acad. Sci. USA **100:** 6216–6220.
64. WEINDRUCH, R., T. KAYO, C.K. LEE & T.A. PROLLA. 2001. Microarray profiling of gene expression in aging and its alteration by calorie restriction in mice. J. Nutr. **131:** 918S–923S.
65. DECABO, R., S.R. FÜRER-GALBAN, R.M. ANSON, et al. 2003. An *in vitro* model of caloric restriction. Exp. Gerontol. **38:** 631–639.

Interventions in Aging and Age-Associated Pathologies by Means of Nutritional Approaches

KENICHI KITANI,[a] TAKAKO YOKOZAWA,[b] AND TOSHIHIKO OSAWA[c]

[a]*National Institute for Longevity Sciences, Aichi, Japan*

[b]*Institute of Natural Medicine, Toyama Medical and Pharmaceutical University, Toyama, Japan*

[c]*Graduate School of Bioagricultural Sciences, University of Nagoya, Nagoya-shi, Japan*

ABSTRACT: So-called antioxidant strategies have not been shown convincingly to be effective in increasing life spans of animals. Thus, the general consensus of experimental gerontology in the last century was that the only reproducible means of prolonging survivals of animals is the calorie restriction paradigm. As a challenge against this dogma, we attempted to examine the effect of two potent antioxidants, one tetrahydrocurcumin (a biotransformed metabolite of curcumin contained in turmeric of Indian curry) and the other green tea polyphenols.

KEYWORDS: antioxidant; aging; mice; tetrahydrocurcumin; green tea polyphenol

INTRODUCTION

The "Free Radical Theory of Aging" (FRTA) initially proposed half a century ago by Harman[1] has been increasingly supported in recent years. However, while there have been a number of studies demonstrating a significant effect of antioxidant treatment in preventing experimentally induced pathologies that are believed to be at least partially caused by oxygen-induced tissue damage, so-called antioxidant strategies have not been shown convincingly to be effective in increasing life spans of animals.[2] Accordingly, the general consensus of experimental gerontology in the last century was as follows: "The only reproducible means of prolonging survival of animals is the calorie restriction paradigm."

As a challenge to this dogma, we attempted to examine the effect of two potent antioxidants, one tetrahydrocurcumin (TC), a biotransformed metabolite of curcumin contained in turmeric of Indian curry, and the other green tea polyphenols (PPs).

Address for correspondence: Kenichi Kitani, National Institute for Longevity Sciences, 36-3 Gengo, Morioka-cho, Obu-shi, Aichi 474-8522, Japan. Voice: +81-5-6245-0183; fax: +81-5-6245-0184.

kitani@nils.go.jp

MATERIALS AND METHODS

Male C57L/6JNia mice (Harlan Sprague Dawley) began to receive treatments at the age of 13 months. In the TC experiment, animals received TC-containing pellets (0.2%) or standard pellets (MF, Oriental Limited, protein 24%). In the experiment with PPs, animals received normal diets (MF) and normal drinking water or water containing green tea water extract product (Sunphenon 100S, Taiyokagaku, Yokkaichi, Japan) containing various PPs (>70%) at a concentration of 80 mg/L, both pasteurized by γ-ray irradiation. Survival of animals were examined until deaths of these animals.

RESULTS

Average life span (days) in TC fed mice was 11.7% longer (882.2 ± 154.6, mean ± SD) than in control mice (797.6 ± 151.2, both $n = 50$) ($P < .01$). The 10% longest survival was also significantly greater (+6.5%, each $n = 5$, $P < .05$) in TC fed animals. The increase in average life expectancy after 24 months of age, calculated by including mice that died before 24 months as negative days, was 125.9%. In mice fed PPs, the average life span increased by 6.4% (801.1 ± 121.5 vs. 852.7 ± 88.2, control vs. PP fed mice, each $n = 50$, $P < .01$). The increase in average life expectancy after 24 months was 72.6%.

Body weights of TC fed animals were slightly (4–6%), but significantly ($P < .05$) lower compared with corresponding values in control mice in the first 6 months of treatments. Thereafter, the difference was totally lost. In PP fed mice, average body weights were almost identical to those in control mice throughout the observation periods.

DISCUSSION

Since the proposal of FRTA by Harman, several attempts have been reported primarily on mice in order to prolong the life spans of animals by feeding animals with different kinds of antioxidants. These earlier attempts used mostly antioxidant preservatives, some of which turned out to be carcinogenic (for review, see Ref. 3). Apparently, a safer and more practical approach to intervene in aging based on antioxidant strategies is needed. Since antioxidants contained in foods (vegetables and fruits) are largely harmless, nutritional antioxidants (so-called nutriceuticals) may justify a further study of this approach. However, most past attempts, including that by Lipman and co-workers,[2] by nutritional means have failed in achieving a statistically significant prolongation of life spans of animals.

In contrast, as shown in the present study, some nutriceuticals appear to have potential of significantly increasing life spans of animals. In the case of TC in the present study, very minor, but significant differences in average body weight are observed between control and TC fed animals. It is conceivable that these differences in body weight have been caused by a slightly lower food intake in TC fed animals, leading to an unintended dietary restriction. However, the difference between the two groups is only 4–6% and also only in the first 6 months of the treatment. In past references, we have been unable to find a study showing a positive effect of dietary restriction on survival of animals that had body weights with such minor differences from control animals.

Accordingly, we judge that the difference in survival between control and TC fed animals was not solely due to the very minor dietary restriction, but that TC feeding significantly affected survival of animals, although an additive (or synergistic) effect of very moderate dietary restriction cannot be excluded. In the case of PPs, body weights were practically identical for both groups, excluding the above possibility, although the effect was milder with PPs compared with TC feeding. Both nutriceuticals have been shown to be effective in preventing a number of experimentally induced age-associated disorders, including cancer, atherosclerosis, and others.[4–10] Furthermore, the advantage of these agents is their lower toxic nature to humans, which has been confirmed in human experimentation over thousands of years.

Since these agents are known to be effective in preventing atherosclerosis that does not involve wild-type rodents, but is the number-one killer of elderly humans, it is expected that supplementation of these agents may be effective for prolonging the life span (at least health span) of humans possibly more effectively than observed in rodents.

CONCLUSIONS

Nutritional approaches in prolonging the health span (if not life span) of humans may be more promising than believed before and deserve further extensive study using nutriceuticals possessing antioxidant properties.

REFERENCES

1. HARMAN, D. 1956. Aging: a theory based on free radical and radiation chemistry. J. Gerontol. **12:** 257–263.
2. LIPMAN, R.D., R.T. BRONSON, D. WU, et al. 1998. Dsease incidence and longevity are not altered by dietary antioxidant supplementation initiated during middle age in C57BL/6 mice. Mech. Ageing Dev. **103:** 269–284.
3. HARMAN, D. 1994. Free radical theory of aging: increasing the functional life span. Ann. N.Y. Acad. Sci. **717:** 1–15.
4. SUGIYAMA, Y., S. KAWAKISHI & T. OSAWA. 1996. Involvement of the β-diketone moiety in the antioxidative mechanism of tetrahydrocurcumin. Biochem. Pharmacol. **52:** 519–525.
5. KIM, J.M., S. ARAKI, D.J. KIM, et al. 1998. Chemopreventive effects of carotenoids and curcumins on mouse colon carcinogenesis after 1,2-dimethylhydrazine initiation. Carcinogenesis **19:** 81–85.
6. KAMADA, Y., T. OSAWA, H. KOBAYASHI, et al. 1999. Chemoprevention by curcumin during the promotion stage of tumorigenesis of mammary gland in rats irradiated with γ-rays. Carcinogenesis **20:** 1011–1018.
7. OKADA, K., C. WANGPOENGTRAKUL, T. TANAKA, et al. 2001. Curcumin and especially tetrahydrocurcumin ameliorate oxidative stress–induced renal injury in mice. J. Nutr. **131:** 2090–2095.
8. YOKOZAWA, T., H.Y. CHUNG, L.Q. HE, et al. 1996. Effectiveness of green tea tannin on rats with chronic renal failure. Biosci. Biotechnol. Biochem. **60:** 1000–1005.
9. YOKOZAWA, T., E. DONG & H. OURA. 1997. Proof that green tea tannin suppresses the increase in the blood methylguanidine level associated with renal failure. Exp. Toxicol. Pathol. **49:** 117–122.
10. YOKOZAWA, T., H. OURA, S. SAKANAKA, et al. 1994. Depressor effect of tannin in green tea on rats with renal hypertension. Biosci. Biotechnol. Biochem. **58:** 855–858.

Absolute versus Relative Caloric Intake

Clues to the Mechanism of Calorie/Aging-Rate Interactions

R. MICHAEL ANSON

Windward Islands Research Institute and St. George's University, St. George's, Grenada, West Indies

ABSTRACT: It has been suggested that the influence of caloric intake on aging rate is not due to the absolute number of calories ingested. Instead, aging rate is altered only when there is a disparity between the actual caloric intake and that which would be ingested if the food supply were unlimited. This review will discuss a few of the studies supporting this viewpoint.

KEYWORDS: caloric restriction; dietary restriction; aging; fasting; energy; calories; life span; longevity; animal models

It has been known since 1935 that caloric intake modulates the rate of aging.[1] In many species, individuals whose caloric intake is limited only by appetite age rapidly, while those with restricted intake age slowly. Whether aging in humans is altered by intake is uncertain. The question may be academic, however, since people worldwide find themselves unable to limit intake even to weight-maintenance levels, let alone to truly restricted levels. Even if people could restrict their intake, it may turn out that chronic undereating is not advantageous to a free-living organism subject to injuries and pathogen exposure. These concerns have led to a quest to understand the mechanism by which caloric restriction (CR) slows the aging rate, with the ultimate goal being the creation of drugs that will mimic a restricted diet without need for deprivation.

There is a growing body of evidence suggesting that the influence of caloric intake on aging rate is not due to the absolute number of calories ingested. Instead, aging rate is altered only when there is a disparity between the actual caloric intake and that which would be ingested if the food supply were unlimited. This brief review will discuss a few of the studies supporting this viewpoint and will suggest ways in which the systems described in these studies may be exploited for testing specific hypotheses regarding the mechanism by which caloric intake modulates aging.

In April 2003, many news services (including CNN, CBS, Yahoo! News, and others) reported that fasting may be good for one's health. This was a slight misinterpretation of a study in which we showed that, for C57BL/6 mice, fasting on

Address for correspondence: R. Michael Anson, Windward Islands Research Institute and St. George's University, St. George's, Grenada, West Indies. Voice: +473-444-4357, ext. 2069; fax: +473-444-1562.
 anson@jhu.edu

alternate days and gorging when food is available mimics caloric restriction, without any net reduction in caloric intake.[2] C57BL/6 mice were not selected by chance. We knew at the outset that the same regimen in other strains was often not beneficial and could even in some circumstances be fatal.[3] The study was important not because it showed that an alternate-day fast might promote longevity, but because it provided a model that can separate a net reduction in caloric intake from the protective effects of CR. By comparing mice fed a limited amount of food daily (LD) with those subjected to every-other-day (EOD) feeding, one can discern which physiological changes are critical for life extension and which are not. Changes not shared by both models are, ipso facto, not necessary for the effect.

The initial event that led to that study occurred at a meeting of the Gerontological Society of America in the mid-1990s. Ruth Lipman reported the results of a study (subsequently published[4]) in which rats were fed a calorically supplemented diet that included corn oil and sweetened condensed milk. To keep the rats from becoming morbidly obese, it was necessary to restrict their access to this food. They were limited to an intake that was 8% higher than that of control animals fed the standard chow. Intriguingly, the speaker noted during the presentation that they "acted restricted," eagerly awaiting food and rapidly consuming it when provided.

If caloric intake could be dissociated from behavior, could it be dissociated from aging rate? The thought seemed far-fetched at first, yet a literature search revealed several studies that suggested that the connection was relative rather than absolute. Indeed, one indication that this might be so is the well-established finding that LD feeding, when begun early in life, lowers body weight. As a result, the actual amount of food consumed per gram body weight is often higher in restricted animals than in ad libitum (AL) controls.[5,6]

Other lines of evidence also exist. In a dramatic test of the effect of excess calories on the rate of aging, rats were trained to wade in a room-temperature, shoulder-high pool for several hours a day. As a result, extra energy was required to maintain body temperature. Rats in the experimental group in this study ate, on average, 44% more than their dry counterparts. Life span, however, was not shortened. (Indeed, the trend was in the opposite direction for both average and maximal life span.)[7]

Another line of evidence is found in the effects of dietary restriction on $ob^{-/-}$ mice in comparison with congenic controls. One group reported that $ob^{-/-}$ mice fed AL consumed 4.2 g of food per day; AL controls consumed 3.0 g per day. CR mice of both genotypes were LD fed at 2.0 g per day. This is equivalent to a 52% restriction for the $ob^{-/-}$ mice and to a 33% restriction for the wild-type mice. Despite a high level of body fat, the longest-lived mice were in the restricted $ob^{-/-}$ group. While not conclusive, the trend supports the thought that it was the relative restriction level rather than the absolute intake that determined longevity.[8]

The most direct (but rather obscure) study addressing this issue was published in 1987.[9] In that report, EOD feeding was found to increase life span in C57BL/6J mice by 56%, while LD feeding (50% of AL intake) increased it by only 36%. In contrast, body weight was decreased by less than 10% in the youngest mice of the EOD group, but by nearly 50% in the LD group. In both groups, these numbers decreased with age. The topic of the study was body weight and aging interactions, and thus the question of food intake was not addressed.

The value of these studies is that they provide us with models that may be used to study the mechanism by which caloric intake modulates the aging rate. Holloszy and Smith showed that there is an increase in AL intake in response to environmental conditions that require increased energy expenditure to maintain body temperature, without an acceleration in aging rate.[7] The effect of CR in combination with this treatment is potentially informative. Harrison et al. showed that mice lacking leptin are extremely responsive to CR.[8] Their findings suggest that ob$^{-/-}$ mice may even be "restricted" at intake levels that are AL for the ob$^{+/+}$ mouse. This model could be useful in studying many factors that have been proposed to play a mechanistic role in the calorie/aging-rate interaction. Perhaps the greatest promise is offered by comparisons of EOD feeding and LD feeding, two commonly used CR paradigms. Ingram and Reynolds showed that, in one strain of mice, both paradigms result in life extension, despite dramatically different effects on body weight.[9] In a follow-up to that study, it was demonstrated that the different effects on body weight were caused by differences in net caloric intake: in the EOD fed mice, net intake approached AL levels.[2] Each of these systems offers innumerable opportunities for contrast and comparison, and promises to allow us to eliminate variables that change coincidentally, not causally, with the alterations in aging rate.

REFERENCES

1. MCCAY, C.M., M.F. CROWELL & L.A. MAYNARD. 1935. The effects of retarded growth upon the length of life span and upon the ultimate body size. J. Nutr. **10:** 63–79.
2. ANSON, R.M. et al. 2003. Intermittent fasting dissociates beneficial effects of dietary restriction on glucose metabolism and neuronal resistance to injury from calorie intake. Proc. Natl. Acad. Sci. USA **100:** 6216–6220.
3. GOODRICK, C.L. et al. 1990. Effects of intermittent feeding upon body weight and lifespan in inbred mice: interaction of genotype and age. Mech. Ageing Dev. **55:** 69–87.
4. LIPMAN, R.D. et al. 1998. Effects of caloric restriction or augmentation in adult rats: longevity and lesion biomarkers of aging. Aging (Milano) **10:** 463–470.
5. MASORO, E.J., B.P. YU & H.A. BERTRAND. 1982. Action of food restriction in delaying the aging process. Proc. Natl. Acad. Sci. USA **79:** 4239–4241.
6. HUBERT, M.F. et al. 2000. The effects of diet, ad libitum feeding, and moderate and severe dietary restriction on body weight, survival, clinical pathology parameters, and cause of death in control Sprague-Dawley rats. Toxicol. Sci. **58:** 195–207.
7. HOLLOSZY, J.O. & E.K. SMITH. 1986. Longevity of cold-exposed rats: a reevaluation of the "rate-of-living theory." J. Appl. Physiol. **61:** 1656–1660.
8. HARRISON, D.E., J.R. ARCHER & C.M. ASTLE. 1984. Effects of food restriction on aging: separation of food intake and adiposity. Proc. Natl. Acad. Sci. USA **81:** 1835–1838.
9. INGRAM, D.K. & M.A. REYNOLDS. 1987. The relationship of body weight to longevity within laboratory rodent species. *In* Evolution of Longevity in Animals, pp. 247–282. Plenum. New York.

Acetyl-L-Carnitine Dietary Supplementation to Old Rats Increases Mitochondrial Transcription Factor A Content in Rat Hindlimb Skeletal Muscles

V. PESCE,[a] F. FRACASSO,[a] C. MUSICCO,[b] A. M. S. LEZZA,[a] P. CANTATORE,[a,b] AND M. N. GADALETA[a,b]

[a]*Department of Biochemistry and Molecular Biology, University of Bari, Bari, Italy*
[b]*Institute of Biomembrane and Bioenergetics, CNR, Bari, Italy*

> ABSTRACT: Acetyl-L-carnitine (ALCAR) fed to old rats has been reported to partially restore mitochondrial function and ambulatory activity. The results of the effect of ALCAR dietary supplementation to 28-month-old rats on mitochondrial transcription factor A (TFAM) content of rat hindlimb skeletal muscles are reported.
>
> KEYWORDS: acetyl-L-carnitine (ALCAR); soleus; extensor digitorum longus (EDL); mitochondrial DNA (mtDNA); mitochondrial transcription factor A (TFAM)

INTRODUCTION

It has been reported that acetyl-L-carnitine (ALCAR) fed to old rats partially restores mitochondrial function and ambulatory activity.[1] We reported previously that ALCAR was able to bring back, 24 hours after injection, in the brain and in the heart of old rats, where they were reduced, transcription[2] and translation of mitochondrial DNA (mtDNA), as well as the phosphate, the pyruvate, the adenine nucleotides, and the carnitine transport, the cardiolipin content of the inner mitochondrial membrane, and cytochrome oxidase activity (for review, see Ref. 3).

Replication and transcription of the mitochondrial genome depend on nuclear DNA-encoded products. One of these products, mitochondrial transcription factor A (TFAM), plays a complex role in the regulation of both processes: it is required for mtDNA maintenance and together with two other factors, TFB1 and TFB2, stimulates mitochondrial transcription.[4]

The content of TFAM and mtDNA increases during aging in human skeletal muscle; since this increase is associated with that of nuclear respiratory factor-1 (NRF-1), it is likely that it is the result of a compensatory response, which acts through nuclear-mitochondrial cross-talk.[5]

Address for correspondence: M.N. Gadaleta, Department of Biochemistry and Molecular Biology, University of Bari, Via Orabona 4, 70125 Bari, Italy.
m.n.gadaleta@biologia.uniba.it

Protein acetylation on the ε-amino group of lysine is an important reversible modification that regulates gene expression. Although acetylation has been described for histone proteins, site-specific acetylation of a growing list of nonhistone proteins has been shown to play an important role in transcriptional regulation and cell proliferation.[6] In particular, HMG1 and other HMG-box proteins are acetylated. TFAM shares most of the characteristics of HMG proteins since it contains two HMG-box-like domains. We reported recently that TFAM isolated from rat liver is acetylated and that its acetyl content does not change with age.[7] The amount of TFAM, in contrast, does change with age in the liver. In liver, cerebellum, and kidney, the TFAM content in 28-month-old rats is from 1.5- to 2.4-fold higher than in 6-month-old rats, whereas its level is unchanged in the heart.[7]

In this paper, results are reported of the effect of ALCAR dietary supplementation to 28-month-old rats on TFAM content of rat hindlimb skeletal muscles soleus and extensor digitorum longus (EDL).

RESULTS AND DISCUSSION

To verify the effect of ALCAR dietary supplementation to aged rats on TFAM content in skeletal muscles, old rats were given a 1.5% (wt/vol) solution of ALCAR in their drinking water[1] for 1 or 2 months before sacrifice at 28 months of age.

To measure TFAM content, total proteins were extracted from about 30 mg of frozen hindlimb soleus and EDL skeletal muscles of male Fischer 344 (Charles River) 28-month-old rats with ALCAR dietary supplementation or not. Total proteins were separated in 12% SDS-polyacrylamide slab minigels and electroblotted onto PVDF membrane. The membrane was subjected to immunoblotting with rat polyclonal antibodies against TFAM and α-actin. Primary antibody for TFAM, a rabbit anti-rat TFAM antiserum, was a gift from H. Hinagaki. Secondary antibodies were labeled with horseradish peroxidase, and detection (ECL-Plus, Amersham) was performed according to the supplier's instructions. The TFAM signals were quantified by densitometry with the Ultrascan-XL laser densitometer (LKB-Pharmacia) and normalized with respect to the α-actin signals.

As reported in FIGURE 1 in soleus of 28-month-old rats, after 1 month of ALCAR dietary supplementation, the TFAM content is 30% higher than in 28-month-old control rats, whereas it remains unchanged in EDL. In 28-month-old rats, after 2 months of ALCAR dietary supplementation, the level of TFAM in the soleus is still 27% higher than in control rats, whereas it has more than doubled in the EDL muscle. In 28-month-old rats, after 2 months of ALCAR dietary supplementation and 1 month of ALCAR withdrawal from the drinking water, the level of TFAM returns to the value of the control animals in the soleus, whereas it remains high in EDL.

The difference in extent and time-responsiveness of the two rat hindlimb skeletal muscles to dietary ALCAR supplementation could be due to their different fiber-type composition and mitochondrial DNA and RNA content, with the soleus being composed of almost all oxidative type I fibers and the EDL composed of almost all glycolytic type II fibers. Reduced mtDNA availability has been reported to be a limiting factor of mitochondrial gene expression in type II, but not type I fibers. Exercise training or chronic electrical stimulation was primarily associated with increased mtDNA content in moderately oxidative type II, but with increased mito-

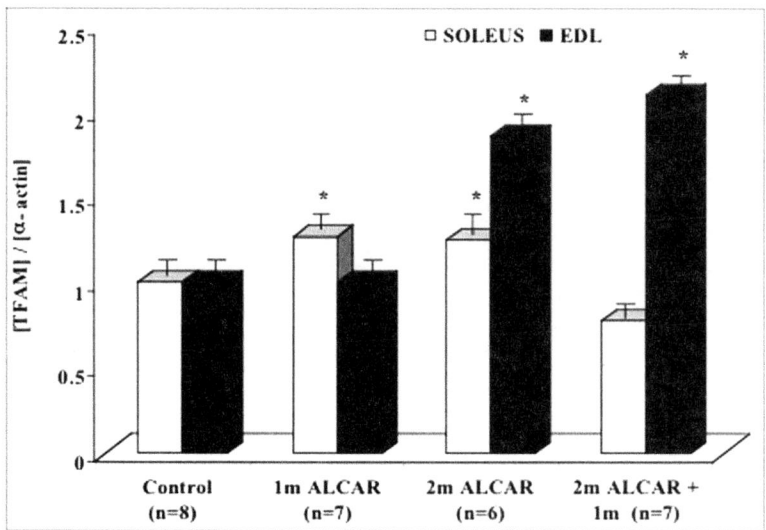

FIGURE 1. TFAM content in soleus and EDL hindlimb skeletal muscles. The data were obtained determining for each muscle the TFAM/α-actin ratio of 28-month-old control rats, 28-month-old rats after 1 or 2 months of ALCAR dietary supplementation, and 28-month-old rats after 2 months of ALCAR dietary supplementation and 1 month of ALCAR withdrawal. Each *bar* represents the average value ± SE from different analyzed animals; n = number of analyzed animals; *statistically significant result ($P < .05$) for ALCAR supplementation diet or not in 28-month-old rats using the ANOVA test.

chondrial transcripts in more highly oxidative type I fibers, suggesting a different regulation of mitochondrial gene expression in different muscles of aged rats.[8]

These results suggest that ALCAR dietary supplementation to old rats might regulate mtDNA transcription and/or replication in the skeletal muscles of old rats by increasing the TFAM level.

It has been recently reported, in fact, that the import of TFAM into rat liver mitochondria increases by 2-fold the incorporation of precursor substrate into rat liver mitochondrial RNAs and stimulates up to 4-fold the RNA synthesis in liver mitochondria from hypothyroid rats.[9] The authors suggested that the low transcription rate associated with the hypothyroid state might be the result of a low TFAM level, which can be recovered by treating animals with T3 *in vivo* or by importing TFAM *in organello*. We reported previously that ALCAR increases cytochrome *c* oxidase subunit I mRNA content in hypothyroid rat liver, showing that ALCAR potentiates the effect of T3 when both substances were administered *in vivo*.[10] It is therefore possible that the ALCAR effect on mitochondrial transcript level in aged and hypothyroid rats previously reported by us might have been mediated by TFAM increase. However, since (as already reported by us[7]) TFAM acetylation level is the same in young and old rats, at least in liver, the signal pathway that can be regulated by ALCAR *in vivo* still remains to be discovered.

ACKNOWLEDGMENTS

We thank H. Hinagaki (Department of Chemistry, National Industrial Research Institute of Nagoya, Japan) for the gift of rat TFAM antiserum. This work has been done with funds from Sigma Tau–Industrie Farmaceutiche Riunite S.p.A. (Contract D.S./2000/C.R./No. 20) and the Italian Space Agency (ASI) (Contract Nos. I/R/064/01 and I/R/322/02). We thank R. Longo for word processing.

REFERENCES

1. HAGEN, T.M., R.T. INGERSOLL, C.M. WEHR, et al. 1998. Acetyl-L-carnitine fed to old rats partially restores mitochondrial function and ambulatory activity. Proc. Natl. Acad. Sci. USA **95:** 9562–9566.
2. GADALETA, M.N., V. PETRUZZELLA, M. RENIS, et al. 1990. Reduced transcription of mitochondrial DNA in the senescent rat: tissue dependence and effect of acetyl-L-carnitine. Eur. J. Biochem. **187:** 501–506.
3. GADALETA, M.N., A. CORMIO, V. PESCE, et al. 1998. Aging and mitochondria. Biochimie **80:** 863–870.
4. FALKENBERG, M., M. GASPARI, A. RANTANEN, et al. 2002. Mitochondrial transcription factors B1 and B2 activate transcription of human mtDNA. Nat. Genet. **31:** 289–294.
5. LEZZA, A.M.S., V. PESCE, A. CORMIO, et al. 2001. Increased expression of mitochondrial transcriptional factor A and nuclear respiratory factor-1 in skeletal muscle from aged human subjects. FEBS Lett. **501:** 74–78.
6. LIU, L., D.M. SCOLNICK, R.C. TRIEVEL, et al. 1999. p53 sites acetylated *in vitro* by PCAF and p300 are acetylated *in vivo* in response to DNA damage. Mol. Cell. Biol. **19:** 1202–1209.
7. DINARDO, M.M., C. MUSICCO, F. FRACASSO, et al. 2003. Acetylation and level of mitochondrial transcription factor A in several organs of young and old rats. Biochem. Biophys. Res. Commun. **301:** 187–191.
8. BARAZZONI, R., K.R. SHORT & K.S. NAIR. 2000. Effects of aging on mitochondrial DNA copy number and cytochrome *c* oxidase gene expression in rat skeletal muscle, liver, and heart. J. Biol. Chem. **275:** 3343–3347.
9. GARSTKA, H.L., W.E. SCHMITT, J. SCHULTZ, et al. 2003. Import of mitochondrial transcription factor A (TFAM) into rat liver mitochondria stimulates transcription of mitochondrial DNA. Nucleic Acids Res. **31:** 5039–5047.
10. GADALETA, M.N., V. PETRUZZELLA, F. FRACASSO, et al. 1990. Acetyl-L-carnitine increases cytochrome oxidase subunit I mRNA content in hypothyroid rat liver. FEBS Lett. **277:** 191–193.

An Appetite for Death

JALAL KOOCHMESHGI

National Research Center for Genetic Engineering and Biotechnology, Tehran, Iran

> ABSTRACT: A diverse array of organisms live longer under dietary restriction. Here, a hypothesis is proposed as a framework for interpreting this phenomenon. Dietary restriction is explained in terms of evolution and antagonistic pleiotropy. Focusing on the decline in reproductive capacity seen in dietary restriction, it is submitted that "normal" appetite is geared toward producing a neuroendocrine and metabolic internal milieu optimized for reproduction, with long-term detrimental effects on health as a by-product. In dietary restriction experiments, the animal is prevented from eating enough to attain this internal milieu and, as a by-product, lives longer.
>
> KEYWORDS: dietary restriction; appetite; aging; reproduction; evolution; antagonistic pleiotropy

A diverse array of organisms live longer under dietary restriction. This phenomenon has been demonstrated in species of rotifers, nematodes, and arthropods, and studied in detail in rodents. It is known as the life-extending effect of dietary restriction and is one of the core components of current research into aging. Indeed, short of drastic measures like genetic manipulation and stem cell therapy, dietary restriction is regarded as the most promising option in the fight against aging.[1,2]

Pervasiveness of this phenomenon across species strongly points to a possible evolutionary explanation, but why and how this "life extension" occurs have been subjects of lively debate. This is an important question. Its answer may point the way toward developing more practical strategies against aging based on the same principles.

Here, we propose a hypothesis as a framework for interpreting this phenomenon across species. We draw attention to an interesting feature of dietary restriction: namely, a concomitant decline in reproductive capacity. This has been shown in several species. For example, in rodents, continued dietary restriction, as well as reduced food availability in the wild, results in delayed onset of puberty and reduced fertility.[3,4] This feature of dietary restriction usually has been relegated to secondary importance in comparison to life extension. Holliday[5] and Harrison and Archer[6] were the first to address it when they interpreted life extension by dietary restriction as an adaptation to carry rodents through extended periods of food shortage to more suitable times for breeding.

We offer a new way of looking at what is happening in dietary restriction experiments. We take interplay of two major evolutionary factors—food intake and reproduction—as the main point, with changes in life span as a by-product.

Address for correspondence: Jalal Koochmeshgi, National Research Center for Genetic Engineering and Biotechnology, P. O. Box 14155-6343, Tehran, Iran.
  jkoochmeshgi@yahoo.co.uk

We submit that, in the unrestricted animal, food intake is geared toward attaining and maintaining optimal reproductive capacity. This level of food intake produces a neuroendocrine and metabolic internal milieu that prepares the body for reproduction. At the same time, some components of this milieu are detrimental to health in the long term as a by-product. This neuroendocrine and metabolic milieu is markedly different from the one seen in the dietary-restricted state (e.g., in hypothalamic-pituitary-gonadal and adrenal axes). In dietary restriction experiments, the animal is prevented from eating enough to attain or maintain reproductive capacity. The neuroendocrine and metabolic internal milieu associated with the normal level of food intake does not materialize, detrimental effects resulting from that milieu do not materialize, and (as a by-product) the animal lives longer, at least in the artificially created environment of the laboratory. In effect, dietary restriction does not extend life; it is "normal" appetite, "normal" food intake, that kills by degrees. One could say "normal" appetite is an appetite for death.

This makes sense in terms of evolution: in the course of evolution, what is selected for is reproductive success and not health in old age. It is conceivable that, in evolution, maintenance of health is compromised for improved reproduction. In fact, this is one of the major themes addressed in the field of life-history evolution.[7–9] Our explanation of dietary restriction experiments is consistent with the notion of antagonistic pleiotropy and enriches this point of view.

This hypothesis also relates dietary restriction to the body of evidence from human studies linking aging and age-associated conditions with reproduction.

ACKNOWLEDGMENTS

The ideas presented here were first formulated during a scientific visit to the Department of Gerontology of the University of Newcastle, United Kingdom. I wish to thank Tom Kirkwood for his support during that visit and the Wellcome Trust for a travel award to attend IABG10.

REFERENCES

1. COMFORT, A. 1979. The Biology of Senescence. Third edition. Elsevier. Amsterdam/New York.
2. ARKING, R. 1998. Biology of Aging. Second edition. Sinauer Associates. Sunderland, MA.
3. MERRY, B.J. & A.M. HOLEHAN. 1979. Onset of puberty and duration of fecundity in rats fed a restricted diet. J. Reprod. Fertil. **57:** 253–259.
4. HOLEHAN, A.M. & B.J. MERRY. 1985. Lifetime breeding studies in fully fed and dietary restricted CFY Sprague-Dawley rats. I. Effect of age, housing conditions, and diet on fecundity. Mech. Ageing Dev. **33:** 19–28.
5. HOLLIDAY, R. 1989. Food, reproduction, and longevity: is the extended lifespan of calorie-restricted animals an evolutionary adaptation? BioEssays **10:** 125–127.
6. HARRISON, D.E. & J.R. ARCHER. 1988. Natural selection for longevity from food restriction. Growth Dev. Aging **52:** 65.
7. RICKLEFS, R.E. & G.L. MILLER. 2000. Ecology. Fourth edition. Freeman. San Francisco/New York.
8. STEARNS, S.C. 1992. The Evolution of Life Histories. Oxford University Press. London/New York.
9. WILLIAMS, G.C. 1957. Pleiotropy, natural selection, and the evolution of senescence. Evolution **11:** 398–411.

Reproductive Switch and Aging

The Case of Leptin Change in Dietary Restriction

JALAL KOOCHMESHGI

National Research Center for Genetic Engineering and Biotechnology, Tehran, Iran

ABSTRACT: We have proposed that normal food intake is geared toward optimizing the internal milieu for reproduction, despite some components of this milieu being detrimental to health. In dietary restriction, the animal is prevented from eating enough to attain or maintain reproductive capacity and this particular milieu does not materialize. Life extension occurs as a by-product. This idea provides a framework for exploring biomolecular changes in dietary restriction and their relevance to aging. Leptin is a case in point: here, a decrease in leptin level in dietary restriction is explored in the light of leptin's role in the complex signaling system of reproductive switch.

KEYWORDS: reproduction; reproductive switch; aging; leptin; dietary restriction

Dietary restriction experiments show that the organism lives longer under sustained restriction of food intake. This phenomenon has been demonstrated in various species and studied in detail in rodents.[1] These experiments provide a model for exploring the phenomenon of aging and possibly intervening in it. Levels of several biomolecules are known to change as a result of dietary restriction and these biomolecules have been considered for their possible role in aging.

We have proposed a hypothesis for interpreting extension of life by dietary restriction [see previous paper by Koochmeshgi in this volume]. It posits that normal food intake is geared toward optimizing the internal milieu for reproduction, despite some components of this milieu being detrimental to health in the long term. In the dietary-restricted state, the animal is prevented from eating enough to attain or maintain reproductive capacity and this particular milieu, with its detrimental effects on health, does not materialize. Life extension occurs as a by-product. This hypothesis can provide a conceptual framework for exploring biomolecular changes seen in dietary restriction and their relevance to aging. Leptin is a case in point.

Leptin, a protein secreted from adipose tissue, has receptors in hypothalamus and is involved in suppressing appetite and activating the hypothalamic-pituitary-gonadal axis. A picture has emerged for the role of leptin in the centrally integrated system

Address for correspondence: Jalal Koochmeshgi, National Research Center for Genetic Engineering and Biotechnology, P. O. Box 14155-6343, Tehran, Iran.
jkoochmeshgi@yahoo.co.uk

monitoring body fat reserve, regulating appetite, and signaling reproductive competence: plasma levels of leptin increase as fat builds up in the body with food intake. Leptin level is monitored through leptin receptors in hypothalamus. Increasing leptin levels signal when the body's fat reserve has reached sufficient mass to meet an organism's needs (e.g., for energy and insulation) and demands of reproduction and offspring care. Appetite is suppressed, the hypothalamic-pituitary-gonadal axis is activated, and the body is switched to reproductive mode. This schema traces leptin's role in tuning reproductive activity to the body's fat reserve, as supported by experimental evidence.[2,3] Admittedly, the full sequence of events involved in this tuning is much more complex and includes a multitude of components and checks and balances.

From an evolutionary point of view, this tuning of reproductive activity to the body's fat reserve, the "reproductive switch," assumes vital importance. If the animal engages in reproductive activity without sufficient fat reserves, it may not be able to sustain itself and carry the burden of reproduction. As a result, survival of both the animal and its offspring will be jeopardized. If, on the other hand, the animal delays reproductive activity in the presence of sufficient fat reserve, it will miss the opportunity for optimal reproductive yield—a serious disadvantage in terms of evolution.

Numerous studies have shown that leptin level decreases in dietary restriction.[4-7] This has led to considerations about its possible role in aging.[8,9] We think that the decrease in leptin level observed in dietary-restricted animals can be explored in the light of leptin's role in the complex and integrated signaling system of "reproductive switch."

In line with our hypothesis on dietary restriction, two broad possibilities present themselves: (1) Leptin by itself has no role in the process of aging. Decreases in leptin levels seen in dietary restriction simply reflect the insufficiency of the body's fat reserve for reproduction, and the observed extension in life is attributable to the fact that reproductive competence is not signaled and downstream events with their detrimental effects on health do not occur. (2) Leptin is involved in the process of aging. With normal food intake, leptin levels build up, signaling the sufficiency of fat reserves for reproduction, and at the same time, by yet undiscovered mechanisms, exert detrimental long-term effects on health. If so, it is interesting to know whether these effects occur only in the context of integrated changes associated with reproductive switch or are independent of them. Experiments aimed at uncoupling components of reproductive switch and downstream events should help in resolving these issues. Such experiments can have practical relevance in developing antiaging interventions.

These questions find parallels in the study of the involvement of other biomolecules in aging, notably investigations on the role of insulin-like growth factor 1 in transgenic models of aging.

ACKNOWLEDGMENTS

The ideas presented here were first formulated during a scientific visit to the Department of Gerontology of the University of Newcastle, United Kingdom. I wish to thank Tom Kirkwood for his support during that visit and Daryl Shanley for fruitful discussions. I also thank the Wellcome Trust for a travel award to attend IABG10.

REFERENCES

1. COMFORT, A. 1979. The Biology of Senescence. Third edition. Elsevier. Amsterdam/New York.
2. CASANUEVA, F.F. & C. DIEGUEZ. 1999. Neuroendocrine regulation and actions of leptin. Front. Neuroendocrinol. **20:** 317–363.
3. BAILE, C.A., M.A. DELLA-FERA & R.J. MARTIN. 2000. Regulation of metabolism and body fat mass by leptin. Annu. Rev. Nutr. **20:** 105–127.
4. MAFFEI, M. et al. 1995. Leptin levels in humans and rodents: measurement of plasma leptin and ob RNA in obese and weight-reduced subjects. Nat. Med. **1:** 1155–1161.
5. TRAYHURN, P. et al. 1995. Effects of fasting and refeeding on ob gene expression in white adipose tissue of lean and obese (ob/ob) mice. FEBS Lett. **368:** 480–490.
6. AHIMA, R.S. et al. 1996. Role of leptin in the neuroendocrine response to fasting. Nature **382:** 250–252.
7. XU, B. et al. 1999. Daily changes in hypothalamic gene expression of neuropeptide Y, galanin, proopiomelanocortin, and adipocyte leptin gene expression and secretion: effects of food restriction. Endocrinology **140:** 2868–2875.
8. SHIMOKAWA, I. & Y. HIGAMI. 1999. A role for leptin in the antiaging action of dietary restriction: a hypothesis. Aging (Milano) **11:** 380–382.
9. SHIMOKAWA, I. & Y. HIGAMI. 2001. Leptin signalling and aging: insight from caloric restriction. Mech. Ageing Dev. **122:** 1511–1519.

Long-Lived αMUPA Transgenic Mice Exhibit Increased Mitochondrion-Mediated Apoptotic Capacity

OREN TIROSH,[a] BETTY SCHWARTZ,[a] IGOR ZUSMAN,[b] GEORGE KOSSOY,[b] SHLOMO YAHAV,[c] AND RUTH MISKIN[d]

[a]*Institute of Biochemistry, Food Science and Nutrition, Hebrew University of Jerusalem, Rehovot 76100, Israel*

[b]*Koret School of Veterinary Medicine, Hebrew University of Jerusalem, Rehovot 76100, Israel*

[c]*Institute of Animal Science, Agricultural Research Organization, Bet Dagan, Israel*

[d]*Department of Biological Chemistry, The Weizmann Institute of Science, Rehovot 76100, Israel*

> ABSTRACT: Caloric restriction (CR) is currently the only therapeutic intervention known to attenuate aging in mammals, but the mechanisms underlying this phenomenon are still poorly understood. To study this issue, the transgenic model of αMUPA mice, which previously were reported to spontaneously eat less and live longer compared with their wild-type (WT) control mice, were used. Currently, two transgenic lines that eat less are available, thus implicating the transgenic enzyme, that is, the urokinase-type plasminogen activator (uPA), in causing the reduced appetite. Recently, several changes in the αMUPA liver were noted, at the mitochondrial and cellular level, which consistently pointed to an enhanced capacity to induce apoptosis. In addition, αMUPA mice showed a reduced level of serum IGF-1 and a reduced incidence of spontaneously occurring or carcinogen-induced tumors in several tissues. Overall, the αMUPA model suggests that long-lasting, moderately increased apoptotic capacity, possibly linked in part to modulation of serum IGF-1 and mitochondrial functions, could play a role in the attenuation of aging in calorically restricted mice.
>
> KEYWORDS: caloric restriction; aging, apoptosis; mitochondria; αMUPA transgenic mice; uPA plasminogen activator

Caloric restriction (CR) can extend the life span of multiple species and is currently the only treatment known to attenuate aging in mammals.[1,2] The underlying mechanisms by which CR exerts its antiaging effects are currently only speculative. To get some insight into these mechanisms, we took advantage of αMUPA transgenic mice. We previously described a line of these mice that showed spontaneously

Address for correspondence: Ruth Miskin, Department of Biological Chemistry, The Weizmann Institute of Science, Rehovot 76100, Israel. Voice: +972-8-9343150; fax: +972-8-9344118.
ruth.miskin@weizmann.ac.il

Ann. N.Y. Acad. Sci. 1019: 439–442 (2004). © 2004 New York Academy of Sciences.
doi: 10.1196/annals.1297.080

TABLE 1. Changes found in αMUPA compared to WT mice[a]

1. Reduced eating, starting spontaneously after weaning (~30% in αMUPA, ~15% in αMUPA/15).
2. Reduced body weight (~30% in αMUPA, ~15% in αMUPA/15).
3. Reduced body length (6%).
4. Increased survival (~20% increased average life span; the age of 10th percentile survivors was 15% longer; 95th percentile—62% longer).
5. Changes of female reproductive parameters (14% reduced litter sizes and 10% reduced birth frequency).
6. Reduced blood sugar (9%).
7. Reduced serum IGF-1 (αMUPA IGF-1 was 70% of the WT level at 5 months of age).
8. Reduced liver/kidney deiodination activity (T4 → T3) (not consistently statistically significant).
9. In αMUPA, the serum corticosterone level was elevated (at 8 A.M.) at 3 months of age, but significantly decreased at 15 months of age.
10. Reduced body temperature [a different diurnal pattern in αMUPA compared with WT; minimal temperature values were seen at 4:00 A.M. (1.8°C reduction) and 12:00 P.M. (0.9°C reduction); indicating a circadian change?].
11. No change in resting metabolic rate (the same in αMUPA and WT when calculated as O_2/h/animal; slightly but significantly increased in αMUPA when calculated as O_2/gram body weight).
12. Age-associated thymus involution occurred normally in αMUPA (in contrast to CR mice).
13. Increased sensitivity to paraquat toxicity (αMUPA and αMUPA/15).
14. Changes indicating a reduced threshold for apoptosis (see text).
15. Reduced incidence of spontaneously occurring or carcinogen-induced tumors.
16. Discolorization of incisor enamel resulting from ectopic transgenic expression in the developing teeth (not related to the reduced eating; αMUPA and αMUPA/15).
17. Reduced capacity to perform in several learning tasks (not yet clear if related to the reduced eating; αMUPA and αMUPA/15).
18. Enhanced transgenic expression in the trigeminal nucleus of the brain stem (αMUPA and αMUPA/15).

[a]Female mice were studied. The comparison relates to the αMUPA line unless the αMUPA/15 line (which so far has been less thoroughly characterized) is specifically mentioned. The changes listed were statistically significant.

reduced eating and increased life span compared with their wild-type (WT) control, thus mimicking calorically restricted (CR) mice[3–6] (see TABLE 1 for more details). An additional transgenic line (αMUPA/15) showing reduced food consumption was generated more recently, thus indicating that the primary causal factor of the reduced eating is the transgenic enzyme, that is, the urokinase-type plasminogen activator (uPA). This extracellular serine protease constitutes a central component of the fibrinolytic system and has also been implicated in events such as tissue remodeling, brain development, and several brain activities (see Refs. 3–7 for a list of references). Since both αMUPA lines spontaneously eat less when fed *ad libitum*, apparently their appetite was reduced. However, it is not yet clear how uPA overexpression could lead to this change. Originally, αMUPA mice were generated in order to investigate the role of uPA in the eye. Therefore, the αMUPA transgene consisted of the full-length uPA cDNA linked to the lens-specific, αA-crystallin promoter.[6] As expected, αMUPA mice expressed uPA mRNA in the ocular lens. Unexpectedly, however, αMUPA mice also showed transgenic expression in several sites that are ectopic with respect to the promoter. For example, the two transgenic lines share a strong transgenic expression, specifically in the trigeminal nucleus of the brain stem, where uPA expression could not be detected in WT mice (unpublished results). Thus, it is possible that the transgenic expression at this unique site, or alternatively, an interference of the transgenic uPA with brain development, could be responsible for the reduced appetite of αMUPA.

Previously, we compared αMUPA and their WT counterpart mice (NIH FVB/N) for parameters that were reported to be altered in calorically restricted mice.[3-5] TABLE 1, which lists previous published and unpublished findings, indicates that αMUPA resembled the CR mice in many respects; however, they also exhibited some differences.

In this study we examined young adult αMUPA mice for several mitochondrial parameters, because mitochondrion-induced oxidative damage is thought to constitute a major driving force in aging.[8,9] Mitochondria also play a critical role in apoptosis, a noninflammatory programmed cell death that occurs in response to a variety of internal insults and external stimuli.[10] Notably, we found that αMUPA and WT mice do not differ in their mitochondrial respiration *in vitro* or in their resting metabolic rate when calculated as O_2/h/animal. In contrast, we found appreciable differences between the mice in several parameters related to apoptosis, as will be discussed next.

The opening of the mitochondrial permeability transition (PT) pore may result in osmotic swelling of the mitochondrial matrix space, which can lead to the release of cytochrome *c*. The latter effect can trigger a cascade of events, resulting in the activation of procaspase into caspase-3, -6, and -7, which are cysteine proteases that can drive the apoptosis process further downstream. To compare the mice for swelling and cytochrome *c* release, we energized mitochondria isolated from the livers of 7-month-old WT and αMUPA mice by supplementing glutamate plus malate (G + M) or succinate plus rotenone (S + R). High-amplitude swelling was initiated by the addition of calcium (60 nmol/mg of mitochondrial suspension). Swelling was evaluated by the decrease in OD 540 nm. To test for the release of cytochrome *c*, we centrifuged energized mitochondria 20 minutes after adding calcium, and conducted Western blots for the supernatants and pellet fractions using cytochrome *c* polyclonal antibodies. The results showed that both swelling and cytochrome *c* release were significantly enhanced in αMUPA (~3-fold and 5- to 20-fold, respectively). Furthermore, the αMUPA mitochondria also showed a diminished capacity to retain calcium.[7]

In view of the results obtained, we further compared αMUPA and WT for additional apoptosis-related parameters, as follows. (a) Because antioxidants can promote the PT pore opening, we compared WT and αMUPA mitochondria for the content of glutathione (GSH), which could constitute one candidate compound that causes the difference in mitochondrial behavior. We found that the GSH level was 31% higher in the αMUPA mitochondria. In contrast, the total GSH level in liver homogenates did not differ between the two mouse types.[7] (b) αMUPA hepatocytes showed an increased level (52%) of propidium iodide (PI) staining and DNA fragmentation (100%), thus indicating that the fraction of apoptotic cells in the liver was roughly twice as high in αMUPA than in WT.[7] (c) Caspase-3 activity (measured as DEVDase activity inhibited by caspase-3 inhibitor II) was enhanced (~35%) in liver homogenates of αMUPA and αMUPA/15 compared with WT.[7] (d) The level of serum IGF-I, an antiapoptotic survival factor, was in αMUPA only 70% of the WT level at 5 months of age.[7] (e) The rate of lung adenomas was higher (about 4-fold) in WT than in the two transgenic lines at 24 to 28 months of age.[7] In addition, young WT mice showed a higher number of premalignant aberrant crypt foci in the colon after diethylhydrazine (DMH) injection, and a higher incidence of tumors in the skin and stomach after dimethylbenzanthracene (DMBA) injection. All the aforementioned changes were statistically significant.

To evaluate whether the reduced eating by αMUPA mice could account for the changes found in their mitochondrial behavior and caspase-3 activity, we conducted similar measurements for WT mice that were either calorically restricted to receive 60% of their *ad libitum* food consumption (CR WT) or were fed *ad libitum* (AL WT). We found that after an 8-week treatment period, mitochondria from the CR WT showed a significantly more enhanced calcium-dependent, high amplitude swelling than the mitochondria of the AL WT mice. In addition, the mitochondrial GSH level and the caspase-3 activity of liver homogenates were significantly higher (17% and 82%, respectively) in the CR WT mice.[7] We therefore concluded that the short-term CR regimen rendered the WT mice similar to αMUPA, at least with regard to the parameters measured here.

In conclusion, this study indicated that CR can enhance the apoptotic capacity at the mitochondrial level in the liver, and apparently also in other mitotic tissues. These results support the view that mitochondria could act as a mediator in the CR-induced antiaging effect. The mitochondrial role emerging from this study, however, appears to be linked to apoptotsis, a process whose fine-tuning toward an optimal threshold could help to continuously maintain tissue homeostasis. Thus, the αMUPA model suggests that a sustained, mild reduction of the threshold for apoptosis, possibly linked in part to IGF-1 and GSH modulation, could play a role in the attenuation of aging in calorically restricted mice.

REFERENCES

1. WEINDRUCH, R. & R.L. WALFORD. 1988. The Retardation of Aging and Disease by Dietary Restriction. Thomas. Springfield, IL.
2. MASORO, E.J. 2000. Caloric restriction and aging: an update. Exp. Gerontol. **35:** 299–305.
3. MISKIN, R. & T. MASOS. 1997. Transgenic mice overexpressing urokinase-type plasminogen activator in the brain exhibit reduced food consumption, body weight and size, and increased longevity. J. Gerontol. **52A:** 3118–3124.
4. MISKIN, R. *et al.* 1999. αMUPA mice: a transgenic model for increased life span. Neurobiol. Aging **20:** 555–564.
5. MEIRI, N. *et al.* 1994. Overexpression of urokinase-type plasminogen activator in transgenic mice is correlated with impaired learning. Proc. Natl. Acad. Sci. USA **91:** 3196–3200.
6. MISKIN, R. *et al.* 1990. Human and murine urokinase cDNAs linked to the αA-crystallin promoter exhibit lens and non-lens expression in transgenic mice. Eur. J. Biochem. **190:** 31–38.
7. TIROSH, O. *et al.* 2003. Mitochondrion-mediated apoptosis is enhanced in long-lived αMUPA transgenic mice and calorically restricted wild-type mice. Exp. Gerontol. **38:** 955–963.
8. HARMAN, D. 1957. The aging process. Proc. Natl. Acad. Sci. USA **78:** 7124–7128.
9. SOHAL, R.S. & R. WEINDRUCH. 1996. Oxidative stress, caloric restriction, and aging. Science **273:** 59–63.
10. RAVAGNAN, L., T. ROUMIER & G. KROEMER. 2002. Mitochondria, the killer organelles and their weapons. J. Cell. Physiol. **192:** 131–137.

Effect of Caloric Restriction on the 24-Hour Plasma DHEAS and Cortisol Profiles of Young and Old Male Rhesus Macaques

H. F. URBANSKI,[a] J. L. DOWNS,[a] V. T. GARYFALLOU,[a] J. A. MATTISON,[b] M. A. LANE,[b] G. S. ROTH,[b] AND D. K. INGRAM[b]

[a]*Division of Neuroscience, Oregon National Primate Research Center, Beaverton, Oregon 97006, USA*

[b]*Laboratory of Experimental Gerontology, National Institute on Aging/ National Institutes of Health, Baltimore, Maryland 21224, USA*

ABSTRACT: Although dietary caloric restriction (CR) can retard aging in laboratory rats and mice, it is unclear whether CR can exert similar effects in long-lived species, such as primates. Therefore, we tested the effect of CR on plasma levels of dehydroepiandrosterone sulfate (DHEAS), a reliable endocrine marker of aging. The study included six young (~10 years) and ten old (~25 years) male rhesus macaques, approximately half of the animals in each age group having undergone >4 years of 30% CR. Hourly blood samples were collected remotely for 24 hours, through a vascular catheter, and assayed for DHEAS and cortisol. Both of these adrenal steroids showed a pronounced diurnal plasma pattern, with peaks occurring in late morning, but only DHEAS showed an aging-related decline. More importantly, there was no significant difference in plasma DHEAS concentrations between the CR animals and age-matched controls. These data fail to support the hypothesis that CR can attenuate the aging-related decline in plasma DHEAS concentrations, at least not when initiated after puberty.

KEYWORDS: dehydroepiandrosterone sulfate; adrenal gland; primate

INTRODUCTION

Dietary caloric restriction (CR) has been shown to extend mean and maximal life span in short-lived rodents. However, it is unclear whether CR can exert similar effects in long-lived species, such as primates.[1–4] To examine this possibility and to gain insights into the underlying neuroendocrine mechanism, this study tested the effect of CR on plasma concentrations of dehydroepiandrosterone sulfate (DHEAS) (i.e., a reliable biomarker of aging), and also on another adrenal steroid, cortisol (i.e., a marker of stress response). In both humans and nonhuman primates, circulating

Address for correspondence: Henryk F. Urbanski, Ph.D., Division of Neuroscience, Oregon National Primate Research Center, 505 N.W. 185 th Avenue, Beaverton, OR 97006. Voice: 503-690-5306; fax: 503-690-5384.

urbanski@ohsu.edu

levels of DHEAS are very high during early adult life, and then show a marked decrease during aging. Previous studies in rhesus macaque monkeys found that long-term CR could significantly attenuate the rate of age-related decline in circulating DHEAS.[4–6] However, these studies focused only on young adults, and so it is unclear whether the effect of CR is maintained through to old age. Also, the determination of circulating DHEAS levels was based on blood samples collected at only one time point during the day. This approach could be problematic, as later studies in rhesus monkeys demonstrated a pronounced circadian pattern of DHEAS release.[6–8] To overcome such limitations, the present study examined the influence of CR on plasma DHEAS levels in both young (10-year-old) and old (26-year-old) adult male monkeys. Moreover, determination of circulating DHEAS levels was based on serial blood samples collected at 1-hour intervals across the whole day. Plasma cortisol also shows a distinct circadian rhythm, and so its concentration in the plasma was similarly based on the serially collected blood samples. Previous rodent studies have shown that corticosterone levels (particularly nighttime levels) are elevated in CR animals, and these results support the view that CR induces a stress response.[4] Thus, our predictions were that plasma DHEAS and cortisol would be significantly higher in the CR animals compared to *ad libitum* fed age-matched controls.

METHODS

Six young (~10 years old) and ten old (~26 years old) male rhesus macaques (*Macaca mulatta*) were obtained from the longitudinal study of CR being conducted by the Laboratory of Experimental Gerontology of the National Institute on Aging (Baltimore). They were transferred to the Oregon National Primate Research Center, and were maintained in accordance with the NIH *Guide for the Care and Use of Laboratory Animals*. They were housed under a 12L:12D photoperiod (i.e., 12 hours of light per day) and used in the following experiment, which was approved by the Institutional Animal Care and Use Committee. For 4 years prior to initiation of the blood sampling, three of the young animals and four of the old animals were subjected to a 30% calorie-restricted diet, as previously described,[8–10] while the controls were fed the same diet at approximate *ad libitum*–fed levels. Subsequently, all of the animals were fitted with an indwelling vascular catheter, and serial blood samples were remotely collected at 1-hour intervals across the day and night.[10] The plasma samples were assayed for DHEAS and cortisol using RIA.[6–8]

FIGURE 1. Effect of 30% calorie restriction (for ~4 years) on the 24-h circulating concentrations of cortisol and DHEAS in young (10-year-old) and old (26-year-old) male rhesus macaques. (NOTE: The hormone profiles are double plotted to facilitate observation of day–night differences.) Each *point* represents the mean plasma hormone level from 3 to 6 animals (shown in *parentheses*); SEM are represented by *vertical lines*. Both of these adrenal steroids showed a distinct 24-h rhythm, which was characterized by an early-morning peak and a late-evening nadir. Overall, mean plasma cortisol concentrations were similar in the young and old animals, regardless of diet (two-way ANOVA). In marked contrast, mean plasma DHEAS concentrations showed a significant aging-related decrease; however, there appeared to be no significant effect of diet.

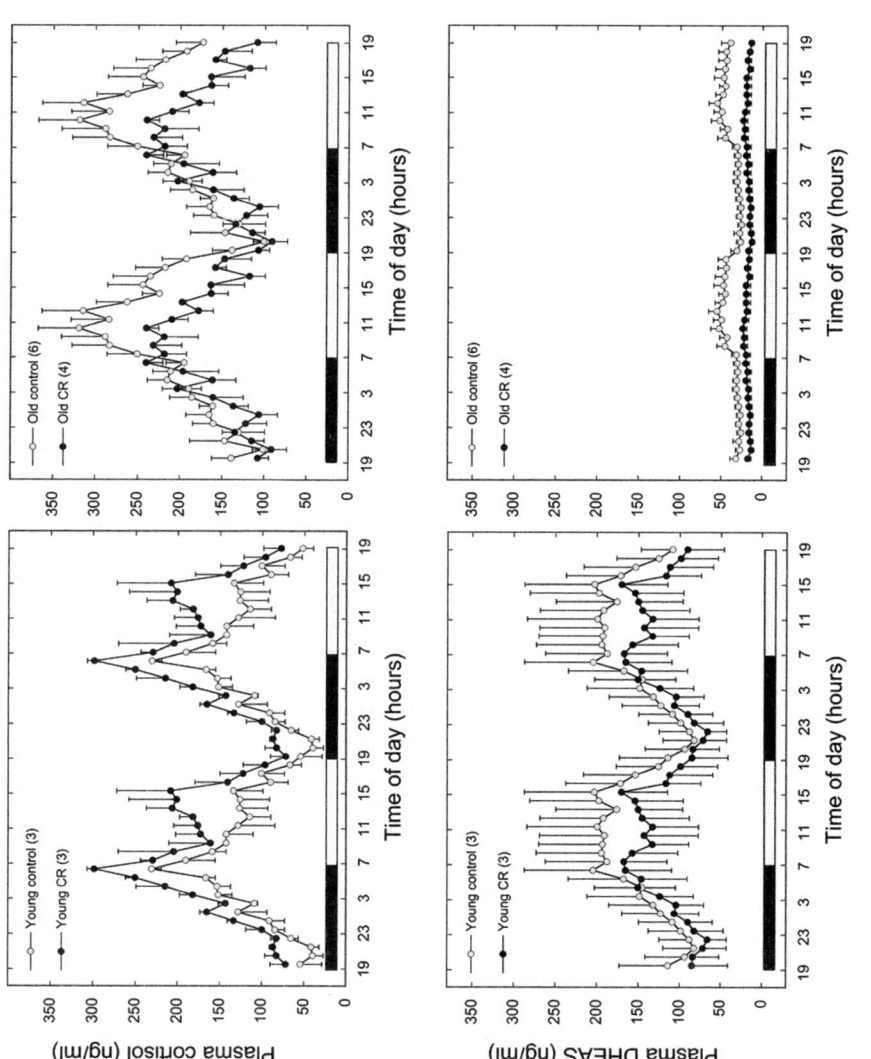

FIGURE 1. See previous page for legend.

RESULTS

Plasma concentrations of DHEAS and cortisol both showed pronounced diurnal patterns (FIG. 1), with peaks occurring during late morning (lights on from 7:00 h to 19:00 h). Mean and maximum plasma cortisol concentrations were similar ($P > .05$) in the young and old animals, regardless of their dietary treatment (two-way ANOVA). Qualitatively, however, the plasma cortisol profile of young CR animals differed from that of the age-matched controls; a second major peak was prominent in the former group (at ~15:00 h) but not in the latter. In the older CR and control animals, a similar qualitative difference between the plasma cortisol profiles was not evident. Mean and maximum plasma DHEAS concentrations showed a significant aging-associated decline ($P < .001$, and $P < .01$, respectively). However, this decrease was not significantly ($P > .05$) attenuated by CR (two-way ANOVA); if anything, plasma DHEAS concentrations appeared to be lower in the CR animals.

DISCUSSION

The collection of serial blood samples across the day and night enabled detailed 24-hour plasma profiles to be established for both DHEAS and cortisol. The data emphasize that in male rhesus monkeys both of these adrenal steroids have a similar clear-cut diurnal pattern, with a peak occurring in the morning around the time when the lights come on. Although the data confirm that plasma DHEAS concentrations decline markedly during aging, they fail to support the hypothesis that short-term (4-year) CR attenuates or delays this decline. Several explanations for this conflict with earlier findings in rhesus monkeys can be proposed.[5,6] One possibility is that the 4-year CR treatment was too short to exert a significant protective effect. Similarly, it is possible that the CR was initiated too late in the old animals (i.e., at ~22 years of age). Alternatively, because only two age groups were examined in the present study (i.e., young and old adults), we cannot exclude the possibility that CR exerts a short-term positive effect on DHEAS levels, but that it is not sustained into old age. Finally, we can acknowledge that the previous reports of a positive CR effect on DHEAS were based on hormonal measurements in blood samples that were collected only once during the day, and thus, could be more prone to the confounding influence of the underlying circadian rhythm.

Regarding plasma cortisol levels, we found no significant age-related change. Although the mean and maximum plasma cortisol levels were similar in the young CR animals and age-matched controls, the CR group displayed a second prominent cortisol peak later in the day. This finding is consistent with the observation that the young CR animals showed enhanced locomotor activity during the evenings (data not shown); it is also in general agreement with results from rodent corticosterone studies.[4] However, when the old monkeys were subjected to CR for the same period of time (4 years), their cortisol response was no greater than in the controls; if anything, plasma cortisol levels were generally lower. This age difference in the cortisol response to CR requires further analysis to elucidate its significance. However, one prediction would be that young monkeys will benefit from CR because stress responses are activated; whereas, older monkeys will not benefit as much.

ACKNOWLEDGMENTS

This work was supported by NIH Grants RR-00163, RR-14451, and AG-19914.

REFERENCES

1. RAMSEY, J.J. et al. 2000. Dietary restriction and aging in rhesus monkeys: the University of Wisconsin study. Exp. Gerontol. **35:** 1131–1149.
2. LANE, M.A. et al. Caloric restriction in primates. Ann. N.Y. Acad. Sci. **928:** 287–295.
3. WEINDRUCH, R. & R.S. SOHAL. 1997. Seminars in medicine of the Beth Israel Deaconess Medical Center. Caloric intake and aging. N. Engl. J. Med. **337:** 986–994.
4. MASORO, E.J. 2000. Caloric restriction and aging: an update. Exp. Gerontol. **35:** 299–305.
5. LANE, M.A. et al. 1997. Dehydroepiandrosterone sulfate: a biomarker of primate aging slowed by calorie restriction. J. Clin. Endocrinol. Metab. **82:** 2093–2096.
6. LANE, M.A., D.K. INGRAM & G.S. ROTH. 1999. Nutritional modulation of aging in nonhuman primates. J. Nutr. Health Aging **3:** 69–76.
7. URBANSKI, H.F. et al. 2002. Influence of calorie restriction on the 24-hour release pattern of cortisol, DHEAS, and testosterone in old male rhesus macaques. Proc. 5th Int. Cong. Neuroendocrinol. Bristol, UK, August 31–September 4, 2002. p.107.
8. URBANSKI, H.F. et al. 2002. Effect of calorie restriction on plasma DHEAS and cortisol concentrations in aging male rhesus monkeys. 84th Annual Meeting of the Endocrine Society. San Francisco, June 19–22, 2002. Endocr. Soc. Abstr. p. 340.
9. INGRAM, D.K. et al. 1990. Dietary restriction and aging: the initiation of a primate study. J. Gerontol. **45:** B148–B163.
10. INGRAM, D.K. et al. 1993. Longitudinal study of aging in monkeys: effects of diet restriction. Neurobiol. Aging **14:** 687–688.
11. URBANSKI, H.F. et al. 1997. Alpha-adrenergic receptor antagonism and N-methyl-D-aspartate (NMDA) induced luteinizing hormone release in female rhesus macaques. Brain Res. **744:** 96–104.

Caloric Restriction Modulates Early Events in Insulin Signaling in Liver and Skeletal Muscle of Rat

MIN ZHU, RAFAEL DE CABO, MARK A. LANE,[a] AND DONALD K. INGRAM

Laboratory of Experimental Gerontology, Gerontology Research Center, Intramural Research Program, National Institute on Aging, Baltimore, Maryland 21224, USA

ABSTRACT: Mutations that extend life span in *C. elegans* suggest that the insulin/IGF-1 signaling (IS) pathway may play a key role in retarding aging and extending life span by caloric restriction (CR). To evaluate this hypothesis, male rats were subjected to either AL (*ad libitum*) or CR (40% from AL) for 2 and 25 months, and then the effects of CR on the early events in the IS pathway in liver and muscle were assessed. The results indicated that aging was accompanied by a significant decline in insulin receptor tyrosine phosphorylation (pY-IR) upon insulin stimulation in both tissues, which was correlated with a significant increase in the activity of protein tyrosine phosphatase 1B (PTP-1B). However, these alterations with age were attenuated by 25CR. Parallel changes observed in liver mRNA of CR rats were upregulated insulin receptor (IR), IGF-1R and IRS-1, but increased expression of IR mRNA was dissociated with the IR protein in 25CR rats. The expression of liver mRNAs involved in lipid metabolism was also analyzed. In contrast to 25AL rats, the expression of mRNAs for PPARs (α, δ, and γ) was significantly increased in 25CR rats. SREBP-1c and fatty acid synthase were reduced, and other genes were increased, including hormone-sensitive lipase and PGC-1 by CR. The data suggest that the normal function of insulin receptor in liver and muscle is required for successful aging. An altered expression of transcription of a number of genes involved in lipid metabolism may also contribute to modulation of the IS pathway by CR.

KEYWORDS: caloric restriction; aging; insulin signaling pathway; PTP-1B

SPECIFIC AIMS

Caloric restriction (CR) is the only nongenetic intervention that has been shown to extend the life span and to retard the development of a broad spectrum of pathophysiological changes in rodents and primates.[1,2] In this study, we addressed the hypothesis that caloric restriction modulates the early events in the insulin/IGF-1

Address for correspondence: Donald K. Ingram, Laboratory of Experimental Gerontology, Gerontology Research Center, National Institute on Aging, National Institutes of Health, 5600 Nathan Shock Dr., Baltimore, MD 21224. Voice: 410-558-8180; fax: 410-558-8323.
doni@vax.grc.nia.nih.gov
[a]Current address: Merck and Co., Inc., RY 34-A576, P.O. Box 2000 Rahway, NJ 07065-0900.

Ann. N.Y. Acad. Sci. 1019: 448–452 (2004). © 2004 New York Academy of Sciences.
doi: 10.1196/annals.1297.082

signaling (IS) pathway, which may play a key role in retarding aging and extending the life span. Using male F-344 rats, we evaluated the effects of CR (40% from *ad libitum* for 2 and 25 months) on the insulin receptor (IR) signaling, and investigated IR signaling regulators such as PTP-1B and genes involved in lipid metabolism.

PRINCIPAL FINDINGS

Caloric Restriction Attenuated an Age-Related Decline in Insulin Receptor Tyrosine Phosphoryation in Response to Insulin Stimulation

First, we measured whether aging and CR altered insulin receptor tyrosine phosphoryation (pY-IR), since these results might reflect alterations of the properties and sensitivity of the receptor to its ligand. Although no difference in pY-IR between CR and AL groups was evident under the basal, without insulin-stimulated condition, a single portal vein injection of insulin (10 U/kg body weight) revealed a significant age-related decline in pY-IR in liver ($P < .01$) and muscle ($P < .01$). However, this age-related decline was attenuated by 25CR (pY-IR/IR: $26.2 \pm 3.5\%$ in AL liver vs. $57.2 \pm 12.3\%$ in CR liver, $P < .01$; $38.7 \pm 5.4\%$ in AL muscle vs. $63.9 \pm 6.1\%$ in CR muscle, $P < .05$). No significant CR effect was observed on pY-IR in 2CR rats. Next, we measured whether the amount of IR protein was altered as a function of CR in both tissues. Results indicated that a significant increase in the amount of IR protein was found in 2CR liver (45% increase, $P < .05$) and 2CR muscle (76% increase, $P < .05$) relative to age-matched AL rats, but did not in those tissues of rats maintained on 25-months CR diets.

Caloric Restriction Improved the Aged-Related Increase in Activity of Protein Tyrosine Phosphatase 1B

Protein tyrosine phosphatase 1B (PTP-1B) is a negative regulator of IR phosphorylation. Overexpression of PTP-1B is known to reduce ligand-stimulated autophosphorylation of the insulin receptor and metabolic responses. Therefore, we investigated whether a CR-induced increase in pY-IR could be attributed to alteration in the enzymatic activity of PTP-1B. Results revealed an age-related increase in PTP-1B activity in liver ($P = .110$) and muscle ($P < .05$) under basal conditions. In contrast to 25AL, 25CR rats exhibited a significant decrease in PTP-1B activity in both tissues, but PTP-1B activity in both tissues of 2CR rats was unaffected.

Caloric Restriction Upregulated mRNAs for Insulin Receptor, IGF-1 Receptor, and IRS-1

We further examined the potential effects of CR on the expression of target mRNAs involved in insulin signaling and whether changes in protein expression, if any, were secondary to changes at mRNA levels. The expression profile of liver mRNAs revealed a significant CR-related increase in IR (70% increase in 2CR and 40% increase in 25CR relative to 2AL rats), IGF-1R (75% increase in 25CR relative to 2AL rats), and IRS-1 (55% increase in 25CR relative to 2AL rats), but increased expression of IR mRNA in the rats maintained on 25 months CR diet was not related to the amount of IR protein.

Caloric Restriction Retarded the Age-Related Decline in the Expression of Transcription Factor mRNAs Involved in Lipid Metabolism

It is possible that altered expression of transcription factors and genes central to lipid homeostasis are likely to contribute to alteration in insulin receptor signaling during aging and CR. To examine this possibility, the expression of genes involved in lipid metabolism was analyzed in liver. The expression of PPARs (α, δ, γ) with several targeted genes was reciprocally regulated during aging and CR. PPARs were barely detected in 25AL rats, but a significant increase was found only in 25CR rats. Sterol regulatory element binding protein (SREBP-1c) mRNA levels were reduced significantly by both 2CR and 25CR, and PPAR-coactivator 1 (PGC-1) mRNA levels were significantly increased 73% in 25CR rats. Fatty acid synthase mRNA levels were decreased in 25CR rats ($P < .001$), and hormone-sensitive lipase mRNA levels were increased 99% in 2CR ($P < .01$) and 127% in 25CR rats ($P < .001$). Increased lipolysis, coupled to decreased lipogenesis, may contribute to adipocytokine production and secretion. For instance, enhancing plasma adiponectin may result in reduced triglyceride accumulation in liver and muscle, thereby improving insulin receptor signaling.

CONCLUSIONS AND SIGNIFICANCE

Alterations in the early steps of insulin signaling have been recognized as an important component of many insulin-resistant states. The present study demonstrates that CR, particularly long-term CR, induces multiple alterations in the early events in the IS pathway, attenuating age-related decline in pY-IR in response to insulin, preventing age-related increase in PTP-1B activity, and upregulating associated mRNAs involved in the IS pathway. The changes that we observed are consistent with the well-known effects of CR on insulin sensitivity, and may contribute to the underlying mechanisms by which this nutritional intervention extends life span and retards aging.

Our findings that long-term CR attenuated an age-related decline in insulin-stimulated pY-IR in insulin-sensitive tissues may account, at least in part, for some of the protective effect of CR toward the development or delay in the onset of type 2 diabetes.[3] An increasing body of evidence suggests that alteration in insulin receptor phosphorylation state is present in insulin-resistant states and type 2 diabetes[4,5] that may lead to a dramatic diminution of the life span. Thus, improving insulin receptor activities in response to insulin may be one way in which potentially detrimental effects of aging on IR function in the animals maintained on an AL diet could be explained. This also suggests that the normal function of the insulin receptor in liver and skeletal muscle is required for healthy aging in mammals. In addition, our data from short-term CR in young animals demonstrated a different mechanism.

We also observed that long-term CR blocked the age-related increase in PTP-1B activity in both liver and skeletal muscle. PTP-1B has been implicated as a negative regulator of insulin receptor signaling and activity of insulin against the β-subunit of insulin receptor.[6,7] Numerous studies have demonstrated that the insulin resistance seen in type 2 diabetes, obesity, and even aging is often accompanied by an increase in PTP-1B activity.[8,9] Similarly, mutant mice lacking PTP-1B exhibit enhanced insulin sensitivity, increased pY-IR, and resistance to obesity,[8,10] consistent with a role of PTP-1B in the insulin receptor signaling. The age-related increase in PTP-1B activity observed in the present study is consistent with reduced insulin receptor function or sensitivity observed in older individuals. The decline we observed in PTP-1B activity in the liver and skeletal muscle of animals maintained on the 25-month CR diet suggests an enhanced insulin response, consistent with our findings that pY-IR was improved in these tissues following insulin stimulation.

When we examined the pattern of aging and changes induced by CR in gene expression related to lipid metabolism, in particular the peroxisome proliferator-activated receptors (PPARs), additional insight emerged regarding possible mechanisms for the observed alterations in insulin receptor signaling. Despite the fact that we did not examine the precise contributions that CR makes to the modulation of insulin receptor signaling, our recent findings[11] provide the molecular evidence that may account for the mechanism by which CR improves insulin receptor signaling. An enhancement in circulating adiponectin levels results in reduced triglyceride levels in plasma and tissues as the concomitants of a concerted modulation in the expression of key transcription target genes involved in fatty acid oxidation and energy combustion, thereby improving insulin receptor signaling.

The significance of this study is severalfold. First, our results provide new insights into the molecular events that may contribute to the mechanism through which CR improves insulin sensitivity and attenuates the age-related increase in glucose intolerance. Specifically, CR improved PTP-1B activity and prevented the age-related decline in pY-IR. Second, our findings suggest that the early events in insulin signal pathway such as PTP-1B may play an important role in aging and its retardation by CR, and that these early events may represent potential targets for other interventions that may mimic the effects of CR without reducing food intake. Finally, an altered expression of transcription of genes that regulate lipid metabolism suggests that lipid mediators may also play an important role in the early events of the insulin signaling during aging and CR.

REFERENCES

1. MASORO, E.J. 2000. Caloric restriction and aging: an update. Exp. Gerontol. **35:** 299–305.
2. ROTH, G.S., D.K. INGRAM & A.M. LANE. 2001. Caloric restriction in primates and relevance to humans. Ann. N.Y. Acad. Sci. **928:** 305–315.
3. HANSEN, B.C. & N.L. BODKIN. 1993. Primary prevention of diabetes mellitus by prevention of obesity in monkeys. Diabetes **42:** 1809–1814.
4. YOUNGREN, J.F., J. PAIK & R.J. BARNARD. 2001. Impaired insulin-receptor autophosphorylation is an early defect in fat-fed, insulin-resistant rats. J. Appl. Physiol. **91:** 2240–2247.
5. FRIEDMAN, J.E., T. ISHIZUKA, S. LIU, et al. 1997. Reduced insulin receptor signaling in the obese spontaneously hypertensive Koletsky rat. Am. J. Physiol. **273:** E1014–E1023.
6. LIU, F. & J. CHERNOFF. 1997. Protein tyrosine phosphatase 1B interacts with and is tyrosine phosphorylated by the epidermal growth factor receptor. Biochem. J. **327:** 139–145.
7. BYON, J.C., A.B. KUSARI & J. KUSARI. 1998. Protein-tyrosine phosphatase-1B acts as a negative regulator of insulin signal transduction. Mol. Cell. Biochem. **182:** 101–108.
8. KLAMAN, L.D., O. BOSS, O.D. PERONI, et al. 2000. Increased energy expenditure, decreased adiposity, and tissue-specific insulin sensitivity in protein-tyrosine phosphatase 1B-deficient mice. Mol. Cell. Biol. **20:** 5479–5489.

9. KENNEDY, B.P. & C. RAMACHANDRAN. 2000. Protein tyrosine phosphatase-1B in diabetes. Biochem. Pharmacol. **60:** 877–883.
10. ELCHEBLY, M., P. PAYETTE, E. MICHALISZYN, *et al.* 1999. Increased insulin sensitivity and obesity resistance in mice lacking the protein tyrosine phosphatase-1B gene. Science **283:** 1544–1548.
11. ZHU, M., J. MIURA, L.X. LU, *et al.* 2004. Circulating adiponectin levels increase in rats on caloric restriction: the potential for insulin sensitization. Exp. Gerontol. In press.

Aging, Exercise, and Phytochemicals
Promises and Pitfalls

LI LI JI[a] AND DAVID M. PETERSON[b]

[a]*Department of Kinesiology and Nutritional Sciences, University of Wisconsin-Madison, Madison, Wisconsin 53706, USA*
[b]*USDA, Agricultural Research Service, Cereal Crops Research Unit, Madison, Wisconsin 53726, USA*

ABSTRACT: Phytochemicals are emerging comprehensive and versatile sources of antioxidants to be consumed to enhance the body's defenses against harmful reactive oxygen species generated endogenously or exogenously. Tocols, favonoids, and phenolic acids compose the majority of this class of antioxidants, although more complex compounds may also be involved, such as ginsenosides. *In vitro* and *in vivo* studies have demonstrated convincingly that dietary supplementation of phytochemicals has beneficial effects against certain types of pathogenesis, disease, cancer, and aging. There is evidence that these effects are related to the ability of phytochemicals to promote the antioxidant defense system and reduce oxidative stress and damage in the cell. However, due to their structural and chemical diversity and complexity, many of the benefits as well as potential adverse effects remain to be examined.

KEYWORDS: aging; antioxidant; exercise; oxidative stress; phytochemical; free radical

Reactive oxygen species (ROS) are generated ubiquitously in aerobic organisms.[1] When these cytotoxic agents overwhelm the endogenous antioxidant defense system, serious oxidative stress and damage occur, as reflected by the oxidative modification of macromolecules such as lipid, protein, and DNA.[2] ROS generation has important implications in the etiology of numerous diseases and in aging.[3,4] Thus, it is critical that cells maintain optimal antioxidant defenses in order to reduce oxidative damage. Dietary supplementation and therapeutic use of antioxidants are emerging measures to prevent and treat oxidative stress-induced diseases.[5,6]

Nature offers an abundance of resources of antioxidants, most of which are present in fruits and vegetables known as phytochemicals.[7] Most of the phytochemicals are in the chemical form of phenolic compounds that have the ability of quenching or reducing ROS due to their redox properties. Tocols (such as tocopherols and tocotrienols), favonoids (such as soy isoflavone, tea catechins, and anthocyanidines), monophenolic acids (such as caffeic acid and ferulic acids), and polyphenolic acids (such as avenathramides) are the most common antioxidant phytochemicals.

Address for correspondence: Li Li Ji, Ph.D., 2000 Observatory Drive, Madison, WI 53706. Voice: 608-262-7250; fax: 608-262-1656.
ji@education.wisc.edu

We have become very interested in exploring this promising field that has great potential in providing effective protection against aging- and exercise-associated oxidative damage. Ginseng and oats are two examples of our recent efforts.[8,9] The purpose of this short communication is to provide highlights of our findings and discuss potential implications.

CHRONIC GINSENG CONSUMPTION ATTENUATES AGE-ASSOCIATED OXIDATIVE STRESS IN RATS

As one of the most popular dietary supplements, ginsengs (*Panax C. A. Meyer*, or Asian ginseng, and *Panax quinquefolius L.*, or North American ginseng) have drawn attention worldwide for their valuable, broad medicinal effects.[10–12] Since 2000, over 900 articles have been published regarding the potential biological effects of ginseng alone. Although the mechanism for ginseng's health-promoting effects is complex and still elusive, it is believed that the primary active ingredients are composed of a mixture of saponin glycosides, known as ginsenosides. Recent research indicates that ginseng has powerful antioxidant properties, which may explain its antiaging and antineoplastic effects.[13] Furthermore, higher ginsenoside content is found in *P. quinquefolius*.[14,15]

Ginseng demonstrates a wide variety of pharmacological effects, probably due to its structural diversity. Phytopanaxadiols, a group of ginsenosides containing two glucose moieties on the C-3 position while differing between glucose and arabinose on C-20, such as Rb1, Rb2, Rc, and Rd, are more abundant in North American ginseng than in Asian ginseng, and exhibit more potent antioxidant properties.[10] Treatment of ginseng extract and dietary supplementation of ginseng has shown a variety of protective effects against oxidative damage *in vitro* and *in vivo*, ranging from isolated low-density lipoprotein (LDL) oxidation, loss of memory, ischemic neuron dysfunction, to heart reperfusion injury.[16–19] A relatively limited amount of literature has investigated the effects of ginseng on aging and age-related health problems.[20–22] Although ginsenosides as a whole appear to have free-radical scavenging and metal-ion chelating abilities, different fractions of phytopanaxadiols appear to exert their antioxidant function via different mechanisms. For example, Rb1 (containing four glucoses) was found to directly interact with hydroxyl radicals and protect ischemic neuron,[18] whereas Rb2 (containing three glucoses and an arabinose in pyranose form) has been shown to stimulate nuclear protein binding to gene regulatory sequences on CuZn SOD promoter.[23,24] Recently, Rh2 and Rh3 have been found to modulate protein kinase C isoforms and differentiation of granulocytes.[25]

Recently, we have performed a study wherein female Fischer 344 rats at 4 ($n = 36$) or 22 ($n = 24$) months of age were randomly divided into three groups, fed either a control diet, or a diet containing 0.5 g/kg (low-dose) or 2.5 g/kg (high-dose) dry ginseng power for 4 months.[8] We used a well-defined Wisconsin ginseng line that contained 12% ginsenosides, among which 9.6% was in the form of phytopanaxadiol. Oxidant generation, measured with 2'7'-dichlorofluorescin (DCFH), was significantly lowered, with ginseng feeding in the homogenates of heart, the oxidative type of skeletal muscle soleus and the deep portion of vastus lateralis (DVL). In the heart young and old rats fed high-dose ginseng diet showed 38% and 18% ($P < .05$) lower oxidant levels compared to control rats, respectively (FIG. 1a).

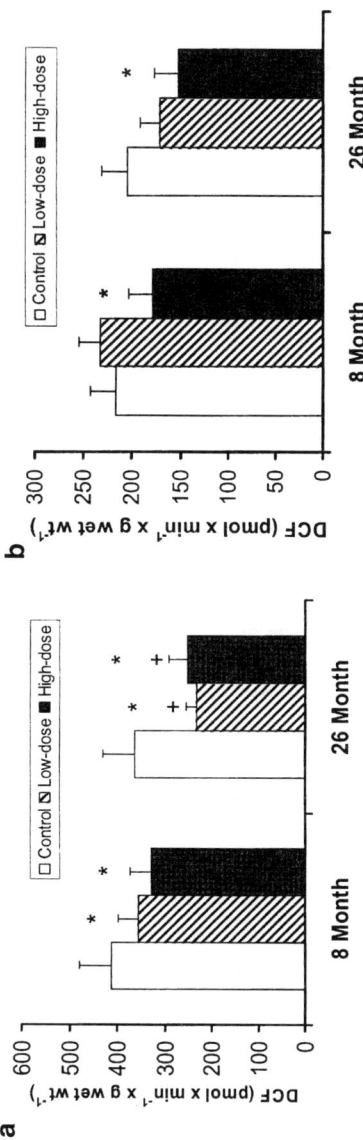

FIGURE 1. Oxidation rate of dichlorofluorescin (DCFH) to dichlorofluorescein (DCF) in the (**a**) homogenate of rat heart, and (**b**) deep portion of vastus lateralis muscle. The assay buffer contained 130 mM KCl, 5 mM MgCl$_2$, 20 mM NaH$_2$PO$_4$, 20 mM Tris-HCl, and 30 mM glucose (pH 7.4) with 5 μM DCFH-diacetate dissolved in 1.25 mM methanol. Each *bar* represents mean ± SEM with number of rats in each group specified in TABLE 2. *$P < .05$, low-dose or high-dose ginseng vs. control. $^+P < .05$, main age effect; $^{++}P < .01$, 26 month vs. 8-month-old rats.

In DVL muscle (FIG. 1b), high-dose ginseng feeding decreased DCF formation by 18% in young rats and by 24% in old rats. Similar effects were found in soleus (not shown). Although ginseng has long been reported to be a scavenger of free radicals *in vitro*, this was the first evidence that steady state ROS concentration might be reduced in chronic ginseng-supplemented animals *in vivo*. Our data showed that the effect of ginseng to reduce ROS generation could be explained by its ability to modulate the endogenous antioxidant defense systems in rat tissues. Rats fed a ginseng-fortified diet generally demonstrated higher levels of SOD and glutathione peroxidase (GPX) activities.[8] SOD activity was elevated in the heart and DVL of young rats by high-dose feeding, and in soleus of both age groups. GPX activity in DVL and soleus muscle was also increased in ginseng-supplemented rats. In addition, citrate synthase activity in the heart of both age groups and DVL of young rats was elevated, suggesting an increased mitochondrial oxidative capacity. Much curiosity remains as to why ginseng feeding led to increased antioxidant enzyme activities. One potential mechanism was that certain structural motifs of phytopanaxadiol (e.g., Rb2) are capable of interacting with specific gene regulatory sequences on antioxidant genes, thereby activating transcription, as was reported for CuZn SOD.[23]

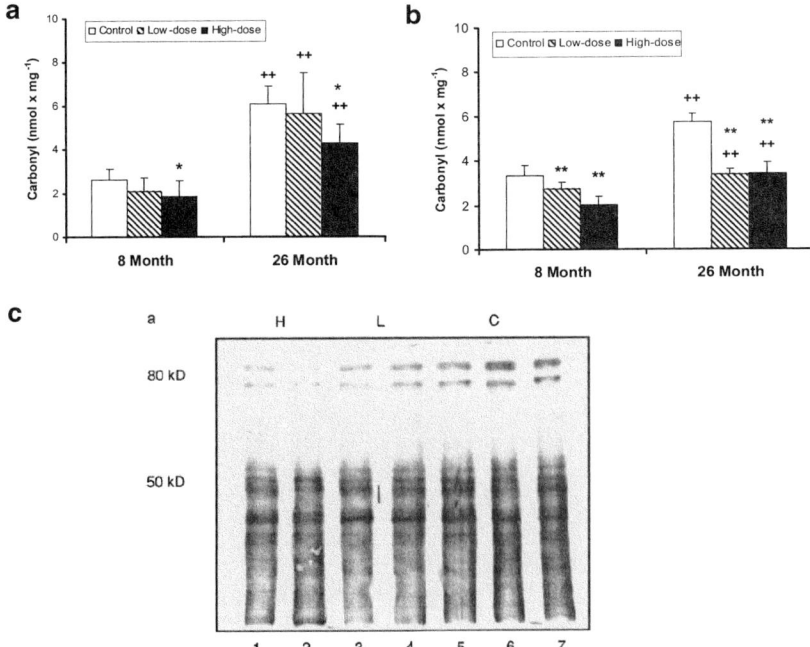

FIGURE 2. Protein carbonyl content in (**a**) rat heart and (**b**) deep portion of vastus lateralis muscle. Each *bar* represents mean ± SEM with 8–14 rats in each group. $^*P < .05$; $^{**}P < .01$, low-dose or high-dose ginseng vs. control. $^+P < .05$; $^{++}P < .01$, 26 month vs. 8-month-old rats. (**c**) Western blot analysis of reactive carbonyl derivatives in the heart of old rats. Samples are pooled from 5 rats randomly selected from each group. *Lanes 1–2*, high-dose ginseng diet; *lanes 3–4*, low-dose ginseng diet; *lanes 5–7*, control diet.

We measured protein carbonyl formation as a marker of oxidative damage in the various tissues. Protein oxidation was more than twofold higher in the hearts and 65% higher ($P < .01$) in the DVL, comparing old vs. young rats (FIG. 2). High-dose ginseng treatment attenuated age-associated protein oxidation in the hearts and DVL muscle. This was confirmed by both chemical assays and Western blot analysis using antibody against protein carbonyl. Taken together, we conclude that North American ginseng supplementation in rats can decrease oxidant production and age-related oxidative damage to protein in the heart and skeletal muscle. Elevated SOD and GPX activities may partially explain these protective effects.

The merit of ginseng consumption has been historically mixed with concerns about potential adverse effects and side effects due to inappropriate dosage.[10–12] In the study just mentioned, high-dose ginseng feeding resulted in a significant reduction of body weight in the aged rats, which was not caused by decreased food consumption. It is uncertain whether the decreased body weight was due to fat or protein loss. However, the significantly increased heart and muscle CS activity resulting from high-dose ginseng feeding argued against a possible retardation of body protein synthesis. Some authors postulated that certain ginsenoside fractions at high doses could behave as prooxidant *in vitro*.[26] Although this possibility could not be ruled out, we did not find any evidence of increased ROS production or oxidative stress as a result of high-dose ginseng feeding. Potential harmful effects of ginseng have been reported in several recent articles. For example, panaxadiol was recently reported to induce apoptotic cell death by depolarization of mitochondrial membrane potential in human hepatoma cells, followed by cytochrome *c* release due to activation of Cdk2 kinase and caspases-9, -3, and -7.[27] Oligosaccharides from ginsenosides could be hydrolyzed in the digestive tract and absorbed into the circulation following oral administration. Some of the major ginsenoside metabolites have been shown to inhibit acetylcholine-induced secretion of catecholamines due to interference of ion channels.[28,29] Yet another report showed that ginsenoside-Rh1 activated the transcription of the estrogen-responsive luciferase reporter gene in MCF-7 breast cancer cells.[30] The effect was blocked by the estrogen receptor antagonist, indicating that Rh1 may act as a weak phytoestrogen. These results led to the suggestion that some of the ginsenoside fractions or ginseng metabolites may serve as prodrugs, the health outcome of which deserve caution and further investigation.

EFFECTS OF AVENANTHRAMIDES ON OXIDANT GENERATION AND ANTIOXIDANT ENZYME ACTIVITY IN EXERCISED RATS

Oats (*Avena sativa* L.) contain several families of phytochemicals that display antioxidant properties, such as tocotrienols, phenolic acids, flavonoids, sterols, and phytic acid.[31–33] Both animal studies and human clinical trials confirmed that oat antioxidants have the potential of reducing cardiovascular risks by lowering serum cholesterol, inhibiting LDL oxidation, and attenuating platelet aggregation and peroxidation. In addition to these well-characterized antioxidants, there is a small fraction of anionic, nitrogen-containing, covalently linked hydroxycinnamic acid compounds, called avenanthramides (AVEN), that have only been identified in oats.[34,35] Among a group of several AVEN that differ in the substituents on the

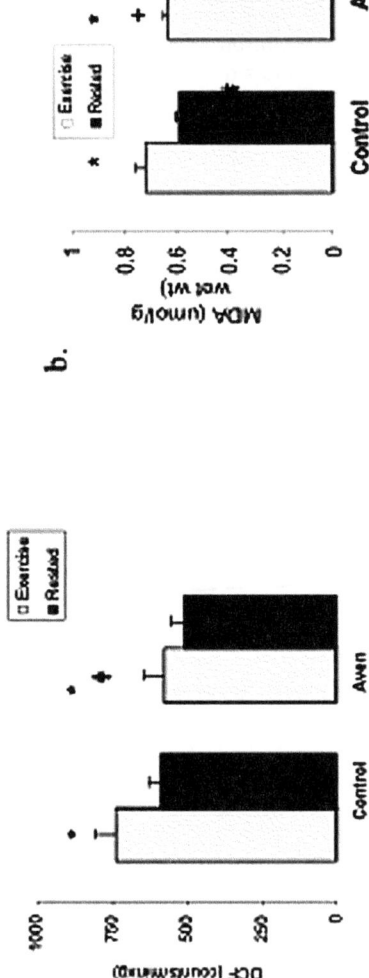

FIGURE 3. (a) Oxidation rate of dichlorofluorescin (DCFH) to dichlorofluorescein (DCF) in the homogenates of soleus muscle from avenanthramide (AVEN)-supplemented and control rats. The assay buffer contained 130 mM KCl, 5 mM MgCl$_2$, 20 mM NaH$_2$PO$_4$, 20 mM tris-HCl, and 30 mM glucose (pH 7.4), plus 2 mM malate and 2 mM pyruvate. Each *bar* represents mean ± SEM (n = 12). *P < .05, exercised vs. rested. +P < .05, AVEN vs. controls. (b) Malondialdehyde (MDA) content in the heart of AVEN-supplemented and control rats. Each *bar* represents mean ± SEM (n = 12). *P < .05, exercised vs. rested. +P < .05, AVEN vs. controls.

cinnamic acid and anthranilic acid rings, three are predominant in oat grain: Bp, Bf, and Bc [N-(3′,4′-dihydroxycinnamoyl)-5-hydroxyanthranilic acid].

In a recent study we examined whether dietary AVEN supplementation increases antioxidant capacity in the biological tissues, thereby reducing steady state ROS formation and oxidative tissue damage.[9] In order to reveal their potential protective effects, we subjected AVEN-supplemented rats to an acute bout of strenuous physical exercise, which is known to increase ROS generation in the heart and skeletal muscle.[36,37] Female Sprague-Dawley rats ($n = 48$, age 6–7 weeks) were fed either an AIN-93-based control diet or the same diet containing 0.1 g/kg AVEN-Bc for 50 days. Each group was further divided into rested and exercised (treadmill running at 22.5 m/min, 10% grade for 1 hour) prior to killing. AVEN supplementation *per se* had no effect on ROS production (using the DCFH method) in most tissues; however, the ROS level was decreased in the oxidative muscle soleus in rats (FIG. 3a). Exercise increased ROS production in the liver, DVL muscle, and soleus muscle, whereas AVEN attenuated exercise-induced ROS in the soleus. AVEN-fed rats showed significantly higher SOD activity in the liver, kidney, DVL muscle, and soleus muscle.[36] AVEN treatment also tended to elevate GPX activity in the heart, kidney, and DVL muscle, compared to control rats. Lipid peroxidation measured by malonaldehyde content in the heart, liver, and DVL muscle was increased as a result of the bout of acute exercise, and AVEN treatment decreased exercise-induced lipid peroxidation in the heart (FIG. 3b). These findings demonstrated for the first time that dietary supplementation of a synthetic avenanthramide selectively attenuated exercise-induced ROS production and lipid peoxidation. The antioxidant effects of AVEN were likely related to its ability to influence tissue antioxidant enzyme systems such as SOD and GPX activities.

CONCLUSION

Phytochemicals are emerging comprehensive and versatile sources of antioxidants to be consumed to enhance the body's defenses against harmful endogenously or exogenously generated ROS. Tocopherols, tocotrienols, favonoids, and mono- and polyphenolic acids compose the majority of this class of antioxidants, although more complex compounds, such as ginsenosides, may also be involved. *In vitro* and *in vivo* studies have demonstrated convincingly that dietary supplementation of phytochemicals has beneficial effects against certain types of pathogenesis, disease, cancer, and aging. There is evidence that these effects are related to their ability to boost the cellular antioxidant defense system and reduce oxidative stress and damage. However, due to their structural diversity and complexity, many of the benefits as well as potential adverse effects remain to be examined.

REFERENCES

1. HALLIWELL, B.H. & J.M.C. GUTTERIDGE. 1999. Free Radicals in Biology and Medicine. Oxford University Press. Oxford.
2. AMES, B.N., M.K. SHIGENAGA & T.M. HAGEN. 1993. Oxidants, antioxidants, and the degenerative diseases of aging. Proc. Natl. Acad. Sci. USA **90**: 7915–7921.
3. FINKEL, T. & N. HOLBROOK. 2000. Oxidants, oxidative stress and biology of aging. Nature. **408**: 239–247.

4. HARMAN, D. 1956. Aging: a theory based on free radical and radiation chemistry. J. Gerontol. **11:** 298–300.
5. YU, B.P. 1994. Cellular defenses against damage from reactive oxygen species. Physiol. Rev. **74:** 139–162.
6. MEYDANI, M. 2002. The Boyd Orr lecture. Nutrition interventions in aging and age-associated disease. Proc. Nutr. Soc. **61:** 165–171.
7. HERTOG, M.G. 1996. Epidemiological evidence on potential health properties of flavonoids. Proc. Nutr. Soc. **55:** 385–397.
8. FU, Y. & L.L. JI. 2003. Chronic ginseng consumption attenuates age-associated oxidative stress in rats. J. Nutr. **133:** 3603–3609.
9. JI, L.L., D. LAY, E. CHUNG, et al. 2003. Effects of avenanthramides on oxidant and antioxidant status in exercised rats. Nutr. Res. **23:** 1579–1590.
10. KITTS, D. & C. HU. 2000. Efficacy and safety of ginseng. Public Health Nutr **3:** 473–485.
11. ATTELE, A.S., J.A. WU & C.S. YUAN. 1999. Ginseng pharmacology: multiple constituents and multiple actions. Biochem. Pharmacol. **58:** 1685–1693.
12. GILLIS, C.N. 1997. Panax ginseng pharmacology: a nitric oxide link? Biochem. Pharmacol. **54:** 1–8.
13. KITTS, D.D., A.N. WIJEWICKREME & C. HU. 2000. Antioxidant properties of a North American ginseng extract. Mol. Cell. Biochem. **203:** 1–10.
14. CHAN, T.W.D., P.P.H. BUT, S.W. CHENG, et al. 2000. Differentiation and authentication of Panax ginseng, Panax quinquefolius, and ginseng products by using HPLC/MS. Anal. Chem. **72:** 1281–1287.
15. WANG, X., T. SAKUMA, E. ASAFU-ADJAYE & G. K. SHIU. 1999. Determination of ginsenosides in plant extracts from Panax ginseng and Panax quinquefolius L. by LC/MS/MS. Anal. Chem. **71:** 579–584.
16. ZHANG, D., T. YASUDA, Y. YU, et al.1996. Ginseng extract scavenges hydroxyl radical and protects unsaturated fatty acids from decomposition caused by iron-mediated lipid peroxidation. Free Radical Biol. Med. **20:** 145–150.
17. CHAN, P., C.S. NIU, B. TOMLINSON, et al. 1997. Effect of trilinolein on superoxide dismutase activity and left ventricular pressure in isolated rat hearts subjected to hypoxia and normoxic perfusion. Pharmacology **55:** 252–258.
18. LIM, J.H., T.C. WEN, S. MATSUDA, et al. 1997. Protection of ischemic hippocampal neurons by ginsenoside Rb1, a main ingredient of ginseng root. Neurosci. Res. **28:** 191–200.
19. JIANG, F., S. DESILVA & J. TURNBULL. 2000. Beneficial effect of ginseng root in SOD-1 (G93A) transgenic mice. J. Neurol. Sci. **180:** 52–54.
20. JAENICKE, B., E.J., KIM, J.W. AHN & H.S. LEE. 1991. Effect of Panax ginseng extract on passive avoidance retention in old rats. Arch. Pharm. Res. **14:** 25–29.
21. NITTA, H., K. MATSUMOTO, M. SHIMIZU, et al. 1995. Panax ginseng extract improves the performance of aged Fischer 344 rats in radial maze task but not in operant brightness discrimination task. Biol. Pharm. Bull. **18:** 1286–1288.
22. YU, S.C. & X.Y. LI. 2000. Effect of ginsenoside on IL-1 beta and IL-6 mRNA expression in hippocampal neurons in chronic inflammation model of aged rats. Acta Pharmacol. Sin. **21:** 915–918.
23. KIM, Y.H., K.H. PARK & H.M. RHO. 1996. Transcriptional activation of the Cu,Zn-superoxide dismutase gene through the AP2 site by ginsenoside Rb2 extracted from a medicinal plant, Panax ginseng. J. Biol. Chem. **271:** 24539–24543.
24. CHANG, M.S., S.G. LEE & H.M. RHO. 1999. Transcriptional activation of Cu/Zn superoxide dismutase and catalase genes by panaxadiol ginsenosides extracted from Panax ginseng. Phytother. Res. **13:** 641–644.
25. KIM, Y.S., D.S. KIM & S.I. KIM. 1998. Ginsenoside Rh2 and Rh3 induce differention of HL-60 cells into granulocytes: modulation of protein kinase C isoforms during differentiation by ginsenoside Rh2. Int. J. Biochem. Cell. Biol. **30:** 327–338.
26. LIU, Z.Q., X.Y. LUO, G.Z. LIU, et al. 2003. In vitro study of the relationship between the structure of ginsenoside and its antioxidative or prooxidative activity in free radical induced hemolysis of human erythrocytes. J. Agric. Food Chem. **51:** 2555–2558.
27. JIN, Y.H., H. YIM, J.H. PARK & S.K. LEE. 2003. Cdk2 activity is associated with depolarization of mitochondrial membrane potential during apoptosis. Biochem. Biophys. Res. Commun. **305:** 974–980.

28. TACHIKAWA, E., K. KUDO, H. HASEGAWA, et al. 2003. In vitro inhibition of adrenal catecholamine secretion by steroidal metabolites of ginseng saponins. Biochem. Pharmacol. **66:** 2213–2221.
29. LEE, J.H., S.M. JEONG, B.H. LEE, et al. 2003. Differential effect of bovine serum albumin on ginsenoside metabolite-induced inhibition of alpha3beta4 nicotinic acetylcholine receptor expressed in Xenopus oocytes. Arch. Pharm. Res. **26:** 868–873.
30. LEE, Y.J., Y.R. JIN, W.C. LIM, et al. 2003. Ginsenoside-Rb1 acts as a weak phytoestrogen in MCF-7 human breast cancer cells. Arch. Pharm. Res. **26:** 58–63.
31. PETERSON, D.M. 2001. Oat antioxidants. J. Cereal Sci. **33:** 115–129.
32. COLLINS, F.W. 1989. Oat phenolics: avenanthramides, novel substituted N-cinnamoylanthranilate alkaloids from oat groats and hulls. J. Agric. Food Chem. **37:** 60–66.
33. DIMBERG, L.H., O. THEANDER & H. LINGNER. 1993. Avenanthramide-A group of penolic antioxidants in oats. Cereal Chem. **70:** 673–641.
34. BRATT, K., K. SUNNERHEIM, S. BRYNGELSSON, et al. 2003. Avenanthramides in oats (*Avena sativa* L.): structure—antioxidant activity relationships. J. Agric. Food Chem. **51:** 594–600.
35. PETERSON, D.M., M.J. HAHN & C.L. EMMONS. 2002. Oat avenanthramides exhibit antioxidant activities in vitro. Food Chem. **79:** 473–478.
36. BEJMA, J. & L.L. JI. 1999. Aging and acute exercise enhance free radical generation in rat skeletal muscle. J. Appl. Physiol. **87:** 465–470.
37. BEJMA, J., P. RAMIRES & L.L. JI. 2000. Free radical generation and oxidative stress with aging and exercise: differential effects in the myocardium and liver. Acta Physiol. Scand. **169:** 343–351.

Aging, Exercise, and Cardioprotection

SCOTT K. POWERS, JOHN QUINDRY, AND KARYN HAMILTON

*Department of Exercise and Sport Sciences and Physiology,
Center for Exercise Science, University of Florida,
Gainesville, Florida 32611, USA*

ABSTRACT: Myocardial ischemia-reperfusion (I-R) injury is a major contributor to the morbidity and mortality associated with coronary artery disease. The incidence of I-R events is greatest in older persons, and studies also indicate that the magnitude of myocardial I-R injury is greater in senescent individuals compared to younger adults. Regular exercise has been confirmed as a pragmatic countermeasure to protect against I-R–induced cardiac injury. Specifically, endurance exercise has been proven to provide cardioprotection against an I-R insult in both young and old animals. Proposed mechanisms to explain the cardioprotective effect of exercise include the induction of myocardial heat shock proteins (HSPs), improved cardiac antioxidant capacity, and/or elevation of other cardioprotective proteins. Of these potential mechanisms, evidence indicates that elevated myocardial levels of heat shock proteins or antioxidants can provide myocardial protection against I-R injury. At present, which of these protective mechanisms is essential for exercise-induced cardioprotection remains unclear. Understanding the molecular basis for exercise-induced cardioprotection is important in developing exercise paradigms to protect the heart during an I-R insult.

KEYWORDS: heart; ischemia-reperfusion; antioxidants; heat shock proteins

INTRODUCTION

Coronary artery disease continues as the major cause of death in developed countries. Although heart disease has an impact on individuals of all ages, the incidence of coronary artery disease is greatest in older populations. A primary pathological manifestation of coronary artery disease is myocardial damage due to ischemia-reperfusion (I-R) injury. The level of I-R–induced myocardial injury can range from a small insult, resulting in limited damage, to a large insult, culminating in major cardiac electrical and mechanical dysfunction. Major I-R injury to the heart can result in permanent disability or death.

Given the worldwide prevalence of coronary artery disease and the associated I-R–induced cardiac injury, developing a countermeasure to protect the heart against I-R–induced damage is important. A pragmatic cardioprotective intervention is physical exercise. Indeed, numerous experimental studies reveal that a regular rou-

Address for correspondence: Scott K. Powers, Department of Exercise and Sport Sciences, Center for Exercise Science, University of Florida, Gainesville, FL 32611. Voice: 352-392-9575, ext. 1343; fax: 352-392-0316.
spowers@hhp.ufl.edu

tine of endurance exercise (i.e., running or swimming) protects the heart from injury during an I-R insult in both young and old animals.[1–5] This review will summarize our current knowledge about the effects of age on myocardial I-R injury and will discuss the evidence indicating that regular exercise is cardioprotective across the life span. Importantly, the potential mechanisms responsible for exercise-induced cardioprotection will also be addressed.

MYOCARDIAL ISCHEMIA-REPERFUSION INJURY: LEVELS OF INJURY

Despite the complexity in the mechanism(s) responsible for I-R–induced tissue injury, essential factors leading to I-R–induced cellular injury have been delineated in recent years. It is now clear that several interrelated factors (e.g., oxidative injury and calcium overload) are responsible for I-R injury.[6] Collectively, these factors promote cellular injury, which can lead to cardiac myocyte death.

Depending upon the duration of both ischemia and reperfusion, three levels of I-R–induced cardiac injury have been described.[7] The lowest level of injury occurs when the ischemic period is <5 minutes (FIG. 1). This level of injury is associated with cardiac arrhythmias, but does not result in ventricular contractile dysfunction or cardiac cell death. The second category of cardiac injury occurs when the ischemic period extends from 5 minutes to 20 minutes. This type of cardiac injury is commonly referred to as myocardial stunning and is characterized by arrhythmias along with a reversible ventricular contractile dysfunction without cardiac myocyte death.[6] The third and most severe level of I-R injury occurs when ischemia is extended beyond 20 minutes. Under these circumstances, cardiac myocytes become irreversibly damaged, resulting in cell death.[7] This is significant because infarcted tissue loses contractility, and therefore the pump function of the heart is diminished. Indeed, the magnitude of myocardial infarction is a major contributor to the mortality associated with myocardial I-R injury.[7]

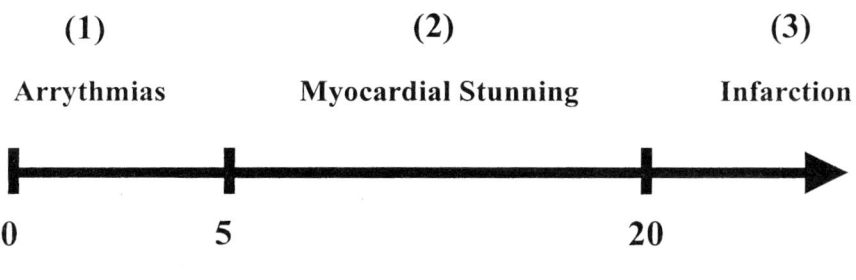

FIGURE 1. An illustration of the three levels of myocardial injury resulting from ischemia-reperfusion. (See text for details.)

AGING AND MYOCARDIAL ISCHEMIA-REPERFUSION INJURY

It is well established that numerous cellular and functional changes occur in the rodent heart over the course of the life span.[8–9] In particular, senescence is associated with (1) alterations in cardiac gene expression;[10] (2) an increased rate of radical production along with unfavorable changes in the glutathione redox status;[9,11] (3) a decrease in mitochondrial cardiolipin and the ratio of mitochondrial membrane omega-3 to omega-6 polyunsaturated fatty acids;[8] and (4) a reduced ability of the heart to respond to stress.[12,13] Given these age-related changes, it is not surprising that I-R–induced myocardial injury is greater in senescent animals compared to young adults.[8,9] The specific mechanisms underlying the increased susceptibility to I-R injury in senescence continues to be an active area of research and debate. Nonetheless, it appears likely that each of the aforementioned age-related changes in the heart could contribute, at least in part, to this increased risk of I-R damage in the heart.

EXERCISE-INDUCED PROTECTION AGAINST MYOCARDIAL ISCHEMIA-REPERFUSION INJURY

It is well known that exercise training improves myocardial tolerance to I-R.[1–5,14] This exercise-mediated protection is observed in both moderate-duration ischemia (i.e,. 5–20 min, resulting in myocardial stunning) and long-duration ischemia (i.e., 40–60 min, resulting in myocardial infarction).[1–5,14] Specifically, recent studies from our laboratory indicate that both long-term (~10 weeks) and short-term (1–5 days) endurance exercise training reduces myocardial oxidative injury and improves myocardial contractile performance in rats following an *in vivo* I-R insult.[1,4,5] Interestingly, short-term exercise training (i.e., 3–5 consecutive days) provides the same cardiac protection as that observed following long-term training (i.e., 10 weeks).[1,3,5]

Mechanism(s) Responsible for the Exercise-Induced Cardioprotection

At present, the mechanism(s) behind the exercise-induced myocardial protection against I-R injury are unknown. In theory, several mechanisms could explain the cardioprotective effect of exercise. These include anatomic changes in the coronary arteries (i.e., collateral circulation), induction of myocardial HSPs, improved myocardial antioxidant capacity, and/or induction of other unknown cytoprotective proteins.

Exercise and Myocardial Collateral Circulation

Although the development of collateral circulation may occur in some animal species following many months of endurance training, evidence indicates that the beneficial effects of short-term exercise are not due to the development of collateral circulation.[15] Hence, by elimination, it appears that the exercise-induced cardioprotection associated with short-duration endurance training is due to the exercise-induced expression of cardioprotective molecules.

Heat Shock Proteins and Myocardial Ischemia-Reperfusion Injury

At the cellular level, proteins play an important role in maintaining homeostasis. Damage to existing proteins or impaired protein synthesis results in a disturbance of cellular homeostasis. To defend against this type of disturbance, cells respond by synthesizing a group of proteins, termed "heat shock proteins." These proteins are induced by a variety of stressful conditions, including prolonged exercise that results in an elevation in body temperature.[3,13,16] Although several heat shock proteins (e.g., HSP10, HSP27, HSP40, HSP60, HSP90) are involved in cellular protection against stress, strong evidence indicates that HSP72 is particularly cytoprotective against protein-damaging stresses such as I-R. The first evidence for HSP72 as a cytoprotective protein during myocardial I-R was correlative in nature.[16] However, recent studies using transgenic animal models have provided more evidence for HSP72 as a cytoprotective protein against I-R injuries.[17]

Although an exercise-induced increase in myocardial HSPs is a potential mechanism to explain the cardioprotection associated with exercise, work by Taylor et al.[14] reveals that exercise training in a cold environment provides cardioprotection during an in vitro I-R insult without elevating myocardial levels of HSP72. These investigators concluded that although HSP72 can promote improved postischemic function in the heart, other mechanisms must be responsible for the exercise-induced cardioprotection.

A recent study in our laboratory supports and expands this work by demonstrating that exercise in a cold environment is associated with cardioprotection without elevating HSP72 or other cytoprotective HSPs (e.g., HSP40, HSP90).[3] These results provide additional evidence that increases in myocardial HSP72, HSP40, and HSP90 are not essential for exercise-induced cardioprotection.[3]

Exercise and Myocardial Antioxidant Capacity

Cells contain several naturally occurring mechanisms of protection from reactive oxygen species injury. Primary enzymatic antioxidant defenses include superoxide dismutase (SOD), glutathione peroxidase, and catalase. Important nonenzymatic defenses include reduced glutathione (GSH) and the vitamins E and C.[18,19] Each of these antioxidants is capable of combining with reactive oxidants to produce other less reactive species. In mammalian cells, SOD exists in two isoforms. One isoform requires CuZn as a cofactor, whereas the second requires Mn as a cofactor. The CuZnSOD is primarily located in the cytosol, whereas the MnSOD is primarily found in the mitochondria.[18] Both isoforms of SOD promote the dismutation of the superoxide radical to form hydrogen peroxide (H_2O_2) and oxygen. Glutathione peroxidase utilizes GSH as a reducing equivalent to reduce H_2O_2 to form oxidized glutathione and water. Similarly, the cytosolic enzyme catalase exerts protection against oxidative injury by converting H_2O_2 to water and oxygen.

An essential duty of GSH is to function with glutathione peroxidase in the removal of H_2O_2. GSH is also able to remove selected ROS directly and assist in the recycling of vitamin C and E. The importance of GSH in protecting cells against oxidant injury has been clearly demonstrated.[18]

The effects of exercise on the activities of primary antioxidant enzymes have been widely investigated. Most studies report that exercise does not elevate myocardial glutathione peroxidase activity in the heart.[1,18,20] Furthermore, the impact of exercise on myocardial catalase activity remains unclear, with some studies reporting an increase,[2] whereas others report that exercise does not elevate cardiac catalase activity.[1,3,4] In contrast, it is widely agreed that exercise-induced expression of myocardial MnSOD occurs rapidly after the onset of exercise training. Indeed, as few as three consecutive days of exercise has been shown to elevate the MnSOD activity in hearts from exercised rats.[1,3,4] It also has been reported that chronic exercise training (i.e., weeks-to-months) elevates cardiac levels of GSH.[5] Unfortunately, at present, limited data exist concerning the effects of exercise on other redox systems in the heart (e.g., thioredoxin).

Based upon the important role that oxidative damage plays in I-R–induced injury in the heart, several investigators have speculated that exercise-induced increases in cardiac antioxidants contribute to exercise-induced cardioprotection.[1,4,5] The strongest evidence to directly link exercise-induced increases in cardiac antioxidants with cardioprotection is the finding that antisense oligonucleotide inhibition of exercise-induced expression of MnSOD in the heart results in a loss of exercise-mediated cardioprotection against myocardial infarction.[15] Although the results appear robust, one study rarely provides a definitive answer to a complex question. Therefore, additional experiments are warranted to explore the role that specific cardiac antioxidants play in exercise-induced cardioprotection at all levels of I-R–induced injury.

Exercise-Induced Cardioprotective Mediators: Future Directions

In addition to the aforementioned cardioprotective molecules, it is possible that exercise promotes the expression of other, yet to be identified, cardioprotective mediators. Historically, the study of gene expression required the analysis of individual mRNA transcripts. However, recent advances in biotechnology, such as microarray analysis, permit the simultaneous measurement of a large number of gene transcripts. Using this technology, our laboratory has taken a discovery-oriented experimental approach using oligonucleotide microarrays (Affymetrix U34A GeneChip containing 8799 probe pairs) to study the impact of exercise on global gene expression in the heart. Our overall objective was to investigate the effect of a single bout of endurance exercise (60 minutes at ~60% VO_2 max) on cardiac gene expression in both young adult (6-month-old) and senescent (24-month-old) male F-344 rats. More specifically, we compared exercise-induced changes in cardiac gene expression across the left ventricle wall (i.e., epicardium vs. endocardium) and determined if exercise-induced changes in cardiac gene expression differed between young-adult and old animals. Based on potential differences in wall stress across the left ventricle during systole, we postulated that exercise-induced alterations in cardiac gene expression would differ between the endocardial and epicardial segments of the left ventricle. Furthermore, we hypothesized that age-related differences would exist in exercise-induced changes in cardiac gene expression.

Our results supported both of these hypotheses. Indeed, in young-adult animals, exercise resulted in a twofold change (i.e., increase or decrease) in the mRNA levels of 166 genes and expressed sequence tags (ESTs) in the epicardium, whereas exercise altered gene expression in 218 genes and ESTs in the endocardium (FIG. 2). Further, age-related differences existed in the number of cardiac genes and ESTs that were differentially expressed in response to exercise (FIG. 2).

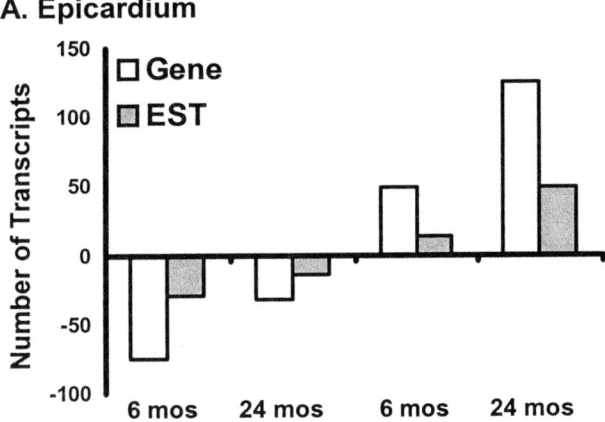

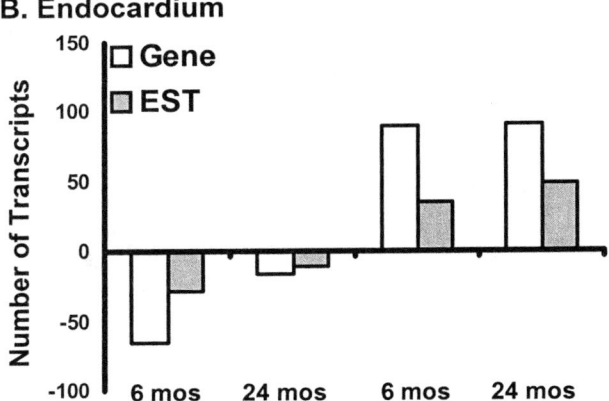

FIGURE 2. Exercise-induced changes in gene and expressed sequence tag (EST) expression in the hearts of young adult (6-month-old) and senescent (24-month-old) F-344 male rats. Exercised animals were compared to age-matched sedentary control animals, and a twofold difference in total gene/EST expression was considered to be significantly different. (**A**) The exercise-induced change in expression of genes and ESTs in the epicardium of both young adult and old rats; (**B**) the alteration in gene and EST expression in the endocardium of both young adult and old rats in response to exercise.

FIGURE 3 illustrates the age-related differences in exercise-induced changes in cardiac gene expression by both functional category and ventricular region. Several age-related differences are noteworthy. First, differences exist between adult and senescent animals in the number of exercise-induced transport genes that were up- or downregulated by exercise (epicardium and endocardium). Second, these age-related differences in exercise-induced alterations in stress response genes are present in both the epicardium and endocardium. Further, age-related differences in exercise-induced gene expression were observed in genes connected with

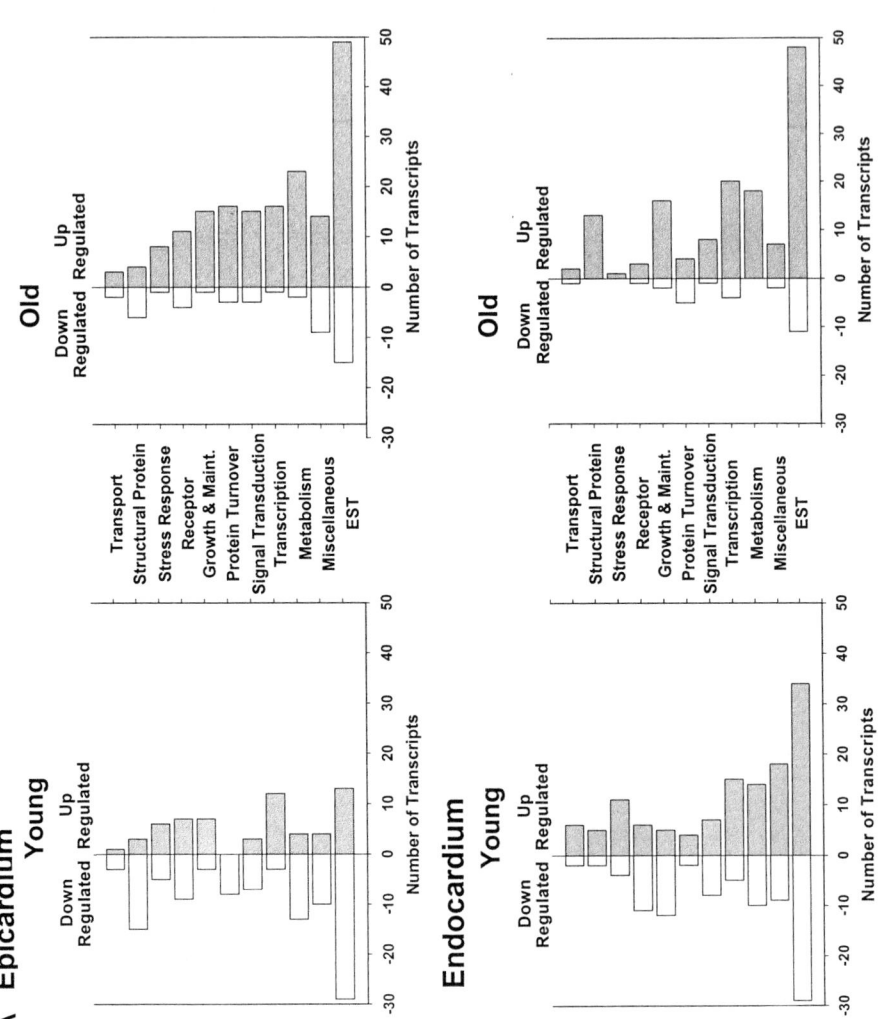

FIGURE 3. *See following page for legend.*

metabolism and structural proteins, as well as genes involved in growth and maintenance. Finally, note the large age-related differences in the up- and downregulation of cardiac ESTs. The large number of exercise-increased cardiac ESTs in both adult and old animals raises interesting possibilities about their potential role as cardioprotective mediators (FIG. 3). Indeed, identifying the function of these proteins in cardiac myocyte function could provide key insights into the mechanisms responsible for exercise-induced cardioprotection. This challenge offers an exciting opportunity for future research in exercise-induced cardioprotection.

SUMMARY AND CONCLUSIONS

It is well established that exercise training decreases myocardial oxidative injury and improves cardiac contractile performance following an I-R insult. The mechanism(s) responsible for this exercise-induced cardioprotection remain unknown and continue to be investigated. Potential mechanisms to explain the protective effect of exercise include induction of cardiac HSPs and/or improved myocardial antioxidant capacity. Although it is clear that elevated levels of HSPs can provide myocardial protection during an I-R insult, new evidence indicates that exercise-induced cardioprotection can be achieved without an increase in HSP72. From recently published work, it appears that the exercise-induced cardioprotection against an I-R–induced myocardial infarction is due, at least in part, to a training-induced increase in myocardial MnSOD activity. Furthermore, it seems possible that one or more unidentified cardioprotective molecules also could play an important role in exercise-induced cardioprotection. Improving our basic understanding of the mechanisms responsible for exercise-induced protection against I-R injury in the heart is important, and will have major implications for improvements in the treatment and management of patients predisposed to I-R injury.

ACKNOWLEDGMENTS

This work was supported by a grant from the National Institutes of Health (NIH R01 HL067855) awarded to Scott K. Powers.

FIGURE 3. Exercise-mediated increase and decrease in left ventricular expression of expressed sequence tags (ESTs) and selected categories of cardiac genes in both young adult (6-month-old) and senescent (24-month-old) F-344 male rats. Exercised animals were compared to age-matched sedentary control animals, and a twofold difference in gene/EST expression was considered significantly different. (**A**) The exercise-induced change, by category, in expression of genes and ESTs in the epicardium of both young adult and old rats; (**B**) the categorical alterations in gene and EST expression in the endocardium of both young adult and old rats in response to exercise.

REFERENCES

1. DEMIREL, H., S.K. POWERS, M.A. ZERGEROGLU, et al. 2001. Short-term exercise improves myocardial tolerance to in vivo ischemia-reperfusion in the rat. J. Appl. Physiol. **91:** 2205–2212.
2. STARNES, J., R. TAYLOR & Y. PARK. 2003. Exercise improves postischemic function in aging hearts. Am. J. Physiol. **285:** H347–H351.
3. HAMILTON, K., S.K. POWERS, T. SUGIURA, et al. 2001. Short-term exercise training can improve myocardial tolerance to ischemia-reperfusion without an elevation in heat shock proteins. Am. J. Physiol. **281:** H1346–H1352.
4. HAMILTON, K., J. STAIB, T. PHILLIPS, et al. 2003. Exercise, antioxidants, and HSP72: protection against myocardial ischemia-reperfusion. Free Radical Bio. Med. **34:** 800–809.
5. POWERS, S., H. DEMIREL, J. COOMBES, et al. 1998. Exercise training improves myocardial tolerance to *in vivo* ischemia-reperfusion in the rat. Am. J. Physiol. **44:** R1468–R1477.
6. BOLLI, R. & E. MARBAN. 1999. Molecular and cellular mechanisms of myocardial stunning. Physiol. Rev. **79:** 609–634.
7. DOWNEY, J. 1990. Free radicals and their involvement during long-term myocardial ischemia and reperfusion. Annu. Rev. Physiol. **52:** 487–504.
8. PEPE, S. 2000. Mitochondrial function in ischemia and reperfusion of the ageing heart. Clin. Exp. Pharmacol. Physiol. **27:** 745–750.
9. LAKATTA, E.G. & S. SOLLOTT. 2002. Perspectives on mammalian cardiovascular aging: humans to molecules. Comp. Biochem. Physiol. **132:** 699–721.
10. BRONIKOWSKI, A., P. CARTER, T. MORGAN, et al. 2003. Lifelong voluntary exercise in the mouse prevents age-related alterations in gene expression in the heart. Physiol. Genomics **12:** 129–138.
11. REBRIN, I., S. KAMZALOV & R. SOHAL. 2003. Effects of age and caloric restriction on glutathione redox state in mice. Free Radical Bio. Med. **35:** 626–635.
12. EDWARDS, M., D. SARKAR, R. KLOPP, et al. 2003. Age-related impairment of the transcriptional responses to oxidative stress in the mouse heart. Physiol. Genomics **13:** 119–127.
13. DEMIREL, H.A., K. HAMILTON, R. SHANELY, et al. 2003. Age and attenuation of exercise-induced myocardial HSP72 accumulation. Am. J. Physiol. **285:** H1609–H1615.
14. TAYLOR, R., M. HARRIS & S. STARNES. 1999. Acute exercise can improve cardioprotection without increasing heat shock protein content. Am. J. Physiol. **276:** H1098–H1102.
15. YAMASHITA, N., S. HOSHIDA, K. OTSU, T. KUZUYA & M. HORI. 1999. Exercise provides direct biphasic cardioprotection via manganese superoxide dismutase activation. J. Exp. Med. **189:** 1699–1706.
16. HUTTER, M., R. SIEVERS, V. BARBOSA & C. WOLFE. 1989. Heat shock protein induction in rat hearts: a direct correlation between the amount of heat-shock protein induced and degree of myocardial protection. Circulation **89:** 355–360.
17. MARBER, M., R. MESTRIL, S.H. CHI, et al. 1995. Overexpression of the rat inducible 70kD heat stress protein in a transgenic mouse increases the resistance of the heart to ischemic injury. J. Clin. Invest. **95:** 1446–1456.
18. POWERS, S., L. JI & C. LEEUWENBURGH. 1999. Exercise training-induced alterations in skeletal muscle antioxidant capacity: a brief review. Med. Sci. Sports Exercise **31:** 987–997.
19. YU, B. Cellular defenses against reactive oxygen species. 1994. Physiol. Rev. **74:** 139–162.
20. POWERS, S., D. CRISWELL, J. LAWLER, et al. 1993. Rigorous exercise training increases superoxide dismutase activity in the ventricular myocardium. Am. J. Physiol. **265:** H2094–H2098.

Regular Exercise

An Effective Means to Reduce Oxidative Stress in Old Rats

SATARO GOTO,[a] ZSOLT RADÁK,[b] CSABA NYAKAS,[b] HAE YOUNG CHUNG,[c] HISASHI NAITO,[d] RYOYA TAKAHASHI,[a] HIDEKO NAKAMOTO,[a] AND RYOICHI ABE[a]

[a]*Department of Biochemistry, Faculty of Pharmaceutical Sciences, Toho University, Funabashi, Chiba, Japan*

[b]*Laboratory of Exercise Physiology, School of Sport Science, Semmelweis University, Budapest, Hungary*

[c]*Department of Pharmacy, College of Pharmacy, Pusan National University, Pusan, Korea*

[d]*Department of Sports Physiology, School of Sports Sciences, Juntendo University, Inba, Chiba, Japan*

> ABSTRACT: A healthy diet and regular exercise are among the major factors that influence quality of life (QOL) in old age. Exercise is believed to be beneficial to improve QOL, retarding age-related decline of physiological functions and preventing age-related diseases. Regular physical exercise can possibly improve age-related functional decline and delay onset of age-related diseases by attenuating potentially harmful oxidative damage and suppressing inflammatory processes even in older age.
>
> KEYWORDS: exercise; oxidative; stress; damage; old; rats; NF-κB

In recent years, the average life span in industrialized countries has increased remarkably, while the quality of life (QOL) and activities of daily living of elderly people are not necessarily satisfactory either for themselves or for their families and society. A healthy diet and regular exercise are among the major factors that influence QOL in old age. Exercise is believed to be beneficial to improve QOL, retarding age-related decline of physiological functions and preventing age-related diseases.

While moderate exercise is obviously healthful, it is often claimed to induce oxidative stress due to an excessive oxygen uptake to meet the high demand of adenosine triphosphate (ATP) that can result in elevated reactive oxygen species (ROS) formation in mitochondria. Other enzymatic systems including xanthine oxidase and NADPH dehydrogenase can also be involved in increasing ROS generation.

Address for correspondence: S. Goto, Department of Biochemistry, School of Pharmaceutical Sciences, Toho University, Miyama 2-2-1, Funabashi, Chiba, 274-8510 Japan. Voice/fax: +81-47-472-1531.

goto@phar.toho-u.ac.jp

Increased utilization of oxygen in mitochondria and in other enzymatic processes would enhance the generation of superoxide anion and hence hydrogen peroxide due to Mn- or Cu,Zn-superoxide dismutase (SOD) activity. As a result of excessive ROS generation, proteins, nucleic acids, and membrane phospholipids may be oxidatively modified, possibly leading to deleterious consequences. Oxidative modification of proteins can influence a variety of cellular functions of many tissues. In fact, a bout of treadmill exercise increased protein oxidation as measured by the carbonyl content in the skeletal muscle[1] as well as in the lung[2] in rat. While a bout of exercise of sedentary animals is likely to cause increased harmful oxidative modifications of proteins, moderate regular exercise can be beneficial by reducing the damage. We have tested this hypothesis using middle-aged and old rats in two different protocols of regular exercise.

EFFECTS OF REGULAR EXERCISE ON COGNITIVE FUNCTIONS AND PROTEIN CARBONYLS IN THE BRAIN OF AGING RATS

Regular swimming exercise for 9 weeks improved cognitive functions in young (4 weeks) and middle-aged (14 months) Wistar rats with a parallel decrease in protein carbonyls of the brain.[3] This finding is consistent with the reports by others that age-related decrease in the cognitive function parallels the decrease in protein carbonyls in the brain of animals treated with a spin-trap compound, N-tert-butyl-α-phenylnitrone (PBN).[4] Beneficial effects of the moderate regular exercise and the PBN treatment appear to be brought about at least in part by upregulation of the activity of proteasome that is believed to be responsible for the degradation of oxidatively or otherwise modified proteins,[3,4] in addition to an increase in the activities of antioxidant enzymes.[5] Upregulation of proteasome activity by the exercise was observed also in the skeletal muscle.[6]

EFFECTS OF REGULAR EXERCISE ON OXIDATIVE STATUS AND TRANSCRIPTION FACTORS RELATED TO INFLAMMATION IN AGING RAT LIVER

Middle-aged (18-month-old) and old (28-month-old) male F344 rats were subjected to regular treadmill exercise for 8 weeks. Training intensity was set at about 75% of VO_{2max} for individual age groups. In both groups, maximal oxygen uptake increased by about 40%.[7] The body weight was reduced by about 10% as compared with sedentary groups. We studied the oxidative status of the liver of the animals.[8] ROS level as measured with dichlorodihydrofluorescein diacetate was significantly higher in the old sedentary groups than in middle-aged counterparts. The regular exercise tended to attenuate the increase, although not significantly, compared with the sedentary controls. Redox status evaluated by glutathione (GSH) showed more than twofold increase in exercised groups, together with decrease in the oxidized form (GSSG). It thus appears that the cellular milieu is shifted to a less oxidative state, suggesting a preventive or reversal effect of the exercise regimen even at old ages. We have also investigated nuclear factor κB (NF-κB) activity. NF-κB is a very important redox-sensitive transcription factor that regulates various inflammatory and immune responses. It forms a complex with the inhibitory protein I-κB, thereby being retained as an inactive form in the cytoplasm. Upon stimulation by oxidative or other stresses, I-κB is phosphorylated and then degraded by proteasome, releasing NF-κB that can move into the nucleus for transcriptional activation of inflammatory protein genes or inactivation of anti-inflammatory protein genes. Binding activity of NF-κB in nuclear extracts to oligonucleotide with the responsive element (electrophoretic mobility shift assay, EMSA) increased with age as expected from the increased oxidative stress mentioned above. Increase in the amount of NF-κB was verified by increase in the amount of p50 and p65 subunits as detected by Western blot. The amount of I-κB in the cytoplasm was higher in the middle-aged animals than in the old. These findings confirm previous reports that NF-κB is activated by increased degradation of I-κB with advancing age.[9] The regular exercise may thus prevent or reverse the age-related changes that promote inflammatory processes.

Glucocorticoids (GC) have anti-inflammatory activities and are used to suppress inflammation in chronic diseases such as asthma and rheumatoid arthritis. GC inhibit gene expression of proinflammatory cytokines including various interleukins and tumor necrosis factor α as well as enzymes or receptors responsible for inflammatory processes such as inducible nitric oxide synthase and cyclooxygenase-2. They also activate gene expression of anti-inflammatory proteins such as lipocortin-1 and β_2-adrenoreceptor. GC receptor (GR) is a transcription factor that influences directly or

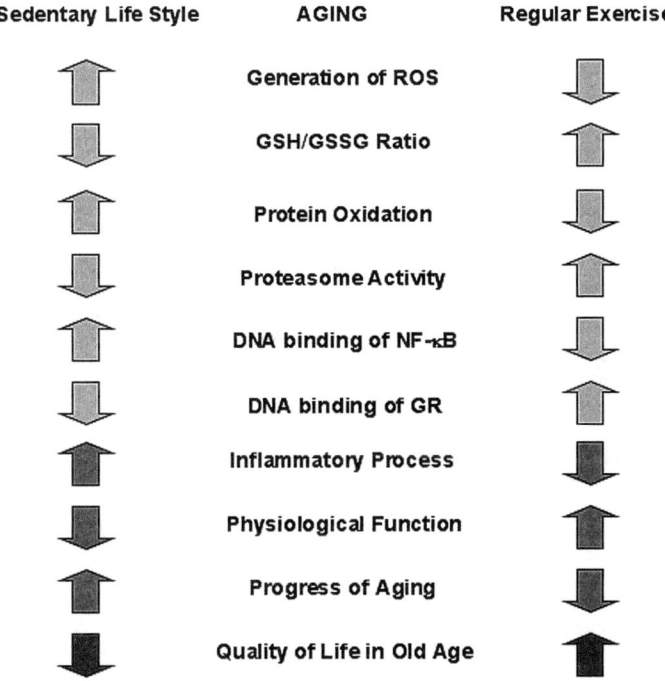

FIGURE 1. Regular exercise can attenuate oxidative status and inflammatory processes, leading to improved quality of life in old age.

indirectly gene expression of the inflammation-related proteins.[10] We showed that activity of GR measured by EMSA is significantly decreased in the liver of aged animals, but 8 weeks of regular exercise was able to reverse the change (Abe et al., in preparation). No significant difference in the amount of GR protein was detected between young adult and old animals, suggesting that the quality rather than the quantity of GR is altered with age. Serum level of GC was significantly higher in the exercised old animals than in the sedentary animals. In view of the anti-inflammatory activities of GC, these observations also support the view that regular exercise has a beneficial effect by reducing inflammation. It is interesting to note that GR can directly interact with NF-κB.[11] It is likely therefore that transcription factors GR and NF-κB synergistically downregulate the expression of inflammation-related genes.

Age-related increase in 8-hydroxy-2′-deoxyguanosine in the nuclear DNA of the skeletal muscle was significantly reduced by the regular exercise with increased DNA repair activity.[7] Although protein carbonyls did not change significantly with age or the exercise, the muscle proteins of exercised old animals were more resistant to oxidative challenge *in vitro* than those of the sedentary counterparts, suggesting increased antioxidative activities in the former.

Thus, regular physical exercise can possibly improve age-related functional decline and delay onset of age-related diseases by attenuating potentially harmful oxidative damage and suppressing inflammatory processes even at old ages (FIG. 1).

REFERENCES

1. REZNICK, A.Z., E. WITT, M. MATSUMOTO & L. PACKER. 1992. Vitamin E inhibits protein oxidation in skeletal muscle of resting and exercised rats. Biochem. Biophys. Res. Commun. **189:** 801–806.
2. RADÁK, Z., A. NAKAMURA, H. NAKAMOTO, et al. 1998. A period of anaerobic exercise increases the accumulation of reactive carbonyl derivatives in the lungs of rats. Pflüg. Arch. **435:** 439–441.
3. RADÁK, Z., T. KANEKO, S. TAHARA, et al. 2001. Regular exercise improves cognitive function and decreases oxidative damage in rat brain. Neurochem. Int. **38:** 17–23.
4. CARNEY, J.M., P.E. STARKE-REED, C.N. OLIVER, et al. 1991. Reversal of age-related increase in brain protein oxidation, decrease in enzyme activity, and loss in temporal and spatial memory by chronic administration of the spin-trapping compound *N-tert-*butyl-alpha-phenylnitrone. Proc. Natl. Acad. Sci. USA **88:** 3633–3636.
5. POWERS, S.K., D. CRISWELL, J. LAWLER, et al. 1994. Influence of exercise and fiber type on antioxidant enzyme activity in rat skeletal muscle. Am. J. Physiol. **266:** R375–R380.
6. RADÁK, Z., T. KANEKO, S. TAHARA, et al. 1999. The effect of exercise training on oxidative damage of lipids, proteins, and DNA in rat skeletal muscle: evidence for beneficial outcomes. Free Radical Biol. Med. **27:** 69–74.
7. RADÁK, Z., H. NAITO, T. KANEKO, et al. 2002. Exercise training decreases DNA damage and increases DNA repair and resistance against oxidative stress of proteins in aged rat skeletal muscle. Pflüg. Arch. **445:** 273–278.
8. RADÁK, Z., H.Y. CHUNG, H. NAITO, et al. 2004. Age-associated increase in oxidative stress and nuclear factor kappaB activation are attenuated in rat liver by regular exercise. FASAB J. **18:** 749–750.
9. CHUNG, H.Y., H.J. KIM, J.W. KIM & B.P. YU. 2001. The inflammation hypothesis of aging: molecular modulation by calorie restriction. Ann. N.Y. Acad. Sci. **928:** 327–335.
10. ADCOCK, I.M. 2000. Molecular mechanisms of glucocorticosteroid actions. Pulm. Pharmacol. Ther. **13:** 115–126.
11. RAY, A. & K.E. PREFONTAINE. 1994. Physical association and functional antagonism between the p65 subunit of transcription factor NF-κB and the glucocorticoid receptor. Proc. Natl. Acad. Sci. USA **91:** 752–756.

Mechanisms in Muscle Atrophy in Immobilization and Aging

MARINA BAR-SHAI,[a] ELI CARMELI,[b] RAYMOND COLEMAN,[a] AND ABRAHAM Z. REZNICK[a]

[a]*Musculoskeletal Research Laboratory, Department of Anatomy and Cell Biology, Rappaport Faculty of Medicine, Technion–Israel Institute of Technology, Haifa 31096, Israel*

[b]*Physical Therapy Program, Sackler Faculty of Medicine, Tel Aviv University, Ramat Aviv 61390, Israel*

ABSTRACT: The purpose of this report was to study the effects of four weeks of hindlimb immobilization on acid phosphatase activity of old rats in comparison with the profile obtained after similar treatment in young rats.

KEYWORDS: immobilization atrophy; muscle wasting; protein breakdown; aging; acid phosphatase activity

The phenomenon of muscle wasting with age is a universal process, sometimes referred to as sarcopenia of old age.[1] In this process, the physiological balance between protein synthesis and breakdown is disturbed, with an increasing shift toward breakdown. Muscles possess both extracellular and intracellular systems of protein degradation. The extracellular degradation systems involve mainly matrix metalloproteinases (MMPs) and lysosomal proteinases such as acid phosphatase (ACP) that are activated in infiltrating macrophages.[2] The intracellular degradation systems are divided into three categories:[3] (1) fast-activated calcium-dependent proteinases (calpains); (2) the ubiquitin-proteasome pathway; and (3) the intracellular lysosomal proteinases. In addition, there are minor local-acting proteinases associated with the sarcolemma and in mitochondria.

In previous studies, we have shown that hindlimb muscles of old rats with disuse atrophy following four weeks of hindleg immobilization display reduced capacities for recovery compared to young rats,[4,5] probably as a result of impaired protein turnover, both synthesis and degradation.

ACP activities have been shown to change considerably both in muscles of immobilized limbs and in aging.[6,7] The purpose of this report was to study the effects of four weeks of hindlimb immobilization on ACP activity of old rats in comparison with the profile obtained after similar treatment in young rats.

Address for correspondence: Prof. A.Z. Reznick, Department of Anatomy and Cell Biology, Rappaport Faculty of Medicine, Technion–Israel Institute of Technology, P. O. Box 9649, Haifa 31096, Israel. Voice: +972-4-8295388; fax: +972-4-8295403.
reznick@tx.technion.ac.il

MATERIALS AND METHODS

Experimental Animals and Immobilization Conditions

The animals used in this project were young (6-month-old) and aged (24-month-old) female Wistar rats. The right hindlegs of the rats underwent external fixation as previously described.[8] The left (contralateral) legs were not immobilized and served as controls. Additional rats without limb fixation served as untreated controls.

Biochemical studies: Animals were divided into four immobilization groups and were immobilized for one, two, three, and four weeks. At the end of each week, a group of four to six animals was sacrificed and their hindlimb muscles (gastrocnemius and quadriceps) were excised. The muscles were frozen in liquid nitrogen for biochemical analysis.

Biochemical Studies

For ACP assay, muscle specimens (200 mg) were thawed and immersed in 1.4 mL of 50 mM Tris (hydroxymethyl) aminomethane buffer, pH 7.4, in the presence of antiproteases: 1 µM phenylmethyl sulfonylfluoride (PMSF) and 1 µM leupeptin. This mixture was homogenized three times for 15 s in a Polytron homogenizer (Kinematica, GmbH, Lucerne, Switzerland). The homogenates were centrifuged for 30 min at 14,000g. The supernatants were separated and used for measuring ACP activity as previously described.[8]

RESULTS AND DISCUSSION

FIGURE 1 shows the specific activity of ACP in immobilized gastrocnemius muscles of old animals compared to controls. In the immobilized muscles, ACP activity increased already after the first week of immobilization, from 17.5 U/mg protein to 26.5 U/mg protein (an increase of 51%), which was statistically significant ($P < .05$). This elevation was observed also for the following three weeks (FIG. 1). In contrast, the contralateral control muscles showed ACP activity increase only in the fourth week of immobilization, when the levels of activity reached values similar to those obtained for the immobilized muscles. The increased levels of ACP at week 4 in the control legs may mean that, at this time, control legs also underwent proteolytic damage. When comparing the patterns of ACP activities in muscles of old rats after limb immobilization with young rats similarly treated, there are noticeable differences in the kinetics of the enzyme activity.[2] In the young rats, ACP activity in immobilized quadriceps increased only after the second week of immobilization and reached a peak of 37 U/mg protein at three weeks. This value is significantly higher than the 30 U/mg protein observed in old rats during the third week of immobilization.[2] In addition, at the end of the fourth week of immobilization, the ACP activity of control legs in young animals remained quite low (23.5 U/mg protein) compared to immobilized muscles of old animals (36 U/mg protein). This may indicate that immobilization in young animals did not result in damage to the control unimmobilized leg.[2] The results presented in this study corroborate previous studies in which it was shown that muscle protein breakdown involves both early and late events.

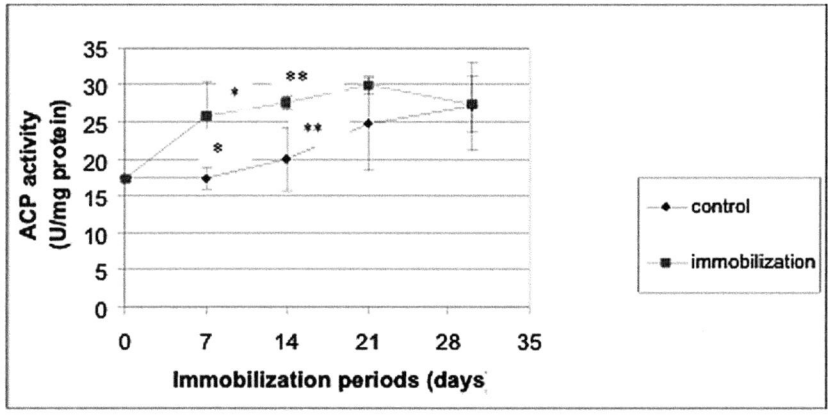

*P<0.05
**P<0.02

FIGURE 1. Acid phosphatase activities in quadriceps muscles of control (contralateral leg) and immobilized hindlimbs of old animals. Each value represents the mean ± SD of 3–4 different animals.

Indeed, studies by Williams *et al.*[9] showed that the early fast events of muscle degradation involved activation of calcium-dependent proteinases, the calpains. The study by Williams *et al.* showed that, in sepsis, the activation of calpains resulted in the initial disintegration of the Z-band proteins, which may be a rate-limiting event resulting in the disturbance of myofilament proteins, actin and myosin. In addition, the increased activities of calpains in immobilization have also been associated with increased oxidative stress and oxidative damage to muscles.[10]

The slow phase of muscle protein degradation involves the activation of the ubiquitin-proteasome pathway and the lysosomal proteinases intracellularly, and lysosomal proteinases and MMPs extracellularly. These proteolytic systems are activated in the later stages of muscle immobilization and involve signaling events initiated by cytokines such as TNF-α, IL-1, and IL-6, secreted by invading macrophages. These extracellular events are followed by intracellular cascades of increased oxidative stress and activation of NF-κB transcription factor, leading to further upregulation of the intracellular proteolytic systems.

In conclusion, the breakdown of muscle proteins involves multisystem and multistep processes that are extremely complicated and require further intensive investigations to decipher their mechanisms in aging animals.

ACKNOWLEDGMENTS

This study was supported by The Krol Foundation of Lakewood, New Jersey. We also would like to express our gratitude to Bilha Pinhasi for her technical assistance.

REFERENCES

1. DUTTA, C. & E.C. HADLEY. 1995. The significance of sarcopenia in old age. J. Gerontol. **50A:** 1–4.
2. REZNICK, A.Z., O. MENASHE, M. BAR-SHAI, *et al.* 2003. Expression of matrix metalloproteinases, inhibitor, and acid phosphatase in muscles of immobilized hindlimbs of rats. Muscle Nerve **27:** 51–59.
3. FURONO, K., M.N. GOODMAN & A.L. GOLDBERG. 1990. Role of different proteolytic systems in the degradation of muscle proteins during denervation atrophy. J. Biol. Chem. **265:** 8850–8857.
4. ZARZHEVSKY, N., E. CARMELI, D. FUCHS, *et al.* 2001. Recovery of muscles of old rats after hindlimb immobilization by external fixation is impaired compared with those of young rats. Exp. Gerontol. **36:** 125–140.
5. ZARZHEVSKY, N., O. MENASHE, E. CARMELI, *et al.* 2001. Capacity for recovery and possible mechanisms in immobilization atrophy of young and old animals. Ann. N.Y. Acad. Sci. **928:** 212–225.
6. WITZMANN, F.A. 1982. Acid phosphatase and protease activities in immobilized skeletal muscles. Can. J. Physiol. Pharmacol. **60:** 1732–1736.
7. SAFADI, A., E. LIVNE & A.Z. REZNICK. 1997. Characterization of alkaline and acid phosphatases from skeletal muscles of young and old rats. Arch. Gerontol. Geriatr. **24:** 183–196.
8. REZNICK, A.Z., G. VOLPIN, H. BEN-ARI, *et al.* 1995. Biochemical and morphological studies on rat skeletal muscles following prolonged immobilization of the knee joint by external fixation and plaster cast: a comparative study. Eur. J. Exp. Musculoskel. Res. **4:** 69–76.
9. WILLIAMS, A.B., G.M. DECOURTEN-MEYERS & J.E. FISCHER. 1999. Sepsis stimulates release of myofilaments in skeletal muscle by a calcium-dependent mechanism. FASEB J. **13:** 1435–1443.
10. KONDO, H., I. NAKAGAKI, S. SASAKI, *et al.* 1993. Mechanism of oxidative stress in skeletal muscle atrophied by immobilization. Acta Physiol. **265:** E839–E844.

Effect of Physical Activity Levels on Bone Strength

KAZUTOSHI KIKKAWA

Department of Health and Physical Education, Hiroshima Prefectural University, Showbara, Hiroshima 727-0023, Japan

ABSTRACT: The present study employs statistical analysis using age as the covariate and seeks to provide cross-sectional data concerning the relationship between bone strength and levels of physical activities among Japanese.

KEYWORDS: age; bone strength; physical activity; SOS

INTRODUCTION

Through four different techniques, Mosekilde[1] emphasized that age by itself is the major determinant of vertebral bone strength, mass, and microarchitecture, although some sex-related differences were also pointed out as factors. Furthermore, a number of studies showed that exercise plays an important role in the prevention of osteoporotic fractures. Espallargues *et al.*[2] through their extensive databases such as MEDLINE conducted investigations of risk factors for osteoporosis and classified them according to their probability into high risk, moderate risk, and no risk groups. Research concerning the degree of bone strength and its related factors has been conducted, but there have been few investigations adjusting for age. Also, guidelines on frequency of exercise are vague. The present study employs statistical analysis using age as the covariate and seeks to provide cross-sectional data concerning the relationship between bone strength and levels of physical activities among Japanese.

METHODS

Speed-of-Sound Measurement

An ultrasound bone density measurement (BMD) apparatus (CM100, Furuno Electronics) was used, and measurements of SOS (speed of sound on bone; units of m/s) were taken. The subjects were 121 women from 18 to 78 years of age (average: 49.7; SD: ±17.6) and 78 men from 18 to 83 years of age (48.7 ± 17.5). They were users of a certain public gymnasium or their acquaintances. SOS was measured with

---

Address for correspondence: Kazutoshi Kikkawa, Ph.D., Department of Health and Physical Education, Hiroshima Prefectural University, Showbara, Hiroshima 727-0023, Japan. Voice: +81-8247-41729.
kikkawa@bus.hiroshima-pu.ac.jp

ultrasound apparatus and, for each subject, the heel of their bare right foot was placed on a footrest for testing. Before and after ultrasound measurements, subjects were questioned as to their age and their levels of sports and/or exercise activity, and their answers were recorded.

Statistical Analysis

In conducting analysis of covariance (ANCOVA), SOS was the dependent variable, the amount of sports/exercise activity (group N, less than once a week; group L, once a week; group H, twice a week or more) was used for the factors, and age was used as the covariate. The software used for statistics was SPSS11.5J for Windows.

RESULTS

Descriptive Statistics

The results for SOS in relation to the level of sports/exercise activity for women were 1520.0 (SD: ±37.7) m/s for group N ($n = 68$), 1543.2 (±31.6) m/s for group L ($n = 35$), and 1525.5 (±36.8) m/s for group H ($n = 18$), with the overall figure for all subjects being 1527.56 (±37.05) m/s.

Test for Parallelism of Regression Lines

Concerning the level of significance for the interaction between the factors and the covariate, $F = 0.866$ shows that there is no significant relationship. In other words, the slopes of the regression lines of the factor levels were equal.

Test of the Hypothesis Related to the Slope ($\beta = 0$)

The results indicated that $\beta = -1.339$ ($t = -9.300$, $\alpha = 0.05$), so it was not the case that $\beta = 0$. Consequently, ANCOVA using the covariate had significance.

Results of Analysis of Covariance

The F value for the factors (degree of sports/exercise activity) was 3.262 ($P = .042$), with the null hypothesis (H0: among the three standards, there was no significant difference) not being supported. Otherwise, for the three groups of men (group N, $n = 32$; group L, $n = 18$; group H, $n = 28$), the same ANCOVA was conducted, but the F value was 0.068; thus, the results were not significant. The observed mean value (±SD) of SOS is 1520.9 (±43.89) for group N, 1523.9 (±30.66) for group L, and 1532.6 (±35.52) for group H. See TABLE 1 for details.

DISCUSSION

A few studies showed that the correlations of BMC (bone mineral content) or BMD and SOS were greater than 0.4, so the validity of this apparatus was supported, but not sufficient.[3,4] In the present study, with women's SOS and age as the covariates, the three levels of frequency of sports/exercise activity were significant as factors

TABLE 1. ANCOVA of physical activity on SOS (bone strength) with age as covariate

Source	df	M.S.	F	P
Women				
Modf. model	3	25,736.4	34.4	.000
Intercept	1	33,341,139	44,570.4	.000
AGE	1	64,699	86.5	.000
ACT	2	2440.2	3.26	.042
Error	117	748.1		
Men				
Modf. model	3	17,342.0	21.49	.000
Intercept	1	29,589,571	36,669.9	.000
AGE	1	49,900.4	61.84	.000
ACT	2	55.0	0.068	.934
Error	74	806.9		

NOTE: ACT is the level of frequency of sports/exercise activity as an independent variable. AGE is the chronological age as covariate.

($P < .05$), but in the case of men they were not. A linear correlation was demonstrated between SOS and chronological age in both the most active ($R = -.578$ in women and $R = -.706$ in men) and the inactive ($R = -.737$ in women and $R = -.772$ in men). As revealed by the results of ANCOVA with age as the covariate, the SOS at a given age was larger in active subjects than in inactive subjects; that is, graphically, the regression line determined for the inactive subjects showed a downward shift. These results suggest that, in the women's case, the level of physical activity affected SOS if the effect of chronological age is ignored; in contrast, in the men's case, the clarified correlations between SOS and frequency of physical activity were not obtained. In order to understand these findings, more research would be necessary concerning the specific types of exercise engaged in.

In the present cross-sectional study, the two findings obtained confirm earlier research involving the effect of physical activity. Both (1) the decline of bone stiffness with aging in both genders and (2) bone strength, BMD, and BMC were affected by whether the subjects had physical activity.

Some sex-related differences concerning bone are generally known. For example, peak bone mass and strength that are higher in men than in women of 20–30 years; an age-related compensatory increment of bone size in men, but not in women; and a higher tendency for disconnection of the trabecular network in women than in men.[1] Other researches demonstrated the same tendencies;[5,6] that is, the diminution in peak vertebral body BMC from young adulthood to old age was less in men than in women. The observed net diminution in BMC during aging was less in men than in women because absolute periosteal bone formation was greater in men than in women and not because absolute bone resorption was less in men. On the contrary, the absolute amount of bone resorbed was greater in men than in women. In particular, the late consequences of estrogen deficiency in elderly women result in abnormalities in calcium homeostasis and increases in parathyroid hormone secretion, leading to increased bone resorption and bone loss.[6]

The results of ANCOVA in the present study seem to be due to two facts: first, the etiology of bone loss in aging men has remained relatively unclear;[7] second, the women's daily living activities were more varied than those of the men.[8]

The present study recommends a frequency of exercise at least once a week in order to maintain bone strength. Khosla et al.[7] suggested that a significantly higher number of vertebral compression fractures occur in patients with postmenopausal osteoporosis who followed a flexion exercise program compared with those using extension exercises. Extension or isometric exercises seem to be more appropriate for patients with postmenopausal osteoporosis. Turner[9] conducted research on BMD and various categories of physical activity. Jogging, swimming, and women's exercises to improve their figure had little predictive value, while cycling, aerobics, walking, and dance had a medium level of influence, and yard work (gardening) and weight lifting had a strong influence.

In order to appropriately carry out exercise prescription, basic studies that analyze various factors such as nutritional state and sports experience[10] are necessary.

CONCLUSIONS

When adjusting for age, the effects of daily physical activity levels on bone strength (SOS) are statistically significant in Japanese women, but not in men. In order to maintain bone strength, we should exercise at least once a week.

REFERENCES

1. MOSEKILDE, L. 2000. Age-related changes in bone mass, structure, and strength—effects of loading. Z. Rheumatol. **59**(Suppl. 1): 1–9.
2. ESPALLARGUES, M., L. SAMPIETRO-COLOM, M.D. ESTRADA, et al. 2001. Identifying bone-mass-related risk factors for fracture to guide bone densitometry measurements: a systematic review of the literature. Osteoporosis Int. **12**: 811–822.
3. YAMAMOTO, A. 1997. Ultrasound apparatus Sound-Scan-2000: a principle of ultrasound apparatus on bone density of tibia. Ultrasound Technol. **97**(6): 56–58.
4. TAKEDA, N., M. MIYAKE, S. KITA, et al. 1996. Sex and age patterns of quantitative ultrasound densitometry of the calcaneus in normal Japanese subjects. Calcif. Tissue Int. **59**(2): 84–88.
5. ROGUCKA, E., T. BIELICKI, Z. WELON, et al. 2000. Variation in bone mineral density in adults in Poland: age and sex difference. Ann. Hum. Biol. **27**: 139–148.
6. DUAN, Y., C.H. TURNER, B.T. KIM & E. SEEMAN. 2001. Sexual dimorphism in vertebral fragility is more the result of gender differences in age-related bone gain than bone loss. J. Bone Miner. Res. **16**: 2267–2275.
7. KHOSLA, S., L.J. MELTON III & B.L. RIGGS. 1999. Osteoporosis: gender differences and similarities. Lupus **8**: 393–396.
8. KIKKAWA, K. 2001. Analysis of covariance of cultivation effect on body size/body composition/bone stiffness of age as covariate among residents living in hilly region. J. Jpn. Assoc. Rur. Med. **49**(5): 719–728.
9. TURNER, L.W. 2002. Influence of yard work and weight training on bone mineral density among older U. S. women. J. Women Aging **14**: 139–148.
10. ILICH-ERNST, J., R.A. BROWNBILL, M.A. LUDEMANN & R. FU. 2002. Critical factors for bone health in women across the age span: how important is muscle mass? Medscape Womens Health **7**: 2.

Naturally Long-Lived Animal Models for the Study of Slow Aging and Longevity

DONNA J. HOLMES

Department of Biological Sciences, University of Idaho, Moscow, Idaho 83844, USA

ABSTRACT: Judicious selection of new animal models for the study of basic aging processes must combine feasibility and good use of the comparative method with evidence of antiaging adaptations, like the ability to combat oxidative damage to cells and tissues. A number of vertebrate species already in use or being developed as new biomedical models lend themselves very well to laboratory studies of aging, including small birds, bats, and mole-rats.

KEYWORDS: aging; antiaging; bats; birds; comparative method; evolution; naked mole-rats

Since the selection of animal models in biogerontology is driven primarily by feasibility considerations, the majority of researchers in the field use short-lived, rapidly aging species. Most also limit their laboratory animals to inbred domestic rodents, invertebrates, or highly specialized, "domesticated" cell lines. This means that our most intensively used animal models (laboratory rodents, flies, worms, and fibroblast cells) not only have life histories quite dissimilar to those of humans and other long-lived animals, but also lack the very trait that we wish to emulate: the ability to resist aging.

The time is now ripe for judicious selection of new animal models for the study of basic aging processes that combines feasibility and good use of the comparative method with evidence of antiaging adaptations, like the ability to combat oxidative damage to cells and tissues. A number of vertebrate species either already in use or being developed as new biomedical models would lend themselves very well to laboratory studies of aging. These include small birds and bats, both of which are surprisingly long-lived for their body sizes, metabolic rates, and lifetime oxygen expenditures.[1,2]

ANIMAL MODELS FOR AGING SHOULD BE SELECTED WITH SOUND EVOLUTIONARY AND COMPARATIVE PRINCIPLES IN MIND

From an evolutionary standpoint, aging is best understood as a consequence of the declining force of natural selection with waning reproductive potential. Specific

---

Address for correspondence: Donna J. Holmes, Department of Biological Sciences, P. O. Box 443051, University of Idaho, Moscow, ID 83844-3051. Voice: 208-882-3055; fax: 208-885-7905.
electric@uidaho.edu

aging processes may then result from either antagonistic pleiotropy (e.g., genes that promote successful reproduction, but have deleterious consequences later in life) or the unmitigated accumulation of harmful mutations. Aging processes arising from pleiotropic genes are predicted to be shared by a wide range of species, while those resulting from mutation accumulation should be idiosyncratic to particular species.[3,4]

In the absence of high mortality rates, natural selection will favor the evolution of long life spans and adaptations for prolonged somatic maintenance.[5] This means that organisms with effective protections against predation, disease, and accident (e.g., hard shells, flight, or a subterranean habit) are expected to evolve long life spans and effective antiaging processes. Studies of species with adaptations for ensuring long-term survival even in the face of repeated insult from damaging metabolic processes are most likely to suggest therapeutic interventions for improving our own health as we age.

Limiting our choice of aging animal models to a narrow taxonomic range of domestic species fails to employ judicious use of the comparative method. Any basic biochemical aging phenomenon shown to be shared by rats and mice (order Rodentia, family Muridae), for example, could be a result of either common ancestry or selection for fecundity during domestication, rather than being generalizable to mammals as a group. Aging processes in short-lived species could conceivably differ qualitatively, as well as quantitatively, from those in much longer-lived organisms. Moreover, distantly related species even within a vertebrate class may have evolved different molecular adaptations in response to the challenge of long-term somatic maintenance.[3]

SOME "NONTRADITIONAL" ANIMAL MODELS FOR AGING

There are, of course, some obvious drawbacks to using "nontraditional" animals in aging studies, including lack of information on husbandry, more genetic heterogeneity, and the fact that some are intimidating to manage in captivity. However, among a number of vertebrates with special potential, there are three warm-blooded examples that stand out: birds, bats, and mole-rats.

Domestic and cage birds, including poultry, small parrots, finches, and pigeons, are already used widely in biomedical research and are inexpensive to maintain. Maximum life spans of birds are generally 2–3 times those of similar-sized mammals. Wild songbirds often exceed 10 years of age; some parrots live over 90 years. Their high lifetime energy expenditures (up to 8 times those of mammals of similar size) and plasma glucose levels (up to more than 3 times higher than those of mammals) suggest that birds have unusually effective adaptations for preventing oxidative and glycoxidative damage. Advanced glycoxidative end products, like pentosidine, accumulate much more slowly in bird than in mammal tissues, and there is growing evidence that bird cells are exceptionally resistant to oxidative damage. Male finches exhibit seasonal regeneration of neurons in brain regions involved in song learning, while male quails retain hypothalamic responsiveness to testosterone during reproductive aging.[6,7]

The domestic laying hen has been used intensively for studies of apoptosis and ovarian cancer. In my laboratory, in collaboration with M. A. Ottinger of the University of Maryland, we are comparing ovarian and neuroendocrine correlates of female aging in short- and long-lived bird species, namely Japanese quail and budgerigar. Our results to date suggest that birds may retain a greater proportion of their primordial oocyte stores at the end of their reproductive life spans than mammals do. Longer-lived birds in the wild, particularly seabirds, have the potential to model very slow or even negligible loss of fertility, but reproductive aging in these species is poorly understood.[6,7]

Bats, as well as birds, are known for achieving long life spans despite high metabolic rates and high lifetime energy expenditures. Results of a new study by Anja Brunet Rossinni are consistent with the free radical theory of aging. Mitochondria of adult little brown bats (*Myotis lucifugus*: documented longevity of 34 years) exhibited similar oxygen expenditures *in vitro* to those of the short-tailed shrew (*Blarina brevicauda*: documented longevity of 3 years); the bat mitochondria, however, produced less than half as much hydrogen peroxide.[8]

Naked mole-rats are subterranean rodents with a eusocial, termite-like social system. A social group normally consists of one reproductive "queen" tended by a number of smaller, nonreproductive "workers." The metabolic rates of mole-rats are low for mammals of their body size; still, their reported life spans of over 25 years in captivity are remarkable for their size. Mole-rats are not difficult to maintain in captivity, and a number of captive research and zoo colonies exist. Studies of aging on mole-rats have only recently been initiated.[9]

The adoption of new and unusual animals for research exploring basic aging mechanisms need not be difficult. At best, however, it will involve careful collaboration between biogerontologists, wildlife biologists, and zoologists well versed in evolutionary principles and judicious application of the comparative method.

REFERENCES

1. HOLMES, D.J. & S.N. AUSTAD. 1995. Birds as animal models for the comparative biology of aging: a prospectus. J. Gerontol. Biol. Sci. **50A:** B59–B66.
2. AUSTAD, S.N. & K.E. FISCHER. 1991. Mammalian aging, metabolism, and ecology: evidence from the bats and marsupials. J. Gerontol. **46(2):** B47–B53.
3. AUSTAD, S.N. & D.J. HOLMES. 1999. Evolutionary approaches to probing aging mechanisms. *In* Methods in Aging Research, pp. 437–452. CRC Press. Boca Raton, FL.
4. MARTIN, G.M., S.N. AUSTAD & T.E. JOHNSON. 1996. Genetic analysis of aging: role of oxidative damage and environmental stresses. Nat. Genet. **13:** 25–34.
5. PARTRIDGE, L. & N.H. BARTON. 1993. Optimality, mutation, and the evolution of ageing. Nature **362:** 305–311.
6. HOLMES, D.J. 2003. Aging in birds. *In* Aging in Organisms, pp. 201–219. Kluwer. Amsterdam/Dordrecht.
7. HOLMES, D.J. & M.A. OTTINGER. 2003. Birds as long-lived animal models for the study of aging. Exp. Gerontol. **38:** 1365–1375.
8. BRUNET-ROSSINNI, A.J. 2003. Reduced free radical production and extended longevity of the little brown bat compared to two non-flying mammals. Mech. Ageing Dev. **125:** 11–20.
9. O'CONNOR, T.P., A. LEE, J.U. JARVIS & R. BUFFENSTEIN. 2002. Prolonged longevity in naked mole-rats: age-related changes in metabolism, body composition, and gastrointestinal function. Comp. Biochem. Physiol. A Mol. Integr. Physiol. **133(3):** 835–842.

The Extreme Aged

Sampling, Measurement, and Statistical Models in Cross-Sectional Estimation and Forecasting

LARRY S. CORDER

Center for Demographic Studies, Duke University, Durham, North Carolina 27798, USA

> ABSTRACT: Little effort has been directed toward studying the relationship between morbidity and mortality at exceptional ages, perhaps for no better reason than it has been difficult to do given available data resources. Two study innovations/adjustments are required to adequately represent count data with reports of health from aged sample persons. These design features are over-sampling of the exceptional group and linkage to detailed administrative reports. The National Long-Term Care Survey (NLTCS) has made it possible to study health and functioning in the context of exceptional longevity.
>
> KEYWORDS: aging; forecasts; pathways; surveys

Substantial attention has been directed toward the description and analysis of exceptional longevity as one expression of mortality dynamics.[1] Little effort has been directed toward studying the relationship between morbidity and mortality at exceptional ages, perhaps for no better reason than it has been difficult to do given available data resources. While mortality dynamics may be studied directly with registry data, the relationship between morbidity and mortality requires development and maintenance of a sample survey apparatus over a sustained period. This is true, in particular, if the relationship is changing quickly. Review and linkage of medical conditions to mortality data are not sufficient under a physical health and functioning measurement model. While various study designs of the population as well as measurement models of health and function are possible, exceptional longevity and the dimensions of health that accompany it are, by definition, rare events. As such, adequate precision is not generally available in national surveys that emphasize health as a study domain, particularly among the aged.[2] Rather, two study innovations/adjustments are required to adequately represent count data with reports of health from aged sample persons. These design features are oversampling of the exceptional group and linkage to detailed administrative reports—in this case, Medicare cost reports. Until recently, few national surveys published estimates for the groups above 75 years of age. Estimation of characteristics for the oldest old (85+) and centenarians (100+) was not readily achievable with extant survey

---

Address for correspondence: Larry S. Corder, Ph.D., Center for Demographic Studies, Duke University, 2117 Campus Drive, Box 90408, Durham, NC 27708-0408. Voice: 919-668-2700; fax: 919-684-5082.
    larrycorder@hotmail.com

designs, while a few local area studies, using sampling and linkage, have produced meaningful research in exceptional longevity.[3]

The National Long-Term Care Survey (NLTCS) study design and measurement model makes it possible to study health and functioning in the context of exceptional longevity. A significant consequence of this fact is the ability to develop pathways[4] to exceptional longevity and calculate active life expectation values for very old ages indeed. The NLTCS is a survey of persons 65 years of age and older in the United States. It has been conducted in 1982, 1984, 1989, 1994, 1999, and 2004 (planned).

A major innovation in the NLTCS study design concerns an additional set of over-samples. After 1989, both healthy persons and persons 95 years of age and older were substantially oversampled. While the "healthy" aging sample does not produce large numbers of exceptionally old persons in the NLTCS, persons of 95+ are available for analysis in both the 1994 and 1999 NLTCS (approximately 700 interviews in each year). This count includes both oversample and regular sample survey persons residing both in the community and in institutions.

Detailed examination of available data sets and ongoing aging research activities suggests the strong potential to study exceptional healthy longevity as part of the study of patterns of health and aging among the exceptionally aged at the population level. Both methods and materials necessary to measure a population's exceptionally healthy longevity are now in place, and recent research suggests that age misreporting for this group is not a serious problem. Research reports suggest minimal impact on results from misreports by whites.[5] Preliminary examination of the combined age distribution across all waves in the NLTCS does not produce many centenarians (275) or supercentenarians (5) in all of the survey waves based on a set of more than 60,000 interviews. Neither white sample persons nor 100+ age reporting appears to produce a more than minimal misreporting problem, leaving a certain amount of nonwhite age misreporting, among exceptionally aged persons.[6] Availability of population registry data, local area studies, mathematical models of population aging, and life table applications are necessary, but not sufficient for development and interpretation of active life expectation measures for the population 95 years of age and older, particularly in light of potential issues with the health and function measurement model normally employed in these studies. The nature of the invariant relationship of measures of health and function to medical expense and death may not be well supported in the exceptional longevity case. Indeed, a rapidly changing pattern of improving age-specific death rates at the oldest ages and rapid change in the achieved characteristics of succeeding cohorts, particularly education, suggest that the means and methods of measuring health levels, via survey data collection, are both an opportunity and a challenge. Local area studies have the advantage of highly focused medically related data collection in a repeated measures environment. Careful attention to the progress of diseases, comorbidity, and susceptibility enables the development of pathways to extraordinary longevity and exceptional healthy longevity as well.[7] Indeed, improvements in treatment of hearing and sight conditions apparently have a very great influence over the level of dementia reporting in population surveys in the most recent decade.[8] The idea or notion of health and function pathways is a direct reflection of the idea that the survival curve can be partitioned for any cohort, synthetic or otherwise, using discrete multivariate techniques to group person years of experience and/or modeled using sets of those time-varying dependent covariates. Changing pathways to disability and death imply changing the relationship between

TABLE 1. Comparisons of the two projection scenarios with Census Bureau projections for 2010, 2025, and 2040

Date	Age	Census Bureau (middle series)	Standard	High education	Ratio high education to census	Ratio high education to standard
2010	65	39,362	40,992	43,771	0.112	0.068
	85	6,115	6,673	8,448	0.381	0.266
	% 85 is of 65	(15.5%)	(16.3%)	(19.3%)		
	95	—	767	1,545	—	1.014
	% 95 is of 65	—	(1.9%)	(3.5%)		
2025	65	59,713	59,950	64,346	0.078	0.073
	85	7,011	7,233	10,161	0.449	0.405
	% 85 is of 65	(11.7%)	(12.1%)	(15.8%)		
	95	—	1,085	2,678	—	1.468
	% 95 is of 65	—	(1.8%)	(4.2%)		
2040	65	68,104	67,425	73,329	0.077	0.088
	85	12,251	11,492	15,538	0.268	0.352
	% 85 is of 65	(18.0%)	(17.0%)	(21.2%)		
	95	—	275	3,170	—	1.486
	% 95 is of 65	—	(1.9%)	(4.3%)		

SOURCE: Reference 11.

morbidity and mortality, the concrete expression of which has been improvement in life expectation at all advanced ages accompanied by improvements in healthy life expectation. Furthermore, recent work on characterizing "frailty" and developing a measurement model suggests additional complexity.[9] Such complexity may be addressed via discrete multivariate analysis (e.g., GoM).

The reality of disease onset, disability, and death patterns appears to have been altered by treatment. People persist in disability-free or disability-reduced disease states for longer periods just as many disease prevalence levels have fallen precipitously in the last century.[10] One result of the changing force of mortality has been the unprecedented growth of the exceptionally aged population. The NLTCS design offers the opportunity to examine its health and function dynamics.

The United States Census Bureau projections (middle series) are compared to standard and high education disability-based projections in TABLE 1.

Two series of projections based on chronic disability data from the 1982, 1984, and 1989 NLTCS were produced. One projection scenario built in disability changes observed from 1982 to 1989. The second examined population changes projected on the basis of the disability and mortality dynamics of the high education subpopulation in the NLTCS. In addition to disability and mortality dynamics, one must also consider the differences in the initial size of the cohorts entering the projections. Those aged 65 in 2010 were born in 1945, with smaller birth cohorts occurring at the end of World War II. Those age 65 in 2025 were born in 1960, or very near the peak size of the postwar baby boom cohorts found in 1963. Those aged 65 in 2040 were born in 1975; those aged 85 in 2040 were born in 1955, again during the rapid increases in the size of the postwar baby boom cohorts. Thus, dynamics of population size and age changes interact with the structure of the disability and mortality dynamics to determine both disability patterns and age distributions over time.

We see the more rapid growth of the 95+ population in the high education projection scenario. In 2010, the high education projections have 3.5% of the total 65+ population above age 95 compared to 1.9% for the standard projection—nearly double. By 2040, there is 4.3% (or 3.2 million persons) of the high education population over age 95, or 149% higher than the standard projection. Thus, it is the aging of the high education female population into more advanced ages that accounts for the rapid relative growth of the institutional population in the high education projection. If these persons were followed to more advanced ages, the proportion disabled might begin to decline as indicated by the life table probabilities due to high rates of death for the severely disabled. The decline would depend on the relative size of the birth cohorts at each date and changes in survival at younger ages.

REFERENCES

1. OLSHANSKY, S.J., B.A. CARNES & A. DESESQUELLES. 2001. Still in search of Methuselah: prospects for human longevity in an aging world. Science **291:** 1491–1492.
2. CORDER, L.S. & K.G. MANTON. 1991. National surveys and the health and functioning of the elderly: the effects of design and content. J. Am. Stat. Assoc. **86:** 513–525.
3. BALTES, P.B. & K.U. MAYER, Eds. 1999. The Berlin Aging Study: Aging from 70 to 100. Cambridge University Press. London/New York.
4. VERBRUGGE, L.M. & A.M. JETTE. 1994. The disablement process. Soc. Sci. Med. **38(1):** 1–14.
5. KESTENBAUM, B. 1992. A description of the extreme aged population based on improved Medicare enrollment data. Demography **29(4):** 565–580.
6. PRESTON, S.H., I.T. ELO, A. FOSTER, *et al.* 1998. Reconstructing the size of the African American population by age and sex, 1930–1990. Demography **35(1):** 1–21.
7. SMITH, J. & P.B. BALTES. 1999. Trends and profiles of psychological functioning in very old age. *In* The Berlin Aging Study: Aging from 70 to 100. Chapter 7, pp. 197–226. Cambridge University Press. London/New York.
8. CORDER, E.H. & K.G. MANTON. 2001. Change in the prevalence of severe dementia among older Americans: 1982–1999. IUSSP conference paper: S01–02.
9. BORTZ, W.M. 2002. A conceptual framework of frailty: a review. J. Gerontol. Med. Sci. **57A(5):** M283–M288.
10. COSTA, D.L. 2000. Long term declines in disability among older men: medical care, public health, and occupational change. NBER working paper: 7605.
11. MANTON, K.G. & L.S. CORDER. 1998. Forecasts of future disabled and institutionalized U.S. populations 1995 to 2040. *In* Ageing, Social Security, and Affordability. Chapter 4.2, p. 345. Ashgate Pub. Brookfield, VT.

Demographics of Human Supercentenarians and the Implications for Longevity Medicine

L. STEPHEN COLES

Department of Surgery, UCLA David Geffen School of Medicine, Los Angeles, California 90095, USA

> ABSTRACT: Demographers have forecast that there are going to be a great many more older adults in the next few decades. This will have great implications for longevity medicine. The Gerontology Research Group, affiliated with the UCLA School of Medicine, has compiled and maintained a Table of Worldwide Living Supercentenarians (persons 110 years or older) for the last 4 years, shedding important light on the biological limits of human morbidity and mortality and providing a realistic perspective on the problem of long-term interventions that can reasonably be achieved in the near future.
>
> KEYWORDS: age; aging; humans; life; longevity; supercentenarians

INTRODUCTION

According to the latest evidence from molecular biologists studying maternally distributed mitochondrial DNA and paternally distributed Y-chromosome linkages, paleontologists studying bone fragments from fossilized skulls, and anthropologists dating the successive migration of hominids over the Earth, we now have an emerging picture of how early humans must have lived. All but one of the hominid subspecies known to have existed over the past 2.5 million years eventually became extinct, making us the sole survivors of a family tree with many branches that just snapped off, sometimes after a million years of apparent success. Neanderthals, for example, lasted only 200,000 years before dying out. Even the largest dinosaurs, which lived much before primates, have been discovered to have numerous teeth marks on their bones as grim testimony to the sort of competitive world they were accustomed to before they fell victim to extinction. Thus, here is our best guess as to how things transpired for *Homo sapiens*.

Perhaps 160,000 years ago, on the shores of a now vanished fresh-water lake somewhere near Addis Ababa, Ethiopia, in Africa, the earliest known *Homo sapiens* were thrust into an intensely competitive high-risk game of chance played according to the rules of an indifferent casino (Darwinian evolution). We can only imagine, from our present vantage point, the sort of harsh world our ancestors endured. The other players in this game of survival (other species), who happened to be in close

---

Address for correspondence: L. Stephen Coles, M.D., Ph.D., Department of Surgery, UCLA David Geffen School of Medicine, Los Angeles, CA 90095-1678.
scoles@ucla.edu

proximity to us in the ecological food chain (or food web when you take microorganisms and parasites into account), did not hesitate to kill and eat their prey, so we imagine that humans were no exception to this law of the jungle.

However, between 10,000 and 15,000 years ago, something new happened. Humans declared the game over. Basically, humans won! There was no way to predict in advance that humans would become the dominant species on the planet, but all other species, especially carnivores, quietly lost. All such predators, possibly including other primates in the genus *Homo*, were effectively neutralized with the introduction of a combination of linguistic collaboration, lethal weapons technology, control of fire, and our seeming willingness to travel long distances. Thus, we afforded ourselves the modest luxury of protecting our tribe's elderly, as much as we spent time caring for our young or even burying our dead in a respectful manner with clear ceremonies for that purpose. The remainder of the wild animals either became pets (we bred wolves to become dogs, while big cats became pet cats) or were adapted to the indignant status of domesticated animals (bred as today's horses, camels, cows, pigs, sheep, goats, chickens, etc., for their economic utility). If these other species were not so inclined, we either exterminated them or else confined them in zoos (a euphemism for "jails"), for which we became the stewards (or self-appointed custodians, depending on one's point of view).

Then, we went on to invent agriculture. This afforded us the luxury of a prodigious food supply, resulting in a relative surplus of leisure time. This, in turn, opened up the possibility of more intellectual pursuits, like writing (recorded history), and allowed for the birth of a new game with a new set of rules, now known as civilization. However, the birth of civilization has been frustratingly uneven, a few steps forward and then some backward steps (as with wars and the frequent burning of libraries throughout human history). Even the veneer of our contemporary civilization may be quite thin when the opportunity arises for vandalism or looting without swift punishment. Nevertheless, most remaining wild habitats were fenced off for our mutual safety. However, even these "protected" habitats may not be 100% safe for wildlife as poachers have been known to sneak into restricted perimeters with modern weapons and kill off wild creatures (like elephants for their tusks or rhinos for their horns).

Ironically, something unexpected happened during the course of inventing civilization. We exposed a novel phenomenon called "aging," something that never was observed before in the jungle. (There are no old animals, except in zoos.) The fact is that all sexually reproducing biological systems must obey the laws of physics and chemistry, and the phenomenon of entropy affects all creatures who live beyond their so-called "biological warranty period" (between 50 and 60 years, or menopause in the case of human females). This phenomenon, related to the Second Law of Thermodynamics, derives from the fact that all creatures are constructed of dynamically changing, stochastic, brittle, fragile, Tinkertoy parts ("molecules"). These molecules are especially susceptible to reactive oxygen species that can cross-link and rearrange morphological structures randomly, mutating even our precious DNA. The mitochondria in old somatic cells (whose own DNA is naked and unprotected by histones) are especially guilty of producing these combustible free radical products over time (especially in the context of excessive caloric intake with reduced demand for ATP linked to a sedentary lifestyle). Conversely, the female germ-cell line (but not the male germ line) is proactive in selecting against primordial germ cells that contain defective (mutated) mtDNA. This guarantees the essential immortality of our species' germ line (but not of particular individuals). Interestingly, mitochondria of paternal origin located in the head of the sperm to provide the ATP energy necessary for tail wiggling/swimming sometimes migrate into the egg during fertilization. However, they are subsequently obliterated by specific enzymes in the egg. Therefore, we have a means to trace our female ancestry back to the original Eve.

Ultimately, this process renders us vulnerable to a random set of age-related diseases once we are no longer protected by the ingenious information programs contained within our DNA that give rise to our "life-history table" (embryogenesis, birth, puberty, and adulthood, with the associated biological imperative of finding a mate and rearing our offspring to reproductive independence, resulting in a next-generation of willing progeny). The evolutionary value of grandparenting is still being debated; however, once our life-history program(s) runs out of creative new things to do, cumulative "molecular infidelity" becomes relentless (as an entomologist once said: "there are no old caterpillars, only old butterflies").

It's not that there were never old people in prehistoric times who didn't have valuable knowledge and wisdom; it's just that they were so rare that selectional pressures favoring old age were undoubtedly low, and we presume that nobody at the time ever thought to describe aging as "undesirable" (or even more presumptuously as a "solvable problem") until now. A prominent gerontologist recently exclaimed, "God never meant for us to see aging!" Conversely, one might hypothetically complain, "God intended for us to die off before we ever witnessed our own aging." Even though these assertions may be true, they suffer from a wealth of presuppositions that render them extremely controversial (theology and teleology [intentionality; purpose; goals]) and are beyond the scope of our present discussion.

To overcome this constraint of aging, concealed but implicit within the old game in order to arrive at a still newer game, we will need to understand what the biological limits are on human life expectancy and maximum life span (the so-called "rectangular curve"). Otherwise, we cannot hope to intervene in ways that do not violate the laws of physics and chemistry and are doomed to fail as either wishful thinking or irrelevant daydreaming. Recall that humans imagined flying for a long time before the Wright brothers, but then again aeronautical engineering is a relatively new discipline within engineering, compared say with civil engineering. Today, most people cannot remember when we did not take airplanes for granted.

SUPERCENTENARIANS

The Gerontology Research Group, affiliated with the UCLA School of Medicine, has compiled and maintained a Table of Worldwide Living Supercentenarians (persons 110 years or older) for the last 4 years. Although an international committee of 30 demographers in various countries has been diligent in helping us to identify such persons with sufficient documentation to validate their claims, the numbers of such distinguished persons has remained relatively stable, ranging from 36 to 46 individuals for the past few years. The current version of this table, updated on a weekly basis, can be found at http://www.grg.org/calment.html/. This Internet Web page also includes over 50 photographs of these oldest-known men and women.

Finally, there are more detailed demographic tables [A–G], which contain lists of past supercentenarians throughout history.

As noted above, we currently have 43 members on the table: 38 females and 5 males. However, the gender ratio (GR) and distribution of nationalities are subject to significant fluctuation with time. The absolute number of individuals in this select class also goes up and down as newly entering members live long enough, while other members pass on. A simple line graph of the numbers of supercentenarians over the last 4 years tends to oscillate like a "stock-market ticker tape," with a moderate upward tendency. However, no reasonable conclusions are yet possible with regard to the regression line that can be calculated using standard statistical methods. In other words, one cannot really say with authority that the maximum life span records of our species will ever be broken systematically in the coming decades as athletic records have been known to fall. Recall that the oldest known *Guinness Book of World Records* case is that of a French woman, Madame Jeanne Louise Calment, who died on August 4, 1997, at the age of 122 years; we are confident that breaking her record will prove to be very difficult. The only thing we can say with certainty about why centenarians live as long as they do is that it's not just because they age more slowly, although that may be true, but because they appear to age more uniformly—without a single "weak link" in any of their more vulnerable systems that might have caused their premature death at an earlier age.

Background of the Table

The data needed to create the table were compiled by an international team of contributors, including professional demographers, university-based centenarian researchers, as well as a number of highly dedicated amateurs who have devoted countless hours over the last 4 years to the task of maintaining its accuracy. Along the way, many journalists from different parts of the world, who normally write human-interest stories on local celebrities, have assisted us in our contacts with family members who, in turn, provide official documentation. Nursing home staff in various parts of the country have also been extremely helpful. Note that the contributors work diligently to meet the challenge of various pretenders-to-membership whose documentation is either forged or lost for a variety of reasons. Many such individuals have been scrupulously deleted. Furthermore, the table is certainly incomplete in that, for less-developed countries, many individuals, who may otherwise have valid claims, have incomplete documentation (like a family Bible) and official documents may never have existed in these countries, if and when they began keeping census records at all. Besides birth certificates, baptismal certificates and marriage certificates are often used when available. Finally, we may not even become aware of many of these individuals since their families, even if they become aware that such a list is being maintained, might have no incentive to inform us or any government officials simply because demographers happen to be gratuitously interested in their personal relatives.

Privacy Statement

For reasons of confidentiality, details of the supporting documentation of those individuals who are filed with the GRG will only be made available to legitimate demographic researchers having a "need to know." An important feature of our research protocol is our focus on persons whose age has been rigorously validated. For a complete validation of the age of a supercentenarian, it is frequently necessary to obtain personal information. For example, in most countries, the precise name of a person is needed to retrieve and match birth and death certificates. Appropriate procedures and rules are designed to protect the confidential nature of personal information, taking into account prevailing data protection laws of many different countries. For example, Germany has different laws from France and the United Kingdom. Data protection procedures and rules adopted by our committee and the IDL (International Database on Longevity) are governed by the general principle that private data about individual persons should not be accessible from information that will eventually be made public unless essential for identification purposes. For example, among these rules is the provision that only specially trained validation personnel will have access to private personal information (such as addresses, phone numbers, names of relatives, and so on). This sort of private personal information shall not be made available to individuals who are external to the validation process and will never be included in a public version of this database.

We believe that these tables shed important light on the biological limits of human morbidity and mortality. Later on, we will attempt to summarize these data in the context of human life-history tables, as well as tables gathered from other species, to provide us with a realistic perspective on the problem of long-term interventions that can reasonably be achieved in the near future.

CONCLUSIONS

In 1889, when he was 72, the eminent French physiologist, Charles Édouard Brown-Séquard, reported that he had rejuvenated himself by injecting himself with the tissue extract of animal testicles. Although a worldwide cult of gullible old men built up around this strange practice over the next two decades, it was finally discredited by legitimate medical scientists [Ref. 4, p. 272]. In recent years, a better understanding of the biochemical and neuroendocrine determinants of aging has put interventions on a somewhat more solid scientific foundation to combat a few of the deleterious consequences of aging. Many theoretical studies are concerned with elucidating the regulatory mechanisms of aging at the cellular level, and we expect that they will also have practical implications that translate into real therapeutic interventions in the coming decades.

After tracking the data in the supercentenarian table above for 4 years, we have seen that the rectangularization of the human longevity curve is increasing. In other words, we are witnessing a natural increase in average life expectancy (but a somewhat slower rate) with no corresponding right-shift in the maximum life span. This compression of morbidity with more healthy years at the end of life was forecast by James Fries more than 20 years ago, when this concept was initially met with skepticism by the medical establishment.[8,9]

It is proposed that we establish an international research agenda as follows: (1) establish an Epidemiology of Aging Database that could be used to forecast trends in aging; (2) understand the fundamental basis of age-associated degenerative conditions and nonfatal chronic illness; and (3) set a priority for documenting and implementing effective programs in prevention that could improve health and perhaps mitigate the economic consequences of unnecessary morbidity among older adults. Demographers have forecast that there are going to be a great many more older adults in the next few decades, and it will be best if we can expect to approach our senior years in the best health that we can hope for.

ACKNOWLEDGMENTS

The GRG Worldwide Living Supercentenarian Table above is the ongoing work product of an international committee with 45 members from over 20 countries, including the United States, Canada, the United Kingdom, France, Germany, Spain, Sweden, Norway, Denmark, the Netherlands, Belgium, Australia, and Japan. The list is regularly compiled for publication by Louis Epstein (New York), our Committee Chairman, and Robert Young (Atlanta, GA), the GRG Senior Claims Investigator.

REFERENCES

1. OLSHANSKY, S.J., B.A. CARNES & A. DESESQUELLES. 2001. Demography: prospects for human longevity. Science **291**(5508): 1491–1492.
2. CARNES, B.A., S.J. OLSHANSKY & D. GRAHN. 2003. Biological evidence for the limits to the duration of life. Biogerontology **4**: 31–45.
3. SHOCK, N.W., R.C. GREULICH, R.A. ANDRES, et al. 1984. Normal Human Aging: The Baltimore Longitudinal Study of Aging. National Institute on Aging. Washington, D.C.
4. HAYFLICK, L. 1994. How and Why We Age. Ballentine Books. New York.
5. OLSHANSKY, S.J., L. HAYFLICK & B.A. CARNES. 2002. No truth to the fountain of youth. Sci. Am. **286**(6): 92–95.
6. DE GREY, A.D.N.J., L. GAVRILOV, S.J. OLSHANSKY, et al. 2002. Antiaging technology and pseudoscience [letter]. Science **296**(5568): 656.
7. WACHTER, K.W. & C.E. FINCH, Eds. 1997. Between Zeus and the Salmon: The Biodemography of Longevity, pp. 269–274. National Academy Press. Washington, D.C.
8. FRIES, J.F. 1980. Aging, natural death, and the compression of morbidity. N. Engl. J. Med. **303**: 130–135.
9. FRIES, J.F. & L.M. CRAPO. 1981. Vitality and Aging: Implications of the Rectangular Curve. Freeman. San Francisco.
10. CAREY, J.R. 2003. Longevity: The Biology and Demography of Life Span. Princeton University Press. Princeton, NJ.

Early-Life Programming of Aging and Longevity

The Idea of High Initial Damage Load (the HIDL Hypothesis)

LEONID A. GAVRILOV AND NATALIA S. GAVRILOVA

Center on Aging, National Opinion Research Center (NORC) and University of Chicago, Chicago, Illinois 60637, USA

ABSTRACT: In this study, we test the predictions of the high initial damage load (HIDL) hypothesis, a scientific idea that early development of living organisms produces an exceptionally high load of initial damage, which is comparable with the amount of subsequent aging-related deterioration accumulating during the rest of the entire adult life. This hypothesis predicts that even small progress in optimizing the early-developmental processes can potentially result in a remarkable prevention of many diseases in later life, postponement of aging-related morbidity and mortality, and significant extension of healthy life span.

KEYWORDS: high initial damage load (HIDL); aging; longevity; early-life; development; programming

INTRODUCTION

In 1991, we suggested a scientific idea that early development of living organisms produces an exceptionally high load of initial damage, which is comparable with the amount of subsequent aging-related deterioration accumulating during the rest of the entire adult life.[1]

This idea of high initial damage load (the HIDL hypothesis) predicts that even small progress in optimizing the early-developmental processes can potentially result in a remarkable prevention of many diseases in later life, postponement of aging-related morbidity and mortality, and significant extension of healthy life span.[1-3] Thus, the idea of early-life programming of aging and longevity may have important practical implications for developing early-life interventions promoting health and longevity.

In this study, we tested the predictions of the HIDL hypothesis. Specifically, the HIDL hypothesis predicts that early-life events may affect survival in later adult life through the level of initial damage. This prediction is confirmed for such early-life factors as paternal age at a person's conception[4] and the month of a person's birth.[4,5]

Address for correspondence: Leonid A. Gavrilov, Center on Aging, NORC/University of Chicago, 1155 East 60th Street, Chicago, IL 60637-2745. Voice: 773-256-6359; fax: 773-256-6313.
gavrilov@longevity-science.org

Ann. N.Y. Acad. Sci. 1019: 496–501 (2004). © 2004 New York Academy of Sciences.
doi: 10.1196/annals.1297.091

Another testable prediction of the HIDL hypothesis is a prevision of an unusual nonlinear pattern of life-span inheritance. This prediction is tested and confirmed: familial transmission of life span from parents to children follows a nonlinear (accelerating) pattern, with steeper slopes for offspring life span of longer-lived parents, as predicted.[6]

DISCUSSION OF THE IDEA OF HIGH INITIAL DAMAGE LOAD

The introductory section presented earlier is written as an abstract briefly summarizing the main ideas, findings, and conclusions of our studies. The purpose of this section is to provide a more detailed discussion of the idea of HIDL.

Reliability theory of aging predicts that a failure rate of simple redundant systems increases with age according to the Weibull (power) law.[1-3] This theoretical prediction is consistent with empirical observations that failure kinetics of technical devices follow the Weibull law.[7] However, biological systems "prefer" to fail according to the Gompertz (exponential) law,[1,8] which calls for explanations.

An attempt to explain exponential deterioration of biosystems in terms of the reliability theory led us to a paradoxical conjecture that biological systems start their adult life with a high load of initial damage.[1-3]

Although this idea may look like a counterintuitive assumption, it fits well with many empirical observations on massive cell losses in early development. For example, the female human fetus at 4–5 months of age possesses 6–7 million eggs (oocytes). By birth, this number drops to 1–2 million and declines even further. At the start of puberty in normal girls, there are only 0.3–0.5 million eggs, just only 4–8% of initial numbers (for review, see Ref. 3).

Massive cell losses in early development are creating conditions for a Poisson distribution of organisms according to the numbers of remaining cells, which in turn produce the exponential (Gompertzian) law of mortality increase.[1] Because the mathematical proof for this statement is already published elsewhere for a more general case of binomial distribution,[1] we can concentrate here on substantive discussion of the idea of HIDL in biological systems.

Biological systems are different from technical devices in two aspects. The first fundamental feature of biosystems is that, in contrast to technical (artificial) devices, which are constructed out of previously manufactured and tested components, organisms form themselves in ontogenesis through a process of self-assembly out of *de novo* forming and externally untested elements (cells). The second property of organisms is the extraordinary degree of miniaturization of their components (the microscopic dimensions of cells, as well as the molecular dimensions of information carriers like DNA and RNA), permitting the creation of a huge redundancy in the number of elements. Thus, we can expect that for living organisms, in distinction to many technical (manufactured) devices, the reliability of the system is achieved not by the high initial quality of all the elements, but by their huge numbers (redundancy).

The fundamental difference in the manner in which the system is formed (external assembly in the case of technical devices and self-assembly in the case of biosystems) has two important consequences. First, it leads to the macroscopicity of technical devices in comparison with biosystems since technical devices are assembled "top-down" with the participation of a macroscopic system (humans) and must be suitable for this macroscopic system to use (i.e., commensurate with humans). Organisms, on the other hand, are assembled "bottom-up" from molecules and cells, resulting in an exceptionally high degree of miniaturization of the component parts. Second, since technical devices are assembled under the control of humans, the opportunities to pretest components (external quality control) are incomparably greater than in the self-assembly of biosystems. The latter inevitably leads to organisms being "littered" with a great number of defective elements. As a result, the reliability of technical devices is assured by the high quality of elements, with a strict limit on their numbers because of size and cost limitations, while the reliability of biosystems is assured by an exceptionally high degree of redundancy to overcome the poor quality of some elements.

It follows from this concept of HIDL that even small progress in optimizing the processes of ontogenesis and increasing the numbers of initially functional elements can potentially result in a remarkable fall in mortality and a significant improvement in life span. This optimistic prediction is supported by experimental evidence of increased offspring life span in response to protection of parental germ cells against oxidative damage just by feeding the future parents with antioxidants.[9] Increased life span is also observed among the progeny of parents with a low resting respiration rate (proxy for the rate of oxidative damage to DNA of germ cells; see Ref. 1). The concept of HIDL also predicts that early life events may affect survival in later adult life through the level of initial damage. This prediction proved to be correct for such early-life indicators as parental age at a person's conception[4] and the month of a person's birth (see FIG. 1, TABLE 1, and earlier publications[4,5]).

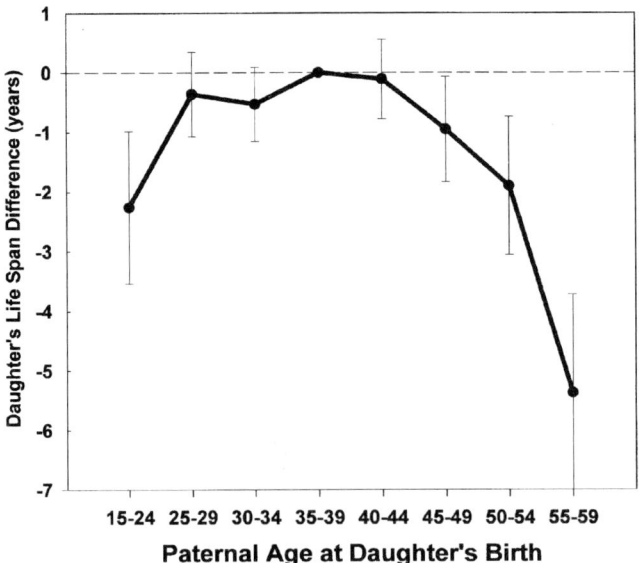

FIGURE 1. Daughters' life span as a function of paternal age at daughter's birth: 5063 daughters from European aristocratic families born in 1800–1880. Both parents lived 50+ years. Details of data analysis are described elsewhere.[4]

TABLE 1. Female life span as a function of month of birth

Month of birth	Net effect, in years (point estimate)	Standard error	P value
February	0.00	Reference level	
March	1.10	0.92	.2331
April	1.72	0.92	.0619
May	2.35	0.90	.0090
June	1.66	0.90	.0665
July	1.86	0.91	.0404
August	1.49	0.90	.0978
September	1.51	0.92	.0986
October	1.95	0.90	.0308
November	2.13	0.93	.0229
December	3.04	0.91	.0009
January	0.94	0.92	.3086
February	0.00	Reference level	

NOTE: Results are obtained through multivariate regression analysis of life-span data (outcome variable) for 6908 women born from 1800 to 1880 (extinct birth cohorts with life span known for each person) who survived to age 30 (focus on analysis of adult life span). The following additional predictor variables are also included in the final model because of their predictive value: (1) calendar year of birth, (2) ethnicity (Russian, British, and others), (3) loss of father during formative years of childhood (before age 15), (4) loss of mother during formative years of childhood (before age 15), (5) cause of death (violent vs. nonviolent), (6) early death of at least one sibling (before age 30), (7) high birth order (7+), (8) nobility rank of the father (indicator of social status), (9) large family size (number of siblings: 9+), (10) maternal life span, (11) paternal life span, (12) paternal age at person's birth, (13) late paternal age at first childbirth (50+ years), (14) birth of the first child by mother after age 30, and (15) death of mother from violent cause of death. The F value for the regression model is 18.12 ($P < .0001$). "Net effect" corresponds to additional years of life gained (or lost) compared to the reference category (life span for those born in February).

Women may be particularly sensitive to early-life exposures because they are mosaics of two different cell types (one with an active paternal X chromosome and another one with an active maternal X chromosome). The exact pattern of this mosaic is determined early in life. If early-life conditions affect the proportion (or distribution pattern) of cells with a given X chromosome, such conditions might have long-lasting effects in later life. Indeed, this conjecture of stronger female response to early-life exposures is confirmed for such early-life predictors of adult life span as paternal age at a person's conception[4] and the month of a person's birth.[4,5]

Another testable prediction of the HIDL hypothesis is a prediction of an unusual nonlinear pattern of life-span inheritance. Traditionally, it is assumed that the dependence of progeny life span on parental life span should follow a linear relationship, which is common to all other quantitative traits in classic quantitative genetics.[10] In other words, for each additional year of parental life span, the children are expected to have some fixed gain in their average life span too, as a result of polygenic inheritance of quantitative traits.[10] However, the HIDL hypothesis leads to a very different prediction of a nonlinear (accelerated) "concave-up" pattern of life-span inheritance. There should be virtually no life-span heritability (a negligible response of progeny life span to the changes in parental life span) when parental life span is below a certain age, and a much higher heritability (an increased response to parental life span) when parents live longer lives. This prediction follows from the hypothesis of HIDL among short-lived parents, whose bodies are damaged during early developmental processes, although their germ-cell DNA might be perfectly normal. (If the germ-cell DNA were damaged too, these short-lived parents would probably produce offspring who also live short lives. This category will thus be unlikely to distort the linear dependence of offspring life span on parental life span by a large amount.) Therefore, the progeny of some short-lived parents may have quite normal life spans, well beyond genetic expectations. This result would thus obstruct the classic linear offspring-on-parent dependence for life span. Only at some high parental life span, when most of the germ-normal/somatically damaged parents are eliminated because of their shorter length of life, will the classic linear pattern of life-span inheritance eventually reveal itself in its full capacity. This prediction of the HIDL hypothesis was tested and confirmed in humans: familial transmission of life span from parents to children proved to follow a nonlinear (accelerating) pattern, with steeper slopes for the life span of offspring born to longer-lived parents, as predicted.[6]

Thus, there is mounting evidence now in support of the idea of fetal origins of adult degenerative diseases, and early-life programming of aging and longevity.[4]

ACKNOWLEDGMENTS

This study was made possible thanks to generous support from the National Institute on Aging (NIH) and a stimulating working environment at the Center on Aging, NORC/University of Chicago. We would like to thank members of the Science Advisory Board (SAB) (http://www.scienceboard.net/) for useful comments on our work made at the SAB discussion group.

REFERENCES

1. GAVRILOV, L.A. & N.S. GAVRILOVA. 1991. The Biology of Life Span: A Quantitative Approach. Harwood Academic. New York.
2. GAVRILOV, L.A. & N.S. GAVRILOVA. 2001. The reliability theory of aging and longevity. J. Theor. Biol. **213:** 527–545.
3. GAVRILOV, L.A. & N.S. GAVRILOVA. 2003 (July 16). The quest for a general theory of aging and longevity. Science's SAGE KE (Science of Aging Knowledge Environment) **2003**(28): 1–10 [available at http://sageke.sciencemag.org].
4. GAVRILOV, L.A. & N.S. GAVRILOVA. 2003. Early-life factors modulating lifespan. In Modulating Aging and Longevity, pp. 27–50. Kluwer. Dordrecht.
5. GAVRILOV, L.A. & N.S. GAVRILOVA. 1999. Season of birth and human longevity. J. Anti-Aging Med. **2:** 365–366.
6. GAVRILOVA, N.S. & L.A. GAVRILOV. 2001. When does human longevity start? Demarcation of the boundaries for human longevity. J. Anti-Aging Med. **4:** 115–124.
7. WEIBULL, W.A. 1951. A statistical distribution function of wide applicability. J. Appl. Mech. **18:** 293–297.

8. GOMPERTZ, B. 1825. On the nature of the function expressive of the law of human mortality and on a new mode of determining life contingencies. Philos. Trans. R. Soc. London **A115:** 513–585.
9. HARMAN, D. & D.E. EDDY. 1979. Free radical theory of aging: beneficial effects of adding antioxidants to the maternal mouse diet on life span of offspring: possible explanation of the sex difference in longevity. AGE **2:** 109-122.
10. FALCONER, D.S. & T.F.C. MACKAY. 1996. Introduction to Quantitative Genetics. Longman. London.

Cardiovascular Disease Delay in Centenarian Offspring

Role of Heat Shock Proteins

DELLARA F. TERRY,[a] MAEGAN McCORMICK,[a] STACY ANDERSEN,[a] JAEMI PENNINGTON,[a] EMILY SCHOENHOFEN,[a] ELIZABETH PALAIMA,[b] MARIA BAUSERO,[b] KISHIKO OGAWA,[b] THOMAS T. PERLS,[a] AND ALEXZANDER ASEA[b]

[a]*Geriatrics Section, Department of Medicine, Boston Medical Center, Boston, Massachusetts 02118, USA*

[b]*Center for Molecular Stress Response, Boston Medical Center and Boston University School of Medicine, Boston, Massachusetts 02118, USA*

ABSTRACT: Cardiovascular disease is a major cause of morbidity and mortality of older Americans. We have demonstrated recently that centenarian offspring, when compared with age-matched controls, avoid and/or delay cardiovascular disease and cardiovascular risk factors. Given recent evidence suggesting that higher circulating levels of HSP70 predict the future development of cardiovascular disease in established hypertensives and a recent study demonstrating a decrease in HSP60 and HSP70 with advancing age, we hypothesized that HSP70 levels would be lower in centenarian offspring compared with controls. The circulating serum concentration of HSP70 in 20 centenarian offspring and 9 spousal controls was analyzed using a modified HSP70 ELISA method. Centenarian offspring showed approximately 10-fold lower levels of circulating serum HSP70 compared with spousal controls ($P < .001$). The exact biological significance of the extremely low levels of circulating serum HSP70 observed in centenarian offspring thus far is not clear. However, circulating HSP has been shown to correlate in diseases or disorders in which there is destruction or damage to target tissues or organs, including cardiovascular diseases and numerous autoimmune disorders. We hypothesize that low levels of circulating serum HSP70 may be an indicator of a healthy state and point to longevity of the host; therefore, our results suggest that levels of circulating serum HSP70 may be a marker for longevity.

KEYWORDS: aging; cardiovascular disease; chaperokine; centenarian; heat shock proteins; longevity

Address for correspondence: Alexzander Asea, Ph.D., Deputy Chief, Center for Molecular Stress Response, Boston Medical Center and Boston University School of Medicine, 650 Albany Street, Boston, MA 02118. Voice: 617-414-1716; fax: 617-414-1697.
aasea@bu.edu

INTRODUCTION

Longevity Runs in Families

Prior research suggests that longevity runs in families. Both the parents and the siblings of centenarians[1] have been shown to have significantly longer life expectancies than the average for their birth cohorts. More recently, we have demonstrated that the children of centenarians, who are typically in their 70s and 80s, have a survival advantage when compared with age-matched controls whose parents died at an average life expectancy. Furthermore, these individuals demonstrate a reduced relative prevalence[2] as well as a delay in the age of onset for heart disease, hypertension, and diabetes.[3] Interestingly, no differences have been found between the offspring of centenarians and controls for several other age-related diseases such as cancer, osteoporosis, and dementia.[2] This suggests that it is perhaps the avoidance or delay of cardiovascular disease and cardiovascular risk factors that facilitate the survival to exceptional old age.

Heat Shock Protein and Its Role in Cardiovascular Disease and Longevity

Heat shock proteins (HSPs) are highly conserved proteins found in all prokaryotes and eukaryotes. The primary role of HSPs is to chaperone, transport, and fold proteins when cells are exposed to a variety of stresses.[4] Under normal physiological conditions, HSP is expressed at low levels; however, a wide variety of stressful stimuli including environmental, pathological, or physiological stimuli can induce a marked increase in intracellular HSP synthesis[4] known as the stress response.

It is now clear that HSP can also exit mammalian cells,[5] interact with cells of the immune system, and exert immunoregulatory effects.[6] The ability of HSP to act as cytokine and chaperone is termed the chaperokine activity of HSP.[7]

The expression of HSP in the early stages of cardiovascular disease might result from one or a combination of factors. For example, risk factors for atherosclerosis such as hyperlipidemia, diabetes, smoking, and hypertension cause oxidative stress. Oxidative stress, in turn, may lead to the induction of HSP expression in vascular smooth muscle cells.[8] In addition, prior research indicates that circulating HSP70 levels predict the development of cardiovascular disease in subjects with established hypertension.[9,10] These authors suggest that HSP70 protects against or modifies the progression of atherosclerosis in this subject group.

With the avoidance and/or delay of cardiovascular disease in centenarian offspring, the evidence suggesting a protective role of HSP70 for cardiovascular disease and a recent study demonstrating an apparent decrease in HSP60 and HSP70 with advancing age,[11] we hypothesized that levels of HSP70 would be lower in centenarian offspring when compared with age-matched controls.

METHODS

The criteria for eligibility, recruitment, and main study outcomes have been published elsewhere.[2]

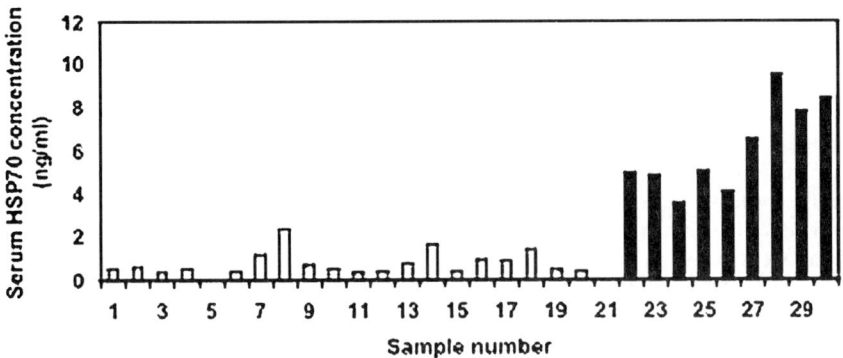

FIGURE 1. Concentration of circulating HSP70. Sera from 20 centenarian offspring (*unfilled bars*; 1–20) and nine spousal controls (*filled bars*; 22–30) were analyzed for the concentration of HSP70 using the HSP70 ELISA kit (StressGen Biotechnologies). Data represent the serum HSP70 concentration and represent two experiments performed with similar results ($P < .001$).

Enzyme-Linked Immunosorbent Assay

Serum from 20 centenarian offspring and 9 spousal controls was analyzed for the concentration of HSP70 using the HSP70 enzyme-linked immunosorbent assay (ELISA) kit (StressGen Biotechnologies, Victoria, BC, Canada) as previously described.[11] The total cell protein content within the serum was determined by Bradford analysis using bovine serum albumin as a standard.

Univariate statistical analysis was done using the Student's t test.

RESULTS

A complete accounting for all potential participants for both groups and a complete description of all enrolled participants have been published elsewhere.[2]

HSP70 levels were measured in convenience subsample of 20 centenarian offspring and nine controls using an HSP70 ELISA kit (StressGen). We demonstrate that circulating HSP70 in centenarian offspring serum (FIG. 1; unfilled bars) is approximately 10 times less than circulating HSP70 found in the serum of spousal controls (FIG. 1; filled bars; $P < .001$).

DISCUSSION

Our prior work has demonstrated that the offspring of centenarians are healthier than age-matched controls.[2] In particular, the delay and/or avoidance of cardiovascular disease may be key for their potential survival to exceptional old age.

The physiological role of circulating heat shock proteins has yet to be defined. However, our results are in agreement with others who have shown that there is a progressive decline in serum Hsp60 and Hsp70 levels with aging.[11] The exact biological significance of the extremely low levels of circulating HSP70 observed in centenarian offspring is not clear. In general, circulating HSP have been shown to correlate in diseases or disorders in which there is destruction or damage to target tissues or organs, including cardiovascular diseases and numerous autoimmune disorders. Low levels of circulating HSP may be an indicator of a healthy state and point to longevity of the host; therefore, we suggest that levels of circulating HSP70 may be a marker for longevity.

Ultimately, further study of circulating HSP70 needs to be performed in a larger sample of individuals to better understand this phenomenon and to account for some of the confounders such as current health status and health habits using multivariate analyses.

REFERENCES

1. PERLS, T.T. *et al.* 2002. Life-long sustained mortality advantage of siblings of centenarians. Proc. Natl. Acad. Sci. USA **99:** 8442–8447.
2. TERRY, D.F. *et al.* 2003. Cardiovascular advantages among the offspring of centenarians. J. Gerontol. A Biol. Sci. Med. Sci. **58:** M425–M431.
3. TERRY, D.F. *et al.* 2004. Cardiovascular disease delay in centenarian offspring. J. Gerontol. A Biol. Sci. Med. Sci. **59:** M385–M389.
4. LINDQUIST, S. & E.A. CRAIG. 1988. The heat-shock proteins. Annu. Rev. Genet. **22:** 631–677.
5. BARRETO, A. *et al.* 2003. Stress-induced release of HSC70 from human tumors. Cell. Immunol. **222:** 97–104.
6. ASEA, A. *et al.* 2000. HSP70 stimulates cytokine production through a CD14-dependent pathway, demonstrating its dual role as a chaperone and cytokine. Nat. Med. **6:** 435–442.
7. ASEA, A. *et al.* 2002. Novel signal transduction pathway utilized by extracellular HSP70: role of toll-like receptor (TLR) 2 and TLR4. J. Biol. Chem. **277:** 15028–15034.
8. LIAO, D.F. *et al.* 2000. Purification and identification of secreted oxidative stress-induced factors from vascular smooth muscle cells. J. Biol. Chem. **275:** 189–196.
9. POCKLEY, A.G. *et al.* 2002. Circulating heat shock protein and heat shock protein antibody levels in established hypertension. J. Hypertens. **20:** 1815–1820.
10. POCKLEY, A.G. *et al.* 2003. Serum heat shock protein 70 levels predict the development of atherosclerosis in subjects with established hypertension. Hypertension **42:** 235–238.
11. REA, I.M., S. MCNERLAN & A.G. POCKLEY. 2001. Serum heat shock protein and anti-heat shock protein antibody levels in aging. Exp. Gerontol. **36:** 341–352.

Testing the Free Radical Theory of Aging in Bats

ANJA K. BRUNET ROSSINNI

Department of Ecology, Evolution and Behavior,
University of Minnesota, Saint Paul, Minnesota 55108, USA

ABSTRACT: The extended longevity of bats, despite their high metabolic rates, may provide insight to patterns and mechanisms of aging. I tested the free radical theory of aging as an explanation for the extreme longevity of the little brown bat, *Myotis lucifugus* (maximum life span potential [MLSP] = 34 years). In a comparative study, I measured whole-organism oxygen consumption and mitochondrial hydrogen peroxide production in brain, heart, and kidney tissues from *M. lucifugus* and short-tailed shrews, *Blarina brevicauda* (MLSP = 2 years). As predicted by the free radical theory of aging, *M. lucifugus* produced approximately half the amount of hydrogen peroxide as *B. brevicauda*. In addition, I compared oxygen consumption and hydrogen peroxide production of adult (~1 year) and juvenile (fully developed and fledged young of the year) *M. lucifugus* to assess oxidative damage to mitochondria (measured as an increase in hydrogen peroxide production) due to the high metabolic rate associated with flight. Contrary to my prediction, juveniles had significantly higher levels of hydrogen peroxide production than adults. I propose that the decreased free radical production in adults is the result of within-individual selection of efficient mitochondria due to selective pressure created by the high energetic demands of flight.

KEYWORDS: aging; free radical theory; long-lived organism; bats; *Myotis lucifugus*; *Blarina brevicauda*

On average, bats live three times longer than nonflying mammals of similar size and basal metabolic rates.[1] However, few studies have focused on explaining the extended longevity of these animals,[2,3] and no studies have attempted to test recent physiological theories of aging in bats. Under the free radical theory,[4] aging is a consequence of damage to cellular constituents caused by reactive oxygen species produced during mitochondrial respiration. Two predictions result from this theory: (1) free radical production is lower in long-lived organisms than in short-lived organisms, and (2) free radical production increases with age as cellular damage accumulates. To test the first prediction, I compared whole-organism oxygen consumption and H_2O_2 production of mitochondria isolated from brain, heart, and kidney tissues of little brown bats, *M. lucifugus*, and short-tailed shrews, *Blarina brevicauda*. Both

Address for correspondence: Anja K. Brunet Rossinni, Department of Ecology, Evolution and Behavior, University of Minnesota, 1987 Upper Buford Circle, Saint Paul, MN 55108. Voice: 763-438-5248; fax: 612-624-6777.
anja.brunet@stanfordalumni.org

species have high metabolic rates, but whereas *M. lucifugus* has a maximum life span record of 34 years in the wild,[5] *B. brevicauda* has a captive life span of 2 years.[6] To test the second prediction, I compared the same measures from adult and fully developed juvenile *M. lucifugus*.

All bats were collected during summer 2002. Adults had visible teats and juveniles were fully developed. Half of the juveniles were not yet capable of flight (prevolant) and the other half were capable of sustained flight (volant). Seven adult *B. brevicauda* were trapped during summer 2002 using standard Sherman traps. I measured metabolic rates of each animal in a closed-chamber respirometer submerged in water at 22°C. I recorded oxygen consumed every 2 minutes for 1 hour. The evening (17:00–20:00 h) after measuring oxygen consumption, I harvested brain, heart, and kidney tissues, isolated intact mitochondria by differential centrifugation and measured H_2O_2 production.[7] I analyzed results using one-way ANOVA and Tukey-Kramer multiple comparison.

Despite consuming similar amounts of oxygen per gram of body mass (4.83 ± 0.30 and 4.19 ± 0.36 mL O_2/h*gr), *M. lucifugus* produced less than half the amount of H_2O_2 produced by *B. brevicauda* in all three tissues (brain: 85.07 ± 6.2 vs. 201.97 ± 5.2 nmol H_2O_2/min*µg mt protein, respectively; heart: 50.63 ± 15.6 vs. 119.07 ± 13.2; kidney: 47.91 ± 9.6 vs. 116.97 ± 8.1; $P \leq .001$). Adult and prevolant juvenile *M. lucifugus* consumed similar amounts of oxygen (4.83 ± 0.30 vs. 4.60 ± 0.36 mL O_2/h*gr, respectively), but volant juveniles consumed significantly less (3.75 ± 0.26 mL O_2/h*gr, $P \leq .01$). Prevolant juveniles produced significantly more H_2O_2 than adults in all three tissues (brain: 112.9 ± 3.97 vs. 85.07 ± 6.2 nmol H_2O_2/min*µg mt protein, respectively; heart: 105.6 ± 10.0 vs. 50.63 ± 15.6, kidney: 73.9 ± 4.5 vs. 47.91 ± 9.6; $P \leq .02$). Juveniles capable of flight produced significantly more H_2O_2 than adults in heart and kidney tissue (heart: 93.3 ± 2.8 nmol H_2O_2/min*µg mt protein; kidney: 69.7 ± 5.9; $P \leq .02$) but similar amounts in brain tissue (81.8 ± 3.1 nmol H_2O_2/min*µg mt protein).

As the free radical theory predicts, *B. brevicauda* produced higher levels of H_2O_2 than *M. lucifugus*. The difference in H_2O_2 between these two species despite similarly high metabolic rates lends support to the free radical theory and to the contention that free radical production is not always proportional to metabolic rate. Contrary to predictions of the free radical theory, the juvenile bats sampled generally produced higher levels of H_2O_2 than the adults, independent of flight ability. I cannot entirely exclude the possibility that this higher H_2O_2 production was because of development, yet I do not believe this is the case because the juveniles had reached adult size and had fully calcified wing bones. I propose that this is an initial decrease in H_2O_2 production, which results from within-individual selection for efficient mitochondria. This selection is caused by the high energetic demands imposed on mitochondria as juvenile bats begin to fly. If there is indeed within-individual selection of efficient mitochondria, one would expect to find heteroplasmy in bats. Recent studies have uncovered evidence of mitochondrial heteroplasmy in a variety of organisms, including bats,[8,9] and this heteroplasmy appears to be heritable in mouse-eared bats[8] and evening bats.[9] I extracted mtDNA from the tested adult and juvenile *M. lucifugus* and amplified a highly variable region of the D-loop. I separated the resulting mtDNA segments by electrophoresis. All tested adults had the same dominant mitotype, whereas there was interindividual variation in mitotype among the juveniles. Although not conclusive, this evidence suggests convergence from various mitotypes in bats with little flight experience to a single mitotype in bats with greater flight experience.

REFERENCES

1. AUSTAD, S.N. & K.E. FISCHER. 1991. Mammalian aging, metabolism and ecology: evidence from the bats and marsupials. J. Gerontol. **46**: B47–B53.
2. BOULIERE, F. 1958. The comparative biology of aging. J. Gerontol. **13**: 16–24.
3. WILKINSON, G.S. & J.M. South. 2002. Life history, ecology and longevity in bats. Aging Cell **1**: 124–131.
4. HARMAN, D. 1956. Aging: a theory based on free radical radiation biochemistry. J. Gerontol. **11**: 298–300.
5. DAVIS, W.H. & H.B. HITCHCOCK. 1995. A new longevity record for the bat *Myotis lucifugus*. Bat Res. News **36**: 6.
6. PEARSON, O.P. 1945. Longevity of the short-tailed shrew. Am. Midl. Nat. **34**: 531–546.
7. HYSLOP, P. & L. SKLAR. 1984. A quantitative fluorometric assay for the determination of oxidant production by polymorphonuclear leukocytes. Anal. Biochem. **141**: 280–286.
8. PETRI, B. *et al.* 1996. Extreme sequence heteroplasmy in bat mitochondrial DNA. Biol. Chem. **377**: 661–667.
9. WILKINSON, G.S. & A. CHAPMAN. 1991. Length and sequence variation in evening bat D-loop mtDNA. Genetics **128**: 607–617.

The Reliability-Engineering Approach to the Problem of Biological Aging

LEONID A. GAVRILOV AND NATALIA S. GAVRILOVA

Center on Aging, NORC and the University of Chicago, Chicago, Illinois 60637-2745, USA

ABSTRACT: We applied reliability theory to explain aging of biological species and came to the following conclusions: (1) Redundancy is a key notion for understanding aging and the systemic nature of aging in particular. Systems, which are redundant in numbers of irreplaceable elements, do deteriorate (i.e., age) over time, even if they are built of nonaging elements. (2) An apparent aging rate or expression of aging (measured as age differences in failure rates, including death rates) is higher for systems with higher redundancy levels. (3) Redundancy exhaustion over the course of life explains the observed *compensation law of mortality* (mortality convergence at later life) as well as the observed late-life mortality deceleration, leveling-off, and mortality plateaus. (4) Living organisms seem to be formed with a high load of initial damage, and therefore their life span and aging patterns may be sensitive to early-life conditions that determine this initial damage load during early development.

KEYWORDS: redundancy; compensation law of mortality; mortality plateaus; reliability theory

INTRODUCTION

Twenty-five years ago, we first applied the reliability theory to explain aging of biological species.[1,2] Since that time, we continued the development of this theory[3–5] and have come to the following conclusions: (1) Redundancy is a key notion for understanding aging and the systemic nature of aging in particular. Systems, which are redundant in numbers of irreplaceable elements, do deteriorate (i.e., age) over time, even if they are built of nonaging elements. (2) An apparent aging rate or expression of aging (measured as age differences in failure rates, including death rates) is higher for systems with higher redundancy levels. (3) Redundancy exhaustion over the course of life explains the observed *compensation law of mortality* (mortality convergence at later life) as well as the observed late-life mortality deceleration, leveling-off, and mortality plateaus. (4) Living organisms seem to be formed with a high load of initial damage, and therefore their life span and aging patterns may be sensitive to early-life conditions that determine this initial damage load during early

Address for correspondence: Leonid A. Gavrilov, Center on Aging, NORC and the University of Chicago, 1155 East 60th Street, Chicago, IL 60637-2745. Voice: 773-256-6359; fax: 773-256-6313.
gavrilov@longevity-science.org

development. The idea of early-life programming of aging and longevity may have important practical implications for developing early-life interventions promoting health and longevity.

The theory also suggests that aging research should not be limited to studies of qualitative changes (such as age changes in gene expression), because changes in quantity (numbers of cells and other functional elements) could be a more important driving force of the aging process.

DISCUSSION OF THE RELIABILITY-ENGINEERING APPROACH TO THE AGING PROBLEM

There may be several different research strategies in attempts to understand the nature of the aging process. The prevailing research strategy now is to focus on the molecular level in the hope of understanding the proverbial nuts and bolts of the aging process. In accordance with this approach, many aging theories explain aging of organisms through aging of organisms' components. However, this circular reasoning of assuming aging to "explain" aging leads to a logical contradiction, because moving in succession from the aging of organisms to the aging of organs, tissues, and cells, we eventually come to atoms, which are known not to age.

Thus, we come to the following basic question on the origin of aging: How can we explain the aging of a system built of nonaging elements? This question invites us to start thinking about the possible systemic nature of aging and to wonder whether aging may be a property of the system as a whole. In other words, perhaps we need to broaden our vision and be more concerned with the bigger picture of the aging phenomenon rather than its tiny details.

To illustrate the need for a broad vision, consider the following questions. (1) Would it be possible to understand a newspaper article by looking at it through an electronic microscope? (2) Would the perception of a picture in an art gallery be deeper and more comprehensive at the shortest possible distance from it?

A good example of a broad vision of the aging problem is provided by the evolutionary theories of aging.[6–8] Evolutionary perspective helps us to stay focused on a bigger picture, and to avoid being overwhelmed by billions of tiny details. Evolutionary theories demonstrate that taking a step back from too close consideration of the details over "the nuts and bolts" of the aging process helps to gain a broader vision of the aging problem.

The remaining question is whether the evolutionary perspective represents the ultimate general theoretical framework for explanations of aging. Or perhaps there may be even more general theories of aging, one step further removed from the particular details?

The main limitation of evolutionary theories of aging is that they are applicable to reproducing organisms only, because these theories are based on the idea of natural selection and on the declining force of natural selection with age.

However, aging is a very general phenomenon—it is also observed in technical devices (such as cars), which do not reproduce themselves in a sexual or any other way and that are, therefore, not subject to evolution through natural selection. Thus, there may exist a more general explanation of aging, beyond the evolutionary theories.

The quest for a general explanation of aging (age-related increase in failure rates) applicable both to technical devices and biological systems invites us to consider the general theory of systems failure known as reliability theory.[1-5] Interestingly, the reliability theory suggests that we reevaluate the old belief that aging is somehow related to limited economic or evolutionary investments in systems' longevity. The theory provides a completely opposite perspective on this issue: that aging is a direct consequence of investments into systems reliability and durability through enhanced redundancy. This is an important statement, because it helps to explain why the expression of aging (age-associated differences in failure rates) might be more profound in more complicated redundant systems, designed for higher durability.[5]

The theory also suggests that research on aging should not be limited to the studies of qualitative changes (such as age-related changes in gene expression), because changes in quantity (numbers of cells and other functional elements) could be an important driving force of the aging process. In other words, aging might be largely driven by a process of redundancy loss.[5,9]

Reliability theory predicts that a system may deteriorate with age even if it is built from nonaging elements with constant failure rates.[3-5] The key issue here is the system's redundancy for irreplaceable elements, which is responsible for the aging phenomenon. In other words, each particular step of system destruction or deterioration may seem to be random (no aging, just occasional failure by chance), but if a system failure requires a sequence of several such steps (not just a single step of destruction), then the system as a whole may have an aging behavior. Why is this conclusion important? Because the significance of beneficial health-promoting interventions often is undermined by claims that these interventions are not proved to delay the process of aging itself, but instead that they simply delay or cover up some particular manifestations of aging.

In contrast with these pessimistic views, reliability theory says that there might be no specific underlying elementary aging process; instead, aging might be largely a property of a redundant system as a whole, because it has a network of destruction pathways, each being associated with particular manifestations of aging (types of failure). Therefore, we should not be discouraged by only partial success of each particular intervention, but instead we can appreciate that we might have many opportunities to oppose aging in numerous different ways.

Thus, the efforts to understand the routes and early stages of age-related degenerative diseases should not be discarded as irrelevant to understanding true biological aging. On the contrary, attempts to build an intellectual firewall between biogerontological research and clinical medicine are counterproductive. After all, the main reason why people are really concerned about aging is because it is related to health deterioration and increased morbidity. The most important age-related changes, with respect to quality of life, are those that make older people sick and frail.

Reliability theory suggests general answers to both the "why" and the "how" questions about aging. It explains why aging occurs by identifying the key determinant of aging behavior: system redundancy in numbers of irreplaceable elements. Reliability theory also explains how aging occurs, by focusing on the process of redundancy loss over time as the major mechanism of aging. It is perfectly compatible with evolutionary theories of aging, and it helps to identify key components, which might be important for the evolution of species reliability and durability (longevity): initial redundancy levels, rate of redundancy loss, and repair potential. Moreover, reliability theory helps evolutionary theories to explain how the age of onset of deleterious mutations could be postponed during evolution, which could be easily achieved by a simple increase in initial redundancy levels. From the reliability perspective, the increase in initial redundancy levels is the simplest way to improve survival at particularly early reproductive ages (with gains fading at older ages). This matches exactly with the higher fitness priority of early reproductive ages emphasized by evolutionary theories. Evolutionary and reliability ideas also help in understanding why organisms seem to "choose" a simple but short-term solution of the survival problem through enhancing the systems' redundancy, instead of a more permanent but complicated solution based on rigorous repair (with the potential of achieving negligible senescence). Thus, there are promising opportunities for merging the reliability and evolutionary theories of aging.

Aging is a complex phenomenon, and a holistic approach using reliability theory may help to analyze, understand, and perhaps control it. We suggest therefore that reliability theory should be added to the arsenal of methodological approaches applied in research on aging.

ACKNOWLEDGMENTS

This study was made possible thanks to a generous support from the National Institute on Aging (NIH, USA) and a stimulating working environment at the Center on Aging, NORC/University of Chicago. We thank members of the Science Advisory Board (SAB) (http://www.scienceboard.net/) for useful comments on our work made at the SAB discussion group.

REFERENCES

1. GAVRILOV, L.A. 1978. A mathematical model of the aging of animals. Proc. Acad. Sci. USSR [Dokl. Akad. Nauk. SSSR] **238:** 490–492.
2. GAVRILOV, L.A., N.S. GAVRILOVA & L.S. YAGUZHINSKY. 1978. The main regularities of animal aging and death viewed in terms of reliability theory. J. Gen. Biol. [Zh. Obshch. Biol.], **39:** 734–742.
3. GAVRILOV, L.A. & N.S. GAVRILOVA. 1991. The Biology of Life Span: A Quantitative Approach. Harwood Academic Publisher. New York.
4. GAVRILOV, L.A. & N.S. GAVRILOVA. 2001. The reliability theory of aging and longevity. J. Theor. Biol. **213:** 527–545.
5. GAVRILOV, L.A. & N.S. GAVRILOVA. 2003. The quest for a general theory of aging and longevity. Science's SAGE KE (Science of Aging Knowledge Environment) for 16 July 2003; Vol 2003, No. 28, 1–10. Available: http://sageke.sciencemag.org.
6. ROSE, M.R. 1991. Evolutionary Biology of Aging. Oxford University Press. New York.
7. GAVRILOVA, N.S. & L.A. GAVRILOV. 2002. Evolution of Aging. In Encyclopedia of Aging. Vol 2. D.J. Ekerdt, Ed.: 458–467. Macmillan Reference USA. New York.
8. GAVRILOV, L.A. & N.S. GAVRILOVA. 2002. Evolutionary theories of aging and longevity. Sci. World J. **2:** 339–356.
9. DE GREY, A.D.N.J. 2003. An engineer's approach to the development of real anti-aging medicine. Science's SAGE KE 2003. http://sageke.sciencemag.org/cgi/content/full/sageke;2003/1/vp1.

Does Exceptional Human Longevity Come with a High Cost of Infertility?

Testing the Evolutionary Theories of Aging

NATALIA S. GAVRILOVA, LEONID A. GAVRILOV,
VICTORIA G. SEMYONOVA, AND GALINA N. EVDOKUSHKINA

*Center on Aging, NORC and the University of Chicago,
Chicago, Illinois 60637-2745, USA*

ABSTRACT: The purpose of this study is to test the prediction of the evolutionary theory of aging that human longevity comes with the cost of impaired reproductive success (higher infertility rates). Our validation study is based on the analysis of particularly reliable genealogical records for European aristocratic families using a logistic regression model with childlessness as a dependent (outcome) variable, and woman's life span, year of birth, age at marriage, husband's age at marriage, and husband's life span as independent (predictor) variables. We found that the woman's exceptional longevity did not increase her chances of being infertile. It appears that the previous reports by other authors of high infertility among long-lived women (up to 50% infertility) are related to incomplete data, that is, births of children not reported. Thus, the concept of the high cost of infertility for human longevity is not supported by the data when these data are carefully cross-checked, cleaned, and reanalyzed.

KEYWORDS: evolutionary theory of aging; higher infertility rates

INTRODUCTION

The purpose of this study was to test the prediction of the evolutionary theory of aging that human longevity comes with the cost of impaired reproductive success (higher infertility rates, see Westendorp & Kirkwood[1]). Our validation study is based on the analysis of particularly reliable genealogical records for European aristocratic families. This data set is appealing to use for two reasons: (1) it has high data accuracy and completeness; and (2) confounding effects of socioeconomic status are minimized in this socially elite group. The data set is comprised of 3,723 married women born from 1500 to 1875 and belonging to the upper European nobility. Every case of childlessness was cross-checked using at least two different sources. Data analyses were based on a logistic regression model using childlessness as a dependent (outcome) variable, and the woman's life span, year of birth, age at marriage,

---

Address for correspondence: Natalia S. Gavrilova, Center on Aging, NORC and the University of Chicago, 1155 East 60th Street, Chicago, IL 60637-2745. Voice: 773-256-6359; fax: 773-256-6313.

gavrilova@longevity-science.org

husband's age at marriage, and husband's life span as independent (predictor) variables. We found that a woman's exceptional longevity does not increase her chances of being infertile. It appears that the previous reports of high infertility among long-lived women (up to a 50% infertility rate, see Westendorp & Kirkwood[1]) are related to incomplete data, that is, births of children not reported. Indeed, data cross-checking revealed that at least in 32% of the cases the allegedly "childless" women did, in fact, have children. Thus, the concept of heavy infertility cost for human longevity is not supported by data, when these data are carefully cross-checked, cleaned, and reanalyzed. Additional relevant information is available at our scientific Web site (http://longevity-science.org/).

THE IMPORTANCE OF DATA QUALITY CONTROL

Previous analysis of childlessness among aristocratic women[1] was made on the assumption that the data was complete. When claims were made that many long-lived women were childless,[1] we found it important to cross-check the data and to make sure that the lack of children was real.

An obvious step was to cross-check the initial data set with other data sources. For example, we examined 335 claims of childlessness in the Bloore's data set used by Westendorp and Kirkwood. When we cross-checked these claims with other professional sources of data, we found that at least 107 allegedly childless women (32%) did have children Thus, at least 32% of childlessness claims proved to be wrong (false-negative claims).

This example demonstrates that extreme caution should be exercised when claims for common childlessness among long-lived women are made. The incompleteness of genealogies can itself generate a spurious increase in the prevalence of allegedly childless women among those who live long lives. This happens because children often are not mentioned in particularly obscure, side branches of genealogical trees (remote relatives). It is also known that long-lived people have more chances of being mentioned in incomplete genealogies, because of their longer paper trail in various archives generated during their long life. Thus, incompleteness of genealogies generates two types of biases—underreporting of children and inflated prevalence of long-lived people, thereby producing a spurious increase in claimed childlessness with increased life span.

Incomplete reporting of children may seriously affect and compromise scientific studies of human fertility. For example, Westendorp and Kirkwood reported: "None of the six women who were born before 1700 and who reached the exceptional age of 90 years and over had more than two children" (p. 745).[1] Our data cross-checking with other data sources revealed that, in fact, none but one of these women had less than three children.

Among these six women was Antoinette de Bourbon (1493–1583) who allegedly had only one child according to the Bloore's database. Study of other data sources revealed that this well-known person (grandmother of Mary Stuart, Queen of Scots) had as many as 12 children! This fact is well known to professional genealogists and is even reported in The Catholic Encyclopedia (Vol. VII, House of Guise, Robert Appleton Company, 1909). Thus, if we compute an average number of children for women who lived 90–99 years with corrected data for Antoinette de Bourbon alone,

TABLE 1. Proportion of childlessness by women's age at death: comparison of our data set with similar data for the historical German population[2] and data for the British aristocracy[1]

Age at death, yr	Proportion of childless women in different data sets		
	Gavrilova data set on European upper nobility	Lycett et al.[2] German data	Westendorp and Kirkwood[1] British aristocracy
20–29	0.17	0.15	0.39
30–39	0.10	0.08	0.26
40–49	0.14	0.08	0.31
50–59	0.13	0.11	0.28
60–69	0.12	0.09	0.33
70–79	0.10	0.09	0.31
80–89	0.15	0.10	0.45
90+	0.12	—	0.49

their average number of progeny would be even higher than average number of progeny for shorter-lived women.

This example demonstrates that genealogical data should be carefully checked against multiple genealogical and historical sources before using them in the scientific studies and making strong conclusions.

RESULTS AND DISCUSSION

This section describes the results obtained with cross-checked, corrected data. TABLE 1 presents the dependence of the frequency of childlessness as a function of the women's life span (univariate analysis).

The data obtained by other researchers are also presented in the same table for comparison. Note the extremely high proportion of childless women in data published by Westendorp and Kirkwood.[1] On the other hand, German data[2] as well as our data for aristocratic women are consistent with each other and do not demonstrate any increase in childlessness for long-lived women. Our estimates of childlessness also are consistent with estimates of childlessness among the British peerage reported by Thomas Hollingsworth in his fundamental historical study.[3]

Results presented in TABLE 1 were obtained using univariate analyses, which do not take into account many important explanatory variables. To avoid the omitted variable bias and to study the true relationship between childlessness and longevity, we need to take into account many other explanatory variables that influence infertility rate. Therefore, we applied multivariate logistic regression with childlessness as a dependent binary variable and calendar year of birth, female age at marriage, husband's age at marriage, female life span, and husband's life span as predictor variables.

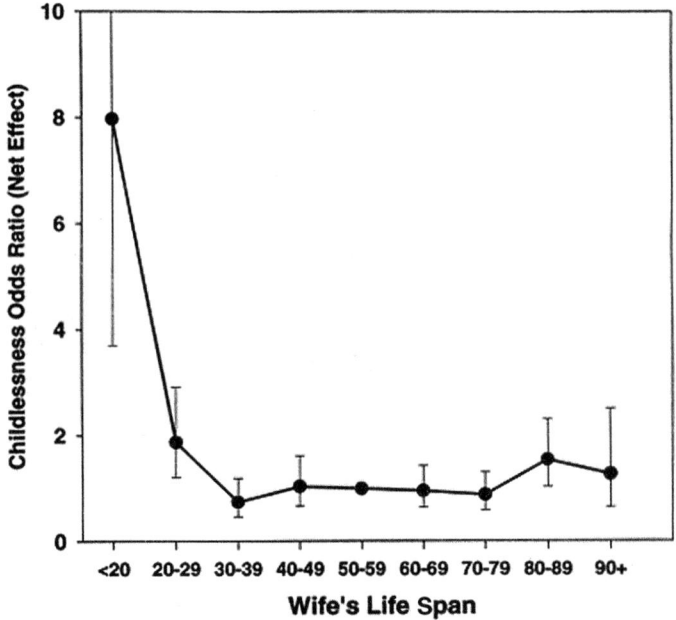

FIGURE 1. Childlessness odds ratio as a function of female life span. Net effects are adjusted for female calendar year of birth, female age at marriage, husband's life span, and husband's age at marriage. Multivariate regression analysis of 3,723 European aristocratic families.

The main result of our study is presented in FIGURE 1. This figure shows odds of being childless as a function of female life span, adjusted for other important confounding variables. The odds of childlessness are particularly high, when the women's life span is too short (under age 30), which is not surprising. What is really important is that the chances of being childless do not demonstrate any increase for long-lived women (life span 90+ years). This result confirms findings from our univariate analyses (TABLE 1) as well as from other studies,[2,4] which demonstrated that long-lived women do not have a higher rate of childlessness even when controlled for other important confounding variables.

Our study does not support the previous published claims that human longevity comes at a high cost of infertility. This conclusion may have both theoretical significance (testing some evolutionary theories of aging), as well as practical implications for the future of life extension. It helps to relax concerns over a question: "Is it morally acceptable to extend human longevity at the cost of infertility?" Some authors have already raised their concerns on the unintended consequences of life span extension: "… increasing longevity through genetic manipulation of the mechanisms of aging raises deep biological and moral questions. These questions should give us pause before we embark on the enterprise of extending our lives."[5] This study helps to alleviate some concerns on these issues.

ACKNOWLEDGMENTS

This study was made possible thanks to a generous support from the National Institute on Aging (NIH, USA) and a stimulating working environment at the Center on Aging, NORC/University of Chicago. We thank members of the Science Advisory Board (SAB) (http://www.scienceboard.net/) for useful comments on our work made at the SAB discussion group.

REFERENCES

1. WESTENDORP, R.G.J. & T.B.L. KIRKWOOD. 1998. Human longevity at the cost of reproductive success. Nature **396:** 743–746.
2. LYCETT, J.E. *et al.* 2000. Longevity and the cost of reproduction in a historical human population. Proc. R. Soc. Lond. **267:** 31–35.
3. HOLLINGSWORTH, T.H. 1964. The demography of the British peerage. Popul. Stud. **18** (Suppl): 3–107.
4. KORPELAINEN, H. 2000. Fitness, reproduction and longevity among European aristocrats and rural Finnish families in the 1700s and 1800s. Proc. R. Soc. Lond. B **267:** 1765–1770.
5. GLANNON, W. 2002. Extending the human life span. J. Med. Philos. **27:** 339–354.

Emerging Area of Aging Research

Long-Lived Animals with "Negligible Senescence"

JOHN C. GUERIN

Centenarian Species and Rockfish Project, Portland, Oregon 97232, USA

> ABSTRACT: Field observations have suggested for quite some time that certain fish, turtles, and invertebrates have extremely long maximum life span potential. Age validation techniques have since confirmed these observations, but scientific analysis to understand the genetic and biochemical basis of this longevity has occurred only recently. The Centenarian Species and Rockfish Project now encompasses 13 pilot research projects, including such diverse investigations as histology, a cDNA library, and mitochondrial mutation analysis. In this document, the term "negligible senescence" is defined, and its background is given; age validation techniques are listed, and the various projects to date, including research results, are summarized.
>
> KEYWORDS: centenarian; long-lived animals; negligible senescence

Aging research has advanced dramatically in the last several years, with much new information available on biochemical and genetic components of aging. However, curiously, one potential area of study for aging research identified at least 70 years ago has not advanced until recently: the analysis of long-lived animals. In the 1930s, it was proposed that some fish do not show signs of senescence.[1] Even though biological tools such as histology existed at that time, no known efforts were made to examine these animals.

The Centenarian Species and Rockfish Project was founded in 1995 to uncover the mechanisms that appear to retard aging in very long-lived animals such as rockfish, turtles, and whales. This new area of study in biomedical gerontology has the potential to reveal the genetic and biochemical processes involved in slow aging that then could be applied for human benefit. The project now incorporates 13 lines of research at several universities and laboratories in the United States and Europe. Although rockfish (genus *Sebastes*) have been the focus to date, biochemical profiling of turtle blood serum has started recently (see the turtle pilot study below), and whales are under consideration. Leonard Hayflick, discoverer of the "Hayflick limit" of cellular senescence and an advisor to this project, states "Guerin's project is not only unique, but probes an area of almost total neglect in biogerontology yet an area with more promise to deliver valuable data than, perhaps, any other."

Address for correspondence: John C. Guerin, Director, Centenarian Species and Rockfish Project, 2345 NE Sandy Boulevard, #25, Portland, OR 97232. Voice: 503-975-4915.
jguerin@agelessanimals.org

Ann. N.Y. Acad. Sci. 1019: 518–520 (2004). © 2004 New York Academy of Sciences.
doi: 10.1196/annals.1297.096

BACKGROUND ON NEGLIGIBLE SENESCENCE

Caleb Finch at USC coined the term "negligible senescence" to describe very slow or negligible aging.[2] He listed several animals exhibiting it, including rockfish, sturgeon, turtles, bivalves, and possibly lobsters. Later in an article from the first Symposium on Organisms with Slow Aging (which the Director of this project also spoke at), Finch further described criteria to test the occurrence of negligible aging. These include no observable age-related increase in mortality rate or decrease in reproduction rate after maturity, and no observable age-related decline in physiological capacity or disease resistance.[3]

Accurate age determination is important in studying long-lived animals. In turtles, determination of minimum age is relatively straightforward with tag and recapture methods. In deep-water fish, the most common technique is growth-zone analysis of the otolith, or ear bone.[4,5] Two recent international symposia have focused entirely on the importance of otoliths in fish life history studies.[6,7] Another technique used by fisheries management to provide an independent age estimate is the radiometric approach, which uses a known radioactive decay series in the core of bones.[8,9] Recent research that showed whales can live over 100 years and possibly over 200 years used aspartic acid racemization.[10]

Zoos also have compiled longevity information. Alligators have been recorded up to 80 years of age, although it is uncertain if death was caused by senescence or environmental factors[11] (Longevity of Reptiles and Amphibians in North American Collections 1992, and personal communication with the Cincinnati Zoo 2001). Green sea turtles have been estimated to take up to a maximum of 50 years to reach maturity in the wild, because of their low-protein diet.[12] Delayed reproduction usually is associated with a very slow rate of aging. A 1994 issue of *Gerontology* was devoted to aging in cold-blooded vertebrates; it compiled research showing that even though some fish are long-lived, many are short-lived and have senescence similar to that seen in mammals.[13]

Many of the animals mentioned above were considered for the best model to study negligible senescence, and rockfish became the first research effort in 1997. The Alaska Fish and Game provided data on randomly sampled Yelloweye rockfish, from commercially caught fish off of Sitka, Alaska. The charts they provided showed that 16% of the fish going to people's dinner tables were 50 years of age or older, with several over 100 years old!

Just recently, the project's fish ecologist, Gregor M. Cailliet, determined that rockfish have both short-lived and long-lived members in the same genus.[14] They range from 12 years for the calico rockfish to 205 years for the rougheye rockfish. Future studies on the project will compare genetic and biochemical measurements between short-lived and long-lived rockfish.

REFERENCES

1. BIDDER, G.P. 1932. Senescence. Br. Med. J. **2:** 583–585.
2. FINCH, C.E. 1990. Longevity, Senescence, and the Genome. University of Chicago Press. Chicago.
3. FINCH, C.E. & S.N. AUSTAD. 2001. History and prospects: symposium on organisms with slow aging. Exp. Gerontol. **36:** 593–597.

4. BAGENAL, T.B., Ed. 1974. The Ageing of Fish. Proceedings of an International Symposium. Unwin Brothers Ltd. Surrey, England.
5. MCFARLANE, G.A. & R.J. BEAMISH. 1995. Validation of the otolith cross-section method of age determination for sablefish (*Anoplopoma fimbria*) using oxytetracycline. *In* Recent Developments in Fish Otolith Research. D.H. Secor *et al.*, Eds.: 319–329. University of South Carolina Press. Columbia, SC.
6. SECOR, D.H. *et al.*, Eds. 1995. Recent Developments in Fish Otolith Research. University of South Carolina Press. Columbia, SC.
7. FOSSUM, P. *et al.*, Eds. 2000. Second International Symposium on Fish Otolith Research & Application, Bergen, Norway, June 20–25 1999, Fisheries Res. (Special Issue) 46.
8. BENNETT, J.T. *et al.* 1982. Confirmation on longevity in *Sebastes diploproa* (Pisces: Scorpaenidae) from $210Pb/226Ra$ measurements in otoliths. Mar. Biol. **71:** 209–215.
9. CAMPANA, S.E. *et al.* 1990. $210Pb/226Ra$ determination of longevity in redfish. Can. J. Fish. Aquat. Sci. **47:** 163–165.
10. GEORGE, J.C. *et al.* 1999. Age and growth estimates of bowhead whales (*Balaena mysticetus*) via aspartic acid racemization. Can. J. Zool. **77:** 571–580.
11. SNIDER, A.T. & J.K. BOWLER. 1992. Longevity of Reptiles and Amphibians in North American Collections. Second edition. Herpetological Circular No. 21. Society for the Study of Amphibians and Reptiles.
12. BJORNDAL, K.A. 1985. Nutritional ecology of sea turtles. Copeia **3:** 736–751.
13. PATNAIK, B.K. 1994. Ageing in reptiles. Gerontology **40:** 200–220.
14. CAILLIET, G.M. *et al.* 2001. Age determination and validation studies of marine fishes: do deep-dwellers live longer? Exp. Gerontol. **36:** 739–764.

Functional Aging and Gradual Senescence in Zebrafish

SHUJI KISHI

Department of Cancer Biology, Dana-Farber Cancer Institute and Department of Pathology, Harvard Medical School, Boston, Massachusetts 02115-6084, USA

ABSTRACT: Zebrafish (*Danio rerio*) has been recognized as a powerful model for genetic studies in developmental biology. Recently, the zebrafish system also has given insights into several human diseases such as neurodegenerative, hematopoietic, and cardiovascular disease, and cancer. Because aging processes affect these and various other human disorders, it is important to compare zebrafish and mammalian senescence. However, the aging process of zebrafish remains largely unexplored, and little is known about functional aging and senescence in zebrafish. In our initial studies to assess aging phenotypes in zebrafish, we have identified several potential aging biomarkers in an ongoing search for suitable ones on zebrafish aging. In aging zebrafish, we detected senescence-associated β-galactosidase activity in skin and oxidized protein accumulation in muscle. On the other hand, we did not observe lipofuscin granules (aging pigments), which accumulate in postmitotic cells, in muscle of zebrafish with advancing age. Consistently, there were continuously proliferating myocytes that incorporated BrdU in muscle tissues of the aged fish. Moreover, we demonstrated that zebrafish have constitutively abundant telomerase activity in adult somatic tissues implicating unlimited replicative ability of cells throughout their lives. Although some stress-associated markers are upregulated and minor histological changes are observed during the aging process of zebrafish, our studies together with other evidence of remarkable reproductive and regenerative abilities suggest that zebrafish show very gradual senescence. By using those biological and biochemical aging markers already characterized in normal zebrafish, transgenic fish analyses and genetic mutant fish screens can be readily performed. These efforts will help to elucidate the role and molecular mechanisms of common or different pathways of aging among vertebrates from fish to humans and also will contribute to the discovery of potential drugs applicable to age-associated diseases in the future.

KEYWORDS: zebrafish; aging; senescence; stress; indeterminate growth; telomerase; telomere

To assess the fundamental biology of growth, aging, and longevity in higher complex organisms, such as vertebrates, it is desirable to expand the range of vertebrate model systems for laboratory studies. In vertebrates, teleost fish represent about half

Address for correspondence: Shuji Kishi, M.D., Ph.D., Department of Cancer Biology, Dana-Farber Cancer Institute and Harvard Medical School, 44 Binney Street, Boston, MA 02115-6084. Voice: 617-632-4227; fax: 617-632-4770.
shuji_kishi@dfci.harvard.edu

of the existing forty to fifty thousand species.[1] Studies on aging in several fish species raised interest on possible novel patterns of senescence.[2–8] Finch categorized senescence into three different types according to the rapid, gradual, and negligible rates of progression, and fish species appear to exhibit each type.[1] For example, pacific salmon and eels exhibit rapid senescence and sudden death almost at first spawning, whereas guppy, platyfish, and medaka and many other teleosts undergo gradual senescence with some similarities to mammalian senescence. On the other hand, other fish including rockfish and carp show indeterminate growth with no indication of increased mortality, consistent with the possibility of very slow or even negligible senescence. Likewise, zebrafish continue growth past sexual maturation with no indication of reproductive senescence given adequate food, space, and conditions.[9,10] Moreover, unlike mammals, zebrafish retain remarkable regenerative abilities in muscle, heart, spinal cord, and other tissues to later advanced ages,[11–15] making them ideal candidates to study aging and senescence.

Zebrafish are the same genus as carp (*Cyprinus carpio*), which potentially reach sizes of more than 100 cm and may live more than 100 years[16,17] but are much smaller (~5 cm) and shorter lived (~5 years).[9] Their relatively small size makes them easier to manage in large numbers in the laboratory environment. Also, they have short generation time of 3–5 months and large clutch sizes of approximately 100–200 eggs per female. Zebrafish are widely used as a powerful model animal in developmental biology, and they are being developed as models for human diseases, contributing to biomedical science. Inventive forward genetic screens in zebrafish are being used to unravel genetic and signaling pathways that control vertebrate development, disease, and behavior.[18] Coupled with gene knockdown and overexpression technologies, and small-molecule–induced phenotypes, large-scale genetic screens in zebrafish provide a powerful system by which to dissect vertebrate gene function and molecular networks.[19,20]

However, the aging zebrafish process of zebrafish has been largely unaddressed, and little is known about age-associated phenotypes and senescence. We surveyed biological and biochemical markers on aging using a wild-type zebrafish strain, and we have presented our initial results of several aging markers in zebeafish.[21] There were two markers that represent age-dependent alterations with upregulation. First, senescence-associated β-galactosidase activity (SA-β-gal), which is a histochemically detectable biomarker of senescence in organismic aging,[22] was increased in skin with the whole zebrafish body at advanced age. Second, oxidized protein, known to accumulate with aging in other organisms,[23,24] also was increased in muscle during the zebrafish aging process. The accumulation of lipofuscin (aging pigment) considered to be a metabolic by-product, particularly of oxidized lipids during the life span, is recognized to increase with age in postmitotic cells.[25] However, we did not detect age-dependent existence of lipofuscin in muscle tissues of zebrafish. Consistently, we demonstrated that many proliferating myocytes incorporated BrdU in aged zebrafish muscle *in vivo*. Telomerase activity that maintains telomere length generally is not detectable in postmitotic cells, but is found in proliferative cells. Intriguingly, we demonstrated constitutively high telomerase activity in muscle throughout zebrafish lives. Finally, we observed some histopathological changes in aging zebrafish and discussed them together with other growth characteristics and aging changes in comparison with previously reported results of guppies that have similar size and life span (TABLE 1).

TABLE 1. Comparison of age-related phenotypes between zebrafish and guppy

	Zebrafish (*Danio rerio*)	Guppy (*Poecilia reticulata*)
	Male/female/unsexed	Male/female/unsexed
Length of development and age at sexual maturity (mo)	3–5 (unsexed)[a] 3–4 (unsexed)[a]	2–4 (unsexed)[b] 2–3 (male)[b] 3–4 (female)[b]
Mean/max life spans (mo)	Mean; 36–42 (unsexed)[c] Max; 58–66 (unsexed)[c]	Mean; ~30 (female)[d] Max; ~48 (female)[d]
Reproductive age	There is no decline in fecundity with 24-month-old male and female fish (wild-type AB strain)[e]	There is no strong decline in fecundity with age, but there is a tendency for females to reproduce less regularly as they age[f]
Aging: Gross pathology	Spinal curvature (unsexed)[g] Neoplasia; the incidence of seminoma increases to ~40% by 2 years of age or more in males[h]	Spinal curvature[i] Thyroid tumor[j] Adenocarcinoma[k] Epidermal cystadenoma[l]
Aging: Tissue pathology	Muscle degeneration (unsexed)[g] Mucous cell hyperplasia in esophagus (unsexed)[m] Small glomerular tufts in kidney (unsexed)[m]	Muscle degeneration[i] Loss of muscle fibers in ventricle (male and female)[n] Degenerative changes in glomeruli and tubules of nephrons (particularly in males)[o]
Aging: Biochemical and molecular changes	Increase of SA-β-gal activity (unsexed)[m] Increase of oxidized protein accumulation (unsexed)[m] Constitutive telomerase activity (unsexed)[m] Existence of BrdU-positive proliferating cells (unsexed)[m] Absense of lipofuscin in certain tissues (unsexed)[m]	Increase of fluorescent age pigments (lipofuscin?) accumulation in brain tissues[p]

[a,b]Information on adult zebrafish (*Danio rerio*) and guppies (*Poecilia reticulata*) was provided by FishBase: World Wide Web Electronic Publication (www.fishbase.org). We also directly measured various adult zebrafish. Adult guppy size information was provided by Reznick.
[c]Gerhardet *et al.*[9]
[d]Mean and maximum life span of guppies (*Poecilia reticulata*) was provided by FishBase: World Wide Web Electronic Publication (www.fishbase.org). Additional information was provided by Reznick.
[e]Upublished observation by Uchiyama and Kishi.[10] There is, however, considerable evidence of decline in fecudity in zebrafish at ~12 to 16 months old. The situation is fairly dependent on each fish husbandry. — *footnotes continued on next page*

TABLE 1 — *Footnotes continued.*
[f]Reznick et al.[6]
[g]Gerhardet al.[9]
[h]Kent et al.; ZFIN Web site (http://zfin.org/zf_info/stckctr/dis_man/Fish_Diseases.html).
[i]Comfort;[26] however, Reznick did not see much spinal curvature in his experiments on aging guppies. In our laboratory we also did not observe spinal curvature (scoliosis), and skinny phenotypes are also sometimes caused by an intracellular parasite, microsporidia infection (http://zfin.org/zf_info/stckctr/dis_man/Fish_Diseases.html).
[j]Woodhead.[27]
[k]Fournie et al.;[28] Fournie et al.[29]
[l]Miller and Aleo.[30]
[m]Kishi et al.[21]
[n]Woodhead.[31]
[o]Woodhead et al.[32]
[p]Strauss.[33]

Based on our initial observation, the zebrafish aging process may be regulated by the balance of at least two cascading events: one is stress-associated catastrophic damage accumulation on organismic elements such as proteins, lipids, and nucleotides, and the other is replicative potential of cells in respective tissues and organs governing growth and regeneration including wound healing ability. The former may be ordinarily regulated in zebrafish as observed in mammals,[5,8] although the results of lipofuscin in aging zebrafish will require further investigation. Thus far, age-dependent increase of SA-β-gal activity and accumulation of oxidized proteins are plausible markers of the aging progression and onset of senescence. Also, regarding SA-β-gal activity in aging zebrafish, we have detected age-dependent increase of staining based on the enzymatic activity irrespective of spinal curvature phenotype, which is a known morphological aging manifestation in zebrafish.[9] On the other hand, zebrafish's remarkable ability of regeneration with cell proliferation in heart, muscle, and nervous systems implies a linkage between regenerative ability and indeterminate growth,[11-15] in relation to abundant telomerase activity throughout their lives.

Along with continuous growth after sexual maturation and lack of clear reproductive senescence, our studies suggest that zebrafish show very gradual or subnegligible senescence, despite the accumulation of some stress-based alterations, and of minor histological changes with advancing age. Because the zebrafish system has been established to readily perform functional genetics and genomics approaches, based on these baseline analyses of the aging process of zebrafish that we have started, systematic genomewide screens for mutations in zebrafish may successfully identify many candidate genes that define life span and senescence specifically in vertebrates, as well as embryological pathways, in the future.

ACKNOWLEDGMENTS

I greatly acknowledge Junzo Uchiyama, Anne Baughman, Tadateru Goto, Mao Lin, and Stephanie Tsai for contribution to this work. I am also very grateful to David Reznick for unpublished information of guppies, and to Mitsuyoshi Matsuo for helpful comments. Finally, I am especially grateful to Thomas Roberts for his support and continuous encouragement. This work was partially supported by A-T Children's Project Research Grant and Ellison Medical Foundation for New Scholar Award in Aging to S.K.

REFERENCES

1. FINCH, C.E. 1990. Longevity, Senescence, and the Genome. University of Chicago Press. Chicago.
2. CAILLIET, G.M., A.H. ANDREWS, E.J. BURTON, et al. 2001. Age determination and validation studies of marine fishes: do deep-dwellers live longer? Exp. Gerontol. **36:** 739–764.
3. EGAMI, N. 1980. Environment and aging: an approach to the analysis of aging mechanisms using poikilothermic vertebrates. Adv. Exp. Med. Biol. **129:** 249–259.
4. MANGEL, M. & M.V. ABRAHAMS. 2001. Age and longevity in fish, with consideration of the ferox trout. Exp. Gerontol. **36:** 765–790.
5. WOODHEAD, A.D. 1998. Aging, the fishy side: an appreciation of Alex Comfort's studies. Exp. Gerontol. **33:** 39–51.
6. WOODHEAD, A.D. 1978. Fish in studies of aging. Exp. Gerontol. **13:** 125–140.
7. REZNICK, D., G. BUCKWALTER, J. GROFF & D. ELDER. 2001. The evolution of senescence in natural populations of guppies *Poecilia reticulata*: a comparative approach. Exp. Gerontol. **36:** 791–812.
8. REZNICK, D., C. GHALAMBOR & L. NUNNEY. 2002. The evolution of senescence in fish. Mech. Ageing Dev. **1237:** 773–789.
9. GERHARD, G.S., E.J. KAUFFMAN, X. WANG, et al. 2002. Life spans and senescent phenotypes in two strains of Zebrafish (*Danio rerio*). Exp. Gerontol. **378–9:** 1055–1068.
10. UCHIYAMA, J. & S. KISHI. 2003. Unpublished observation.
11. POSS, K.D., L.G. WILSON & M.T. KEATING. 2002. Heart regeneration in zebrafish. Science **298:** 2188–2190.
12. ROWLERSON, A., G. RADAELLI, F. MASCARELLO & A. VEGGETTI. 1997. Regeneration of skeletal muscle in two teleost fish: *Sparus aurata* and *Brachydanio rerio*. Cell Tissue Res. **2892:** 311–322.
13. REIMSCHUSSEL, R. 2001. A fish model of renal regeneration and development. ILAR J. **424:** 285–291.
14. BECKER, T., M.F. WULLIMANN, C.G. BECKER, et al. 1997. Axonal regrowth after spinal cord transection in adult zebrafish. J. Comp. Neurol. **3774:** 577–595.
15. POSS, K.D., M.T. KEATING & A. NECHIPORUK. 2003. Tales of regeneration in zebrafish. Dev. Dyn. **2262:** 202–210.
16. AMANO, M. 1971. How to Breed Nishiki Koi. Kashima Shoten. Japan.
17. ALLEN, G.R. 1991. Field guide to the freshwater fishes of New Guinea. Christensen Research Institute. Madang, Papua New Guinea.
18. PATTON, E.E. & L.I. ZON. 2001. The art and design of genetic screens: zebrafish. Nat. Rev. Genet. **212:** 956–966.
19. SHIN, J.T. & M.C. FISHMAN. 2002. From Zebrafish to human: modular medical models. Annu. Rev. Genomics Hum. Genet. **3:** 311–340.
20. DODD, A., P.M. CURTIS, L.C. WILLIAMS & D.R. LOVE. 2000. Zebrafish: bridging the gap between development and disease. Hum. Mol. Genet. **9:** 2443–2449.
21. KISHI, S., J. UCHIYAMA, A.M. BAUGHMAN, et al. 2003. The zebrafish as a vertebrate model of functional aging and very gradual senescence. Exp. Gerontol. **387:** 777–786.
22. DIMRI, G.P., X. LEE, G. BASILE, et al. 1995. A biomarker that identifies senescent human cells in culture and in aging skin in vivo. Proc. Natl. Acad. Sci. USA **9220:** 9363–9367.
23. OLIVER, C.N., B.W. AHN, E.J. MOERMAN, et al. 1987. Age-related changes in oxidized proteins. J. Biol. Chem. **26212:** 5488–5491.
24. STARKE-REED, P.E. & C.N. OLIVER. 1989. Protein oxidation and proteolysis during aging and oxidative stress. Arch. Biochem. Biophys. **2752:** 559–567.
25. BRUNK, U.T. & A. TERMAN. 2002. Lipofuscin: mechanisms of age-related accumulation and influence on cell function. Free Radic. Biol. Med. **335:** 611–619.

26. COMFORT, A. 1964. Aging: The Biology of Senescence. Routledge and Kegan Paul, London.
27. WOODHEAD, A.D. 1979. Thyroid tumours in the senile guppy, *Lebistes reticulatus* peters. Exp. Gerontol. **144:** 211–215.
28. FOURNIE, J.W., W.E. HAWKINS & W.W. WALKER. 1992. Adenocarcinoma of the retinal pigment epithelium in the guppy *Poecilia reticulata* Peters. J. Comp. Pathol. **1064:** 429–434.
29. FOURNIE, J.W., W.E. HAWKINS & W.W. WALKER. 1999. Proliferative lesions in swimbladder of Japanese medaka *Oryzias latipes* and guppy *Poecilia reticulata*. Dis. Aquat. Organ. **382:** 135–142.
30. MILLER, A.S. & J.J. ALEO. 1970. Spontaneous epidermal cystadenoma in a guppy *Lebistes reticularis*. J. Pathol. **1004:** 317–318.
31. WOODHEAD, A.D. 1984. Aging changes in the heart of a poeciliid fish, the guppy *Poecilia reticulatus*. Exp. Gerontol. **196:** 383–391.
32. WOODHEAD, A.D., V. POND & K. DAILEY. 1983. Aging changes in the kidneys of two poeciliid fishes, the guppy *Poecilia reticulatus* and the Amazon molly P. Formosa. Exp. Gerontol. **183:** 211–221.
33. STRAUSS, R.E. 1999. Brain-tissue accumulation of fluorescent age pigments in four poeciliid fishes (cyprinodontiformes) and the estimation of "biological age." Growth Dev. Aging **634:** 151–170.

Immortal Ethics

JOHN HARRIS

*Institute of Medicine, Law and Bioethics, School of Law,
University of Manchester, Manchester M13 9PL, United Kingdom*

> ABSTRACT: This article draws on ideas published in my "Intimations of Immortality" essay in *Science* (Vol. 288, No. 5463, p. 59, April 7, 2000) and my "Intimations of Immortality—The Ethics and Justice of Life Extending Therapies" in editor Michael Freeman's *Current Legal Problems* (Oxford University Press 2002: 65–97). This article outlines the ethical issues involved in life-extending therapies. The arguments against life extension are examined and found wanting. The consequences of life extension are explored and found challenging but not sufficiently daunting to warrant regulation or control. In short, there is no doubt that immortality would be a mixed blessing, but we should be slow to reject cures for terrible diseases that may be an inextricable part of life-extending procedures even if the price we have to pay for those cures is increasing life expectancy and even creating immortals. Better surely to accompany the scientific race to achieve immortality with commensurate work in ethics and social policy to ensure that we know how to cope with the transition to parallel populations of mortals and immortals as envisaged in mythology.
>
> KEYWORDS: ethics; life-extending therapy; aging

Life-extending therapies and optimistic discussions of their promise and probable effect are an increasing dimension of serious scientific and philosophical discussion.[a] If such therapies ever become reality,[1,2] and if our bodies could repair damage caused by disease and aging "from within,"[3] the effects not only on personal health and survival but also on society and on our conceptions of ourselves and of the sorts of creatures we are would be profound.[4–6] If we could switch off the aging process[7,8] we could then, in Lee Silver's words, "write immortality into the genes of the human race" (these possibilities were rehearsed in the BBC TV *Horizon* program[9]).

FAMILIARITY WITH IMMORTALS

Increased longevity and its logical extension, some would say its *reductio ad absurdum,* immortality, have a long history. The human imagination is familiar with the idea of immortals and mortals living alongside one another and interacting. The *Iliad*, the *Odyssey*, the Bible, the Koran, the Ramayama, and Shakespeare's plays all

---

Address for correspondence: John Harris, Institute of Medicine, Law and Bioethics, School of Law, Williamson Building, University of Manchester, Oxford Road, Manchester M13 9P, United Kingdom. Voice: +44-161-275-3473; fax: +44-161-275-7704.
john.m.harris@man.ac.uk
[a]I have benefited from the incisive comments of my colleague Søren Holm.

have made such ideas familiar, and even modern classics have taken seriously the possibility of immortality. In his celebrated trilogy in five parts *The Hitchhiker's Guide to the Galaxy*, Douglas Adams imagines a man who had achieved immortality by accident:

> To begin with it was fun, he had a ball, living dangerously, taking risks, cleaning up on high-yield long-term investments, and just generally outliving the hell out of everybody.
>
> In the end it was the Sunday afternoons that he couldn't cope with, and that terrible listlessness which starts to set in at about 2.55 when you know that you have had all the baths you can usefully have that day, that however hard you stare at any given paragraph in the newspapers you will never actually read it ... and that as you stare at the clock the hands will move relentlessly on to four o'clock, and you will enter the long dark teatime of the soul.[10,b]

Despite the apparent pessimism of this passage many people would be prepared to endure "the long dark teatime of the soul" in exchange for immortality.[c] Indeed, there is much evidence both from literature, and in the literature, that suggests that many people are willing to trade off quality of life for longevity.[11] From the pact of Faust, celebrated by writers from Marlowe to Goethe, to Bram Stoker's vampires,[d] to choices made by cancer patients with a terminal diagnosis,[12] the evidence is strong that people want extra life time even at substantial costs in terms of pain and quality of life, even when outcomes are highly uncertain.

IMMORTALITY IS NOT INVULNERABILITY

Note that immortality is not the same as invulnerability, and even "immortals" could die or be killed. Accidents, infectious diseases, wars, and domestic violence would all take their toll, and although we might hope for progress in combating existing diseases, the development of new threats, such as HIV/AIDS and the emergence of variant Creutzfeldt–Jakob disease have demonstrated, may increase rather than reduce human vulnerability over time. If we add to this the diminishing effect of proven therapies such as antibiotics through the emergence of resistant strains of bacteria, it is difficult to predict the likely levels of "premature" deaths in a future in which increased life expectancy was developing and spreading through the human population.

LIFE EXTENSION SAVES LIVES

When we save a life, by whatever means, we simply postpone death. Life saving is just death postponement. This is a truth from which it follows that life-extending therapies are, and must always be, life-saving therapies and must share whatever priority life saving has in our morality and in our social values. So long as the life is of acceptable quality (acceptable to the person whose life it is),[13] we have a powerful, many would claim an overriding, moral imperative to save the life, because to

---

[b]For the record, the immortal's name was Wowbagger (p. 9).
[c]And we should note that Wowbagger himself did find something meaningful to do through all eternity.
[d]I am grateful to Simon Woods for insights into the un-dead.

fail to do so when we can would make us responsible for the resulting death (this claim is defended in detail in Harris[13,14]).

Three main sorts of philosophical or ethical objections have been leveled at life extension. It has been claimed that life extension would be unjust; it would be pointless and ultimately unwanted because of the inevitable boredom of indefinite life and would in any event be nugatory or self-defeating because personal identity could not survive long periods of extended existence. I may wish to be immortal but in the end it wouldn't be "me" so the project fails. Finally it is claimed that life extension would be prohibitively expensive in terms in increased healthcare costs. We will look at all these issues now, but necessarily briefly.

GLOBAL JUSTICE

One thing we do know is that the technology required to produce such results will be expensive. For existing people with multiple interventions probably required, the costs will be substantial. To make modifications to the embryo or even to the gametes before conception, people will have to be determinedly circumspect about procreation and will probably need to use reproductive technologies to have their immortal children. Even in technologically advanced countries therefore, "immortality" or increased life expectancy is likely to be confined to a minority of the population. In global terms, the divide between high-income and low-income countries will be increased, with low-income countries effectively denied access to the technology that might make some of their citizens immortal. The issue of the citizens of rich countries gaining further advantages over the poor will rightly disturb many. How are we to understand the demands of justice here?

Parallel Populations

A feature of life-extending treatments, which seldom has been thought through, is the fact that as treatments become available we will face the prospect of parallel populations, of "mortals" and "immortals" existing alongside one another.[15] Thus, the problems of global justice will be repeated in those societies able to implement life-extending therapies. Just as there will exist parallel societies, some able to provide immortalizing therapies and some not, so within those societies that have the technology and the resources required there would exist parallel populations of mortals and immortals. This of course is precisely the destiny for which the poetic imagination has prepared us, literally from "time immemorial."

Although such parallel populations seem inherently undesirable and even unfair, it is not clear that we could, or even that we should, do anything about such a prospect for reasons of justice. If immortality or increased life expectancy is a good, it is doubtful ethics to deny palpable goods to some people because we cannot provide them for all. And this unfairness is not simply contingent, a function of a regrettable, but, in principle, removable lack of resources. There will always be circumstances in which we cannot prevent harm or do good to everyone, but surely no one thinks that this affords us a reason to decline to prevent harm to anyone in particular. If twins suffer from cancer and one is incurable and the other not, we do not conclude that we should not treat the curable cancer because this would in some sense be unjust to the incurable twin. We don't refuse kidney transplants to some patients unless and until we can provide them for all with renal failure. We do, however, have a clear ethical responsibility to ensure that the question of which of those who could benefit receives the treatment should be decided according to some just principle of distribution.

We don't usually regard ourselves as wicked in Europe or North America because we perform many transplants (this claim is defended in detail in my *Violence and Responsibility*[e] and in *The Value of Life*), whereas low-income countries perform few or none at all. The solution, however, is certainly not to say that we will outlaw transplantation unless and until equitable distribution on some agreed principles can be guaranteed. The introduction of any new complex and/or expensive technology raises these problems. The impact on global justice or on justice within societies is important and must be addressed; it is a principled objection, but not an objection in principle to the introduction of life-extending therapies. The principle requires that strenuous and realistic efforts be made to provide the benefits of the technology justly and as widely as possible, not that the benefits be denied because of the impossibility of ensuring adequate justice of provision.

Immortality as the Side Effect of Therapy?

Remember that immortality is not unconnected with preventing or curing a whole range of serious diseases. It is one thing to ask the question "Should we make people immortal?" and answer in the negative; it is quite another to ask whether we should make people immune to heart disease, cancer, dementia, and many other diseases and decide that we should not, because a "side effect" of the treatment would be increase in life expectancy. We are then unlikely ever to face the question: Should we make people immortal, "yes" or "no"? We may rather be called upon to decide whether we should treat a particular disease when we know an effective treatment will extend life span.

It might then be appropriate to think of immortality as the side effect of treating or preventing a whole range of diseases. Could we really say to people "You must die at the age of thirty or forty or fifty, because the only way we can cure you is to extend your life span?" Faced with such a choice, an individual might well say, "Let me have my three score and ten and then let me die." Given the quite pervasive and irrational hostility to euthanasia, whether societies would be willing to allow such bargains to be made is doubtful.

LONGEVITY IS A RATIONAL GOOD

Given that people want life and fear death, it is difficult not to see longevity, and perhaps immortality, as a palpable good. Many have taken issue with this claim on two main grounds: either that indefinite life eventually would become terminally boring or that over long periods of survival personal identity could not be maintained and so the survival of a particular individual would prove illusory. Elsewhere (see p. 282 in Ref. 16) I have criticized, and I believe decisively refuted both these

---

[e]Although still many too few.

objections. Suffice it to say that only the terminally boring are in danger of being terminally bored, and perhaps they do not deserve indefinite life. Those who are bored can, thanks to their vulnerability, opt out at any time. But those of us who do not have terminal failure of the imagination should be left to create new ways of enjoying life and doing good. It is easy to see that that personal identity is not required for a coherent desire for indefinite survival. Suppose "Methuselah" has three identities, A, B, and C, and that C can remember nothing of A's life. But suppose the following is also true: A will want to be B who will remember being A, B will want to become C who will remember being B but possibly not remember being A. It is not irrational for A to want to be B and not irrational for A to want to be B partly because he or she knows that B will be able to look forward to being C, even though by the time she is C she won't remember being A. Thus, even if personal identity in some strict sense fails over time, it is not clear that a sufficiently powerful motivation for physical longevity fails with personal identity. This would remain true however many selves "Methuselah" turns out to be.

Prominent among recent denigrators of the idea of life extension has been Leon Kass, who identifies the core question as the following: "Is it really true that longer life for individuals is an unqualified good?" Kass has many arguments against life extension, all of which fail disastrously.[16] We have space to consider only his main objection: "For to argue that human life would be better without death is, I submit, to argue that human life would be better being something other than human .... The new immortals, in the decisive sense, would not be like us at all. If this is true, a human choice for bodily immortality would suffer from the deep confusion of choosing to have some great good only on condition of turning into someone else." [17] Insofar as this claim of Kass's relies on claims about psychological continuity, over time it has the problems we have already considered. However, Kass's argument seems to be suggesting a more simple objection: that since the (current) essence of being human is to be mortal, immortals would necessarily be a different type of being and therefore have a different identity. There is a sense in which this is true, but not, I think, any sense in which it would be irrational to want to change identity to the specified extent. Someone who had been profoundly disabled from birth (blind say, or crippled) and for whom a cure became available in his or her mid-forties would become in a sense a different person. They would lead a different type of life in many decisive ways. It does not follow that the blind or crippled individual has no rational motive to be cured. It would be both odd and cruel say to them, as Kass presumably would have us do, "it is deeply confused to want to cease to be disabled because then you will no longer exist."

POPULATION POLICY

Many people addressing the question of life extension have assumed that such a possibility will have a disastrous effect on the world's population with the present generation living indefinitely and a procession of subsequent generations adding to the congestion.[18] However, this is by no means either a likely or even the most likely scenario. The effect of life extension on population will be a function of several different factors, the outcomes of which are all difficult to predict. The first is the degree of uptake, which itself will be heavily dependent on cost and availability of the therapies. Granting, as we have, that life-extending therapies gradually will become available, cost, risk, and uncertainty will mean that for a very long time the numbers of people availing themselves of such therapies will be a tiny proportion of the world's population. We already have noted a possibly increasing human vulnerability due to new infectious diseases or antibiotic resistant strains of bacteria. Again it is difficult to predict the continuing effect of these on population or how the advent of some immortals would affect the equation. Disease may well continue to be an effective leveler, improving its own technology as we improve ours. And of course immortal but vulnerable people will continue to die in accidents and from injuries received.

THE END OF REPRODUCTION

Should we assume the necessity for, or desirability of, the creation of future generations? Is there a moral difference between a future that will contain x billion people succeeded by another x billion different people and so on indefinitely, or x billion people living indefinitely and replacing themselves on the (rare?) occasions when they are killed? Although, as we have noted, this is an unlikely scenario, posing the question in this stark form enables us to ask an important question. That question is whether what matters morally is that life years of reasonable quality exist or that different people with lives of reasonable quality exist. Put in this way the problem assumes a familiar form—should we maximize life years or individual lives? (There is an enormous literature on this. See, e.g. Refs. 19–21.) From the life years perspective, it ought not to matter how many new people the world would contain but simply how many life years of acceptable quality it will contain. Those who, like me, find the life years approach unsatisfactory will be inclined to think that individual lives matter. But even so, it could consistently be held that it is the individual lives of existing people that matter, not how many new individual lives there will be.

However, the argument for making sure that there will be new generations is not settled by the outcome of the debate between those who think that future lives count equally with existing lives and those who do not. One group of such reasons has to do with the desire to procreate and the pleasures of having and rearing children.[22,23]

The second set of reasons has to do with the advantages of fresh people, fresh ideas, and the possibility of continued human development. If these reasons are powerful, and I believe they are, and if the generational turnover proved too slow for regeneration of youth and ideas and for the satisfactions of parenting, we might face a future in which the fairest and the most ethical course might be to contemplate a sort of "generational cleansing."[f] This would involve deciding collectively how long it is reasonable for people to live in each generation and trying to ensure that as many as possible live healthy lives of that length. We then would have to ensure that, having lived a "fair innings," they died at the appropriate time to make way for future generations. Achieving this result by voluntary or ethical means might be difficult; attitudes to suicide and euthanasia might change, but probably not overnight.

---

[f] I deliberately choose the term "generational cleansing" for its obvious unpalatable connotations.

Christine Overall, in her recent book *Ageing, Death and Human Longevity*,[24] has found it difficult to be sure of Harris's attitude toward "generational cleansing" (p. 85). For the record, I think it would be unjustifiable, and therefore it is difficult to see how we could resist death-postponing therapies.

IMMORTALITY IS COST-EFFECTIVE

Søren Holm[g] has suggested that immortality so far from increasing health costs per individual actually might dramatically reduce them; there might be in short an economic discounting argument for the public funding of "immortality" interventions.

Let us assume the following: (1) for both mortals and immortals, there is the same period of old age with increased healthcare costs (say 10 years, but the length does not matter for the argument) and the same costs of treatment during those years (let's say £10,000 on average); (2) the mortals will reach this period in 70 years and the immortals in 1,000 years; (3) there is a 1% per year rate of real economic growth. The present-day discounted costs of treating a person in 70 years will be £4,948, whereas the present-day cost of treating the same person in 1,000 years will be 43 pence! It thus makes economic good sense to invest now and postpone healthcare costs from 70 years into the future to 1,000 years into the future, and as is evident from the figures, it makes sense even if immortals would have a much longer and more costly old age (because of the discounting, even a 10-fold increase in costs would not matter).[h] Add to this the probability that a greater number of immortals would die as the result of accidents rather than long drawn out illnesses and the economic arguments grow stronger still.

CONCLUSION

For the first time in human history we face the prospect of a truly open future, involving sequential as well as simultaneous opportunities, and stretching, open-ended before the individual in an unprecedented but truly liberating pathway. We should be slow to reject cures for terrible diseases even if the price we have to pay for those cures is increasing life expectancy and even creating immortals. Better surely to accompany the scientific race to achieve immortality with commensurate work in ethics and social policy to ensure that we know how to cope with the transition to parallel populations of mortals and immortals as envisaged in mythology.

---

[g]In a personal communication. The calculations are those of Søren Holm.

[h]Douglas Adams used a similar argument to show that the cost of traveling in time to eat at "the Restaurant at the end of the universe" would bring the price of eating at the most expensive restaurant of all time easily within reach of the most humble budget. "All you have to do is deposit one penny in a savings account in your own era, and when you arrive at the End of Time the operation of compound interest means that the fabulous cost of your meal has been paid for." See his *The Restaurant at the End of the Universe*. Pan Books. London. 1980: 81.

REFERENCES

1. BODNAR, A.G., M. OUELLETTE, M. FROLKIS, et al. 1998. Extension of life-span by introduction of telomerase into normal human cells. Science **279:** 349–352.
2. WEINRICH, S.L., R. PRUZAN, L.B. MA, et al. 1997. Reconstitution of human telomerase with the template RNA component hTR and the catalytic protein subunit hTRT. Nat. Genet. **17:** 498–502.
3. MCBREARTY, B.A., L.D. CLARK, X.M. ZHANG, et al. 1998. Genetic analysis of a mammalian wound-healing trait. Proc. Natl. Acad. Sci. USA **95:** 11792–11797.
4. THOMSON, J.A., J. ITSKOVITZ-ELDOR, S.S. SHAPIRO, et al. 1998. Embryonic stem cell lines derived from human blastocysts. Science **282:** 1145–1147.
5. PEDERSEN, R.A. 1999. Embryonic stem cells for medicine. Sci. Am. **280:** 68–73.
6. MOONEY, D.J. & A.G. MIKOS. 1999. Growing new organs. Sci. Am. **280:** 60–65.
7. LANZA, R.P., J.B. CIBELLI & M.D. WEST. 1999. Prospects for the use of nuclear transfer in human transplantation. Nat. Biotechnol. **17:** 1171–1174.
8. LANZA, R.P., J.B. CIBELLI & M.D. WEST. 1999. Human therapeutic cloning. Nat. Med. **5:** 975–977.
9. BBC TV HORIZON PROGRAMME. 2000. Life and Death in the 21st Century. Broadcast, January 2000.
10. ADAMS, D. 1982. Life, The Universe and Everything. Pan Books. London.
11. WEISS, K.M. 2000. The Biology of Ageing and the Quality of Later Life. In Ageing 2000: Our Health Care Destiny. Vol. 1. Biomedical Issues. Gates & Samorajski, Eds.
12. SLEVIN, M.L., L. STUBBS & H.J. PLANT. 1990. Attitudes to chemotherapy comparing views of cancer patients with those of doctors and the general public. Br. Med. J. **300:** 1458–1460.
13. HARRIS, J. 1987. The Value of Life. Routledge. London.
14. HARRIS, J. 1980. Violence and Responsibility. Routledge & Kegan Paul. London.
15. SILVER, L.M. 1999. Remaking Eden. Phoenix Giant. London.
16. HARRIS, J. 2002. Intimations of immortality—the ethics and justice of life extending therapies. In Current Legal Problems. Michael Freeman, Ed.: 65–97. Oxford University Press. Oxford.
17. KASS, L.R. 2001. L'Chaim and Its Limits: Why Not Immortality? First Things **113:** 17–24.
18. GLANNON, W. 2002. Identity, prudential concern, and extended lives. Bioethics **16:** 266–283.
19. HARRIS, J. 1987. QALYfying the value of life. J. Med. Ethics **13:** 117–123.
20. HARRIS, J. 1997. The rationing debate: maximising the health of the whole community. The case against: what the principal objective of the NHS should really be. Br. Med. J. **314:** 669–672.
21. MCKIE, J., J. RICHARDSON, P. SINGER & H. KUHSE. 1998. The Allocation of Health Care Resources—An Ethical Evaluation of the "QALY" Approach. Ashgate Pub. Aldershot, UK.
22. HARRIS, J. 1998. Rights and reproductive choice. In The Future of Human Reproduction: Choice and Regulation. J. Harris & H. Søren, Eds.: 5–37. Oxford University Press. Oxford.
23. HARRIS, J. 1999. Clones, genes and human rights. In The Genetic Revolution and Human Rights: The Amnesty Lectures 1998. J.C. Burley, Ed.: 61–95. Oxford University Press. Oxford.
24. OVERALL, C. 2003. Ageing, Death and Human Longevity. University of California Press. Berkeley, CA.

Collective Suttee

Is It Unjust to Develop Life Extension if It Will Not Be Possible to Provide It to Everyone?

JOHN K. DAVIS

*Brody School of Medicine, East Carolina University,
Greenville, North Carolina 27858-4354, USA*

ABSTRACT: If we can anticipate that life extension will be too expensive to provide to everyone, is that a reason not to research and develop it? *Collective suttee* is the policy of inhibiting or prohibiting life extension on such grounds: just as widows are killed on their husbands' funeral pyres, potential Methuselahs would not be allowed to outlive everyone else. However, in other contexts we judge that taking from the haves is unjustified when doing so confers a merely marginal benefit—or no benefit—to the have-nots. By this standard, collective suttee is probably unjustified, for the burdens borne by the have-nots are likely to be too small to justify denying extra decades or centuries to those who can afford it.

KEYWORDS: access; antiaging; anti-aging; extended life; equality; immortality; justice; life extension; prolongevism; prolongevity

If we cannot make life extension available to everyone, is that a reason not to research and develop it? The nightmare is this: a wealthy gerontocracy of near-immortals who live on and on in endless summer, looking down with indifference as commoners come and go in a passing spectacle of mortality, like ranchers watching an ever-changing herd of cattle. Leonard Hayflick warns that "those involved in the discovery and the rich and powerful will have earliest access or, depending on availability, even the only access," and Leon Kass believes it would "be the ultimate injustice if … the world were divided not only into rich and poor but into mortal and immortal."[1,2] Similar warnings can be found in Harris.[3]

Whether people have a moral right to publicly subsidized life extension will be controversial, but the point may be moot. Life extension may well be too costly for the world's haves to provide it for all the world's have-nots even if they really try. Developed countries might offer it to their citizens through government-guaranteed loans; extended life is extended time for repayment. Moreover, if aging is halted, there is less need to save for retirement and end-of-life care. However, even if developed countries can subsidize it for all their citizens, many in the developing

---

Address for correspondence: John K. Davis, J.D., Ph.D., Department of Philosophy, University of Tennessee, 816 McClung Tower, Knoxville, TN 37996-0480. Voice: 865-974-7216; fax: 865-974-3509.

jdavis95@utk.edu

world will miss out. After all, according to the World Bank, 54.7% of the human race lives on less than $2 per day.[4]

If we cannot provide life extension to everyone, should we *deny* it to everyone? Daniel Callahan suggests that, on grounds of limited access and other reasons, "[w]e can make [life-extension] socially despicable. Just like nuclear testing, we can decide we don't want it."[5] Walter Glannon is more explicit:

> Of course, we could allow people to pay for life-extending technology. But this would be unfair to those who could not afford to pay because it would preclude them from having the same choice as those who are financially better off. [This provides some] moral grounds for not allowing people to extend their lives beyond the present norm.[6]

I call this *collective suttee*: just as widows in traditional India were not allowed to outlive their husbands, so potential Methuselahs must not outlive everyone else. Even when opponents of life extension do not cite unequal access *alone* as grounds for prohibition or inhibition, many will cite it as *a* ground.

Collective suttee can be achieved through a policy of *prohibition*, in which life extension is outlawed, or *inhibition*, in which life-extension research and development is delayed and hindered. The alternative is *free choice*, in which life-extension research and development is unhindered and adequately funded, and life extension is not prohibited. Collective suttee consists of imposing prohibition or inhibition on the grounds that it is wrong for some to have access when it is not possible to give it to everyone. (I will not consider in this article whether prohibition or inhibition are justified when it *is* possible to make life extension available to at least some have-nots, yet the haves fail to do so—that is a different problem.) Is collective suttee justified?

One might argue for it on egalitarian grounds, reasoning that, if we cannot extend the life spans of all have-nots, we should achieve equality of life span by curtailing the life spans of the haves. However, philosophers generally believe that justice does not permit "leveling-down": making some people worse off when doing so does not make anyone else better off.[7,8] Most also believe that redistribution from those who are better off to those who are worse off *can* be justified by improving the condition of those who are worse off, even if doing so reduces the total amount of good in that society.[7–11] On what I call the *consensus view* of justice and equality, redistribution is not justified by merely marginal improvements for some at a dramatic cost to those who are better off. Most readers probably agree; for example, few of us would endorse massive redistributions of wealth from the developed countries to the undeveloped countries when doing so does not noticeably improve conditions in the undeveloped countries. Is collective suttee justified if the consensus view is correct?

On the consensus view, collective suttee is justified only if the availability of life extension imposes a more than marginal burden to the have-nots. There are several possible burdens. First, the have-nots may be taxed for government-subsidized life-extension research ("No taxation without elongation!"). Second, the haves might use their extra life-years to improve their privileged positions, making it harder for the have-nots to catch up. Third, the have-nots will suffer distress as they watch the haves cheat death.[12,a] Fourth, life extension might have Malthusian consequences as the death rate plummets and more people demand space and resources. This problem

---

[a]Contrary to John Rawls (and probably most other philosophers), Richard Hare has argued that envy can, depending on the circumstances, be the kind of burden that justifies redistribution.

is somewhat disjunct from the access problem, for Malthusian consequences will be worse the more people who have access, yet the wider the access the weaker the access objection.[b] However, even nonuniversal access might be enough to significantly increase the world's population.

Which is worse—living through a century of increased crowding, distress, and watching the haves pull further ahead, or being denied centuries of additional life? Comparing 1 year for a have to 1 year for a have-not, collective suttee seems far more burdensome to the have than free choice is to the have-not.

To compare the entire *lives* of these two, we must entertain some assumptions. These assumptions are very speculative, but they suffice to illustrate the trade-offs. Suppose an average person would be indifferent between 20 years of the burdens suffered by a have-not and 19 years as a have-not free of those burdens. If so, each year of burdens should be discounted by 95% (a year of burdens is equivalent to .95 quality-adjusted life-years; for a good introduction to QALYs, see Nord[13]). Suppose also that the have-nots enjoy an average life span of 100 (for ease of calculation), that life extension effectively halts aging, and that the accident rate is such that life extension adds an average of 500 years of life to the original 100. On these assumptions, free choice burdens the have-nots by the equivalent of 5 life-years each (5% of 100 years) even though their lives are not any shorter, whereas collective suttee denies 500 years of life to each have. At 500 years versus the equivalent of 5 years, collective suttee seems unjustified on a life by life comparison too.

What about comparing entire *populations* of haves and have-nots? As I articulated the consensus view, it is an open question whether the appropriate comparison is between two representative individuals or between entire populations of haves and have-nots. Without taking a position on that question, let us compare populations. According to a World Bank study, 22% of the world's population is "middle class" (defined as having US $3470 or more in yearly purchasing power parity).[14] For discussion, let us assume that these people are haves, and that they can afford to subsidize another 8% of the human race, so that 30% of the human race has access to life extension. Free choice then produces this distribution for a population of 100:

30 haves × 500 each = **+15,000** (extra years)

70 have-nots × 5 each = **−350** (equivalent in years).

Readers may differ in their judgments on this point, but on the consensus view, this trade-off does not seem to justify restricting life extension.

But there is another burden. Suppose life extension will become available to all citizens in developed countries by the year 2053. Someone living in Madagascar in 2053 would have access to extended life *if only* he or she lived 5000 miles to the northwest, and *we* would have access to extended life *if only* we lived 50 years in the future. The have-nots include both most Third-world poor in 2053 and most adults

---

[b]In "Life-Extension and the Malthusian Objection," forthcoming in *The Journal of Medicine and Philosophy*, I argue that anticipated Malthusian consequences do not justify restricting the availability of life extension. That paper concerned people who do have access and must suffer Malthusian consequences but prefer not to, and the relative benefits and burdens of haves who want and haves who do not want access. The present article, by contrast, concerns whether people who must suffer such consequences but do *not* have access have a right not to bear that burden, even if imposing that burden on them produces more total benefit than otherwise.

today—*you* are probably a have-not. On reflection, you may feel somehow worse off—not only worse off than the haves, but worse off than thought you were in some noncomparative sense that cannot be fully explained by reference to taxes, equal opportunity, and Malthusian concerns. Why?

The answer concerns why it is bad to die. If death is nonexistence, then there is nothing unpleasant about *being* dead. Instead, death is a *comparative* harm for the deceased; it is bad by comparison with continued life. Some philosophers argue that death is bad by *comparison* with continued life.[15] Others argue that death is bad because it *deprives* one of continued life.[16] When I speak of "comparison," I do not take sides in this controversy; I simply mean that philosophers are agreed that nonexistence is not a bad state or experience, but bad by contrast with what might have been. Moreover, *how* bad it is to die at a particular time depends on comparison with the length and quality of life you would have if you did not die then.[17,c] It is sad to die at 97; it is tragic at 17.

Life extension changes the comparison. If you anticipate living into your nineties, your future death seems less bad than most. However, if life extension becomes available to people wealthier than you, then death at 97 seems far worse than it used to. Life extension makes you worse off by making your death worse. True, this is a comparative harm—your life is not any shorter—but death has always been harmful only in a comparative sense. This is not simply a matter of distress, for how you feel about a given harm is a separate, different harm. Distress about impending death is like distress about slander: you are distressed when you find out you were slandered because being slandered is harmful independently of the distress it causes—otherwise you would have no reason to feel distressed about it.[18,d]

Of course, people who lived 1000 years ago had no access to life extension, so they were have-nots, but their deaths do not seem as tragic as those of 21st-century have-nots. How bad life extension makes your death is a matter of degree. Your death is bad in proportion to, among other things, your odds of avoiding death for a significant time. The better the odds that you could obtain life extension, the worse it is to die at 97. For example, death at 97 is far worse for a have who received life extension than for a have-not who never had a real chance at access, just as it is much worse to buy the winning lottery ticket and lose it than to buy one of the losing tickets (if you bought a losing ticket, it is not very likely that you would have bought the winning one instead). It was not completely impossible for humans to achieve life extension 1000 years ago, just astronomically unlikely. It is still very unlikely that a have-not in 2053 can pay for life extension, but much more likely than obtaining it 1000 years ago. Therefore, it is worse to be a have-not in 2053 (or now) than one who died 1000 years ago, or even 10 years ago. It has always been unfortunate that we could not slow or halt aging, but the possibility of life extension in the near future increases that misfortune. If life extension is available to others but not to you, then the better the odds that you *could* otherwise have had access, the worse your death, and the worse the odds, the better your death.

With this in mind, suppose life extension becomes possible and society adopts free choice. How much worse would this make death for the have-nots? A have-not

---

[c]My approach to this issue is inspired in part by Chapter Two of McMahan.[17]
[d]This argument is the converse of Bishop Butler's famous argument that we do not desire things for the pleasure they give us, but get pleasure from obtaining what we desire.

might become a have by succeeding in business, or winning a lottery, or a breakthrough might drastically lower the cost of treatment. Suppose the odds of one of these developments (most likely the breakthrough) is 10%. The badness of a have-not's death at 97 is a function of 500 lost years discounted by 90% to reflect the 10% odds of getting access, for a total harm equivalent to 50 life-years. Her life is no shorter, but it is as if she died at 97 when she could have lived to 147. If we add the other burdens earlier estimated as equivalent to 5 life-years per have-not, her total loss attributable to being a have-not in a world with life extension is equivalent to 55 life-years. Here are the trade-offs under free choice when we include death-related burdens:

30 haves × 500 = **+15,000** (extra years)

70 have-nots × 55 = **−3,850** (equivalent in years).

Now, instead of a total burden equivalent to 350 life-years, the have-nots are worse off by a total of 3,850.

But would the have-nots be substantially better off under prohibition and/or inhibition? Prohibition is not completely feasible; black markets will occur, so a have's odds of access under prohibition are not much less than under free choice. Therefore, a have-not's death is almost as bad under prohibition as it is under free choice. Inhibition, however, is very feasible; arguably it is happening now through indifference and inadequate research funding. Right now life extension is *medically* impossible for everyone. Once life extension is developed, free choice makes it only *financially* impossible for the have-nots, and therefore more possible overall. By delaying the development of life extension, inhibition extends the time of medical impossibility. For have-nots during this period of extended medical impossibility, inhibition makes life extension not only financially impossible but medically impossible as well, and therefore less possible overall. Therefore, during this period, death is not as bad for the have-nots as it would be under free choice, for their odds of access are worse.

How much inhibition helps a have-not depends on the odds that life extension will become medically possible during that person's lifetime despite inhibition. Those odds are unknowable, but if we assume for discussion that inhibition cuts in half the odds that life extension will become medically possible during one's lifetime, then inhibition reduces a have-not's odds of access from 10% (under free choice) to 5%. Multiplied by 500 life-years per have-not, the burden of being a have-not under inhibition is equivalent to 25 life-years. Adding the other burdens equivalent to 5 life-years, a have-not's burden under inhibition is equivalent to 30 life-years—25 fewer life-years than under free choice, whereas 70 have-nots of 100 are burdened equivalent to 2100 life-years—1750 less than under free choice. The trade-offs under inhibition are 500 years per have versus (the equivalent of) 25 years per have-not and 15,000 life-years for 30 haves versus (the equivalent of) 1750 years for 70 have-nots. This is hard to justify on the consensus view.

We have entertained some very speculative assumptions; is my argument undermined by different assumptions? Suppose life extension gives only 50 extra years, and that only 6% of the human race has access:

6 haves × 50 = **+300** (extra years)

94 have-nots × 1 = **−94** (equivalent in years).

The burden per have-not is estimated at the equivalent of one life-year partly because, with one-fifth as many haves, a have-not's odds of becoming a have are one-fifth less: 5% odds becomes 1%, and 1% of 50 years is half a year. The nondeath burdens are reduced to another half a year because there will be few or no discernible Malthusian consequences with so few haves and so few extra years, because there is less to envy, and because an extra 50 years does not provide haves with as much advantage.

On a life by life comparison, this does not seem to justify collective suttee, for each have would lose 50 years to reduce a have-not's burden by (the equivalent of) 1 year. On a comparison of *populations*, things are less clear; whether a trade-off of 300 years for 6 haves versus (the equivalent of) 94 years for 94 have-nots justifies collective suttee must be left to the reader's judgment. In my judgment, it is not. Let me conclude by reviewing what it would take to justify collective suttee. First, one might claim that justice requires taking away from the more fortunate even when this does not make anyone better off. However, this has rarely, if ever, been advocated in other contexts. Second, one might also claim that a year of burdens for a have-not are much worse than I have supposed, perhaps equivalent to a 50% discount. I believe most readers will find that implausible, though I may be mistaken. Third, one might claim that a have-not's odds of access under inhibition are far, far worse than under free choice. However, that supposes that life extension is not likely to be developed without government support, and that too seems false. Finally, one might judge both that the appropriate comparison is between populations, not persons, and that a trade-off of 300 years for 6 haves versus (the equivalent of) 94 years for 94 haves justifies collective suttee. I do not share the belief that only population comparisons are relevant, and I am uneasy about the judgment that this trade-off justifies collective suttee. If those of us who are skeptical about all four claims are correct, then the anticipated impossibility of providing life extension to everyone does not justify *denying* it to everyone.

REFERENCES

1. HAYFLICK, L. 2001. Anti-aging medicine: hype, hope, and reality. Generations **25:** 20–26.
2. KASS, L. 2001. L'Chaim and its limits: why not immortality? First Things **11:** 17–24.
3. HARRIS, J. 2001. Intimations of immortality. Science **288:** 59. Kevles, D. 1999. Life on the far side of 150. *New York Times*, March 16, 1999, Op-Ed: 27. Juengst, E., *et al.* 2003. Antiaging research and the need for public dialog. Science **299:** 1323.
4. TIMMER, H. 2003. The international economy and prospects for developing countries. *In* Global Economic Prospects and the Developing Countries. U. Dadush & R. Newfarmer, Eds.: 31. Office of the Publisher of the World Bank. Washington, D.C. Available at: http://www.worldbank.org/prospects/gep2003/chap1.pdf.
5. FISCHER, J. 2000. The cells of immortality: scientists are tinkering with natural limits on the human life span. Is that a good idea? U.S. News & World Report **128:** 58–59.
6. GLANNON, W. 2002. Reply to Harris. Bioethics **16:** 292–293.
7. ARNESON, R.J. 1993. Equality. *In* A Companion to Contemporary Political Philosophy. R. E. Goodin & P. Pettit, Eds.: 489–507. Blackwell. Oxford.
8. POJMAN, L.P. & R. WESTMORELAND. 1997. Introduction: the nature and value of equality. *In* Equality: Selected Readings. L. P. Pojman & R. Westmoreland, Eds.: 5. Oxford University Press. Oxford.
9. RAWLS, J. 2001. Justice as Fairness: A Restatement. Harvard University Press. Cambridge, MA.
10. RAWLS, J. 1971. A Theory of Justice. Harvard University Press. Cambridge, MA.

11. FRANKFURT, H. 1987. Equality as a moral ideal. Ethics **98:** 22.
12. HARE, R.M. 1978. Justice and equality. *In* Equality: Selected Readings. L P. Pojman & R. Westmoreland, Eds.: 225. Oxford University Press. Oxford.
13. NORD, E. 1999. Cost-Value Analysis in Healthcare: Making Sense of QALYs. Cambridge University Press. Cambridge.
14. MILANOVIC, B. & S. YITZHAKI. 2001. Decomposing world income distribution: does the world have a middle class? Available from: http://econ.worldbank.org/files/1423_wps2562.pdf/.
15. SILVERSTEIN, H.S. 1980. The evil of death. J. Philos. **77:** 401–424.
16. NAGEL, T. 1979. Death. *In* Mortal Questions. T. Nagel, Ed.: 1–10. Cambridge University Press. Cambridge.
17. MCMAHAN, J. 2002. The Ethics of Killing: Problems at the Margins of Life. Oxford University Press. Oxford.
18. BUTLER, B. 1726. Sermon XI—Upon the love of our neighbor. *In* British Moralists: 1650–1800. D. D. Raphael, Ed.: 364–373. Hackett. Indianapolis, IN.

Biogerontologists' Duty to Discuss Timescales Publicly

AUBREY D. N. J. DE GREY

Department of Genetics, University of Cambridge, Cambridge CB2 3EH, United Kingdom

ABSTRACT: Aging is unpopular with the general public—but, it would seem, only up to a point. Treatments that claim (sometimes justifiably) to extend the total and/or healthy life span of elderly people, or even just make them look younger, are welcomed with open wallets throughout the world. If, however, one suggests to the typical nonbiologist—or even to the typical nongerontologist biologist—that we should therefore aim, in due course, to take this desire to its logical conclusion and bring aging under the same degree of control that we currently have over most infectious diseases, one is nearly always met with strong and sometimes strident opposition. I argue here that the prevalence of this outright irrationality is largely the fault of gerontologists themselves. Most people harbor a deep-seated fear of profound change in their lives and embrace it only after extensive soul-searching to convince themselves of its benefit. It cannot and should not be denied that a postaging world would be as profoundly different from today's as we can imagine. Hence, when given the opportunity to postpone sober consideration of its pros and cons, most people leap at that opportunity. It is provided to them by the nearly universal refusal of gerontologists to speculate about the timescales within which truly effective rejuvenation therapies may be developed. I suggest that this reticence, while appropriate in purely scientific fields, is hugely irresponsible in a biomedical discipline, because of its potential to delay the development of such therapies by denying them the funding that would be forthcoming if society had greater optimism concerning their foreseeability. Arguments that such funding, and/or the public's trust in scientists, would be short-lived if timescale predictions were not borne out are too flimsy to outweigh this. A further danger is the avoidable loss of life following the development of rejuvenation therapies that would result from inadequate ability to provide them universally; here again, scientists today can minimize this loss of life by agitating for forward planning by government, which will only occur when policymakers' minds are concentrating on timescale predictions.

KEYWORDS: human healthy life extension; public debate; timescales

The market for products that stave off the ravages of old age to a modest degree, perhaps making one look and/or feel ten or even twenty years younger than one thinks one would without them, is huge in all industrialized nations, particularly the United

Address for correspondence: Aubrey D.N.J. de Grey, Department of Genetics, University of Cambridge, Downing Street, Cambridge CB2 3EH, UK. Voice: +44-1223-765665; fax: +44-1223-333992.
ag24@gen.cam.ac.uk

Ann. N.Y. Acad. Sci. 1019: 542–545 (2004). © 2004 New York Academy of Sciences.
doi: 10.1196/annals.1297.100

States. Similarly, the enormous amount spent on medical care to combat—again only to a modest degree—age-related diseases is apparently considered money well spent, including in countries in which it is mostly derived from taxation. But the idea of improving very considerably on present-day therapies, to the extent of doubling or perhaps even extending indefinitely the human life span potential, is not greeted with such enthusiasm: indeed, it generally elicits outright hostility in those who feel uninhibited from showing such a response and a robust effort to change the subject in those who do not. Since it cannot for a moment be denied that the defeat of aging is the logical extension of treatments whose desirability the public so assiduously demonstrates, something very odd is going on in the minds of the large majority of the developed world who regard putting off aging a little as wonderful, but putting it off a lot as ghastly. Why?

This paradox becomes even starker when the views of the relevant scientists are examined. With very few exceptions, biogerontologists do not subscribe to the public consensus concerning the more ambitious goal: they regard human aging as a wholly undesirable phenomenon whose postponement and cure would be of incalculable benefit to humanity, albeit at the (hopefully temporary) cost of considerable turbulence as civilization adjusts to its new circumstances. When society regards the views of the scientific community so highly in other walks of life, how can this dislocation be explained? And is it legitimate for us as biogerontologists to leave it to others to seek such an explanation, as most of us habitually do, or is it our responsibility to explain it?

Many biogerontologists appear to feel that they do not have such a responsibility. Perhaps this is due more to psychological than to conscious factors: the prevalence of comments from laypeople along the lines of "Who would want to spend all that time being old?", "Wouldn't we get terribly bored?", or "How would we pay for all those pensions?" fills many of us with such awe at their breathtaking stupidity that any ardor to persist in a patient explanation of what success in this endeavor would actually mean is rapidly sapped. But this is not a legitimate reaction to such inanity, in my view. To put it simply, it is just not plausible that people are really that dumb. Hence, before we abandon our fellows to their misconceptions, we as biogerontologists are duty bound to seek a more satisfactory basis for the persistence of these extraordinarily transparently flawed opinions.[1]

On doing so we are forced, it seems to me, to acknowledge that one very simple reason fits the facts: denial. Nonbiogerontologists are not equipped to evaluate reliably the likely rate of progress toward a cure for aging, and they know it. They also know, therefore, that once they let themselves believe that aging might truly be cured in time to let them (or their children) live for many centuries, they will become susceptible to possibly the greatest disappointment that we can imagine if progress is slower than they anticipate. Hence they prefer to pretend, however absurdly, that such an advance would not be so great anyway; this provides a modest protective barrier against the terror of thinking of aging as we really should, that is, as the greatest scourge to which mankind remains universally exposed. Only a modest one, however—certainly, I claim, inadequate to maintain such denial in the face of authoritative statements of realistic timescales for the advent of real antiaging medicine. This is why we biogerontologists, who are acutely aware of our responsibility not to suggest unrealistically optimistic timescales for the defeat of aging, must also be aware—which, by and large, we are evidently not—of our converse responsibility not to suggest (or imply, by silence) unrealistically *pessimistic* timescales. We possess unique influence over society's willingness to continue to condemn people to a (by future standards) hugely premature death in decades to come by delaying the defeat of human aging.

I should stress that I do not consider biogerontologists to have been at fault in this matter for very long—arguably for no more than about five years. This is because until quite recently there was no such thing as an unrealistically pessimistic timescale for the advent of real antiaging medicine: it was too far off to be foreseeable. Since the turn of the millennium, however, such a stance has not been justifiable. To be sure, there remain aspects of age-related decline that we do not have a detailed understanding of how to repair—in fact, when it comes to the *fine* details, this applies to most, if not all, such aspects. But we do now have a thorough understanding of what those aspects are—a list, which we can be fairly confident is exhaustive, of the things that give a healthy 40-year-old a shorter remaining life expectancy than a healthy 20-year-old—and a specific description of already-feasible ways to reverse large parts of them, sufficient, if implemented, to be highly likely to double or treble the remaining life expectancy of middle-aged mammals.[2,3]

Let us be clear about the scale of all this. Fixing aging is tricky, to be sure, and will take time, but the sooner we start seriously trying to do it, the sooner we will succeed. It is simply incorrect to suppose that serendipitous discoveries in years to come will entirely determine the date at which aging is cured: just as fortune favors the prepared mind, scientific luck is partly made by those who benefit from it. To deny this presents two huge and immediate dangers to humanity. One is that funding will continue not to be adequately targeted to the translational research that can make real antiaging medicine a reality as soon as possible; the simple fact that over 100,000 people die every day of causes that kill virtually no one under 30 demonstrates the gravity of that error. The second danger is that the laboratory breakthroughs that convince society that real antiaging medicine is on the way, and which therefore turn our lives upside-down overnight, will occur before governments have had time to make long-range plans to make the transition to a postaging world as smooth and rapid as possible.

Both these dangers are exacerbated by biogerontologists' perpetuation of their once-justifiable stance of refusing to discuss timescales. It is not good enough to say that we will *eventually* control aging: "eventually" is not a word that makes people change their pension or life insurance plans, or politicians their spending priorities. Hence, alien though it may be to the basic scientist's way of thinking, we as specialists in the biology of aging can no longer shrink from publicly estimating the time-frame for the arrival, if not of real antiaging medicine itself, then at least of the laboratory breakthroughs mentioned earlier. I consider it highly likely that within ten years from now, if the rather modest necessary funding is forthcoming, we will have the ability to take a mouse cohort with a three-year life expectancy, when it is already two years old, and treble its remaining life expectancy (that is, give it a total life expectancy of five years). I also consider it highly likely that the announcement of that degree of control over mouse aging will almost instantly overturn society's prevailing fatalism concerning any chance of personal benefit from real antiaging medicine. The sooner that moment comes, and the readier we are to exploit it when it does, the better—and we had better do all we can to expedite it, or it is we, the scientists of aging, who will bear the greatest blame.

REFERENCES

1. DE GREY, A.D.N.J. 2003 The foreseeability of real anti-aging medicine: focusing the debate. Exp. Gerontol. **38:** 927–934.
2. DE GREY, A.D.N.J., B.N. AMES, J.K. ANDERSEN, *et al.* 2002. Time to talk SENS: critiquing the immutability of human aging. Ann. N.Y. Acad. Sci. **959:** 452–462.
3. DE GREY, A.D.N.J. 2003. An engineer's approach to the development of real anti-aging medicine. Sci. Aging Knowledge Environ. **2003:** VP1.

The Pitfalls of Planning for Demographic Change

GREGORY B. STOCK

Program on Medicine, Technology, and Society, UCLA School of Public Health, Department of Health Services, Los Angeles, California 90024-1759, USA

ABSTRACT: As we begin to understand the biology of aging, it will be ever more tempting to try to plan for the social consequences of the coming biomedical interventions in this arena. However, this will remain a daunting task, because the larger consequences of the arrival of antiaging interventions will greatly depend on the relative character and timing of the specific procedures that emerge. Three basic classes of interventions are likely: ones that slow aging in adults, ones that reverse aging in adults, and embryonic interventions that modify the overall trajectory of human aging. The consequences of each will differ significantly in the time required before noticeable demographic shifts begin to manifest in the human population, and in the social and political changes the interventions evoke. The specific societal consequences generally will arrive long before the demographic ones, and will hinge on the technical details of the interventions themselves—their complexity, physiological targets, modes of delivery, costs, unpleasantness, and the character and frequency of side effects.

KEYWORDS: demographic change; antiage; life-span extension; reversing aging; retarding aging

The trajectory of life is brutal. It is difficult for a youngster to go to a nursing home and fully appreciate that the frail elderly there were once as vital and full of life as he or she is. And it is even more difficult for the young to comprehend that one day they too will be as old and frail—if they are lucky enough to make it that far. Everything we love eventually will be taken from us as we grow old, our senses diminish, our friends and loved ones pass away, and finally we die.

Dealing with this truth has always been challenging, and we see several different basic approaches to the task. Some people ignore it, pretending that they will somehow be spared. This is particularly easy for the young, who haven't begun to manifest any noticeable symptoms of decline. Others simply deny their mortality, claiming that death is not real and that their souls will live eternally, or that they will live on in their creations or in the hearts of others. Still others accept this process of decline as inevitable and natural, or they may even maintain that it is best, because death is what gives meaning to life. And finally, there are those who battle against

Address for correspondence: Dr. Gregory B. Stock, Director, Program on Medicine, Technology, and Society, UCLA School of Public Health, Department of Health Services, 760 Westwood Boulevard, Los Angeles, CA 90024-1759. Voice: 310-825-9715; fax: 413-487-7512
gstock@signumbiosciences.com

the process, trying to escape its seeming inevitability. Ponce de Leon slogged through the jungles of Florida searching for the fountain of youth. And today, cryonicists contract to freeze their bodies (or merely their heads) in the hope of eventual resurrection by future medical science equipped with nanotechnology and other breakthrough devices.

Regardless of how we face the prospect of our own eventual decline, however, in this era of breathtaking medical advances, aging is grist for a horde of charlatans peddling elixirs of vitamins and hormones. A clutter of pitches ring out on the Internet: *Unleash Your Youth with Professional Strength Human Growth Hormone! Aging—Don't accept it, turn back the clock now!* But medical science has yet to bring us much in this realm. The sad truth is that what Shakespeare wrote in 1598 still applies today.

> And so from hour to hour we ripe and ripe
> And then from hour to hour we rot and rot;
> and thereby hangs a tale.
>
> —*As You Like It*, Act ii. Scene 7

But what if biogerontology makes real progress? What if science's unraveling of the workings of life brings us not warmed over Ponce de Leon, but true breakthroughs in our understanding of aging? What if we learn to retard or even reverse key aspects of the process?

Some say this will never happen, so we should keep our eyes on the real diseases that afflict us. Others think it will happen, and feel it's reckless not to plan for the enormous dislocations ahead.[1] I maintain that breakthroughs in the biology of aging are quite plausible, but that any social planning for broad life-span extension at this point would be nearly worthless, except for a few relatively obvious actions that would be of value anyway.

It is important to understand up front that the project to dramatically extend human life span is greatly at odds with the present goals of biogerontology, which are not to buy more life, but to condense our morbidity.[2] Ostensibly, success would mean that we would live long, healthy lives, and then rapidly deteriorate like a salmon that has spawned. Initially, such a project might seem reasonable, but push it to its logical conclusion, and it would be a nightmare, profoundly at odds with our true aspirations.

Imagine how unprepared we would be to die even at 80 if we had been fit and vital until a few weeks earlier. Wrenched from our prime without ever-worsening debilities to make us disengage from the world would not only be excruciating personally, it would leave a gaping void behind. Sickness and decline are unwelcome visitors, but at least they prepare us and those around us for our departure.

If human life span proved immutable, of course, more health and less sickness would seem pretty good. But when push comes to shove, most people would prefer a healthier *and* a longer life. Our true aspiration is not compressed morbidity, but more and better years.

The real question, though, is not what we want, but what is possible, and one need go no further than the other articles in this volume to see that such possibilities are not implausible. The potential of any particular intercession to alter aging can easily be disputed, but not that medical science is following many plausible paths toward controlling key aspects of aging. So, let's consider the likely consequences of controlling the aging process.

There can be little doubt that meaningful health-span extension would be widely embraced if it became possible. The popularity of cosmetic surgery and nutritional supplementation attest to that. Some people, of course, insist that it would be a huge mistake to extend human life span. They worry that already there are too many people, that environmental problems would deepen, that life would lose its meaning, that reaching for more life would be selfish, or even that the extra years would be boring. Yet even they will sometimes whisper, "but put me on your list."

If regenerative medicine conquered aging, the breakthrough would without question bring profound shifts in the way we live. Virtually every facet of human society would change: family relationships, educational structures, the passage of wealth and power from one generation to the next, the very shape of our institutions. Truly, the collapse of social security would be the least of our problems.

Questions and concerns about the new directions we would take are easy to find: Would antiaging interventions fragment society, erode our values, ignite a population explosion, pit one generation against the next? But definitive answers are hard to come up with. They depend too much on unknowable details of the technology itself. Aging is multifaceted, and various aspects of it are sure to be addressed with differing success and at differing rates.

A future with the elderly having youthful bodies and ossifying brains would be vastly different from one with sharp-minded oldsters whose immune systems were failing. And both would differ completely from one in which we simply halved the pace of aging, thereby doubling our life spans.

Three distinct categories of antiaging interventions are possible: ones that slow aging in adults, ones that reverse aging in adults, and ones that must take place in embryos (or perhaps young children) to be effective.

One obvious question about these interventions is how quickly they would shift the age distribution of our population if they became broadly available. Another question is how long it would take them to provoke meaningful social and political challenges.

Each of these intervention categories would lead to very different delays before the age distribution of the human population would shift in a significant way. Reversing aging would have immediate, massive effects, because it would sharply reduce the numbers of frail and elderly by rejuvenating them. Retarding aging would bring a gradual shift that would take decades to affect the population's age distribution, and even then, would merely mute the consequences of current graying by slowing the decline brought by added years. Embryonic interventions would have almost no effect on the population until 60 or 70 years after they were broadly embraced, because diseases of aging virtually by definition are reserved for the old, and it would take a long time for the first treated cohort to emerge from youth and middle age.

In contrast to these differential effects, massive social and political shifts would come quickly regardless of the intervention category. That society would react strongly to effective interventions that retard or reverse aging is obvious. But effective antiaging interventions in embryos or young children would bring a strong response as well, because the success would ignite public hopes for adult interventions. Indeed, success with antiaging interventions even in mice would probably lead to a *war on aging* as adults increasingly decided that they'd rather be part of the first generation to enjoy extended life spans than part of the last to miss out.

Once human aging was seen as potentially malleable, I suspect we might quickly come to see it not simply as *a* disease, but as *the* disease—an affliction that affects everyone, that cripples and kills as it progresses, and that might be treatable. The idea of aging as a disease is not yet mainstream, but in 2001 Temple argued that, in the genomic era, we would need to view disease not as a cluster of symptoms but as a *state* that places individuals at *increased risk* of *adverse consequences.*[3] He was thinking of preventive treatment for genomic factors that place individuals at heightened risk for various known diseases, but aging satisfies his criteria as well.

Aging is the critical underlying factor in cancer, arthritis, Alzheimer disease, atherosclerosis, and other conditions of advancing years. Quite simply, aging is what makes us "old" and brings on these diseases. It is a diffuse, late-onset genetic disorder that we all suffer.

Any meaningful antiaging interventions will rapidly bring large social and political consequences, but what will those consequences be? That is the crucial question for budding social planners. And the answer is, "it depends."

One major determinant of these consequences will be cost. Any intervention or cluster of interventions will have both fixed costs, such as those for R&D and various equipment, and variable costs, outlays that are directly proportional to the number of people using the technology. These variable costs are what will most shape the implications of the technology. If the variable costs are low, for example, such as with drugs, enormous pressure will arise to provide government funding to make them available to everyone, regardless what their development costs were.

If variable costs are high, however, such as would be the case for complex ongoing, individualized procedures that are labor and equipment intensive, it would be too expensive to provide the procedures to everyone. Conflicts thus would be bound to arise over how to distribute and ration the interventions. And the more they were reserved for the wealthy, the sharper the class conflict would likely be.

Many other factors besides price will be critical as well. Our response to such technology will depend on the modality of the treatments, whether they have harsh side effects, need frequent repetition, are arduous, take long to act, are risky, must begin before a certain age, and, of course, whether they reverse or merely slow aging. Each factor will influence the public's embrace of, and response to, the technology. The modality of intervention, for instance, will greatly influence the ability of the government to regulate the technology. Drugs would be virtually impossible to regulate even if significant risks were associated with them, whereas equipment-intensive clinical procedures might be more controllable. And we must not forget that none of these various factors will be static, because any such technology is bound to evolve over time.

Such specifics also will affect the nature of the social adjustments required by the technologies and the character of the social conflicts provoked. Daunting intergenerational conflicts might be sparked by imbalances of wealth and power. Difficulties may result from social ossification too, as more and more people become invested in stability. Revolutionary change often waits until a new generation can grab the reins of power from the previous one, and that process might be altered considerably.

Developing new visions of the human life trajectory would be challenging as well, because it is far from obvious how marriage, jobs, education, childbearing, and the other of life's passages would be best integrated into much longer lives. New life strategies would have to evolve as they did with the arrival of birth control, the emancipation of women, or the 30-year increase in life expectancy in the developed world during the 1900s, and the shifts would not be easy ones.

The benefits from extending human life span, however, would be more than personal. William Nordhaus at Yale University estimates that half the standard-of-living increase in the United States during the past century rests upon the 30-year increase in longevity in that period.[4] Today, it takes decades of education and experience to teach us to handle ourselves effectively in the world, and people often are just beginning to hit their groove when they begin to tire and fade. Extending our prime even a few decades would act as a remarkable infusion of talent and energy into the world.

Without question, effective antiaging interventions would change society in many ways, but advance preparation can't help much, simply because there are so many possible paths before us. And I haven't even looked at how antiaging technology might interact with other coming technological advances outside of the life sciences. Any preparations we make today are mere guesswork, but there are a few adjustments we can and should make.

We should, for example, root out systemic social rigidities that are sensitive to demographic and longevity shifts. To have social security benefits kick in at a certain age is unnecessarily rigid. Retirement and benefits instead should be keyed to health or performance indices. And wherever possible, choices should be placed in the hands of the individual. For example, the private social security accounts pioneered by Jose Pinera in Chile[5] and now used in nearly 20 countries is a far more robust way of supporting retirement than the social security monoliths of Western Europe and the United States. With these buckling under today's changes in family size and demographics, what would they do with real antiaging medicine?

Even the idea of striving to extend our lives, however, is discomforting to many. The goal seems so unworthy and narcissistic. It is the nobility of self-sacrifice and the heroism of risking death for the common good that we celebrate. Reaching for longevity evokes images of cowards on the deck of the Titanic pushing aside women and children to reach the lifeboats, hypochondriacs counting their vitamins and avoiding anyone with a cough, or even vampires sucking the blood of innocents.[6]

However, we must look more deeply at the source of our repugnance, because the context that brings extended life spans may soon change. Today, struggling for more life involves intense self-focus and is largely futile in any event. But meaningful breakthroughs in the biology of aging might alter this.

Taking a pill to extend our years—an intervention vastly different from the self-starvation of caloric restriction—would be neither selfish nor self-absorbed. It would be common sense. And if we could alter embryos or children to double their expected life span, the added years would not tarnish these beneficiaries any more than we've been tarnished by antibiotics and vaccines.

We are at the start of a new millennium, and at the end of this millennium, when future humans look back at our era, they will see it as a unique, extraordinary moment that reshaped the meaning and trajectory of human life. Machine intelligence, nanotechnology, genetic engineering, and space exploration are among the seminal developments taking place today. But the ragged frontiers of aging will be where the real action is, because our next frontier is not space, but our own biology, and we care so much about aging and death.

Of all the things that advancing technology may bring us, the most consequential would be to roll back the limits of our own life spans. When your brain is turning to mush from Alzheimer disease or when cancer is sucking away your life, all the telecommunications, artificial intelligence, and special effects in the world will seem of little consequence. We are creatures of flesh and blood, and, ultimately, it is the health and vitality of this tissue that will shape our lives.

REFERENCES

1. DE GREY, A. *et al.* 2002. Is human aging still mysterious enough to be left only to scientists? Bioessays **24:** 667–676.
2. PARTRIDGE, L. & D. GEMS. 2002. Mechanisms of ageing: private or public? Nature Rev. Genet. **3:** 165–175.
3. TEMPLE, L. *et al.* 2001. Defining disease in the genomics era. Science **293:** 807–808.
4. NORDHAUS, W. 1999. The Health of Nations: The Contribution of Improved Health to Living Standards. NBER Working Paper No. w8818, February 2002, National Bureau of Economic Research.
5. PINERA, J. 1995. Empowering workers: the privatization of social security in Chile. Cato J. **15:** 155–166
6. STOCK, G. 2002. Redesigning Humans: Our Inevitable Genetic Future. Page Houghton Mifflin. New York.

Report on the Open Discussion on the Future of Life Extension Research

AUBREY D. N. J. DE GREY

Department of Genetics, University of Cambridge, Cambridge CB2 3EH, United Kingdom

> ABSTRACT: Following a highly stimulating series of talks on the social and ethical implications of greatly extended life spans, a discussion of the issues was held, in which a series of straw polls was conducted. An alarming conclusion from these polls was that most participants thought it either probable or "not improbable" that comprehensive functional rejuvenation of middle-aged mice would be possible within 10–20 years, but also felt that biogerontologists should not yet discuss timescales (either for mouse rejuvenation or similar progress in humans) in society at large. This combination of views may be very dangerous, as it assumes that humanity will need little forward planning to transition smoothly from its current almost universal fatalism concerning the defeat of aging to a widespread appreciation of its foreseeability or even imminence.
>
> KEYWORDS: life extension research; public debate; timescales

The "nonbiology" (ethics, sociology, and politics) session of IABG10 concluded with a short open discussion about the issues raised during the session and earlier in the conference. This discussion (like the rest of the session) was bravely chaired by Tom Kirkwood, to whom much thanks is due.

The bulk of the discussion consisted of a series of straw polls, arising largely from a suggestion by Patrick Dixon following my short talk[1] that began the session. First, delegates were asked whether they favor or oppose open public debate about the direction of biomedical gerontology, and there was virtual unanimity in favor. The next poll asked whether such discussion should emphasise the possible life extension resulting from such work or the possible health extension; here again the vote was nearly unanimous, with health extension being the favored emphasis. I noted that the difficulty with making a stark contrast between the two was that they were almost certain to occur hand in hand—that being frail is risky and being robust is not, so that extending healthy life span will tend to extend total life span, too. Donald Ingram pointed out that the healthy/total distinction was closely related to the context of publicly funded biogerontology work in the United States, given that (to take the most explicit example) the National Institute on Aging is a part of the National Institutes of Health, and its inauguration was made difficult by the perception that aging is not a disease.

Address for correspondence: Aubrey D.N.J. de Grey, Department of Genetics, University of Cambridge, Downing Street, Cambridge CB2 3EH, UK. Voice: +44-1223-765665; fax: +44-1223-333992.
  ag24@gen.cam.ac.uk

The remaining straw polls and discussion centered on timescales and were extremely instructive with regard to optimism about rates of progress compared to what is generally stated by biogerontologists in more public forums. The first poll asked whether it was probable that "robust mouse rejuvenation" (RMR) would be developed within a decade. (I had defined this term quantitatively earlier as a treatment of mice of a strain with a natural life expectancy of three years, starting when they were already two years old, which trebles their remaining life expectancy—i.e., gives them an average age at death of five years.) A remarkable 30% of the audience considered that this was probable, with 15% or so disagreeing and the majority abstaining. This poll was followed by one asking the same question with a two-decade timescale, and on this vote very few said the prospect was improbable; the vote was split roughly equally between those saying it was probable and those abstaining.

The value of these polls might be questioned: after all, as has been said, you do not resolve a scientific question by voting. However, in this case the polls were given very considerable significance by their juxtaposition with the remaining poll, in which delegates were asked how they viewed the public discussion of timescales (for robust mouse rejuvenation or for any level of human life extension) by experts in the field. There was a large majority opposed to the pursuit of such topics in public forums at this time. Michael Rae opined that it would be reasonable to discuss timescales for human life extension as and when we had achieved robust mouse rejuvenation, but not until then. I protested that delaying such a debate until that time would be foolish, despite the acknowledged limits of our confidence in any such predictions, first, because the achievement of RMR could be greatly accelerated by a widespread public awareness of its relevance to human life extension, and second, because that awareness would become very widespread overnight once something like RMR was reached, with consequently huge social turbulence that might have been greatly diminished by forward planning on the part of policymakers—something that is unlikely while they remain oblivious of the possible timescales. William Bains rejoined that this was not a plausible scenario and that talk of timescales was likely to do more harm than good in the long run, as anticipated timelines failed to materialize (as they so often do). I noted the conspicuous counterexample of the war on cancer, whose funding has seen consistent increases since Nixon's 1971 speech, despite the much more modest progress that was predicted then.

Kirkwood closed the discussion with a prediction on which there was no likelihood of dissent: that this debate will be with us for some time to come. Doubtless it will resurface at the 11th IABG, as well as many times before and after.

REFERENCE

1. DE GREY, A.D.N.J. 2004. Biogerontologists' duty to discuss timescales publicly. Ann. N.Y. Acad. Sci. **1019**: 542–545.

Mechanisms of Hormesis through Mild Heat Stress on Human Cells

SURESH I. S. RATTAN

Danish Centre for Molecular Gerontology, Department of Molecular Biology, University of Aarhus, DK-8000 Aarhus–C, Denmark

ABSTRACT: In a series of experimental studies, it was shown that repetitive mild heat stress has antiaging hormetic effects on growth and various other cellular and biochemical characteristics of human skin fibroblasts undergoing aging *in vitro*. We have reported the hormetic effects of repeated challenge at the levels of maintenance of stress protein profile; reduction in the accumulation of oxidatively and glycoxidatively damaged proteins; stimulation of the proteasomal activities for the degradation of abnormal proteins; improved cellular resistance to ethanol, hydrogen peroxide, and ultraviolet-B rays; and enhanced levels of various antioxidant enzymes. Detailed analysis of the signal transduction pathways to determine alterations in the phosphorylation and dephosphorylation states of ERK, JNK, and p38 MAP kinases as a measure of cellular responsiveness to mild and severe heat stress is in progress. Furthermore, comparative studies using nonaging immortal cell lines, such as SV40-transformed human fibroblasts, spontaneous osteosarcoma cells, and telomerase-immortalized human bone marrow cells are also in progress for establishing differences in normal and cancerous cells for their responsiveness to mild and severe stresses.

KEYWORDS: aging; antiaging; heat shock; signal transduction; proteasome

INTRODUCTION

Because aging is characterized by a decrease in the adaptive abilities due to progressive failure of maintenance and repair mechanisms, it has been hypothesized that if cells and organisms are exposed to brief periods of mild stress, one should observe antiaging, health-improving, and longevity-promoting effects. Such a response to low doses of otherwise harmful conditions improving the functional ability of cells and organisms is known as hormesis. However, the harmful effects of high doses have long shadowed the hormetic effects of low-level stress.[1] Although most of the work on hormesis has been driven by pharmacological and toxicological studies, applying hormesis in aging research and therapy is a recent development.[2,3]

Using a mild stress protocol of exposing serially passaged human fibroblasts to 41°C for 1 h twice a week throughout their replicative life span *in vitro*, we have re-

Address for correspondence: Dr. Suresh I.S. Rattan, Department of Molecular Biology, University of Aarhus, Gustav Wieds Vej 10C, DK-8000 Aarhus–C, Denmark. Voice: +45-8942-5034; fax: +45-8612-3178.
   rattan@imsb.au.dk

ported several beneficial antiaging effects. These effects included the maintenance of youthful morphology, reduced accumulation of damaged proteins,[2,4–6] increased levels of various heat shock proteins (Hsp), increased proteasomal activities, increased antioxidative abilities, and increased resistance to ethanol, hydrogen peroxide, and UV-A irradiation.[7] The available data so far are proving highly valuable in understanding the molecular mechanisms of antiaging hormetic effects of repeated mild heat stress (RMHS) on human and other systems.

HEAT SHOCK RESPONSE

Heat shock (HS) response is one of the primordial intracellular defense mechanisms against stressful conditions. Optimal HS response for Hsp synthesis and activity is essential for cell survival. The cellular stress response can be viewed as an adaptative or "survival instinct" response for the defense and maintenance of its structural and functional integrity.[8] Signaling pathways involved in HS response are still largely unknown. However, some kinases, such as stress activated protein kinase (SAPK) c-Jun terminal kinase (JNK or SAPK1) and p38 (SAPK2), are suggested to play an important role. HS activates mitogen-activated protein kinase (MAPK), extracellular signal-regulated kinase (ERK), and SAPK.[9] These kinases are involved in both survival and death pathways in response to other stresses and therefore may contribute significantly to the HS response.[10] Activation of p38 occurs very early during stress and leads to the phosphorylation of Hsp27. It is triggered by a highly specific HS sensing pathway and requires the activation of upstream kinases such as the MAPKK MKK3/6 and the MAPKKK apoptosis signal-regulating kinase-1 (ASK1). HS is also thought to activate the epidermal growth factor (EGF) receptor in an agonist-independent way.[9]

It is suggested that JNK is preferentially associated with the protective effects of HS against severe stress. A major mechanism for HS-induced JNK appears to be the direct inhibition of the JNK phosphatase that normally inactivates JNK. An early and transient activation of the JNK and p38 pathways usually is associated with survival and differentiation, whereas a late and sustained activation might point to apoptosis.[9] Our studies are in progress for the detailed analysis of the signal transduction pathways as a measure of cellular responsiveness to mild and severe heat stress.

ACTIVATION OF HEAT SHOCK FACTORS

The induction of the HS response is through heat shock factors (HSFs) working as molecular links between environmental stresses and the stress response.[8] The four vertebrate HSFs are expressed constitutively and cooperate functionally. HSFs have a nuclear localization sequence that is necessary both for the transition of HSFs from inactive to active state and for nuclear import. Using electrophoretic mobility shift assay, we have observed that RMHS at 41°C activates HSF1 and facilitates its nuclear translocation and DNA binding in human skin fibroblasts, thus initiating the HS response.[7] No studies have yet been performed on other HSFs, and also it is not known whether mild stress activates HSFs to the same extent as a severe stress at higher temperatures.

HEAT SHOCK PROTEINS

Genes encoding Hsp are highly conserved, and, in mammals, many Hsp families comprise multiple members that differ in inducibility, intracellular localization, and function.[8] Hsp play diverse roles as chaperones and/or proteases. In unstressed cells, Hsp act in successful folding, assembly, intracellular localization, secretion, regulation, and degradation of other proteins. Under conditions in which protein folding is perturbed or proteins begin to unfold and denature, Hsp have been shown to assist in protein refolding, to protect cellular systems against protein damages, to dissolve protein aggregates to some extent, to sequester overloaded and damaged proteins into larger aggregates, to target damaged proteins to degradation, and to interfere with the apoptotic program.

We have shown that the basal levels of the constitutive Hsc70 and stress-inducible Hsp70 and Hsp27 proteins increase during cellular aging of human skin fibroblasts even without any HS[7] and is interpreted as an adaptive response to increased intracellular stress during aging. Increased levels of Hsp27, Hsc70, and Hsp70 in senescent cells are indicative of their failed attempt to maintain structural and functional ability and to survive for as long as possible. In comparison, exposing these cells to repeated bouts of mild stress stimulates the synthesis of these Hsp, maintains their levels high, and helps to improve the functional ability and survival of cells without interfering with their replicative life span.[7] In contrast, the basal levels of Hsp90 decreased significantly during cellular aging with and without RMHS treatment.[7] Although the exact mechanisms for the decrease of Hsp90 are not understood, it is known that Hsp90 during stress binds to partially unfolded proteins and is degraded together with them in a manner similar to what can be observed for Hsp70 after HS. Furthermore, Hsp90 is a powerful modulator of HSF1, and the deletion of Hsp90 has been shown to promote the ability of yeast cells to launch a stress response. It therefore is possible that a decrease in the level of Hsp90 during cellular aging and after RMHS treatment is also an adaptive response resulting in the activation of HSF1, which then stimulates the transcription and translation of other HSP.

PROTEIN DEGRADATION

One of the main effects of RMHS on human cells is the reduction in the extent of accumulation of oxidatively and glycoxidatively damaged proteins.[4,5] Although this may be caused by an increase in cellular resistance of RMHS-treated cells to glucose and other protein damaging agents,[6] another possibility is the enhanced removal of abnormal proteins by increased turnover. The bulk of ATP-dependent proteolysis is conducted by the ubiquitin-proteasome system, which is a multisubunit, multicatalytic proteinase complex (MCP), or 20S proteasome. During aging, there is a decline in the activities of the proteasome, including a decreased activity of the proteasome toward artificial peptide substrates as well as the ability to preferentially degrade oxidized proteins. We have found that human skin fibroblast cells exposed to RMHS had 20–100% increased proteasome activities, without any accompanied increase in the 20S proteasomal content. Furthermore, this increase in proteasomal activities was related to a significant increase in the amount of the proteasome activator 11S, which is an adaptor between the 20S proteasome and some of the chaperones in the cytosol. Although we have not yet determined the extent of transcription and translation of 11S activator, we have observed that the number of 11S units bound to the 20S proteasome were significantly higher in RMHS-treated cells.[11] Such an increased binding makes it possible for the RMHS-treated cells to activate the proteasome faster than the unstressed cells.

Lysosome is the other major cellular proteolytic system affected by aging. The Hsc73-specific lysosomal-proteolytic pathway is inhibited in senescent fibroblasts.[12] Accumulation of lipofuscin, which is an aggregate of oxidized proteins and lipids, affects the lysosomal activities. However, no studies have yet been done on the effects of RMHS on lysosome-mediated protein degradation.

Finally, antiaging hormetic effects of mild heat shock appear to be facilitated by reducing protein damage and protein aggregation by activating internal antioxidant, repair, and degradation processes. Hsp are involved in preventing the accumulation of highly damaged proteins during aging, because they govern both the repair of weakly damaged proteins and the catabolism of highly damaged proteins. Thus, hormetic pathways are suggested to activate several key proteins involved in the stress response. Indeed, hormesis leads to the maintenance of the HS response during aging, and the concomitant transitory and moderate overexpression of Hsp in cells and organisms is greatly beneficial.

ACKNOWLEDGMENTS

This project is a part of the shared cost action programme FUNCTIONAGE under the EU Biomed & Health Programme and Quality of Life Projects. Research grants from the Danish Medical Council (SSVF), Danish Research Council (SNF), and Senetek PLC are also acknowledged.

REFERENCES

1. CALABRESE, E.J. & L.A. BALDWIN. 2003. Toxicology rethinks its central belief. Nature **421:** 891–892.
2. RATTAN, S.I.S. 1998. Repeated mild heat shock delays ageing in cultured human skin fibroblasts. Biochem. Mol. Biol. Int. **45:** 753–759.
3. RATTAN, S.I.S. 2001. Applying hormesis in aging research and therapy. Hum. Exp. Toxicol. **20:** 281–285.
4. VERBEKE, P., B.F.C. CLARK & S.I.S. RATTAN. 2000. Modulating cellular aging in vitro: hormetic effects of repeated mild heat stress on protein oxidation and glycation. Exp. Gerontol. **35:** 787–794.
5. VERBEKE, P., B.F.C. CLARK & S.I.S. RATTAN. 2001. Reduced levels of oxidized and glycoxidized proteins in human fibroblasts exposed to repeated mild heat shock during serial passaging in vitro. Free Radic. Biol. Med. **31:** 1593–1602.
6. VERBEKE, P., M. DERIES, B.F.C. CLARK, et al. 2002. Hormetic action of mild heat stress decreases the inducibility of protein oxidation and glycoxidation in human fibroblasts. Biogerontology **3:** 105–108.
7. FONAGER, J., R. BEEDHOLM, B.F.C. CLARK, et al. 2002. Mild stress-induced stimulation of heat shock protein synthesis and improved functional ability of human fibroblasts undergoing aging in vitro. Exp. Gerontol. **37:** 1223–1238.
8. VERBEKE, P., J. FONAGER, B.F.C. CLARK, et al. 2001. Heat shock response and ageing: mechanisms and applications. Cell Biol. Int. **25:** 845–857.

9. DORION, S. & J. LANDRY. 2002. Activation of the mitogen-activated protein kinase pathways by heat shock. Cell Stress Chaperones **7:** 200–206.
10. GABAI, V.L. & M.Y. SHERMAN. 2002. Interplay between molecular chaperones and signaling pathways in survival of heat shock. J. Appl. Physiol. **92:** 1743–1748.
11. BEEDHOLM, R., B.F.C. CLARK & S.I.S. RATTAN. 2004. Mild heat stress stimulates proteasome and its 11S activator in human fibroblasts undergoing aging in vitro. Cell Stress & Chaperones **9:** 49–57.
12. HALLÉN, A. 2002. Accumulation of insoluble protein and aging. Biogerontology **3:** 307–315.

The Arrest of Biological Time as a Bridge to Engineered Negligible Senescence

JERRY LEMLER, STEVEN B. HARRIS, CHARLES PLATT, AND TODD M. HUFFMAN

Alcor Life Extension Foundation, Scottsdale, Arizona 85260, USA

ABSTRACT: Biological systems can remain unchanged for several hundred years at cryogenic temperatures. In several hundred years, current rapid scientific and technical progress should lead to the ability to reverse any biological damage whose reversal is not forbidden by physical law. We therefore explore whether contemporary people facing terminal conditions might be preserved well enough today for their eventual recovery to be compatible with physical law. The ultrastructure of the brain can now be excellently preserved by vitrification, and solutions needed for vitrification can now be distributed through organs with retention of organ viability after transplantation. Current law requires a few minutes of cardiac arrest before cryopreservation of terminal patients, but dogs and cats have recovered excellent brain function after 16–60 min of complete cerebral ischemia. The arrest of biological time as a bridge to engineered negligible senescence, therefore, appears consistent with current scientific and medical knowledge.

KEYWORDS: cryopreservation; vitrification; cryonics; cryogenics

In 1971, the eminent gerontologist, Dr. George Martin, made the following observations:[1]

> a comparatively modest investment in research could theoretically provide man with a partial and interim solution to the "terrible problem of death awareness" recently discussed by Sir John Eccles.... I must confess that the only solution which appeals to me is one which preserves the central nervous system. The spectacular success of cryobiological procedures in the long-term preservation of viability at the cellular level suggests that, in principle, satisfactory whole organ preservation may yet be achieved.... Of course,... preservation will of necessity have to be carried out *in situ*, presumably using perfusion techniques.

This suggestion, based on an original proposal by R. C. W. Ettinger,[2] is based on one fact and two assumptions. The fact is that at the boiling point of liquid nitrogen, changes in biological systems generally are agreed to be negligible for periods of hundreds to thousands of years. The first assumption is that it is possible to cool a human being to such a temperature without fundamentally destroying the essential information underlying memory and personality in the brain. The second assumption is that medical and scientific progress will continue until medical resuscitation tech-

---

Address for correspondence: Jerry Lemler, Alcor Life Extension Foundation, 7895 E. Acoma Drive, Scottsdale, AZ 85260. Voice: 480-905-1906; fax: 480-922-9027.
jlemler@alcor.org

nology is limited only by physical law. If these assumptions are correct, the memories and personalities of people preserved by today's methods should be intact after revival by future technology, and medical time travel can be used as a bridge to a time in which senescence can be controlled. Let us now briefly consider evidence pertaining to the validity of the two assumptions underlying the possibility of medical time travel.

REACHING SAFE HAVEN

Technology in the field of cryopreservation is currently undergoing revolutionary change. In 1971, the only method available for preserving viability for indefinite periods involved freezing, but today a radically different preservation method, vitrification, is available. As the name implies, vitrification allows systems to be preserved in the vitrified or glassy (noncrystalline solid) state, which eliminates the structural disruption caused by ice crystals.[3] Studies that are still ongoing have shown, using both transmission and scanning electron microscopy, that the ultrastructure of rabbit brains is well preserved using current methods to both vitrify and rewarm entire cephalic preparations (FIG. 1). The extension of similar techniques to clinically dead human beings at the Alcor Life Extension Foundation has indicated, based on visual inspection and other observations, that the human brain indeed can be vitrified even after extended periods of clinical death. Furthermore, recent studies (Y. Pichugin et al., submitted for publication) have shown that not only the ultrastructure but also the viability of rat hippocampal slices can be preserved by vitrification. In addition, rabbit kidneys transplanted after being perfused with advanced vitrification solutions have supported life with little injury (G.M. Fahy et al., submitted for publication). These observations in combination with the fact that human synapses are hardy enough even to survive after freezing and thawing[4] provide powerful support to the proposition that the essential information content of the human brain can now be kept intact during the processes required to reach low and stabilizing temperatures.

OVERCOMING LEGAL OBSTACLES

To actually implement medical time travel, the preservation process must currently be applied after the declaration of legal death. However, legal death is normally pronounced upon the cessation of heartbeat and breathing, and in our experience never involves the criteria for brain death required for organ donation. Although a brief period of cerebral ischemia is necessitated to permit the declaration of legal death, this is not an obstacle in view of recent observations that it is possible to completely resuscitate dogs after 16 minutes of unpretreated normothermic cardiac arrest with no lasting neurological deficits (TABLE 1; S.B. Harris et al., in preparation). Furthermore, it was demonstrated many years ago that damage induced by 60 min of complete normothermic cerebral ischemia in the cat could be reversed using simple methods, resulting in the permanent survival of the cat with retained locomotor, self-cleaning, and purring behaviors and with recognition of laboratory personnel.[5] Modern methods of cardiopulmonary bypass can be applied shortly after legal

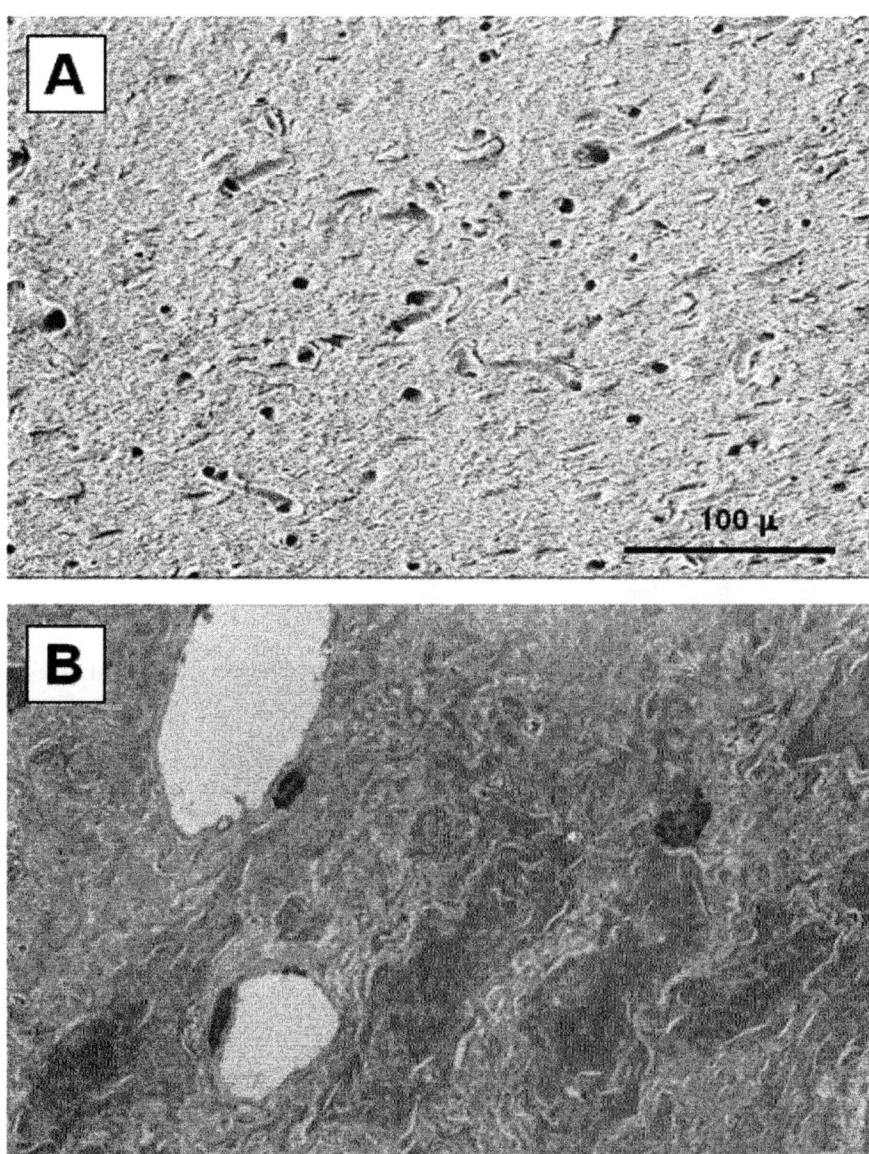

FIGURE 1. (**A**) Scanning electron microscopic image of the cerebral cortex of a New Zealand white rabbit after perfusion with M22 vitrification solution, cooling to below the glass transition temperature, and slow rewarming. Note dilated but normal capillary structure, smooth neuropil, and absence of large (~20–200 μm) disorganized cavities in the tissue that normally result from ice formation. (**B**) Transmission electron microscopic image of the hippocampal dentate gyrus, showing shrunken but preserved features. The brain was fixed with a solution containing cryoprotectant and then slowly diluted in low-osmolality Karnovsky's fixative until all cryoprotectant was removed before being processed for scanning or transmission electron microscopy.

TABLE 1. Dogs surviving with no neurological deficit after prolonged normothermic cardiac and circulatory arrest induced by ventricular fibrillation[a]

Dog number and name	Tympanic temperature[b]	Time with MAP below 30 mmHg
2 (Cerberus)	35.9	14 min 15 s
5 (Scroffy)	37.3	14 min 45 s
6 (Claudia)	38.0	14 min 48 s
10 (Maude)	37.7	15 min 45 s
14 (Bob)	37.7	15 min 25 s
16 (Stuart)	37.6	16 min 15 s

[a]Dogs were resuscitated after the periods shown by immediate cardiopulmonary bypass, rapid postinsult cooling to 34°C, and a complex pharmacological support protocol that will be described elsewhere (Harris *et al.*, in preparation). All dogs were allowed to survive for at least 6 months after resuscitation.

[b]Temperature just before electrically induced ventricular fibrillation. Tympanic temperature closely approximates intracerebral temperature in canines. Courtesy of Critical Care Research, Inc.

NOTE: MAP, mean arterial pressure (objective marker of circulatory arrest).

(clinical) death and are unequivocally able to maintain the biological viability of both the brain and the body for extended periods until cryopreservation is initiated. Therefore, application of advanced vitrification methods to human beings after legal death is not medically invalidated by warm ischemic injury.

THE LIMITS OF REPAIR

Once cooled to safely below the glass transition temperature, there is no known time limit beyond which safe storage cannot continue.[6] Therefore, the possibility of successfully reviving would-be time travelers must be considered in the light of technological advances of the indefinite future. Assuming technological progress continues until fundamental physical limits are reached, any required repair process that is consistent with physical law should become available to rescue contemporary people.

In considering the possibility of repair, we can distinguish between two fundamentally different kinds of injury. The first kind of injury involves, in essence, the rearrangement, misfolding, or chemical modification of the molecules constituting the patient, but especially of molecules constituting the patient's brain. The reversal of this kind of injury will require the ability to recognize and correct molecular changes. The fact that biological systems already perform these functions on a continuous basis implies that repairs of this nature are consistent with physical law, and detailed engineering calculations and designs for molecular recognition and manipulation systems of the kind that would be capable of effecting the required repair processes are available.[7–9] Quantitative descriptions of possible repair scenarios also have been described.[10]

The second kind of injury involves the outright loss of biological information, such as might be induced by major gunshot wounds to the brain or several days of postmortem autolysis. Although any injury may be repairable in which the original state of the patient can be inferred from the damaged state, there are clearly modes of death in which complete or even partial inference of the correct structure will be impossible, and in this case no repair technology, no matter how advanced, can be successful. Complete erasure of the patient's identity in this way has been called "information theoretic death"[10] and, unlike "clinical death," represents true death of the individual. Unfortunately, current knowledge is insufficient to determine whether information theoretic death has taken place in some cases, or whether partial loss of information is sufficient to render future repair pointless. However, in most cases, these uncertainties and dilemmas need not arise.

CONCLUSIONS

Medical time travel is consistent with current medical and scientific knowledge and may offer a bridge to the future for those who cannot wait for the development of engineered negligible senescence. Information on the many facets of this procedure that cannot be discussed in this short space can be obtained at <http://www.merkle.com/cryo/techFeas.html>, <http://www.nanomedicine.com/NMI.htm>, <http://www.nanomedicine.com/NMIIA.htm>, and <http://www.alcor.org>.

REFERENCES

1. MARTIN, G.M. 1971. Brief proposal on immortality: an interim solution. Perspect. Biol. Med. **14:** 339–340.
2. ETTINGER, R.C.W. 1964. The Prospect of Immortality. Doubleday. New York.
3. FAHY, G.M., D.R. MACFARLANE, C.A. ANGELL & H.T. MERYMAN. 1984. Vitrification as an approach to cryopreservation. Cryobiology **21:** 407–426.
4. ANONYMOUS. The cryobiological case for cryonics. <http://www.alcor.org/Library/html/caseforcryonics.html>.
5. HOSSMANN, K.A., R. SCHMIDT-KASTNER & P.B. GROSSE. 1987. Recovery of integrative central nervous function after one hour global cerebro-circulatory arrest in normothermic cat. J. Neurol. Sci. **77:** 305–320.
6. MAZUR, P. 1984. Freezing of living cells: mechanisms and implications. Am. J. Physiol. **247:** C125–C142.
7. DREXLER, K.E. 1992. Nanosystems: Molecular Machinery, Manufacturing, and Computation. Wiley. New York.
8. FREITAS, R.A. 1999. Nanomedicine. Vol 1. Basic Capabilities. Landes Bioscience. Austin, TX.
9. FREITAS, R.A. 2003. Nanomedicine. Vol 2. Biocompatibility. Landes Bioscience. Austin, TX.
10. MERKLE, R.C. 1992. The technical feasibility of cryonics. Med. Hypotheses **39:** 6–16.

Apolipoprotein E Genotype and Age at Menopause

JALAL KOOCHMESHGI, SEYED MEHDI HOSSEINI-MAZINANI, SEYED MORTEZA SEIFATI, NASRIN HOSEIN-PUR-NOBARI, AND LADAN TEIMOORI-TOOLABI

National Research Center for Genetic Engineering and Biotechnology, Tehran, Iran

ABSTRACT: We tested the hypothesis that there is a connection between apolipoprotein E (*APOE*) genotype and age at menopause. A sample of women aged between 50 and 60 years who had reached natural menopause was studied. Survival analysis of data showed a significant relationship between *APOE* genotype and age at menopause, carriers of the *APOE*4 allele reaching menopause at an earlier age. Our findings can have a bearing on the question of the evolution of this major human polymorphism and human life history. These findings are also relevant to the question of the connection between reproductive parameters and age-associated diseases.

KEYWORDS: apolipoprotein E; menopause; life history

INTRODUCTION

Apolipoprotein E (APOE) is produced mainly in the liver and found in plasma as a constituent of very-low-density lipoprotein (VLDL) and chylomicrons. It was first recognized for its important role in extracellular lipid transport and metabolism, but later also emerged as a major determinant in several biological processes not obviously related to its role in lipid transport, including Alzheimer disease.[1]

APOE is a polymorphic gene and has three variants, E2, E3, and E4. Case–control association studies have widely implicated E2/E3/E4 polymorphism in several age-associated diseases and conditions, notably coronary heart disease, Alzheimer disease, and osteoporotic fractures, with *APOE*4 allele being associated with these conditions.[2–4]

In an interesting parallel, age at menopause in women shows a connection with the same age-associated diseases and conditions, an early age at menopause being a major risk factor.[5] Noticing this parallel, we proposed that there may be a relationship between *APOE* genotype and age at menopause.

In a broader context, life-history studies lend substance to this hypothesis: several studies have connected *APOE* genotype and life span, with *APOE*4 allele being associated with a shorter life span.[6] Remembering that life span is linked to reproductive schedule across species,[7] one wonders whether this gene may influence

Address for correspondence: Jalal Koochmeshgi, National Research Center for Genetic Engineering and Biotechnology, P.O. Box 14155-6343, Tehran, Iran.
jkoochmeshgi@yahoo.co.uk

reproductive parameters (age at menopause among them) as well as life span in humans.

MATERIALS AND METHODS

We studied a sample of retired female teachers aged between 50 and 60 who had reached natural menopause. Menopausal status was defined as absence of menstrual cycles for 12 consecutive months, first beginning at over the age of 40 and in the absence of iatrogenic causes.

Subjects were recruited using the registry of the Association of Retired Teachers, Tehran, Iran. Female members of the association who fell within the age frame were randomly contacted by phone through the association. The study was explained to them and they were invited to participate. To control for possible sources of bias in sampling, we asked those who declined whether they could share the grounds for their decision.

Those who consented to participate in the study answered a subject selection phone questionnaire administered by female physicians. At this stage, individuals who had not reached menopause and also those whose age at menopause could not be determined due to hysterectomy and/or ovariectomy, introduction of hormone replacement therapy before menopause, or continuous use of oral contraceptive pills, were excluded.

After signing the consent form, the subjects who were selected sat for a detailed interview. Age at menopause was meticulously determined during the process of gathering clinical history. Major factors known to influence age at menopause also were investigated. These included history of smoking, marital status, and handedness. To avoid ethnicity bias, we established geographical origin of both parents.

Venous blood (2–5 mL) was obtained for DNA analysis. *APOE* genotyping was performed by the standard PCR-RFLP method. Survival analysis for the age at menopause was performed by Kaplan-Meier and Cox regression tests using SPSS statistical software.

RESULTS AND DISCUSSION

To date, 242 subjects have been selected for interview. No compliance bias and no ethnicity bias could be discerned. In 161 of these subjects, age at menopause could be determined to half a year. This is expected in a retrospective study in which problems with recollection make it difficult to verify age at menopause in many subjects. Nonetheless, because of the convenience of retrospective studies, most studies on factors affecting the age at menopause follow this design.

In most human populations studied, relative scarcity of E2 and E4 alleles make E2/E2 and E4/E4 homozygotes very rare; therefore, following an established procedure, we assigned subjects to three genotype groups: genotype group E2 (genotypes E2/E2 and E3/E2), genotype group 3 (E3/E3), and genotype group 4 (E4/E4 and E3/E4). In our sample, among those with a verified age at menopause, genotype group 2 comprises 22 subjects (13.7%), genotype group 3 includes 113 subjects (70.2%), and genotype group 4 consists of 26 subjects (16.1%). This distribution is consistent

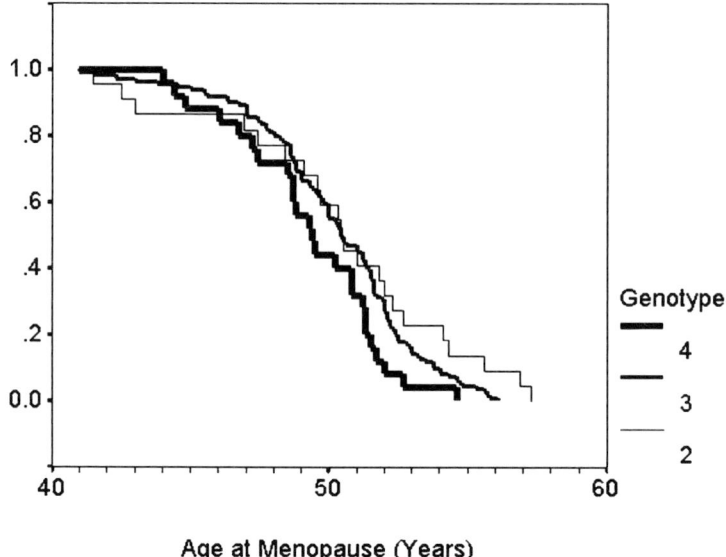

FIGURE 1. Survival curves for age at menopause according to apolipoprotein E genotype.

with data available on the distribution of APOE variants in the general Iranian population from studies of our group (unpublished data).

Survival curves for the age at menopause in three genotype groups are shown in FIGURE 1. The effect of *APOE* genotype on the age at menopause was examined using the multivariate Cox regression method. Three main factors known to influence age at menopause—smoking, marital status, and handedness—were taken into account. *APOE* genotype affected age at menopause as an independent predictor. *APOE* genotype group E4 predicted an earlier age at menopause compared with the two other genotype groups ($P = .049$).

It has been well established that age at menopause is a complex trait influenced by genes and environment. However, study of specific genes influencing age at menopause is in its infancy. We are continuing our study and complementing it with several other candidate genes.

Phylogenetic studies have suggested that *APOE*4 is the ancestral human apolipoprotein E allele, from which the E2 and E3 alleles have evolved.[8] Finch and Sapolsky were the first to consider APOE variants in the context of life history.[9] They argued that *APOE*3 may have been selected during the evolution of the unique role of grandmothering in early humans and that the advantages of grandmothers who are mentally and physically fit by the minimization of Alzheimer disease and coronary artery disease would select for the spread of the *APOE*3 allele.[9] Our findings, though, suggest that at some time during human evolution, age at menopause actually moved forward concurrent with the increase in *APOE*3 and *APOE*2 allelic frequencies (whether at that time humans lived long enough for this time shift—or the phenomenon of menopause itself—to materialize is another question worth contemplating). To gain a more comprehensive view of the subject, we have included other reproductive parameters (e.g., age at menarche and number of offspring) in our ongoing study. We interpret our findings in the context of the evolution of human life history in response to changes in environment, diet, and lifestyle, as well as social structures. These findings are also relevant to the question of the connection between reproductive parameters and age-associated diseases.

ACKNOWLEDGMENTS

We thank the members of the Association of Retired Teachers, Tehran, Iran, for their kind and valuable assistance. Special thanks are due to Yadollah Pooyan, director, and Fahimeh Farzanegan, secretary of the Association. One of the authors (J.K.) thanks Mohammad Hossein Sanati for his crucial support of this research project, and the Wellcome Trust for a travel award to attend the IABG10.

REFERENCES

1. MAHLEY, R.W. & S.C. RALL. 2000. Apolipoprotein E: far more than a lipid transport protein. Annu. Rev. Genomics Hum. Genet. **1:** 507–537.
2. DE KNIJFF, P. & L.M. HAVEKES. 1996. Apolipoprotein E as a risk factor for coronary heart disease: a genetic and molecular biology approach. Curr. Opin. Lipidol. **7:** 59–63.
3. CEDAZO-MINGUEZ, Z. & R.F. COWBURN. 2001. Apolipoprotein E: a major piece in the Alzheimer's disease puzzle. J. Cell. Mol. Med. **5:** 254–266.
4. CAULEY, J.A., J.M. ZMUDA, K. YAFFE, *et al.* 1999. Apolipoprotein E polymorphism: a new genetic marker of hip fracture risk—the study of osteoporotic fractures. J. Bone Miner. Res. **14:** 1175–1181.
5. MASSART, F., J.Y. REGINSTER & M.L. BRANDI. 2001. Genetics of menopause associated diseases. Maturitas **40:** 103–116.
6. SCHACHTER, F., L. FAURE-DELANEF, F. GUENOT, *et al.* 1994. Genetic associations with human longevity at the APOE and ACE loci. Nat. Genet. **6:** 29–32.
7. RICKLEFS, R.E. & G.L. MILLER. 2000. Ecology. 4th ed. Freeman. New York.
8. MAHLEY, R.W. 1988. Apolipoprotein E: cholesterol transport protein with expanding role in cell biology. Science **240:** 622–630.
9. FINCH, C.E. & R.M. SAPLOSKY. 1999. The evolution of Alzheimer disease, the reproductive schedule, and apoE isoforms. Neurobiol. Aging **20:** 407–428.

ns and the
The Molecular Chaperones and the Phenomena of Cellular Immortalization and Apoptosis *in Vitro*

JENS KRØLL

Hafnia Unit of Biogerontology, Frederiksberg, Denmark

ABSTRACT: The molecular chaperones are housekeeping molecules that assist in the folding and prevention of the aggregation of proteins and nucleotides, as well as participating in the elimination of ubiquitinated molecules. Evidence is reviewed to suggest that the Werner protein is a DNA chaperone and also that an increase in the expression of the molecular chaperones is the common denominator in the extension of cellular and species longevity as well as in the process of cellular immortalization, the inherent immortality of germ cells, and the inhibition of cellular apoptosis. It is possible that the immortalization of normal somatic cells is caused by an accidental reprogramming of the genome, recreating the chaperone expression of the germ cells. It is suggested that the molecular chaperones are evolution facilitators determining the life span of individual cells as the evolution of longevity in species.

KEYWORDS: protein chaperones; RNA chaperones; DNA chaperones; Werner protein; heat shock proteins; cellular immortalization; apoptosis; cancer; aging

HOUSEKEEPING CHAPERONES

The molecular chaperones are highly conserved proteins that participate in such "housekeeping" functions as assisting in the folding of proteins and nucleotides, prevention of aggregation of polymers, disaggregatiion of misfolded molecules, facilitation of polymer transport across biological membranes, and participation in the degradation of ubiquitinated molecules.[1]

CHAPERONE SPECIES

Protein Chaperones

The protein chaperones often cooperate in more or less complex chaperone machines as, for example, Hsp90, Hsp70, Hop, Hsp40, and p23 in association with the steroid receptor, or Hsp90 and p23 in association with telomerase.

Address for correspondence: Jens Krøll, Hafnia Unit of Biogerontology, Godthåbsvej 111,3, DK-2000 Frederiksberg, Denmark. Voice: +45-38862220.
krollj@danbbs.dk

Ann. N.Y. Acad. Sci. 1019: 568–571 (2004). © 2004 New York Academy of Sciences.
doi: 10.1196/annals.1297.106

Nucleotide Chaperones

The DEAD box proteins, for example, SV40T and the human homologue p68, are RNA-dependent ATPases and RNA helicases that were recently shown to be RNA chaperones.[2] The Werner protein (WRN) is a DNA-dependent ATPase and DNA helicase covalently associated with the SUMO-1 ubiquitin. WRN is active in unwinding alternate DNA structures, such as DNA–RNA hybrids and triplexes and tetraplexes, that may cause genomic instability;[3] WRN is a possible DNA chaperone.

Hsp90 is unique among the protein chaperones from a highly conserved nucleotide binding pocket, shared by DNA gyrases and DNA repair proteins. It is possible that Hsp90 includes nucleotides in its chaperoning activities, as, for example, in cooperation with p23 to serve as a chaperone for telomeric DNA.

CHAPERONES AND LONGEVITY

Longevity of Cells

Transfection with individual chaperones as, for example, Hsp70 or SV40T, extends the life span of fibroblasts *in vitro*; hormetic procedures do this by increasing the expression of Hsp70. The drastic reduction in the level of Hsp90 during aging *in vitro*[4] suggests a possible antagonistic effect of this chaperone on replicative senescence.

Longevity of Species

The molecular chaperones also influence the longevity of species. Thus, an upregulation of Hsp70 extends the life span of *Caenorhabditis elegans* and of senescence-accelerated mice. Also, the extension of mammalian life span due to caloric restriction correlates with an increase in the expression of Hsp70

CHAPERONES AND CELLULAR IMMORTALIZATION

Although the extension of the cellular life span *in vitro* after transfection with individual chaperones occurs with high frequency, the frequency of immortalization of normal human somatic cells is exceedingly low, approximately 10^{-7}, although this can vary, depending on tissue and immortalization procedure. An increase in chaperone expression is a common feature of immortalized cells. A further indication that heat shock proteins are causally involved in the process is the observation that cellular immortalization can be induced by heat shock procedures, by selecting cells with a high inherent chaperone defense. An obvious advantage of this approach for the generation of immortalized cell lines is the avoidance of transfection with viral carriers, as used in other immortalization procedures.

Cellular immortalization observed after exposure to mutagens is, in addition to hyperexpression of the chaperones, accompanied by genomic instability. Changes are also observed after transfection with oncogenes, such as c-*myc* and SV40T, where the interference with tumor-suppressor gene products, such as p53, p21, p16, and pRb, predisposes to neoplastic transformation. The cellular immortalization phenomenon probably occurs not because of, but despite, this interference. In fact, the unimportance of these changes for the immortalization phenomenon is demonstrated from the cellular immortalization induced by transfection with h-TERT. Here, the immortalization of normal differentiated cells is not a consequence of telomerase activity *per se*, but is possibly related to an increase in the expression of the functionally associated chaperones Hsp90 and p23.

Cellular immortalization by "alternative lengthening of telomeres" (ALT) depends on the associated promyelocytic leukemia (PML) bodies, the described functions and structure of which highly resemble that of a Hsp60 chaperonin complex.[5] Immortalization induced by overexpression of VEGF also involves the ALT mechanism.[6]

The chaperone expression is increased in immortalized cancer cell lines, but cellular immortalization is not a precondition for malignant cell growth. In fact, most mammary carcinoma explants succumb to replicative senescence *in vitro*; also, cell lines immortalized by transfection with h-TERT shows no signs of invasive growth after transplantation *in vivo*.

CHAPERONES AND INHERENT CELLULAR IMMORTALITY

A support for the suggestion that the molecular chaperones are of crucial importance for cellular immortality *in vitro* is the fact that the expression of the molecular chaperones is relatively high in inherently immortal cells. Thus, the level of Hsp70 is relatively high in the immortal cell lines of catfish; similarly, the level of Hsp90 is relatively high in the inherently immortal mammalian germ cell lines.[7,8] Although the transfection of individual chaperones enables an extension of the life span of normal somatic cells *in vitro*, immortalization of the cells may require a coordinated up-regulation of protein and nucleotide chaperones, creating a chaperone matrix resembling that of the inherently immortal germ cells.

CHAPERONES AND APOPTOSIS

The molecular chaperones have antiapoptotic effects. This is illustrated by the observations that the elimination of Hsp70 by antisense procedures, or the inactivation of Hsp90 by specific blocking of the ATPase module of the nucleotide binding pocket by geldanamycin, induces massive cellular apoptosis.[9,10] Similarly, an apoptotic response results from inactivation of the SV40T chaperone in cells immortalized by transfection with this oncogene. Also, the apoptotic effect of p53 may result from its preferential sequestration of Hsp90.

CONCLUSIONS

The level of expression of the molecular chaperones correlates to cellular and species longevity, as well as to cellular immortalization and apoptosis. The rare event of cellular immortalization of normal somatic cells *in vitro* probably results from the clonal selection of cells with a high inherent chaperone defense or possibly from an accidental reset of the genome, recreating the nucleotide, and protein chaperone matrix of the inherently immortal germ cells, with possible emphasis on Hsp90. It has been suggested that the Werner protein is a DNA chaperone.

The molecular chaperones may be evolution facilitators, responsible for the survival of individual cells as for the evolution of longevity in species.

REFERENCES

1. KROLL, J. 2002. Molecular chaperones and the process of cellular immortalization in vitro. Biogerontology **3**: 183–185.
2. LORSCH, J.R. 2002. RNA chaperones exist and DEAD box proteins get a life. Cell. **109**: 797–800.
3. BROSH, R.M. & V.A. BOHR. 2002. Roles of the Werner syndrome protein in pathways required for maintenance of genome stability. Exp. Gerontol. **37**: 491–506.
4. FONAGER, J., R. BEEDHOLM, B.F. CLARK & S.I. RATTAN. 2002. Mild stress-induced stimulation of heat-shock protein synthesis and improved functional ability of human fibroblasts undergoing aging in vitro. Exp. Gerontol. **37**: 1223–1228.
5. HENSON, J.D., A.A. NEUMANN, T.R. YEAGER & R.R. REDDEL. 2002. Alternative lengthening of telomeres in mammalian cells. Oncogene **21**: 598–610.
6. BAIS, C., A. VAN GEELEN, P. EROLES, et al. 2003. Kaposi's sarcoma associated herpesvirus G protein-coupled receptor immortalizes human endothelial cells by activation of the VEGF receptor-2/ KDR. Cancer Cell **3**: 131–143.
7. MATSUMORI, M., H. ITOH, I. TOYOSHIMA, et al. 2002. Characterization of the 105-kDa molecular chaperone. Identification, biochemical properties, and localization. Eur. J. Biochem. **269**: 5632–5641.
8. MCLAREN, A. 2001. Mammalian germ cells: birth, sex, and immortality. Cell Struct. Funct. **26**: 119–122.
9. NYLANDSTED, J., W. WICK, U.A. HIRT, et al. 2002. Eradication of glioblastoma, and breast and colon carcinoma xenografts by Hsp70 depletion. Cancer Res. **62**: 7139–7142.
10. NIMMANAPALLI, R., E. O'BRYAN, D. KUHN, et al. 2003. Regulation of 17-AAG-induced apoptosis: role of Bcl-2, Bcl-xL, and Bax downstream of 17-AAG-mediated downregulation of Akt, Raf-1 and Src kinases. Blood **102**: 259–275.

Cirrhosis Progression as a Model of Accelerated Senescence

Affecting the Biological Aging Clock by a Breakthrough Biophysical Methodology

G. MARINEO, F. MAROTTA, AND G. SISTI

Delta Research and Development, Research Center for Medical Bioengineering, Tor vergata University, Rome, Italy

ABSTRACT: To test new treatment modalities, a pilot study with a novel noninvasive biophysical methodology (Delta-S DVD) that can artificially exert a "decrease of entropy" through the patented electromagnetic-driven delivery of "energy clusters" was designed. This process has been modulated and integrated by the body as a "self" source to support the energy-dependent functional stores, thus modifying reparative into regenerative mechanisms of liver parenchyma. Seven long-standing hepatitis C virus–positive (Child A-B) cirrhosis patients with overt symptoms and portal hypertension and failure or side effects of antiviral drug treatment underwent 40-min sessions of Delta-S DVD daily for six months and were followed up monthly. At the end of the first month, rapid improvement of symptoms and a decrease of portal hypertension were noted. At the end of treatment, all patients showed either a complete (80%) or a partial (20%) regression of fatigue (FISK score), peripheral edema, pruritus, and palmar erythema. As observed, despite having stopped beta-blockers, F1 esophageal varices disappeared (60%), whereas F2 decreased to F1. The Doppler ultrasound aspect of partial (40%) or total (20%) atrophy was either reduced (60%) or reverted to normal (20%), and the respiratory dynamics of the portal vein improved (80%) or normalized (20%), whereas gross scarring nodules disappeared in 40% of cases. These promising data pave the way for an innovative physiopathological approach with extensive clinical applications.

KEYWORDS: entropy; cirrhosis; regeneration; aging

INTRODUCTION

Thermodynamically speaking, the cell is an open system, because it is constantly exchanging material with the surrounding environment in a dynamic equilibrium between the continuous breakdown and parallel synthesis of molecules, although the constituents are apparently constant in concentration and spatial arrangement. Thus, the cell has the property of evolving toward more complex forms of organization/

Address for correspondence: Dr. Giuseppe Marineo, Delta Research and Development, Via di Mezzocammino, 85, 00187 Roma, Italy. Voice: +39-065237-1173; fax: +39-065237-1171.
g.marineo@mclink.it

Ann. N.Y. Acad. Sci. 1019: 572–576 (2004). © 2004 New York Academy of Sciences.
doi: 10.1196/annals.1297.107

differentiation, during which the system changes from a more to a less probable state; that is, entropy decreases at the expense of available energy, which clearly plays a vital role not only in maintaining life, but also in allowing proper regenerative processes. When the biochemical signals on which homeostasis of tissues depends are altered, a rapid modification occurs in the rate of renewal, which may take one of two different forms: (1) regulated enhancement of the normal rate aimed at specific purposes, such as fibrous tissue turnover; and (2) pathological enhancement uncoupled with the needs of adaptation/compensation, as in the case of cirrhosis.

Besides organ transplantation for selected cases and winning out against overcrowded waiting lists, there are no valid therapeutic options for liver cirrhosis, and a relentless progression of degenerative complications remains the dismal prospect for most patients. Although the underlying viral-associated phenomena are likely to play a relevant role in such disease, there is strong evidence that self-maintained mechanisms are taking place within the liver matrix that invariably lead to a severe morphofunctional derangement. Moreover, quite recently, it has been shown that healthy livers also undergo an age-related functional decay.[1] Thus, the biophysical approach to the treatment of liver cirrhosis was based on the theoretical possibility of treating a biological system at higher levels of complexity than is needed to perform biochemical action. The main principle of such a noninvasive technique is the "decrease of entropy," which can be artificially obtained through an electromagnetic-driven delivery of "energy clusters." This has been modulated to be highly compatible with the biological target, that is, can be used by it to support or reactivate deficient energy-dependent processes, thus modifying reparative into regenerative mechanisms of liver parenchyma. This variation is artificially induced by using electromagnetic induction to transfer "energy packets" that are generated by using such a methodology. However, using a device dedicated to dermal tissue, we had already obtained remarkable remodeling of keloids and heavy scarring abnormalities secondary to severe burns with unaltered benefit in patients who had been followed up for up to 4 years.[2,3]

MATERIALS AND METHODS

Our study population consisted of six patients with cirrhosis associated with hepatitis C virus, who showed overt symptomatology and portal hypertension. Under careful medical control, all patients were instructed to stop any vitamin or disease-specific medication (such as potassium-sparing diuretics, furosemide, β-blockers, bile acids, or albumin infusion). All patients underwent a careful clinical assessment together with validated scoring of fatigue (Fisk) and depression (Hamilton), gastroscopy, abdominal ultrasound, and Doppler ultrasound (done by experienced physicians who were unaware of the treatment), routine biochemistry, and lymphocyte subset analysis. Except for gastroscopy (done upon entry and again in 3 and 6 months), all evaluations were repeated on a monthly basis for 6 months during which daily 40-minute sessions (5 days/week) of Delta-S DVD 5.0 were performed. The "DVD 5.0" system generates nonionizing electromagnetic fields whose region is very distant from the bands "suspected" of being harmful to humans (extremely low frequency, ultrahigh frequency, microwave), whereas the power used was very low (<7 W peak-to-peak). The fields are generated by digital synthesis and dynam-

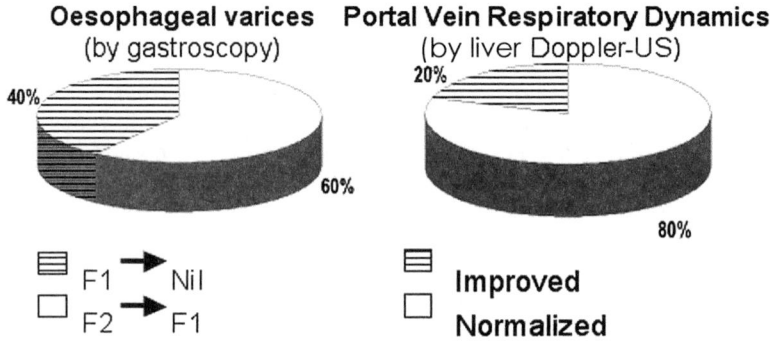

FIGURE 1. Effect of 6-month treatment with Delta DVD 5.0 in patients with cirrhosis in the absence of any medication.

ically structured in such a way so as to interact correctly with the specific application and to be transmitted through flexible irradiators surrounding the parts of the patient's body to be treated. Such fields are used to "query" the target biological system and to transfer the "energy packets," the contents of which vary as a function of the preceding query. This feedback allows a self-guidance system, because each energy transfer is analyzed iteratively by checking out several characteristics of the field using an expert system that governs in real time the dynamic modification of the fields. Further details concerning the technology may be obtained by consulting patent 01282820 registered in Rome on November 12, 1995 by the owner, G. Marineo.

RESULTS

After six months, patients showed either a complete (80%) or a partial (20%) regression of fatigue (Fisk score), a complete reversion of depression (Hamilton score), peripheral edema, and pruritus. The Doppler-ultrasound aspect of partial (40%) or total (20%) atrophy were either reduced (60%) or reverted to normal (20%), whereas overt scarring nodules disappeared in 40% of cases. Portal vein respiratory dynamics improved (80%) or normalized (20%), and, as assessed by independent observers, despite having stopped β-blockers, F1 varices disappeared (60%), whereas F2 ones were reduced to F1 levels (FIG. 1). A significant increase of active B lymphocytes and natural killer cells (mean increase: +71.2%; $P < .002$) also occurred.

CONCLUSIONS

The process of recovery may be of the reparative and/or the regenerative type, although only the latter ensures the full "restitutio ad integrum" of the pristine tissue, including its functional efficiency. In its energetic and homeostasis-maintaining aspects, biological life respects the laws of thermodynamics. Regenerative/reparative processes are energy dependent, and so they have an energy cost on which the qualitative level of the healing process presumably depends, that is, the state of the functional reserve. Thus, under a thermodynamic interpretation of the repair processes, the biological data of the form–function correspondence of a tissue or an organ or a more complex biological system may be redefined as follows: (1) Form: Maintained at the expense of usable energy. The energy that actually can be used to maintain homeostasis inevitably decreases with time, and so the form is degraded toward a more disordered state (higher entropy), because it happens during normal aging processes and after chronic disease activation of the functional reserve. (2) Function: This is also an energy-dependent process closely linked to the entropy of the tissue/organ/body, which represents an indirect measure of the latter's efficiency (the greater the entropy, the lower the function, the greater the structural disorder). It follows that if a variation of negative entropy can actually be introduced by a favorable modification from an external source, it is to be expected that an anticlockwise process will occur, namely, a regenerative event. This could conceivably be achieved by using electromagnetic induction to transfer useful energy, that is, energy that can be converted into work, an event that is apparent in the reparative processes that express the corresponding decrease in entropy in the tissues concerned. Our preliminary data show that all patients had a significant improvement in clinical, biochemical, and instrumental parameters of liver cirrhosis and despite stopping any medication. This novel biophysical technique seems to positively affect "biologically irreversible" parameters, thus representing a promising new modality to effectively treat cirrhosis and challenge aging mechanisms. On a wider scale, such a noninvasive entropy variation treatment modality, devoid of any side effects, opens a new multidisciplinary approach to age- and disease-associated organ failure, as suggested in preliminary studies,[4–7] in which extensive use is made of theoretical tools capable of rationalizing basic research procedures. A larger controlled clinical study with patients with liver cirrhosis, which also uses the gold standard measurement of portal hypertension (hepatic vein wedged pressure), is ongoing at the moment.

REFERENCES

1. CICCIOCIOPPO, R., M. CANDELLI, D. DI FRANCESCO, et al. 2003. Study of liver function in healthy elderly subjects using the ^{13}C-methacetin breath test. Aliment. Pharmacol. Ther. **17:** 271–277.
2. MARINEO, G. 1995. Application of thermodynamics in treatment of unaestheticism. V World Congress of International Society of Dermatology. October 26–29, 1995. Montecatini, Italy.
3. MARINEO, G., E. INDRIZZI, G. GASPARINI, et al. 2002. Biophysics-induced tissue regeneration. A pilot study using "Delta-S" Entropy Variation System on Burns Sequelae and Keloids. 19th Kumamoto Medical Bioscience Symp. on Cellular, Molecular and Genetic Aspects of Biological Response to Planned and Unplanned Injury. Kumamoto, Japan. (This work was awarded the Outstanding Paper Prize.)
4. MARINEO, G. & F. MAROTTA. 2002. Physiological aging process and functional reserve. Preliminary study with an experimental biophysical anti-aging treatment. 1st Asia Pacific Conf. on Anti-Ageing Medicine. Singapore.
5. MARINEO, G. & F. MAROTTA. 2002. Biophysics and aging of immune system. A pilot study on functional recovery of immunodeficiency due to aging and chronic activation-induced stress. 1st Asia Pacific Conf. on Anti Ageing Medicine. Singapore.

6. MARINEO, G. & F. MAROTTA. 2003. An innovative biophysical approach to aging of immune system. A pilot study on functional recovery of secondary immunodeficiency. 4th Annual Conf. on Regenerative Medicine. Washington, DC.
7. MARINEO, G. & F. MAROTTA. 2003. Physiological aging process and functional reserve. Preliminary study with a non-invasive biophysical anti-aging approach. Anti-Aging World Conf. Paris, France.

How an Individual Fecundity Pattern Looks in *Drosophila* and Medflies

V. N. NOVOSELTSEV,[a,b] R. ARKING,[c] J. R. CAREY,[d] J. A. NOVOSELTSEVA,[a] AND A. I. YASHIN[b,e]

[a]*Institute of Control Sciences, Moscow, Russia*

[b]*Max-Planck Institute for Demographic Research, Rostock, Germany*

[c]*Wayne State University, Detroit, Michigan, USA*

[d]*Department of Entomology, University of California, Davis, California, USA*

[e]*Sanford Institute of Public Policy, Duke University, Durham, North Carolina, USA*

ABSTRACT: Reproduction usually is characterized by a mean-population fecundity pattern. Such a pattern has a maximum at earlier ages and a subsequent gradual decline in egg production. It is shown that individual fecundity trajectories do not follow such a pattern. In particular, the regular individual fecundity pattern has no maximum so that experimentally observed maximums are average-related artifacts. The three-stage description of individual fecundity, which includes maturation, maturity, and reproductive senescence, is more appropriate. Data are presented for *Drosophila* and Mediterranean fruitfly females that clearly confirm this hypothesis. A systematic error between egg-laying scores and the regular individual pattern allows for evaluation of how close the random scores are to the pattern. The first finding of the analysis of the systematic errors is that they are consistent with the three-stage hypothesis and do not contradict the absence of the maximum in the regular individual pattern. The other finding is the existence of obvious dynamic properties of the systematic error. The slow decrease in egg-laying at the maturity stage might be the result of a cost of mating. It can also be a consequence of "structural" senescence, that is, a slow rate accumulation of oxidative damage in the gonads.

KEYWORDS: fruitfly; structural senescence; Medfly population

Each individual fly can be characterized by the set of fecundity-related traits. The first one is the onset of reproduction, x_{onset}, after which the egg-laying rises step by step to the genotype-endowed reproductive capacity (RC). Then, the constant egg-laying rate is maintained in the organism, depending on environmental conditions, until the onset of senescence occurs at age x_s. This means that the rate of egg-laying is constant at the time interval $T = (x_s - x_{onset})$. Only at $x = x_s$, when senescence occurs, does the egg-laying curve start to decrease exponentially with the time constant, τ_{tail}.

Address for correspondence: V. N. Novoseltsev, 117997 Profsoyuznaya 65, Institute of Control Sciences, Moscow, Russia.

novoselc@ipu.rssi.ru

We present data for *Drosophila* and Mediterranean fruitfly females that clearly confirm this hypothesis. To demonstrate it, we use two sets of data. The first set is a control strain of Wayne State *Drosophila* (R-strain, 493 flies) in an artificial selection experiment for increased longevity,[1,2] and the second set is a 1000-fly Medfly population.[3–5] In both cases, a flat individual fecundity pattern exists, having a constant-rate plateau period replaced by an exponential "senescent part" at some critical age.

Thus, all regular individual fecundity patterns are flat and have no maximum. The mean-population maximum in fecundity rate arises as a by-product of averaging of individual fecundity patterns across the population.[6] An individual fecundity pattern, randomly repeated, yields the "normal" mean-population pattern with a maximum at early ages, after averaging by a population.

Egg scores in each individual represent a "noisy" component, which is superimposed over the regular pattern. A systematic error of such a presentation allows for evaluation of how close, in general, the random signals are to their regular patterns. To calculate such errors, one needs to average the individual errors by the members of the population, which are at the distinct stage of their life, maturity, or senescence. The errors at the maturation stage obviously equal zero because there is no egg-laying.

The resulting averaged value of a systematic error is conditional, with a condition that at the day of averaging the flies are at the corresponding stage of their life. This means that at each day of maturity, one averages only the errors of the mature individuals. At each day of senescence, only those flies are averaged that already achieved the senescent stage. Such patterns reflect heterogeneity in egg-laying, because their final parts mirror the errors in those flies who spend the longest time at that stage, sometimes much longer than the average value for the population.

To calculate systematic errors, one needs to separate the errors related to the maturity stage from the errors related to the senescence stage. Thus, in each individual fly, we "move" the first day of her senescence to the origin of a new graphic. It becomes

$$SEM_i = \frac{1}{N_i} \sum_{j=1}^{N_i} (x_{ij} - RC_j),$$

$$SEM_i = \frac{1}{N_i} \sum_{j=1}^{N_i} (x_{ij} - RC_j \cdot \exp[-i/\tau_{j,\text{tail}}])$$

(1)

where SEM_i is a systematic error at the ith day of maturity, and SES_i is a systematic error at the ith day of senescence. In SEM_i, $(x_{ij} - RC_j)$ is an individual error of a fly j at day i, and x_{ij} is the number of eggs laid by the fly, $j = 1, ..., N_i$. Finally, N_i is the number of flies still being at the plateau at day i, and RC_j is the height of the plateau in the jth fly. For a senescence stage, SES_i, $\tau_{j,\text{tail}}$ is the time constant of the senescence "tail" for the jth fly. At the maturation stage, when there is no egg-laying, the systematic error equals zero by definition.

The results of testing the three-stage hypothesis for 493 control R-strain females in the *Drosophila* population are presented in FIGURE 1. The errors SEM_i and SES_i are given for $i = 0, 1, 2 ...$, until the last fly leaves the corresponding stage. The flies

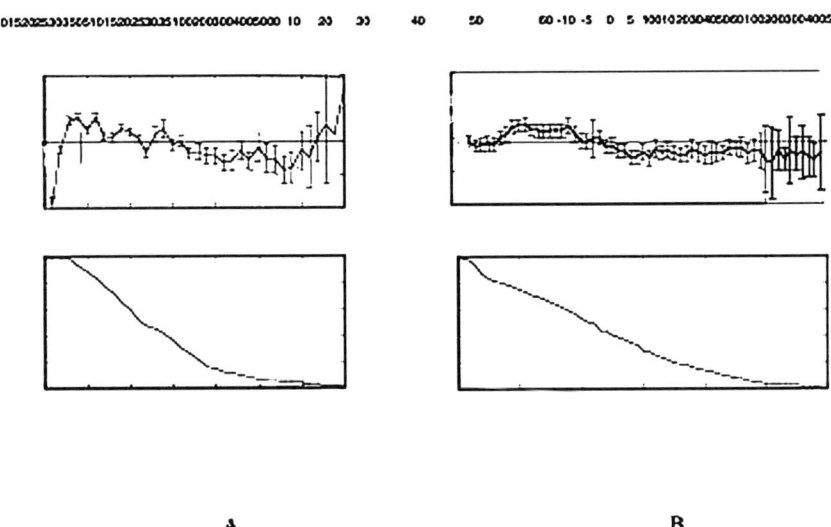

FIGURE 1. Systematic errors in Wayne State *Drosophila* population. (**A**) Maturity period. (*top*) The scores for the first, second, etc., day of maturity are compared with the corresponding level of individual fecundity plateau, *RC*, in each individual fly. The errors are averaged and the results are plotted against days of maturity. (*bottom*) The number of flies at the maturity stage. (**B**) Reproductive senescence. (*top*) The scores at reproductive senescence stage (zero day is the last day of maturity). (*bottom*) The number of flies at the senescence stage.

leaving the maturity stage join the flies at the senescence stage, and those who leave the senescence stage die.

The main finding is that the left pattern is consistent with the three-stage hypothesis and does not contradict the absence of a maximum in the regular pattern of individual fecundity. This means that there may be individual maximums in the egg-laying scores, but in this case they are randomly scattered along the plateau. After averaging, only the small excess is observed.

The second finding is the obvious dynamic property of the averaged fecundity pattern. This pattern accelerates during the first days of maturity, and at the fourth day is 7.2 eggs/day higher than the averaged level. Then, the number of eggs per day starts to decrease at a rate of ~0.6 eggs/day^2 until day 28. At the first day of maturity, all 493 flies are living and thus present in the left plate below. Then, the number of mature flies smoothly diminishes because some of them achieve the onset of senescence and leave the "steady-state" group.

The systematic errors at the senescence stage demonstrate a very smooth sliding along the exponential curve until the end of life. At the onset of senescence, the same 493 flies are alive, because no flies die at the maturity stage. Even flies that die prematurely[6] have a short senescence tail, ~1 day long. Although natural mortality decreases the number of senescing flies, the new flies, arriving from the maturity stage, slow the diminution. The process is continued until the death of the last fly.

The 1000-fly Medfly population demonstrates similar characteristics. For 4 days, the counts increase to a level that is above the prediction by four eggs per day. Then, at days 8–16, the decrease in the egg-laying rate is seen as analogous to that in *Drosophila*. This fact might be used as an argument for a reproductive senescence at the maturity stage, analogous to that in *Drosophila*. However, the subsequent increase in fecundity rate contradicts this hypothesis.

In Novoseltsev et al.,[7] it was hypothesized that a constant rate of egg-laying must be maintained at the maturity stage, but this decrease probably makes the question disputable. In particular, this decrease might be the result of a cost of mating.[8–10] It can also be a consequence of "structural" senescence at the ages of maturity, that is, a slow rate of accumulation of oxidative damage in the gonads.

REFERENCES

1. ARKING, R. 1987. Successful selection for increased longevity in *Drosophila:* analysis of the survival data and presentation of a hypothesis on the genetic regulation on longevity. Exp. Gerontol. **22:** 199–220.
2. ARKING, R., V. BURDE, K. GRAVES, et al. 2000. Identical longevity phenotypes are characterized by different patterns of gene expression and oxidative damage. Exp. Gerontol. **35:** 353–373.
3. CAREY, J.R. 1997. What demographers can learn from fruit fly actuarial models and biology. Demography **34:** 17–30.
4. CAREY, J.R., P. LIEDO, H.-G. MÜLLER, et al. 1998. Relationship of age patterns of fecundity to mortality, longevity, and lifetime reproduction in a large cohort of Mediterranean fruit fly females. J. Gerontol. Biol. Sci. **53A:** B245–B251.
5. MÜLLER, H.-G., J.R. CAREY, D.Q. WU, et al. 2001. Reproductive potential predicts longevity of female Mediterranean fruitflies. Proc. R. Soc. Lond. Ser. B **268:** 445–450.
6. NOVOSELTSEV, V.N., J.A. NOVOSELTSEVA & A.I. YASHIN. 2003. What does a fly's individual fecundity pattern look like? The dynamics of resource allocation in reproduction and ageing. Mech. Ageing Dev. **124:** 605–617.
7. NOVOSELTSEV, V.N., R.J. CAREY, J.A. NOVOSELTSEVA, et al. 2004. Systemic mechanisms of individual reproductive life history in female Medflies. Mech. Ageing Dev. **125:** 77–87.
8. PARTRIDGE, L. 1986. Sexual activity and life span. *In* Insect Aging. Strategies and Mechanisms. K.-G. Collatz & R.S. Sohal, Eds.: 45–54. Springer-Verlag. New York.
9. PITNICK, S. & F. GARSIA-GONZALES. 2002. Harm to female increases with male body size in *Drosophila melanogaster*. Proc. R. Soc. Lond. B Biol. Sci. **269:** 1821–1828.
10. PROWSE, N. & L. PARTRIDGE. 1997. The effects of reproduction on longevity and fertility in male *Drosophila melanogaster*. J. Insect Physiol. **43:** 501–512.

Mitochondria, Sex, and Mortality

IAN K. ROSS

Department of Molecular, Cellular and Developmental Biology, University of California, Santa Barbara, California 93106-9610, USA

ABSTRACT: It has been proposed that prior to the evolution of sex, the endosymbiotic relationship between mitochondria and nuclear genomes would have selected mechanisms that maintained the optimum interaction between the two genomes. Once sex evolved, mating would introduce *different, competitive*, mtDNA and/or nDNA gene products that could well upset the balance. Mechanisms, such as the specific degradation of one mitochondrial genome that is known to occur, could have been selected to prevent part of such competition. Unlike most protein complexes in the cell, the proteins of the multienzyme complexes of the ox-phos system are derived from both nuclear-genome-coded genes and mito-chondrial-genome-coded genes. Minor mutations in either mtDNA or nDNA coding for these proteins are known to lead to major and catastrophic diseases of humans, suggesting that very tight and precise interactions are required. To maintain the evolutionarily established balance after mating, *monoallelic* expression of the nuclear-coded genes would be advantageous and prevent subtly different competitive proteins from interacting with the resident mitochondria. This would require regulation of the expression of those specific nuclear genes, possibly under the control of the resident mitochondria. It is possible that *aging cells* could lose the requisite tight regulation and allow expression of proteins derived from the formerly repressed nuclear alleles that would compete for mitochondrial complex sites. With age, random failure of this control could lead to increasingly inefficient mitochondria in different tissues and organs and eventually to senescence and death.

KEYWORDS: mitochondria; mortality; aging; gene regulation

What is the evolutionary pressure behind uniparental inheritance of mitochondria? What is the basis of the random nature of death among clones (e.g., identical triplets)? Is there any connection between these phenomena? These questions have yet to be answered despite the plethora of work on mitochondria and aging mechanisms, but the work in my lab and others may suggest a testable connection and rationale for mitochondrial inheritance and random causes of death.

Mitochondria play very dynamic roles in cell behavior, affecting programmed cell death, numerous diseases, and possibly cell aging and senescence leading to Alzheimer disease and cancer, and Olson and Stenlid[1] have shown that mitochondria affect fungal virulence as plant pathogens. Current investigations center on the role

---

Address for correspondence: Ian K. Ross, Dept. of Molecular, Cellular and Developmental Biology, University of California, Santa Barbara, CA 93106-9610. Voice: 805-893-2784; fax: 805-893-4724.

ross@lifesci.ucsb.edu

of nuclear genes in regulating mitochondrial genes or physiological function, or on the affect mitochondrial gene mutations have on cell function. Considering that mitochondria are endosymbionts and that all known cases of endosymbiosis involve strict regulation of both entities—a two-way street—there has been little attention paid to the possibility of a two-way street of gene regulation.

Mitochondria in nearly all organisms from protozoa to humans are almost always inherited from only one parent. If mitochondria are carried into the zygote by the sperm[2] or where both gametes may bring mitochondria into the zygote, as in slime molds,[3] one set of mitochondria is selectively destroyed. This suggests an evolutionary necessity to have only one mitochondrial type in association with the nuclear genomes. In higher fungi, in which mating results in not one zygote but two distinct individual mycelia with identical nuclei but different mitochondria, studies have shown that the phenotypes may depend on the particular mitochondria present.[4,1] In searching for an explanation for this phenomenon, I have focused on the oxidative–phosphorylation–enzyme complexes in the mitochondria that are composed of proteins coded by both mitochondrial and nuclear genomes.

For example, the NADH dehydrogenase complex (Complex I) is a mixture of nuclear-coded proteins and mitochondrial-coded proteins that have to assemble precisely in order to operate at optimum efficiency. The numbers of nuclear/mitochondrial-coded proteins in the complex varies with species, for example, in the fungus *Neurospora* there are 25 nuclear-coded proteins and 7 mitochondrial-coded proteins, and in humans ~35 nuclear-coded proteins combine with 7 mitochondrial-encoded proteins, thus requiring appropriate interactions of far more proteins than in most protein–protein recognition systems. The complexity is such that it can be postulated that irregularities in alignment could affect the efficacy of the interaction. That these proteins must interact with structural precision is made clear by the discoveries that single base mutations in mtDNA coding, for the proteins that compose these complexes are known to lead to major and catastrophic diseases of humans.[5] It also has been reported recently that single amino acid changes in nuclear-coded proteins of Complex I can result in lethal childhood diseases.[6]

If such "minor" changes can cause such damage, it is logical to assume that mechanisms may have been selected to prevent such misalignments occurring too frequently in nature. Blier *et al.*[7] proposed that during the evolution of the relationship between mitochondria and nuclear genomes mechanisms would have been selected that maintained the optimum interaction between the two genomes. Successful interactions would have been maintained by asexual, mitotic, multiplication to form populations of cells with compatible mitochondria and nuclei.

Because mating brings two sets of haploid nuclear genes into the zygote, two alleles of each of the proteins in question could theoretically be expressed. If maternal and paternal alleles differed in base sequence affecting amino acid sequence, the two allelic proteins in zygotes could have different abilities to interact with the mitochondrial-gene–coded proteins of the complexes. Competition, therefore, could lead to adverse interactions and less than optimal mitochondrial efficiency.

Mitochondrial exclusion at zygote formation would thus effectively prevent a foreign set of mitochondria from competing with the nuclear-coded gene products. It has been postulated that phenomena such as polar body formation and mitochondrial proliferation during oocyte maturation and reduction in numbers after fertilization are means of matching mitochondria to nuclear genomes, and that failure of such matching leads to unsuccessful conceptions. This could stem from the fact that every meiosis would rearrange genes; consequently, in the gametes or haploid state, what was a paternal allele now could be in the environment of the female mitochondrion—would this be a viable mixture, and if not, could this explain in part the tortuous behavior of oocytes, polar bodies, nonfunctioning sperm, and that the majority of conceptions do not mature?[8]

The nuclear interaction is more complex because it involves transport of many nuclear-coded proteins to the mitochondria that play vital roles in mitochondrial function, maintenance, and multiplication. Significantly, unlike the ox-phos proteins, most of these operate without the need to interact structurally with proteins of mitochondrial origin and could easily function regardless of their nuclear origin. In the ox-phos complexes, however, allelic differences among homologous proteins could prevent optimum efficiency, and it would be to the advantage of the cell to keep such interactions restricted to evolutionary compatible proteins, such as the maternal alleles and the maternally inherited mitochondria. Consequently, it is possible that during evolution there might have been the selection of mechanisms that regulated which set of alleles coding for these proteins would be expressed—resulting in monoallelic expression of specific genes—possibly a form of imprinting. Of significant interest to this hypothesis is that two of the Complex I proteins that are coded for by nuclear genes in all animals and fungi so far examined are found in the mitochondrial genome of plants, algae, and protozoa.[9] As part of the mitochondrial genome, gene expression would of necessity be monoallelic in plants. In recent years several reports have appeared on monoallelic expression of several different kinds of genes, by different and imperfectly understood regulatory mechanisms.[10,11]

Until recently it was thought unlikely that the postulated regulation of the mitochondrial/nuclear interaction could exist, though there is a report of a possible mitochondrial protein fragment influencing a nuclear gene expression,[12] and a report that small fragments of mitochondrial DNA are transferred to yeast chromosomes and are involved in the repair of double-stranded breaks.[13] It is therefore possible that the mitochondria in a cell may be capable of influencing the expression of nuclear genes whose products are intimately associated with mitochondrial proteins in the electron transport system.[7]

My laboratory is currently exploring the hypothesis that nuclear genes coding for proteins that form the oxidative-phosphorylation pathway are expressed monoallelically and that the allelic expression is related to the particular mitochondria present in the cytoplasm. Most current model organisms, being diploid with no multiplying haploid stage, do not permit the kind of analysis needed, and I am developing a novel model system utilizing the unique mating behavior of certain higher fungi that places nuclei in different mitochondrial backgrounds as a normal function of mating. Both haploid and functional diploid strains can be maintained indefinitely, mating results in two diploid thalli, and multiple mating type alleles permit crossing any strain with many others. This permits ready identification of genes being expressed in the haploids and subsequent determination of which allele(s) is(are) being expressed in the diploids and the correlation of such expression with particular mitochondria. The use of this system also permits studying what phenotypic changes result from the induced expression of both alleles in a common cytoplasm.

There are many important implications involved, in that any failure of the regulation could well lead to cell malfunctions generating cell environments conducive to cancer and cell aging. To be effective over the life of an organism, the control of gene expression would have to be a tight regulation. It is possible that aging cells could lose the requisite tight regulation and allow expression of nuclear-DNA–derived proteins competing for mitochondrial complex sites. Random failure with age of this control could lead to increasingly inefficient mitochondria and eventually to senescence and death in different tissues and organs, suggesting that one part of the onset of aging in cells, and possible diseases resulting from cell malfunction, may be a result of failure of mitochondrial influence on nuclear genes.

REFERENCES

1. OLSON, A. & J. STENLID. 2001. Mitochondrial control of fungal hybrid virulence. Nature **411**: 438.
2. SUTOVSKY, P. et al. 2000. Ubiquitinated sperm mitochondria, selective proteolysis, and the regulation of mitochondrial inheritance in mammalian embryos. Biol. Reprod. **63**: 582–590.
3. MORIYAMA, Y. & S. KAWANO. 2003. Rapid, selective digestion of mitochondrial DNA in accordance with the *matA* hierarchy of multiallelic mating types in the mitochondrial inheritance of *Physarum polycephalum*. Genetics **164**: 963–975.
4. RAYNER, A. & I.K. ROSS. 1991. Sexual politics in the cell. New Sci. **129**: 30–33.
5. LINNANE, A.W. et al. 1989. Mitochondrial DNA mutations as an important contributor to ageing and degenerative diseases. Lancet **1**: 642–645.
6. LOEFFEN, J. et al. 2001. Mutations in the complex I NDUFS2 gene of patients with cardiomyopathy and encephalomyopathy. Ann. Neurol. **49**: 195–201.
7. BLIER, P.U. et al. 2001. Natural selection and the evolution of mtDNA-encoded peptides: evidence for intergenomic co-adaptation. Trends Genet. **17**: 400–406.
8. CUMMINS, J. 1998. Mitochondrial DNA in mammalian reproduction. Rev. Reprod. **3**: 172–182.
9. RASMUSSON, A.G. et al. 1998. Physiological, biochemical and molecular aspects of mitochondrial complex I in plants. Biochim. Biophys. Acta **1364**: 101–111.
10. BIX, M. & R.M. LOCKSLEY. 1998. Independent and epigenetic regulation of the Interleukin-4 alleles in CD4[+] T cells. Science **281**: 1352–1354.
11. TANAMACHI, D.M. et al. 2001. Expression of natural killer receptor alleles at different Ly49 loci occurs independently and is regulated by major histocompatibility complex Class I molecules. J. Exp. Med. **193**: 307–316. Published on-line January 29, 2001.
12. CHELSTOWSKA, A. et al. 1999. Signalling between mitochondria and the nucleus regulates the expression of a new D-lactate dehydrogenase activity in yeast. Yeast **15**: 1377–1391.
13. RICCHETTI, M. et al. 1999. Mitochondrial DNA repairs double-strand breaks in yeast chromosomes. Nature **402**: 96–100.

Ultrasound as an Alternative to Aspiration for Determining the Nature of Pleural Effusion, Especially in Older People

HAMIDREZA SAJADIEH, FARZAD AFZALI, VAHAB SAJADIEH, AND AMIRREZA SAJADIEH

Esfahan University of Medical Sciences, Esfahan, Iran

ABSTRACT: Sonography was performed by two expert radiologists separately after selecting 80 patients (45 men and 35 women) whose pleural fluids had been aspirated and examined by the lab. The radiologists were given no clinical information concerning the patients, and the result compared with lab results. The radiologists evaluated three criteria in determining the nature of the pleural effusion: septation, echogenicity, and thickening of pleura by more than 3 mm. The study showed that the pleural effusion with septation or internal echogenicity is always an exudate. Also sonographic evidence of thickened pleura (more than 3 mm) is highly suggestive of an exudate. Although an anechoic effusion is more probably evidence of a transudate, we have seen it in 14% of patients with exudates. The lab results showed that there were 29 patients with transudates and 51 with exudates, and in ultrasound results there were 34 with transudates and 46 with exudates. A transudate is always without echogenicity, while exudates can be with or without echogenicity. It was therefore concluded that sonography is useful in determining the nature of pleural effusion.

KEYWORDS: ultrasound; transudate; exudates; pleural effusion

INTRODUCTION

Many diseases, such as cardiac diseases, nephrotic syndrome, and malignancies, cause pleural effusion. It is important for a physician to know the nature of pleural effusion: Is it a transudate or an exudate? The answer determines the individual diagnosis and treatment.

For years there has been no way except aspiration of the pleural fluid to discover what kind of effusion we have encountered. This invasive method is unacceptable for many of the patients, especially in older people because of their concomitant diseases and their concomitant medications. In addition, aspiration causes some important complications, such as pneumothorax or probably infection.

Address for correspondence: Hamidreza Sajadieh, Esfahan University of Medical Sciences, Salmanfarsi St., Behesht Ave., Num 45, 15888-63154, Esfahan, Iran.
hamidsajadieh@yahoo.com

TABLE 1. Results of sonography reports in patients with pleural effusion

				Pleural effusion		
	Number of patients	Without separation, pleural thickening, echo	With separation or pleural thickening, and without echo	Pleural effusion with internal echo	With separation	With pleural thickening
Exudate						
Infectious disease	17	2	6	9	4	4
Malignancy	26	4	6	16	7	11
Collagen disease	8	1	3	4	2	3
Total	51	7	15	29	13	18
Transudate						
Cardiac disease	11	1	10	0	0	1
Renal disease	15	1	14	0	0	1
Hepatic disease	3	0	3	0	0	0
Total	29	2	27	0	0	2

In this study, we introduce a new method of treatment—ultrasonography—which may offer an easier, less expensive, and more acceptable approach in this regard, especially in old age. Also, chest ultrasound can supplement other imaging modalities of the chest, and guides a variety of diagnostic and therapeutic procedures. This latter mehod can easily and accurately detect pleural effusion, pleural thickening, pleural tumors, tumor extension into the pleura, as can the chest wall, pleuritis, and pneumothorax. Many ultrasound features and signs of these diseases have been well characterized and widely applied in clinical practice.

Under the guidance of real-time ultrasound the success rates of invasive procedures on pleural diseases increase significantly, whereas the risks are greatly reduced. The advantages of low-cost, bedside availability, and no exposure to radiation have made ultrasound an indispensable diagnostic tool in modern pulmonary medicine.

METHODS AND MATERIALS

After 80 patients (45 men and 35 women) were selected, their pleural fluids were aspirated and examined by sonography performed by two expert radiologists separately. The radiologists had no clinical information concerning the patients, and the result wa scompared with lab results. The nature of the effusions was established on the basis of chemical, bacteriologic, and cytological examination of the pleural fluid:

(1) Pleural effusion with septation;
(2) Pleural effusion with echogenicity;
(3) Thickening of pleura by more than 3 mm.

When we see one or more of these criteria we report it as an exudative pleural effusion. Sonography was performed in two positions: supine and sitting upright.

RESULTS

In this study, pleural effusions with septation or internal echogenicity are always exudates. Also sonographic evidence of thickened pleura (more than 3 mm) is highly suggestive of exudate. Although an anechoic effusion is more probably evidence of a transudate, we have seen it in 14% of patient with exudates.

In lab results we had 29 patients with transudates and 51 with exudates, and in ultrasound results we had 34 patients with transudates and 46 with exudates.

DISCUSSION

Transudate is always without echogenicity, but exudates may or may not be without echogenicity (see FIGS. 1–6).

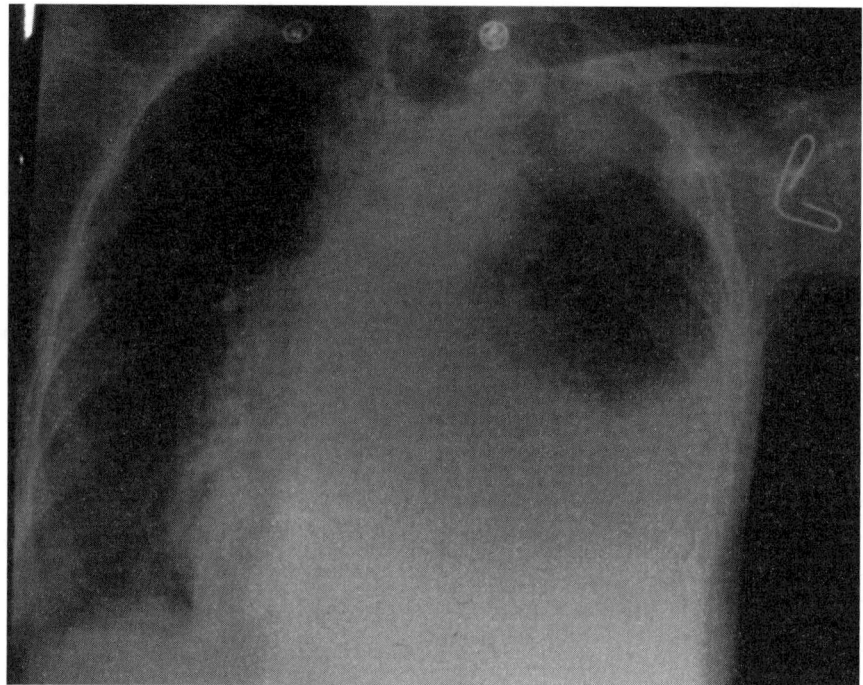

FIGURE 1. Chest X ray shows exudative pleural effusion, lobulation of pleura, fibrosis, and pleural thickening.

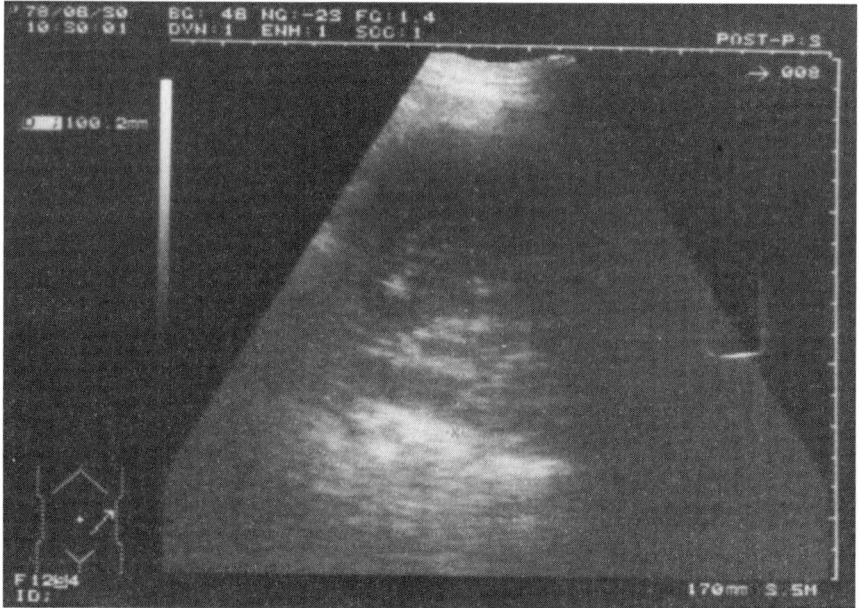

FIGURE 2. Ultrasound exam of the same patient: exudative pleural effusion can be seen in the floating debris.

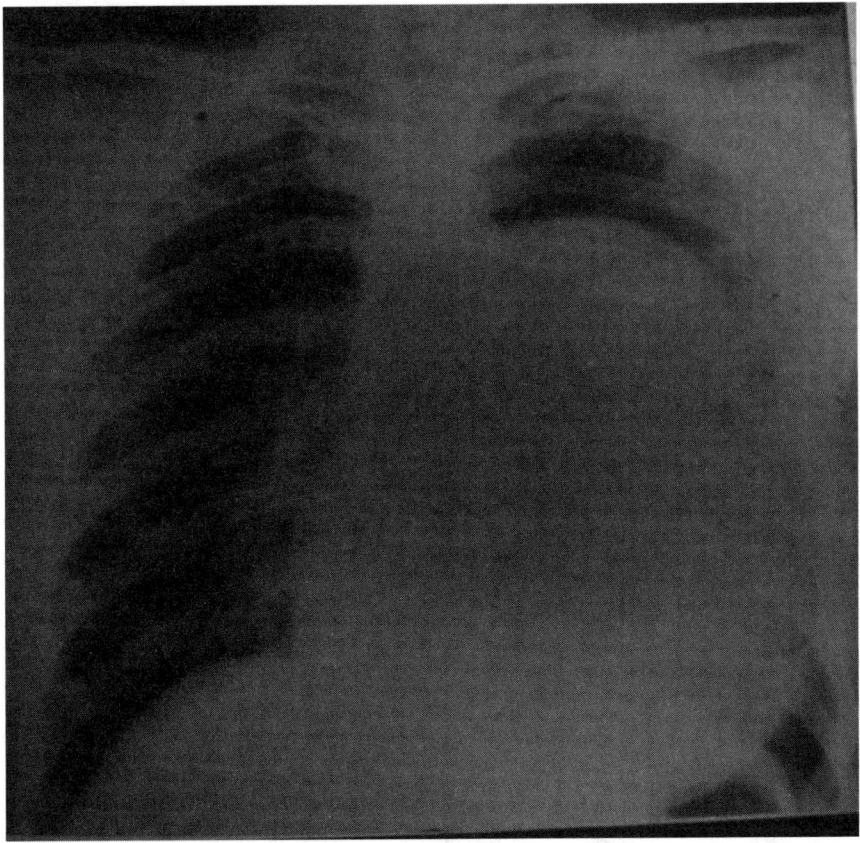

FIGURE 3. Local pleural effusion in PA chest X ray. Note large round opacity that is superimposed on the heart at *right*.

If we see a parenchymal lesion in association with pleural effusion, we can more probably report it as an exudate. Pleural nodules are hypoechoic and they have sharp borders. We can find them on both visceral pleura and parietal pleura, but pleural thickening is hyperechoic, it has no sharp borders, and it can be found on parietal pleura. Pleural thickening can be diffused or localized (plaque). Diffused pleural thickness may be due to fibrosis or malignancy. Circumferential thickening of pleura and thickening of pleura of more than 10 mm are highly indicative of malignancy. We can see irregular pleural thickening in both fibrosis and malignancy, but again

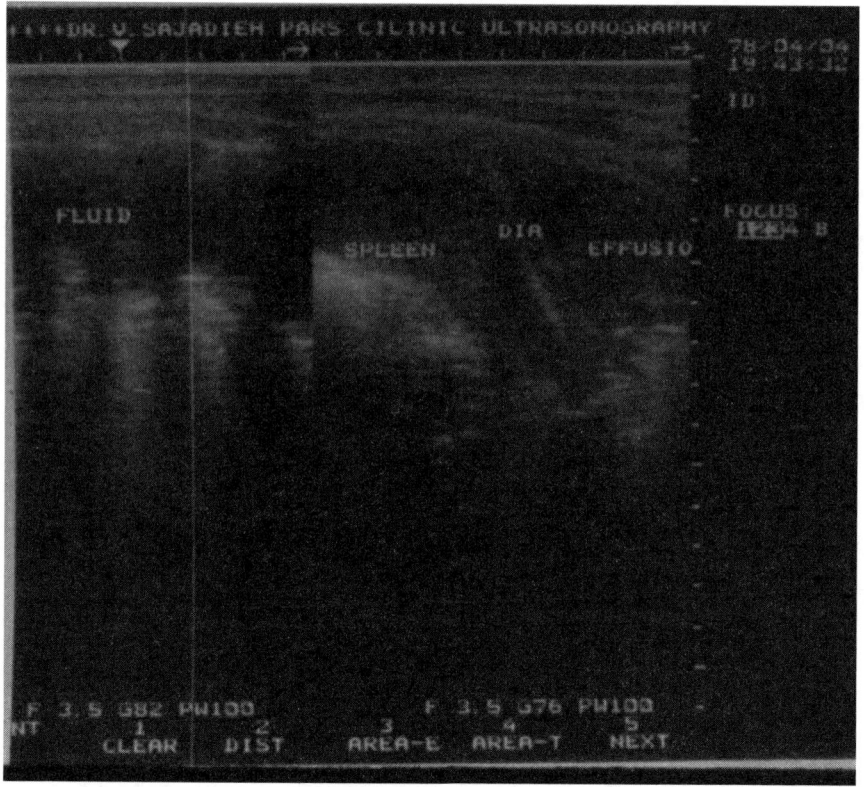

FIGURE 4. Exudative pleural effusion: the echogenicity of the pleural effusion has increased. It is comparable to the liver near the pleural effusion.

irregularity in pleural thickening is highly indicative of malignancy. Fibrosis causes the pleural effusion to be solid and lobulated.

Homogenous echogenic pleural effusion was due to hemorrhagic effusion or empyema. Also, when we see a normal pleura with pleural effusion, we cannot rule out malignancy. Malignant pleural effusion is second only to congestive heart failure as the most common cause of pleural effusion in patients over 50.

We conclude that sonography is useful in determining the nature of pleural effusion. Sonography also has the ability to show other findings associated with effusions, such as metastasis to pleura, pleural nodules, and some intraparenchymal lung lesions, which is more common in older people, and in this regard its use is more beneficial for them than any other method. Finally, when sonography cannot diagnose the differentiation between exudates and transudates exactly, at least it can show us the best site for aspiration.

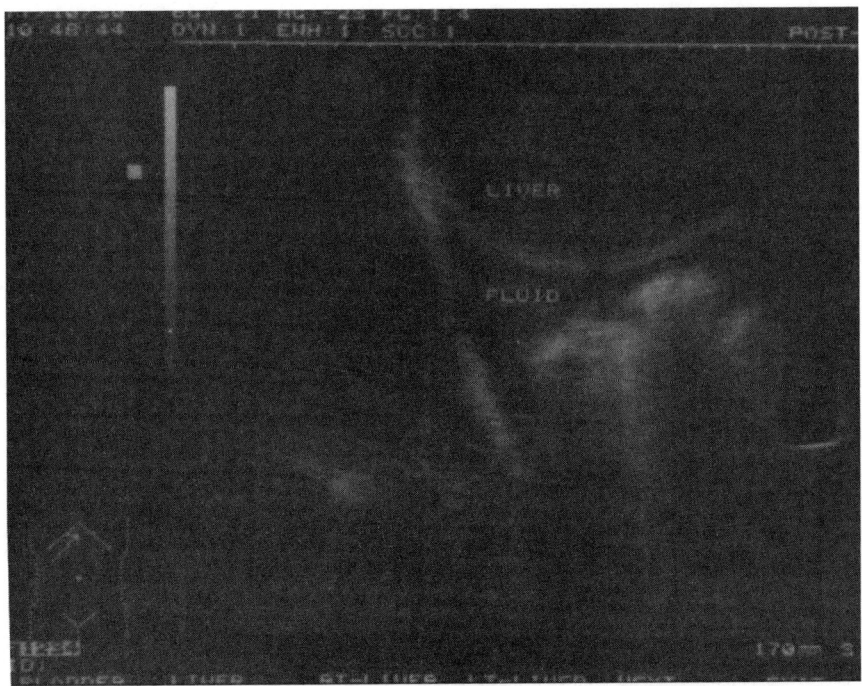

FIGURE 5. Exudative pleural effusion with pleural thickening.

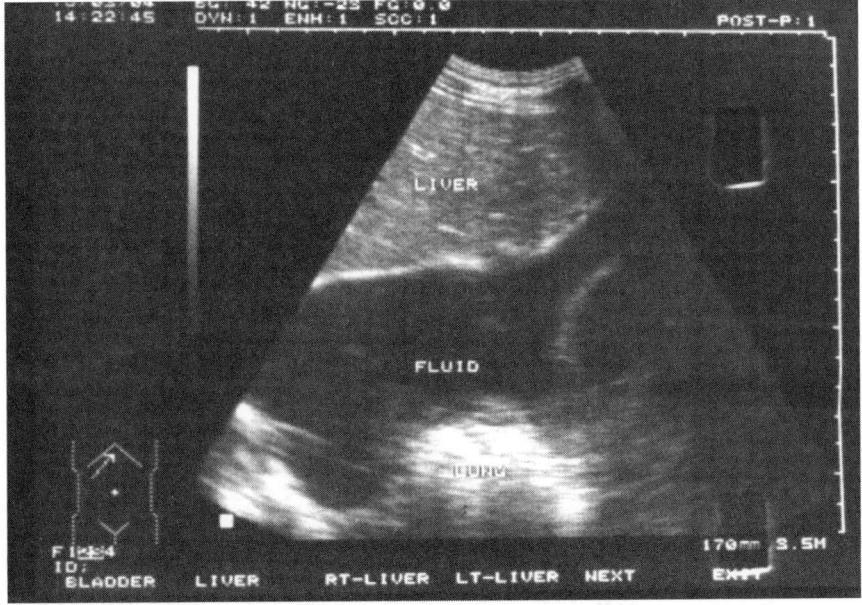

FIGURE 6. Transudative pleural effusion.

REFERENCES

1. BRANT, W. 2001. Chest ultrasound. *In* The Core Curriculum Ultrasound. W. Brant, Ed.: 437–443. Williams & Wilkins. Philadelphia, PA.
2. TSAI, T. & P. YANG. 2003. Ultrasound in diagnosis and management of pleural disease. Curr. Opin. Pulm. Med. **9:** 282–290.
3. MATHIS, G. 1997. Thorax sonography: Part 1, Chest wall and pleura. J. Ultrasound Med. **23:** 1131–1139.
4. WERNECKE, K. 1997. Sonographic features of pleural disease. AJR **168:** 1061–1066.
5. MAFFESSANTI, M., P. BORTOLOTTO & M. GROTTO. 1996. Imaging of pleural disease. Arch. Chest Dis. **51:** 138–144.
6. LEVIN, D. & J. KLEIN. 1999. Imaging techniques for pleural space infections. Semin. Respir. Infect. **14:** 31–38.
7. EIBENBERGER, K. 1994. Quantification of pleural effusion: sonography versus radiography. Radiology **191:** 681–688.
8. TARGHETT, R. 1992. Sonographic approach to diagnosing pleural effusion pulmonary consolidation. J. Ultrasound Med. **11:** 667–677.
9. DYNES, M. 1992. Imaging manifestation of pleural tumors. Radiographics **12:** 1191–1199.
10. TARGHETTA, R. 1992. Ultrasonographic approach to diagnosing hydropneumothorax. Chest **101:** 931–943.
11. WERNECHE, K. 1987. Pneomothorax evaluations by ultrasound: preliminary results. J. Thorax Imaging **2:** 76.

Index of Contributors

Abe, R., 471–474
Afanas'ev, I.B., 343–345
Afzali, F., 585–592
Aiken, J.M., 289–293
Alberti, E., 48–52
Almeida, H., 135–140
Ames, B.N., 365–367, 406–411
Andersen, S., 502–505
Annable, L., 326–329
Anson, R.M., 412–423, 427–429
Aquino, A., 141–146
Arbeev, K.G., 64–69
Aringer, M., 178–185
Arivazhagan, P., 350–354
Arking, R., 577–580
Asea, A., 502–505
Aspinall, R., 116–122
Atamna, H., 365–367

Baird, D.M., 265–268
Bakala, H., 211–214
Baldelli, B., 379–382
Balietti, M., 29–32, 33–36, 44–47
Barja, G., 333–342
Barnett, Y., 178–185
Barretto, R., 195–199
Bar-Shai, M., 475–478
Bartling, B., 228–231
Bausero, M., 502–505
Bauza, J.Y., 48–52, 53–57
Behrstock, S., 5–14
Ben-Yehuda, A., 178–185
Bertoni-Freddari, C., 29–32, 33–36, 37–40, 44–47, 379–382
Bertuccelli, J., 195–199
Beyers, M., 215–218
Bird, J., 256–259
Bogdanova, V., 106–110
Braak, H., 24–28
Bracci, M., 127–134
Brand, M.D., 388–391
Brown-Borg, H.M., 317–320
Brun, J., 215–218
Brunet Rossinni, A.K., 506–508
Brunk, U.T., 70–77, 285–288

Bulteau, A.-L., 219–222
Burton, D., 256–259
Busuttil, R.A., 245–255

Cahaya, H.S., 365–367
Campbell, F.C., 147–170
Campisi, J., 245–255
Candore, G., 141–146
Cantatore, P., 269–273, 430–433
Carey, J.R., 577–580
Carmeli, E., 475–478
Caruso, C., 141–146
Casadesus, G., 1–4
Casoli, T., 29–32, 33–36, 37–40
Cassano, P., 269–273
Castellanos, M.R., 53–57
Chen, C., 355–359
Cho, K.A., 309–316
Chung, H.Y., 471–474
Cipriano, C., 127–134
Claros, M.G., 232–239
Coleman, R., 475–478
Coles, L.S., 490–495
Collazo, J., 48–52, 53–57
Colonna-Romano, G., 141–146
Contreras, R., 355–359
Corder, E.H., 24–28
Corder, L.S., 486–489
Crespo, D., 41–43

Dalen, H., 70–77
Davidson, E., 232–239
Davis, J.K., 535–541
Davis, T., 274–277
de Cabo, R., 412–423, 448–452
de Grey, A.D.N.J., xv–xvi, 147–170, 542–545, 552–553
De Magalhães, J.P., 375–378
Delfino, A., 37–40
Di Stefano, G., 29–32, 33–36, 37–40
Dobson, C.B., 15–18
Dokal, I., 147–170
Dollé, M., 245–255
Donehower, L.A., 171–177

Donnelly, J., 392–395
Downs, J.L., 443–447
Dumble, M., 171–177

Eaton, J.W., 70–77
Ebralidse, K., 240–244
Edwards, M.G., 85–95
Effros, R.B., 123–126
Erusalimsky, J.D., 111–115
Evdokushkina, G.N., 513–517

Fairbairn, L.J., 147–170
Fakan, S., 379–382
Faragher, R.G.A., 256–259, 274–277
Fattoretti, P., 29–32, 33–36, 37–40, 44–47, 379–382
Feng, D., 360–364
Fernández, C.I., 48–52, 53–57
Fernandez-Viadero, C., 41–43
Ferreira, J., 135–140
Fesce, E., 195–199
Fracasso, F., 430–433
Friguet, B., 211–214, 219–222
Frostholm, A., 58–63
Fülöp, T., 178–185
Funes, S., 232–239

Gadaleta, M.N., 269–273, 430–433
Garyfallou, V.T., 443–447
Gatza, C., 171–177
Gavrilov, L.A., 496–501, 509–512, 513–517
Gavrilova, N.S., 496–501, 509–512, 513–517
Gazzanell, G., 379–382
Ghebremedhin, E., 24–28
Giacconi, R., 127–134
Giorgetti, B., 29–32, 33–36, 44–47
Goldspink, G., 294–298
Goncharova, N.D., 321–325
Gonos, E.S., 206–210
González-Halphen, D., 232–239
Gorgoulis, V.G., 330–332
Goto, S., 471–474
Graham, G.J., 147–170
Gray, D.A., 215–218
Gredilla, R., 333–342

Green, M.H.L., 256–259
Guerin, J.C., 518–520

Hadj, A., 78–84
Hagen, T.M., 346–349
Hamilton, K., 462–470
Handa, S., 383–387
Harman, S.M., 299–308
Harris, J., 527–534
Harris, S.B., 559–563
Haussmann, M.F., 186–190
Henson, S., 116–122
Heusèle, C., 219–222
Hiona, A., 96–105
Holmes, D.J., 483–485
Hong, Y., 111–115
Hosein-Pur-Nobari, N., 564–567
Hosseini-Mazinani, S.M., 368–369, 564–567
Huang, H.-L., 111–115
Huffman, T.M., 559–563
Huntington, C.E., 186–190

Imasawa, T., 383–387
Ingram, D.K., 412–423, 443–447, 448–452
Ishigami, A., 360–364, 383–387
Itzhaki, R.F., 15–18

Jahoda, C.A.B., 147–170
Jang, I.S., 309–316
Jennert-Burston, K., 256–259
Ji, L.L., 453–461
Jones, C.J., 274–277

Kasahara, Y., 383–387
Kawanishi, S., 278–284
Kendaiah, S., 333–342
Khrapko, K., 240–244
Kikkawa, K., 479–482
Killilea, D.W., 365–367
Kim, K.T., 309–316
Kin, N.M.K.N.Y., 326–329
King, M.P., 232–239
Kipling, D., 265–268, 274–277
Kishi, S., 521–526

INDEX OF CONTRIBUTORS

Kitani, K., 424–427
Kletsas, D., 330–332
Klipp, E., 370–374
Klopp, R., 85–95
Kondo, Y., 360–364
Koochmeshgi, J., 368–369, 434–435, 436–438, 564–567
Kossoy, G., 439–442
Kowald, A., 370–374
Kraytsberg, Y., 240–244
Krøll, J., 568–571
Kubo, S., 383–387
Kuramoto, M., 360–364, 383–387
Kurz, D.J., 111–115
Kurz, T., 285–288

Ladonni, S., 368–369
Lane, M.A., 412–423, 443–447, 448–452
Lapin, B.A., 321–325
Leake, A., 285–288
Lee, H.-G., 1–4
Leeuwenburgh, C., 96–105, 269–273, 333–342
Lemler, J., 559–563
Lezza, A.M.S., 269–273, 430–433
Lio, D., 141–146
Liu, H., 346–349
Liu, R.-M., 346–349
López, O., 53–57
Lowe, J., 256–259
Lynch, M.D., 191–194

Machida, T., 360–364
Mahé, C., 219–222
Mainfroid, V., 375–378
Malatesta, M., 379–382
Malavolta, M., 127–134
Mamczarz, J., 412–423
Marasco, S., 78–84
Mariani, E., 178–185
Mariatos, G., 330–332
Marineo, G., 572–576
Marotta, F., 195–199, 572–576
Martínez, L., 48–52
Maruyama, N., 360–364, 383–387
Mary, J., 211–214
Mattison, J.A., 412–423, 443–447
McCormick, M., 502–505

McGrath, L.T., 392–395
McLeod, J., 178–185
McMaster, D., 392–395
Megias, M., 41–43
Mendoza, Y., 48–52
Michalsky, A.I., 64–69
Migeot, V., 375–378
Miller, F., 78–84
Miskin, R., 439–442
Miwa, S., 388–391
Mocchegiani, E., 127–134
Moreau, M., 219–222
Morrow, J.D., 85–95
Musicco, C., 430–433
Muti, E., 127–134
Muzzioli, M., 127–134

Nagley, P., 78–84
Nair, N.P.V., 326–329
Naito, H., 471–474
Nakamoto, H., 471–474
Neuzil, J., 70–77
Neves, D., 135–140
Ngom, P.T., 116–122
Nisbet, I.C.T., 186–190
Nizard, C., 219–222
Novoseltsev, V.N., 577–580
Novoseltseva, J.A., 577–580
Nyakas, C., 471–474

Ogawa, K., 502–505
Ohm, T.G., 24–28
Oikawa, S., 278–284
Osawa, T., 424–427
Ostler, E.L., 256–259

Pak, J.W., 289–293
Palaima, E., 502–505
Panneerselvam, C., 350–354
Park, S.C., 309–316
Partridge, L., 388–391
Pawelec, G., 178–185
Pennington, J., 502–505
Pepe, S., 78–84
Pérez-Martínez, X., 232–239
Perls, T.T., 502–505
Perry, G., 1–4
Pesce, V., 430–433

Peterson, D.M., 453–461
Phaneuf, S., 333–342
Pido-Lopez, J., 116–122
Platt, C., 559–563
Poggioli, S., 211–214, 219–222
Popesco, M.C., 58–63
Porter, A.C.G., 147–170
Powers, S.K., 462–470
Pratsinis, H., 330–332
Prolla, T.A., 85–95

Quick, D., 78–84
Quindry, J., 462–470

Radák, Z., 471–474
Rakoczy, S.G., 317–320
Rattan, S.I.S., 554–558
Rea, I.M., 392–395
Rejniak, K., 58–63
Remacle, J., 375–378
Reyes-Prieto, A., 232–239
Reznick, A.Z., 475–478
Riga, D., 396–400, 401–405
Riga, S., 396–400, 401–405
Riyahi, K., 388–391
Rogo, C., 127–134
Rosenfeldt, F., 78–84
Rosillo, J.C., 48–52
Ross, I.K., 581–584
Roth, G.S., 412–423, 443–447
Rotter, A., 58–63
Ryu, S.J., 309–316

Safran, P., 195–199
Sajadieh, A., 585–592
Sajadieh, H., 585–592
Sajadieh, V., 585–592
Sarkar, D., 85–95
Saunois, A., 219–222
Schnebert, S., 219–222
Schneider, F., 396–400, 401–405
Schoenhofen, E., 502–505
Schwartz, B., 439–442
Schwartz, G., 326–329
Scola, L., 141–146
Seifati, S.M., 564–567
Selman, C., 333–342
Semyonova, V.G., 513–517

Seyama, K., 383–387
Sheeran, F., 78–84
Sheerin, A., 256–259
Shenvi, S., 346–349
Shimosawa, T., 383–387
Shipley, S.J., 15–18
Shtereva, N., 106–110
Silber, R-E., 228–231
Simm, A., 228–231
Singh, K.K., 260–264
Sisti, G., 572–576
Smith, M.A., 1–4
Solazzi, M., 29–32, 33–36, 44–47
Stock, G.B., 546–551
Svendsen, C.N., 5–14

Tajiri, H., 195–199
Takahashi, R., 471–474
Takeda, A., 1–4
Taneva, E., 106–110
Tang, M., 215–218
Taylor, M.G., 24–28
Teimoori-Toolab, L., 564–567
Terman, A., 70–77
Terry, D.F., 502–505
Thal, D.R., 24–28
Thavundayil, J.X., 326–329
Tirosh, O., 439–442
Toescu, E.C., 19–23
Toussaint, O., 375–378
Trivier, E., 111–115
Trougakos, J.P., 206–210
Tsirigotis, M., 215–218
Tyner, S., 171–177

Ukraintseva, S.V., 64–69, 200–205
Urbanski, H.F., 443–447
Uthus, E.O., 317–320

Venkatachalam, S., 171–177
Verduga, R., 41–43
Vijg, J., 245–255
Vleck, C.M., 186–190
von Zglinicki, T., 285–288

Wang, H., 346–349
Weindruch, R., 85–95

INDEX OF CONTRIBUTORS

Winkler, D.W., 186–190
Wong, S.L., 365–367
Woulfe, J., 215–218
Wowk, M., 78–84
Wozniak, M.A., 15–18

Xiong, J., 19–23

Yahav, S., 439–442
Yashin, A.I., 64–69, 200–205, 577–580

Yokozawa, T., 424–427
Yoshida, C., 195–199
Young, I.S., 392–395

Zacharatos, P., 330–332
Zatta, P., 44–47
Zhang, M., 215–218
Zhu, M., 412–423, 448–452
Zhu, X., 1–4
Zusman, I., 439–442